"Most first aid books descr[...]
ultimately end up with the [...]
or hospital or ambulance is right around the corner. But what about [...]
of a lifetime—in the wilds of Mongolia or the mountains of Tibet or several days out to sea? 'Seek medical advice' helps not a bit. In these situations, there is no better resource (including having a direct line to your hospital ER) than Medicine for the Outdoors. Dr. Paul Auerbach is to wilderness medicine what Bill Gates is to computers; he is the source, and so this book is a treasure trove of information not only for untrained laypeople but for most physicians. There [...] more understandable or complete collection of information on what to do for anything that might befall an adventure traveler—from high altitude cerebral edema to soapfish dermatitis to cougar attack to how to stitch a laceration. Even better, Medicine for the Outdoors provides essential guidance in advance of an adventure to help with planning and prevention—from immunizations to equipment and clothing to dietary precautions. The handy appendices include a drug reference, conversion tables, and definitions of common medical terms. Contemplating an adventure? The old adage 'Seek medical attention' has been replaced with 'Get Medicine for the Outdoors.'"
Luanne Freer, MD, FACEP, FAWM, Past President, Wilderness Medical Society; Medical Director, Yellowstone National Park; Founder/Director, Everest ER, Nepal

"This book has the information you need to prevent, recognize and treat medical emergencies in any environment. Primarily a medical guide for outdoor, wilderness and remote areas, it is also an excellent reference for home and disaster situations. Most importantly, it is written by one of the foremost experts in this field, so you can trust this information."
Howard Backer, MD, MPH, FACEP, Director, California Emergency Medical Services Authority

"The sixth edition of Medicine for the Outdoors is more impressive and indispensable than ever. The uncomplicated clear writing and illustrations are delightfully easy to understand, and the book is remarkably thorough and superbly detailed. I highly recommend it to anyone who is serious about working and playing in the outdoors."
Donald C. Cooper, PhD, MBA, Editor, Fundamentals of Search and Rescue; Chair, National Fire Protection Association Technical Search and Rescue Committee

"When a crisis occurs in the backcountry, punching in 911 may not even get you a dial tone—you're on your own. This book is your wilderness 911. Take the time to read it and know the principles of care provided within it. Medicine for the Outdoors just might save your life."
Frank Hubbell, DO, Founder of Stonehearth Open Learning Opportunities (SOLO); President, New Hampshire Osteopathic Association; Member, New Hampshire Medical Control Board; Director, Conway Walk-In Clinic

"Students with a broad range of experience take wilderness medicine courses. It's not easy to find a comprehensive text that accommodates all their needs. Medicine for the Outdoors engages the non-professional while keeping the most seasoned provider informed in the latest techniques for backcountry medical practice. Dr. Auerbach has written another book that is a gold standard for anyone with an interest in health and safety outdoors."
William Fred Baty, WEMT-P, Retired Fire Chief, City of Knoxville Fire Department; Lead Wilderness Medicine Instructor, The Wilderness Medicine Program, Roane State Community College, Knoxville, Tennessee

"This manual contains a wealth of succinct, up-to-date, and practical advice. It is an indispensable medical guide for wilderness enthusiasts and health professionals."
Kent R. Olson, MD, Clinical Professor, UCB-UCSF Joint Medical Program; Clinical Professor of Medicine & Pharmacy, UCSF; Medical Director, San Francisco Poison Control System

"You always hope for the best and plan for the worst. Being well prepared for the unexpected in the wilderness is greatly enhanced by our 'survival bible,' namely, Medicine for the Outdoors. Our guides, trip leaders, and clients never adventure without this well-written and easy-to-understand book, and we invariably benefit from it. The common sense approach and complete coverage have helped us mitigate situations and avoid greater emergencies. In all reaches of the globe, with Medicine for the Outdoors, we're much closer to definitive care."
Laurence Alvarez-Roos, Co-founder, Bio Bio Expeditions World Wide

"Auerbach's Medicine for the Outdoors continues to serve as an ideal portable reference. Whether you are in the front country, exploring tropical reefs, or trekking at high altitude, Medicine for the Outdoors rapidly guides to solutions for the most important medical problems. I strongly recommend this reference as a primary source for laypersons as well as a supplement for individuals with advanced wilderness medicine training."
Brad L. Bennett, PhD, NREMT-P, FAWM, Captain, US Navy (Retired); Adjunct Faculty, Military and Emergency Medicine Department, Uniformed Services University of the Health Sciences; President, Wilderness Medical Society

"Traveling in the wilderness or abroad can be punctuated by unexpected illness or injury. If you plan to travel where medical care is not readily available, Medicine for the Outdoors is the resource you want to have with you. Dr. Auerbach, one of the foremost experts on wilderness medicine, covers topics from basic first aid to major medical illnesses, trauma, medications, and medical kits. Medicine for the Outdoors provides knowledge that can help you survive until further assistance is available."
Albert R. Wheeler III, MD, Emergency Medicine of Jackson Hole; Medical Director, Grand Teton National Park EMS; Medical Director, Teton County Search and Rescue

"From first aid for minor wounds to treating altitude sickness, from poisonous mushrooms to hazardous aquatic life, Medicine for the Outdoors covers all the information an adventurer might need for emergency care in the wilderness. My previous editions are well-read and dog-eared. Auerbach's book is a must-read on any explorer's list."
Bill Clendenen, CEO, Health & Safety Institute

"Marine research takes me to remote corners of the globe, often distant from immediate rescue and medical care. Medicine for the Outdoors is packed as an essential item along with oxygen and first aid kit should my diving team need emergency field care. It is by far the most comprehensive, well-written and useful reference available—a must-have for remote field work."
Dr. Michael A. Lang, Senior Vice President, OxyHeal Health Group; Adjunct Faculty, UC San Diego–Emergency Medicine

"Curiosity entices us to places on this planet where there are neither 911 nor emergency rooms. Whether we hike in a forest, climb along the frozen edge of a mountain top, trek deep within a rainforest, or dive in the rich waters of a coral reef, the most valuable asset to that trip is emergency preparedness. In my travels around the globe, I have seen first-hand the life-saving value of proper first aid. Paul Auerbach's encyclopedic knowledge, vision, advice and instructions offer priceless preparation for that moment we hope never comes. Paul's sixth edition of Medicine for the Outdoors is an essential read before any expedition, and should be the first item to go into the gear bag."
David Doubilet, Contributing Photographer, National Geographic Magazine

MEDICINE FOR THE OUTDOORS

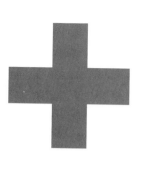

THE ESSENTIAL GUIDE TO FIRST AID AND MEDICAL EMERGENCIES

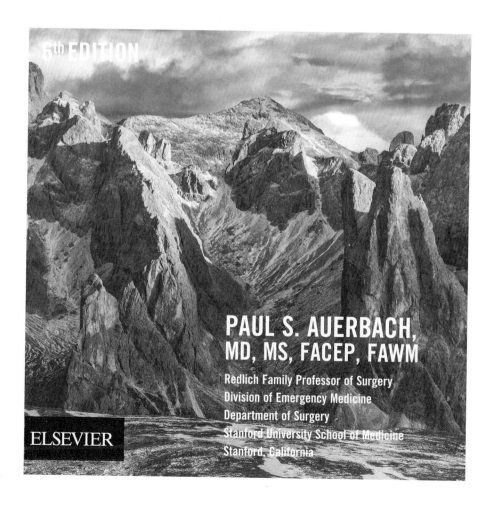

6th EDITION

PAUL S. AUERBACH, MD, MS, FACEP, FAWM

Redlich Family Professor of Surgery
Division of Emergency Medicine
Department of Surgery
Stanford University School of Medicine
Stanford, California

ELSEVIER

ELSEVIER

1600 John F. Kennedy Blvd.
Ste 1800
Philadelphia, PA 19103-2899

MEDICINE FOR THE OUTDOORS, SIXTH EDITION

ISBN: 978-0-323-32168-6

Notices

Library of Congress Cataloging-in-Publication Data

Auerbach, Paul S.
  Medicine for the outdoors : the essential guide to first aid and medical emergencies / Paul S. Auerbach, MD, MS, FACEP, FAWM, Redlich Family Professor of Surgery, Division of Emergency Medicine, Department of Surgery, Stanford University School of Medicine, Stanford, California.—Sixth edition.
     pages cm
  Includes index.
  ISBN 978-0-323-32168-6 (pbk. : alk. paper)   1. Outdoor medical emergencies.   2. First aid in illness and injury.   I. Title.
  RC88.9.O95A94 2016
  616.02′52—dc23

2014047120

Executive Content Strategist: Kate Dimock
Content Development Manager: Lucia Gunzel
Content Development Specialist: Gabriela Benner
Publishing Services Manager: Catherine Jackson
Project Manager: Rhoda (Bontrager) Howell
Design Direction: Amy Buxton

Printed in the United States of America

Last digit is the print number: 9   8   7   6   5   4   3   2   1

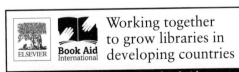

Working together
to grow libraries in
developing countries

www.elsevier.com • www.bookaid.org

PREFACE

The outdoor environment is miraculous, but it is ever-changing and can become hostile in a moment. Good fortune favors the well prepared, and there are no more important considerations for a successful outdoor experience than safety and first aid. Severe weather, rugged terrain, wild animals, and equipment failure all conspire to create or complicate medical hardships that must be diagnosed swiftly and remedied with certainty. The therapies can be integral to survival. Medical education is thus as compelling as any other category of learning.

This revised sixth edition of *Medicine for the Outdoors* has been thoroughly updated and rewritten based on advances in medical knowledge, suggestions from readers, and reviews of the previous edition. I am indebted to my family, professional colleagues, and friends, who always support me in my medical activities and writing endeavors. Brian, Lauren, and Danny share the outdoor spirit and have each put this book to good use. As always, *Medicine for the Outdoors* is dedicated to all the wonderful people who have given generously of their time to the Wilderness Medical Society and other reputable organizations, and thereby advanced the specialty of wilderness medicine.

With as much effort as we seek to maintain our personal well-being, let each of us seek to maintain the wilderness. It is my fervent hope that we can approach preservation of planet Earth with the same passion that we devote to our vital medical missions; for without the wilderness, there can be no wilderness medicine.

Paul S. Auerbach, MD
Spring, 2015

INTRODUCTION

The purpose of this book is to provide you with brief explanations of a wide variety of medical problems and to offer practical solutions. *Medicine for the Outdoors* is arranged to make information easy to retrieve. Part One outlines basic principles of health care that should be applied to all outdoor travel. Parts Two and Three describe medical situations, beginning with life threats and covering, in turn, major and minor medical problems you might encounter. Part Four discusses disorders related to various wilderness settings from both medical and safety perspectives. Part Five covers additional practical information, such as evacuation guidelines and techniques, water disinfection, useful knots and hitches, drug injection techniques, and recommendations for immunization. Appendix One lists medications and doses, with an emphasis on medications mentioned elsewhere in the book. Conversion tables for common measurements are found in Appendix Two. Appendix Three outlines guidelines for prevention of hepatitis, acquired immunodeficiency syndrome (AIDS), and other diseases transmitted by human body fluids. Appendix Four describes and illustrates commonly used applications of the SAM Splint. Appendix Five offers advice about personal safety in an age of global conflict, kidnapping, and terrorism. Appendix Six is a brief description of emergency canine medicine. The glossary defines medical and technical terms. The index will guide you swiftly to any topic.

To keep the book to a manageable size, I assume that you have a basic understanding of how your body works. Thus, explanations are brief and to the point. This is neither a survival manual nor an outdoor sports medicine encyclopedia. Rather, the book is meant to be carried on a journey as a ready reference for a layperson who needs to medically rescue or aid an ill or injured victim. I have included information that is necessary to make simple, accurate diagnoses and to act on them.

This book does not transform a layperson into a physician, but we all recognize that there are times when medical help is miles or even days away. No intervention is completely without risk; however, some familiarity with diseases and injuries can minimize that risk. Although some of the techniques and drugs described could worsen a situation if misapplied or incorrectly administered, the treatments presented are current and well accepted. Still, *the recommendations should not be considered substitutes for prompt evaluation by a trained medical professional.* If at any time a diagnosis is uncertain, or a victim appears to be more than minimally ill, all efforts should be directed at seeking a professional medical opinion.

The basic therapies recommended do not include all those that could be rendered by a physician with advanced equipment and a large armamentarium of drugs. I have not described every infectious or tropical disease that could possibly be contracted during a journey abroad. However, the diagnosis and management of illnesses such as schistosomiasis, malaria, Lyme disease, anaplasmosis, Ebola virus disease, yellow fever, dengue fever, West Nile viral disease, and Rocky Mountain spotted fever are relevant to many people who travel domestically and overseas in wilderness areas, and have therefore been included. Because we live in an age of biohazards, information has been added to include a few of these entities, such as anthrax.

In addition to "Western medicine," there exists "complementary and alternative" (from the Western perspective) medicine, sometimes referred to as "naturopathic" medicine. While many of the recommendations of naturopathic doctors are appropriate and effective, I personally do not have the expertise upon which to make such recommendations. However, in a wilderness setting, and certainly when being treated by healers in non-Western countries, you may wish to be the beneficiary of such remedies. If so, you will need to perform your own validation of remedies, such as *Melaleuca alternifolia* (tea tree) oil as a topic antiseptic or anti-itch preparation.

To use this or any medical reference to best advantage, review the pertinent sections before your expedition. Practice the manual skills, such as the application of splints and slings, until you are confident.

I have also provided information that is as important as medical knowledge. This includes such topics as how to avoid being struck by lightning, drowning prevention, and what to do if you fall through the ice or are caught in a flood zone or near a forest fire.

I hope that you are enlightened, and that good luck prevails.

CONTENTS

PART ONE

General Information

HOW TO USE THIS BOOK

To use this book to best advantage, read the appropriate sections *before* you embark on a trip. In this way, you'll remember where to find information in case of an emergency. Use the index to locate specific topics, such as bee stings, frostbite, or choking. When reading about different problems, you may be referred to general instructions for medical aid, which are presented in Parts One and Two. All readers are encouraged to participate in organized first-aid and outdoor safety programs, such as those offered by the National Ski Patrol, American Red Cross, Outward Bound, National Outdoor Leadership School, Stonehearth Open Learning Opportunities, Kling Mountain Guides, Wilderness Medicine Outfitters, Advanced Wilderness Life Support, Wilderness Medical Associates, and Out-doorSafe. Cardiopulmonary resuscitation (CPR) training that conforms to American Heart Association standards is available through multiple venues. Automated external defibrillator (AED) training should be completed.

Many drugs recommended in the book are available only through prescriptions provided by physicians. A physician or pharmacist should explain each drug's use and side effects. All pregnant women should consult a physician before any expedition for current advice on the advisability of activities, immunizations, and the use of particular drugs. Many of the drugs mentioned in the book are listed in Appendix One. Unless a particular dose and/or duration are specified, the reader is referred to Appendix One. Recommended doses of drugs are adult doses, unless otherwise noted.

I have simplified the recommendations for administration of antibiotics. I sometimes note recommended medications and the dose and duration for which they should be given. Again, further details on dosages may be found in Appendix One. If not otherwise specified, the default duration for administration of an antibiotic is 7 days.

The group of nonsteroidal antiinflammatory drugs (NSAIDs) comprises a very common type of medication. Examples include ibuprofen and naproxen. Throughout the book, when I recommend using an NSAID, these may be used interchangeably, unless a specific drug is mentioned. Doses are given in Appendix One, notably in the section entitled *"For relief from muscle aches or minor arthritis."*

For estimation of body weight, 1 kilogram (kg) equals 2.2 pounds (lb), so each pound equals 0.45 kilogram. For temperature conversion (when reading thermometers) between Fahrenheit and Centigrade (Celsius), use the following formula:

Degrees Fahrenheit = (9/5 times degrees Centigrade) plus 32

or

Degrees Centigrade = 5/9 times (degrees Fahrenheit minus 32)

A temperature conversion table is found on page 476. Volume and weight conversion tables are found on pages 478 and 479. For practical purposes, 1 "liter" of liquid as a measurement can be used interchangeably with 1 "quart." I have provided metric equivalents (sometimes approximate) for most of the measurements given.

Although most people don't have ready access to oxygen tanks and face masks, I sometimes recommend oxygen administration for the benefit of persons so equipped. Information about oxygen administration is found on page 405.

When administering an injection, *never* share needles between people. Appendix Three briefly discusses guidelines for prevention of hepatitis, acquired immunodeficiency syndrome (AIDS), and other diseases transmitted via contact with human blood and other bodily fluids. Whenever possible, always *observe blood and bodily fluid precautions* (see page 481).

BEFORE YOU GO

BE IN GOOD HEALTH

To the extent possible, be in good health:

1. Maintain the proper weight for your height, age, and body type.
2. Exercise regularly. Be aware of your body's condition. Build strength, flexibility, and endurance.
3. Eat a healthy diet and learn to love fruits, vegetables, fiber, nuts and seeds, and complex carbohydrates (e.g., whole grains). Pay particular attention to ingesting sufficient amounts of calcium, iron, and other nutrients essential to metabolism, growth, and preservation of your eyesight, bones, and joints. Don't eat much processed meat, fast food, or junk food. Don't be obese.
4. Complete proper screening examinations for treatable diseases such as breast, cervical, colon, testicular, and prostate cancer. Think about your heart and brain, and test at appropriate intervals for high-density lipoproteins, low-density lipoproteins, and total cholesterol. Maintain your blood pressure below a worrisome value. Pay attention to your blood glucose to maintain an acceptable fasting value.
5. If you are pregnant, don't take chances with your baby's health.
6. Maintain all recommended immunizations against such diseases as tetanus and pertussis (whooping cough), and get an annual flu shot.
7. Wear your seat belt when driving and wear a helmet when riding a bicycle or motorcycle. Never attempt dangerous maneuvers if you're tired or intoxicated.
8. Give up tobacco. Drink alcohol only in moderation. Be aware that using marijuana can cause reduced awareness, hallucinations, impaired decision making, slowed reflexes, and decreased peripheral vision.
9. Brush and floss your teeth at least once each day.
10. Get enough sleep. This is important for your physical and mental health. Attempt to obtain 8 to 9 hours per each 24 hours in synchrony with your normal circadian rhythm ("biological clock"). Avoid potentially dangerous activities if you are sleep-deprived.

BE PREPARED

There is no substitute for preparedness. Adherence to this basic rule will prevent or ease the majority of mishaps that occur in the wild. Proper education before situations of risk allows you to cope in a purposeful fashion, rather than in a state of fear and panic. At least two, and prefer- ably all, members of a wilderness expedition should understand first aid and medical rescue. On a casual family outing, at least one responsible adult should be skilled in first aid. Manual skills, such as mouth-to-mouth breathing, cardiopulmonary resuscitation (CPR), and the application of bandages and splints, should be practiced beforehand. Become familiar with technical rescue techniques pertinent to the environment you will be in (e.g., high-angle rock, swift water, or avalanche-prone areas). Be certain to carry appropriate survival equipment, such as maps, a global positioning system (GPS) or compass, waterproof matches, firestarter materials, a knife, nonperishable food, a flashlight, AvaLung in avalanche territory, and adequate first-aid supplies. Minimize the need for improvisation.

Be prepared for the harshest environmental conditions you might expect to encounter. To the best extent possible, become familiar with the setting and possible survival scenarios, particularly should you become stranded or lost. If you will be traveling in avalanche country, consider taking a level 1 avalanche certification course recognized by the American Avalanche Association or other reputable organization.

Before undertaking a trip where you will be far from formal medical assistance, it's wise to attend to any obvious medical problems. If you have not done so within the past 6 months, visit a dentist. Make certain that all of your immunizations are up to date (see page 420). If you have a significant medical problem, you should carry an information card, a MedicAlert bracelet or tag, or something similar. If you will be traveling abroad, be certain to have insurance that will cover you for medical evacuation from the location and specific environment in which you plan to adventure.

A common question asked of wilderness medicine physicians is whether a person can engage in certain activities or travel in a particular environment, depending on the person's state of health and medical history. Given the number of persons with preexisting conditions, especially those who are part of a growing senior population, these are very important considerations. Whether a person has coronary artery disease, diabetes, rheumatoid arthritis, sickle cell anemia, or any other of numerous conditions, it's important to understand what situations are felt to be safe and what situations are felt to be risky. Preexisting conditions are sometimes classified as "unstable." If they are unstable, they can be worsening. In general, persons with unstable conditions should not travel to high altitude, because resultant low blood oxygen levels may impair or prevent recovery from the condition. If you have a preexisting condition, consult with your physician before undertaking any activity, such as that in extreme cold, heat, or high altitude, or travel remote from medical care, that might put you or your companions at (unacceptable) risk. People with specific medical disabilities, such as chronic severe lung disease, may be advised by a physician to avoid certain stressful environments, such as high altitude.

A sexually active woman of childbearing age should have a test for early pregnancy detection before a wilderness expedition. Any pregnancy under 8 weeks' gestation has a 25% chance of miscarriage. Furthermore, it might be sensible to confirm (by an ultrasound examination) that the fetus is properly situated within the uterus and that there is not a risk for an ectopic (outside-the-uterus) pregnancy (see page 126), which could rupture and threaten the mother's life.

COMMON SENSE

Many accidents occur because people ignore warning signs or don't anticipate problems. Swimmers are stung by jellyfish outside protective net enclosures; nonswimmers drown while participating in hazardous whitewater rafting adventures. *Pay heed to rangers, posted warnings, weather reports, and the experience of seasoned guides.* Prepare for situations of risk by developing your skills in less challenging conditions. Wear recommended personal safety equipment, such as a flotation jacket, safety harness, or climbing helmet. Don't tolerate horseplay in dangerous settings.

RULES OF THE ROAD

When abroad, remember that most injuries occur while traveling on roadways, so be particularly careful. Although it may be tempting to participate in the local modes of transportation, this may be hazardous. If you're a driver or passenger in or on a motor vehicle, remember that roadways in developing nations are often dangerous. If there are traffic rules, they often are not enforced. Here are important safety rules:

1. Don't ride in the back of a truck or on the roof of a bus.
2. Always wear a seatbelt. For children, have them travel in the back seat in correctly positioned age- and size-appropriate restraints.
3. Wear a helmet when on a motorcycle or moped (if you must use these conveyances).
4. Avoid nighttime travel.
5. Don't travel alone.
6. Watch for pedestrians, particularly when visibility is low.
7. Don't exceed the posted speed limit.
8. Slow down at intersections and crosswalks. Don't pass another vehicle at an intersection or crosswalk.

Here are important safety rules for pedestrians:

1. When possible, walk on paths or sidewalks. Stay off roads that prohibit pedestrians.
2. Wear bright or reflective clothing.
3. If you must walk on the road, walk on the shoulder facing traffic. Be careful if you're on unstable ground or next to a drop-off. Try to make eye contact with the driver approaching you.
4. Look both ways, twice, before crossing a road or path. Try to do so at crosswalks or intersections. Cross in good lighting.

CONDITIONING AND ACCLIMATIZATION

Many health hazards of wilderness travel, such as falls, can be avoided by a reasonable degree of fitness, which can be acquired only by conditioning. Every expedition member should begin from a state of maximum fitness (aerobic exercise capacity, agility, and muscle strength, power, and endurance). Conditioning may make a person more capable in a situation of rescue, including performing CPR. Other health hazards, such as temperature extremes and high-altitude disorders, can in certain circumstances be avoided by acclimatization to the environment. Acclimatization is a physiologic adaptation that's often different from, and may be unrelated to, physical fitness. For instance, see the discussion on acclimatization to high altitude on page 307.

EQUIPMENT

Be prepared for foul-weather conditions. Always assume that you will be forced to spend an unexpected night outdoors. Carry warm clothing and waterproof rain gear. Know how to dress properly for all types of weather using a layered approach. Break in all footwear, and take care to pad rough edges and exposed seams. Consider carrying a compact emergency position-indicating radio beacon (EPIRB).

Persons who wear eyeglasses with multifocal (bifocal, trifocal, or progressive) lenses tend to be elders. It has been shown that wearing lenses with appropriate single-distance focus decreases the incidence of falls during outdoor activities. This may be because multifocal eyeglasses diminish depth perception and cause blurred contrast.

Before each use and after any collision or impact, a safety helmet of any sort (ski, bicycle, etc.) should be inspected for integrity. If there are cracks, dents, or other damage, the internal structure of the helmet may be altered in such a way as to lessen its ability to protect the wearer. If that is the case, replace the helmet. Helmets should fit comfortably and snugly and be worn properly. Pads should contact the cheeks and forehead, and the back of the helmet should not contact the nape of the neck. The edge of the forehead opening should rest approximately two fingers-breadth above the eyebrows. The chin strap should be tightened to the point that one finger can slide between it and the underside of the chin. If extra insulation is needed under the helmet for thermal protection, use a thin garment, not a thick hat. When wearing goggles, size them so that the top edge rests snugly and comfortably against the edge of the helmet forehead opening.

All expedition leaders should carry safety and first-aid supplies for the most likely mishaps. Medical supplies must be arranged so that they can be rapidly located and deployed and be available during all phases of the expedition, including travel to and from the adventure area. Each person on an adventure trip or expedition should carry a personal medical kit, including essential medications. Recommended first-aid items are listed in Part Five.

Become familiar with the safety profile of all equipment. For instance, be aware of the flammability of tents, clothing, sleeping bags, and so forth if you will be in the vicinity of a campfire. Certain inflatable air mattresses may be comfortable and convenient, but pose a suffocation hazard for small children if they become entrapped between the mattress and the fabric sides of a tent. Knives with spring-loaded actions and/or without a safety latch must be handled with great caution.

COMMUNICATION

Prepare a trip plan (itinerary) and record it in a location (trailhead, ranger station, marina, or the like) where someone will recognize when a person or party is overdue and potentially lost or in trouble. Similarly, determine beforehand a plan for getting help in an emergency, whether it involves radio communication, ground-to-air or ship-to-shore signals, cellular telephone, or knowing the location of the nearest pay telephone, ranger station, or first-aid facility. If mobile rescue-grade equipment is to be used, it should be checked and double-checked before departure, and regularly scheduled communications should be prepared. At least two members of any expedition should be able to fashion standard ground-to-air distress markers. Make sure children wear an item of bright clothing and carry a whistle that they know to blow if they are frightened or lost. If you carry a radio, know how to tune in to a weather information channel. The National Weather Service issues a "watch" when conditions are right for development of a concerning weather pattern, and a "warning" when its arrival is imminent.

If you will be traveling within an area with telephone or radio communication, whether on land or at sea, carry precise instructions for persons to be able to communicate in an emergency. For instance, a diver should know how to contact the Divers Alert Network (www.diversalertnetwork.org). An expedition may wish to establish a relationship with an organization such as Global Rescue (www.globalrescue.com) for medical consultation or evacuation.

TRIP PLANS

In most stories of miraculous ocean or wildland survival, the first chapter includes the account of how the victim lost his way. All wilderness travelers should carry maps, be proficient with a global positioning system (GPS) or compass routing, understand how to signal for help, and know in advance where they intend to explore. If you're traveling in snow country, you should know how to avoid being caught in an avalanche and consider carrying an avalanche rescue beacon (transceiver) that operates on the frequency of 457 kilohertz (kHz). The signal carries 100 to 150 ft (30 to 46 m) and is received by the rescuers' units. In avalanche country, also carry a shovel and a collapsible probe pole. Consider wearing an AvaLung or an ABS Avalanche Airbag System. A technology for locating an avalanche victim is the RECCO harmonic radar-based detector.

MEDICINES

There is no need to carry a drugstore on a day hike. In general, it's best to avoid administering new (to the user) drugs in a wilderness setting unless they are absolutely necessary, because untoward side effects may be more difficult to manage when distant from urban medical care. On the other hand, drugs necessary to treat established medical problems (such as nitroglycerin tablets or spray for a person with angina) should always be on hand. It is the responsibility of the trip leader to be aware of any potential significant medical problems and to insist that people in obviously poor physical condition not undertake activities that might endanger themselves or others. Any person with allergies, diabetes, epilepsy, or special medical instructions should wear an identification bracelet or carry a medical information card. Anyone who takes medications should carry a list of drugs and doses. If you travel abroad, it's wise to carry an adequate supply of routine medications, as well as a note from a physician stating their necessity, should you be questioned or need refills. All people should receive adequate antitetanus and other locally required immunizations before the trip. Basic medical supplies are listed in Part Five.

NUTRITION

Anyone who undertakes vigorous physical activity should consume adequate calories in a well-balanced diet. A debilitating weight-reduction program should not be continued in the wilderness, where a rescue might depend on extraordinary effort and endurance.

To avoid dehydration and exhaustion, take adequate time to eat, drink, and rest. Don't plan to live off the land unless you are a survival expert. Most adult men require 3500 to 5000 food calories each day to sustain heavy physical exertion. This may add 2 to 3 lb for each day's food to your backpack. Women require 2000 to 3500 calories. A nutritious diet for any activity can easily be maintained with proper planning. For instance, for backpackers, it has been suggested that the diet should be composed of 50% carbohydrates achieved by constant "carbohydrate snacking," 35% fat, and 15% protein. To calculate the number of calories worth of food to carry, multiply your ideal body weight in pounds times 22. For example, a 150 lb (68 kg) person would carry $150 \times 22 = 3300$ calories, divided into the food group ratios mentioned previously.

Consider carrying a supply of energy bars, such as the Clif Bar, NuGo, Luna Bar, Lärabar, Balance Bar, Promax Bar, or PowerBar. For a less nutritious energy boost of carbohydrates, sodium, and potassium, carry Clif Shot Energy Gel or Gu Energy Gel. However, don't count on food bars to maintain you.

People who become patients need to maintain a decent nutrition status. This is important for medical and psychological reasons. Here are some factors to consider:

1. Plan ahead. Everyone needs to eat.
2. Even if a victim is not hungry, he needs nourishment. He should consume at least 30 g of carbohydrate every 30 minutes if he is physically active. This is necessary to maintain blood sugar in an acceptable range for continued exertion. Common symptoms of low blood sugar are shakiness, hunger, sweating, sudden moodiness or behavior changes, confusion, headache, pale skin color, dizziness, and fatigue.
3. Food and drink can be emotionally reassuring.

FLUID REQUIREMENTS

Fluid requirements have been well worked out for all levels of exercise. They are highlighted in the section on heat illness (see page 296). Most people underestimate their fluid requirements. Although there is variation, the following is a hydration requirement based on an average minimal recommendation of 2 to 3 liters of liquid per day for an adult man: minimal water loss—2300 mL; water loss in hot environmental temperature—3300 mL; and water loss during heavy exercise with significant sweating—6600 mL. Other factors that increase fluid loss are activities at high altitude or in cold, dry air (increased loss during breathing), anything that increases sweating, and ingestion of drugs (e.g., alcohol or diuretics) that increase urinary losses.

Encourage frequent rest stops and water breaks. If natural sources of drinkable water (springs, wells, ice-melt runoff) will not be encountered, you should carry at least a 48-hour supply. Carry supplies for water disinfection (see page 406). Inspect your urine to be certain that it is light-colored, rather than dark-colored. Dark coloration usually indicates that you are not adequately hydrated.

PERSONAL HYGIENE AND BODILY WASTE DISPOSAL

Personal hygiene can have an effect on preventing disease transmission. The most obvious activity is washing hands effectively before eating or preparing foods. Soap and water scrubbing, followed by an application of an alcohol-based (at least 60%) gel, is the most effective technique. To wash hands properly, wet them with clean water, then lather with soap. Take care to wash bottom and top of hands, between the fingers, and under the nails. Scrub for at least 20 seconds, then rinse with clean, running water before drying with a clean cloth or towel or air drying. Sharing a contaminated towel can spread germs, so if conditions and time permit, consider air drying. Washing skin in bacteria-laden areas, such as underarms, in the groin, and around genital areas, may decrease infections in these locations. Tampons should not be retained in place for prolonged periods of time, in order to avoid toxic shock syndrome. Brushing teeth and flossing will diminish dental decay and gum infections.

Defecation is a common cause of spreading infections, in particular, various diarrheal diseases. If an outhouse is available, use it. If provision has not been made to carry wastes out of wilderness areas, they can be buried in holes (minimum depth 6 in [15 cm]) and covered tightly with soil, sand, or leaf litter, at least 100 yards from natural water sources. Toilet paper should be carried out, be biodegradable and buried, or carefully burned. Urinate far from camp and trails, preferably on rocks or bare ground. Treat animal waste like human waste.

GENERAL INJURY PREVENTION: RISK FACTORS

Injuries occurring in outdoor settings have associated risk factors. Here they are, with some of them repeated elsewhere in the book in the appropriate locations, because injury prevention is the name of the game:

Before the Activity

1. Poor mental and/or physical conditioning
2. Lack of education on proper skills and techniques to use in the field
3. Lack of appropriate equipment
4. Use of recreational drugs
5. Equipment not properly maintained
6. Poor trail/trek/route planning (natural hazards, unstable terrain, bad weather conditions, etc.)
7. Lack of awareness of risks and types of injuries

During the Activity

1. Poor physical status (fatigue, injured, etc.)
2. Refusal to wear and use safety protective gear
3. Lack of awareness of personal skills limitation
4. Lack of knowledge of the terrain
5. Equipment failure
6. Lack of safety devices integrated into equipment
7. Poor trail/trek/route maintenance

After the Event

1. Lack of appropriate injury management
2. Lack of knowledge how to contact and relay information to emergency services
3. Difficult-to-remove equipment
4. Poor trail/trek/route conditions and directions for rescue personnel

DISASTER PREPAREDNESS

If there is a chance that you may be called on to assist during a disaster, it's important to be prepared. At a minimum, you should be prepared to be self-sufficient:

1. Be physically and emotionally fit.
2. Be vaccinated for any diseases endemic to the region in which you will be a rescuer.
3. Carry a kit that will allow you to survive for a few days. This kit should contain at least the following items:
   a. Water disinfection supplies sufficient to generate 2 liters of water per day. It is better to be able to prepare 4 liters of water per day.
   b. Food that requires little or no preparation.
   c. An improvised shelter, such as a plastic sheet, cord, garbage bags, "space" blanket, and sleeping bag. A small tent with mosquito screens or netting is optimal. Include a rain fly.
   d. Fire preparation supplies (e.g., tinder and firestarter).
   e. Maps, a compass, and a GPS unit.
   f. Emergency lighting, including a headlamp and extra batteries.
   g. Cell phone or satellite phone. Also carry a whistle, survey tape, a mirror, and pad and pencil.
   h. First-aid kit.
   i. Insect repellent and sunscreen.
   j. Extra prescription glasses, extra clothing, and a multi-tool with a sharp knife.

If you are involved in a disaster response, be aware that there are many methods of "tagging" (for the purpose of triage, or sorting) patients according to their medical status. The most commonly employed method designates patients as:

1. *Green:* Minimally significant medical condition; "walking wounded"; able to care for self or with minimal assistance.
2. *Yellow:* "Delayed"—may need significant medical attention, but is expected to survive if immediate care is not rendered.
3. *Red:* "Immediate"—requires immediate life-saving intervention(s).
4. *Gray:* "Expectant"—survival is highly unlikely, even with advanced care; requires comfort measures.
5. *Black:* Dead.

In the event of a disaster, real tags may be placed on patients to indicate their categories. Another method is to use an illuminated triage light, such as a chemical light or a weather-proof battery-powered light (e.g., the E/T light [www.triagelights.com]).

The military also follows Air Evacuation (MEDEVAC) Priorities:

1. *Priority I:* Urgent—needs to be evacuated as soon as possible, with a maximum delay of 2 hours, in order to save life, limb, or eyesight, to prevent complications of serious illness, or to avoid permanent disability
2. *Priority IA:* Urgent Surg—needs surgical intervention to save life and stabilize for further evacuation
3. *Priority II:* Priority—sick or wounded and requiring prompt medical care within 4 hours or condition could deteriorate to "Urgent," where special treatment is not available, or who will suffer unnecessary pain or disability
4. *Priority III:* Routine—condition not expected to deteriorate significantly, can wait for up to 24 hours
5. *Priority IV:* Convenience—evacuation by vehicle is a matter of convenience rather than necessity

THE SCENE

When you come across a victim in need of help, he or she often is part of an accident scene, and so you must "size up" the scene and establish priorities. A structured approach will help keep you and everyone else calm and will maximize the chances for a successful outcome. Your priorities in any significant medical situation are to maintain emotional self-control; ensure the safety of yourself, your team, and the victim(s); and try to determine a reasonable overview of the situation to allow yourself to be rational and effective.

1. Don't rush in until you have had an opportunity to look over everything—the physical setting, any obvious hazards, and the victim(s).
2. Eliminate any physical dangers to the victims and rescuers. This is often referred to as "securing the scene." For instance, if you're assisting an injured hunter, be certain that no one is in the firing line of a loaded weapon, or if you are near the edge of a cliff, move to a safe location. Move out of an obvious avalanche path and away from falling rocks, and distance yourself from hazardous animals. Take shelter from lightning. Retreat from a venomous snake, swarm of stinging insects, or edge of a swiftly flowing river.
3. Don't assume that you appreciate how sick or injured the victims are until you have had a chance to examine them or take a report from a reliable examiner.
4. Protect yourself and other rescuers as best possible from exposure to contaminated blood and bodily fluids (see page 481).
5. Examine the victim(s). This first examination is called a "primary survey" and is intended to first identify any life threats. ABCDE stands for airway (see page 22); breathing (see page 28); circulation (see page 30); disability and neurologic status (including neck injury—see page 59); and exposure to the environment.
6. Treat any immediately life-threatening illnesses or injuries. If possible, explain to the victim what you're doing.
7. Make an initial call for help as soon as you are able, and try to include as much information about your location, the conditions of the victims, and what you need (supplies, food, etc.) as possible. If necessary, activate emergency medical services (e.g., call 911: EMS).
8. Perform a "secondary survey" (complete examination—see page 14) and then continue treatment. Communicate effectively with the patient. Whenever possible, explain what you're doing while maintaining a calm, supportive demeanor. Persons who are seriously ill or injured need reassurance.
9. Think about shelter and assign someone to that task, particularly in bad weather.
10. Create a treatment plan.
11. Create a plan for evacuation.
12. Prepare the victim for transportation.

DUTY TO ASSIST

In most circumstances, a person is not legally obligated (unless by employment) to assist someone in medical need. You may feel a moral obligation, but this is your decision. Good Samaritan statutes require you to follow accepted guidelines and to act as would any prudent person with similar training under the same set of circumstances. So, if you have not been trained to administer first aid, you're not expected to be able to accomplish that. You are not expected to put your or another person's life in danger in order to perform a rescue or other-wise assist a victim. Whenever possible, introduce yourself and ask the victim for permission (consent) to treat. You may attempt to persuade the victim to accept your assistance to the extent that you're comfortable doing so. If the victim is medically incompetent or is a minor (without an available parent or guardian) you're generally looked upon favorably by the law. If you begin to treat a victim, you're obligated to stay with him until you transfer care to another person.

GENERAL FIRST-AID PRINCIPLES

In all first-aid situations, the rescuer must remain calm. If you panic, you will lose control of the victim, as well as of yourself. To establish authority, speak and act calmly and purposefully. Introduce yourself to the victim and ask his permission for you to assist. Allow the victim to discuss the incident, his situation, and his fears. If you can involve the victim in his rescue and treatment, it's often good for his morale. Try not to be judgmental, and save criticism for after the event. Avoid laying any blame on people; they may get hurt emotionally or become argumentative as a result. When communicating with a victim and bystanders, remember that you are not only caring for the victim, but in many ways, for family and friends. It is important to communicate frequently, honestly, and in a manner that is reassuring and inspires cooperation and hope. Promote communication and teamwork. If you need assistance in handling a situation, ask for and be willing to accept it. If a situation or medical leader is needed, try to establish this position and be clear about who is in charge.

Examine the victim for a medical bracelet, wallet card, or other medical record.

Don't endanger additional inexperienced rescuers. If you cannot get to the victim easily, send for help. Approach all victims safely; don't allow the sense of urgency to transform a sensible rescue into a series of risky, or even foolhardy, maneuvers. If it appears that the victim is too ill to be moved, set up camp immediately. In all cases, protect the victim from the elements from above and below.

If you have paper and a writing instrument, record your observations. If you send someone for help, have him carry a piece of paper that states the victim or victims' location, nature of the emergency, number of people needing help, condition of the victim(s), what is being done to treat the victim(s), and any specific environmental conditions or physical obstacles. Accident report forms are available from organizations such as The Mountaineers.

Always assume the worst. Assume that each victim you encounter has a broken neck or has had a heart attack until proved otherwise. Always be conservative in your treatments and recommendations for further evaluation or rescue.

Never move a seriously injured victim unless he is in danger from the environment or needs to be moved for medical reasons. Don't encourage a victim to get up and "shake it off" until you have examined him for a potentially serious problem. If you must remain in a wilderness location for a prolonged period of time caring for a victim who has become your patient, remember to attend to the basic survival requirements, which include air (oxygen) for breathing, shelter, water, food, psychological support, and human waste disposal. If possible, change dressings applied to wounds every 24 hours.

Never administer medicines or perform procedures if you're not sure what you are doing. The Good Samaritan has certain legal protections for his actions so long as he operates within prudent limits and takes reasonable care. This book will not make you a doctor. A good rule to follow is *primum non nocere*: "First of all, do no harm." If you're not certain what to do and the situation isn't worsening, don't interfere. Explain to the victim that you are not a physician, but will do your best to get him through whatever crisis he has encountered, to the best of your knowledge and ability. If you encounter a victim who may be seriously ill, seek an expert opinion as soon as possible. Even if your treatment seems successful, it's wise to consult a physician if you would have ordinarily done so.

Listen to the patient. The story of what happened and the medical history can be extremely important in making swift and appropriate medical decisions. Let the victim tell you what happened in his or her own words, and try not to interrupt unless it's important. If a victim has a sprained ankle, a comprehensive discussion may not be necessary, but if it is appropriate, try to elicit the following:

Current illness: What happened? When did it happen? Why did it happen? If the victim is suffering pain, describe its location, time of onset, whether it came on suddenly or gradually, whether it comes and goes, its quality (dull, sharp, cramping, etc.), how it is made worse or relieved, and whether the victim has suffered anything similar before (and if so, whether there was a medical diagnosis). Have the victim describe all symptoms, such as nausea, vomiting, diarrhea, blurred vision, shortness of breath, fatigue, cough, and so on.

Prior illnesses and preexisting conditions: Have the victim describe any previous illness (heart attack, asthma, pneumonia, meningitis, etc.) and any current conditions (diabetes, anemia, abnormal heart rhythms, etc.) and how they have been and are currently being treated.

Surgeries: Have the victim list any surgical operations, such as appendectomy or knee surgery.

Medications: Have the victim list any current medications.

Allergies: This includes allergies to food, plants, insects, and medication(s) and the nature of the allergic reaction(s).

Immunizations, exposure to communicable diseases, recent foreign travel, occupation, recent dietary history: Any of these may be appropriate if the victim is perhaps suffering from an infectious disease, including food poisoning or toxic ingestion.

Review of systems: This is a comprehensive questioning about each organ system to determine if the victim has or has ever had symptoms referable to each system:

- *General:* Fever, chills, fatigue, weakness, unintentional weight loss or gain, excessive thirst or urination, hot or cold temperature intolerance, excessive sweating, easy bruising, loss of appetite, dizziness, history of intravenous drug use
- *Head:* Headache, dizziness
- *Eyes:* Blurred vision, double vision, decreased vision, discharge, itching, pain
- *Ears:* Decreased hearing, ringing or buzzing in the ears, discharge from the ears, pain
- *Nose:* Nosebleeds, difficulty breathing, nasal discharge, sinus infection
- *Throat:* Sore throat, foreign body sensation, tonsillitis, hoarseness or difficulty talking, painful swallowing, difficulty swallowing
- *Dental:* Tooth loss, abscess, dentures, bleeding from gums
- *Neck:* Pain, decreased range of motion, arthritis
- *Chest (lungs):* Difficulty breathing, chest pain when breathing, shortness of breath, wheezing, cough (productive of sputum or nonproductive), coughing blood, history of tobacco use
- *Heart:* Palpitations, pressure-like sensation in the chest, chest pain, fainting
- *Abdomen:* Pain, mass
- *Gastrointestinal:* Nausea, vomiting (describe what is vomited), diarrhea (describe color and consistency), red blood in stools or dark black stools, yellow skin (jaundice), perianal itching, constipation, excessive gas, bloating, belching
- *Hematologic/immune:* Anemia, frequent infections, exposure to human immunodeficiency virus (HIV) or Ebola virus
- *Genitourinary:* Change in frequency of voiding, incontinence, painful urination, discolored or malodorous urine, back pain, blood in urine, history of sexual contacts, penile or vaginal discharge, testicular pain, date and character of last menstrual period (normal, abnormal), vaginal bleeding

- *Neurologic:* Seizure, weakness in any body part, numbness or tingling of any body part, difficulty with coordination or walking, difficulty with speech or comprehension, fainting
- *Muscular/skeletal:* Muscle cramps, weakness, incoordination, muscle pain, joint pain or swelling
- *Psychiatric:* Abnormal thinking, hallucinations (visual or auditory), desire to hurt self or others, inappropriate crying or laughing, depression, nervousness, insomnia, mood changes

EVALUATE THE VICTIM

Your goal is to eventually examine the entire victim, unless the situation precludes the examination or it's completely obvious that you're dealing with an isolated body part, such as a hand injury. To begin, immediately determine if the victim is breathing, if his heart is beating, and if he has any obvious major injuries. Techniques and procedures for treatment are covered in Part Two.

Vital Signs by Age Group

When you examine a person, you will usually be able to count the pulse rate in beats per minute, count respirations in breaths per minute, and sometimes obtain the blood pressure. Here are normal values for these "vital signs":

Age	Weight	Breaths/Min	Pulse/Min	Systolic Blood Pressure (mm Hg)
Newborn	6-9 lb (3-4 kg)	30-50	120-160	60-80
6 mo-1 yr	16-22 lb (8-10 kg)	30-40	110-140	70-80
2-4 yr	24-34 lb (12-16 kg)	20-30	100-110	80-95
5-8 yr	36-55 lb (18-26 kg)	14-20	90-100	90-100
8-12 yr	55-100 lb (26-50 kg)	12-20	80-100	100-110
12-18 yr	>110 lb (50 kg)	12-20	60-90	100-120
Adult	>110 lb (50 kg)	12-18	55-90	120

Look, listen, and feel for breathing (Figure 1). Put your ear close to the victim's mouth and nose, and try to detect if he is moving air into and out of his lungs. Watch for chest wall motion. Determine if a victim is breathing by listening and feeling for air movement around the mouth and nose and observing the chest for unassisted rise and fall. In cold weather, look for a vapor cloud or feel for warm air moving across your hand. If the victim is not breathing well (or at all), you must manage the airway (see page 22) and begin to breathe for him (see page 28), *taking care to maintain the position of the neck if there is any chance of a cervical spine injury* (see page 35). Observe the number of breaths per minute; normal is 12 to 18 per minute for adults, 20 to 30 per minute for small children, and 30 to 50 per minute for infants.

Characterize the nature and effort of breathing. Look to see if breathing is effective—the chest expands, and air movement is appreciated. Observe if the victim is laboring to breathe. In an adult, if the breathing rate is less than 10 or greater than 30 breaths per minute, the skin color is blue, or the victim is confused or unconscious, be prepared to assist breathing (see page 28).

If the breathing is noisy, rattling, or "musical" and high-pitched, suspect an airway obstruction (see page 22), particularly if the victim is lying on his back. If the victim has a loose denture

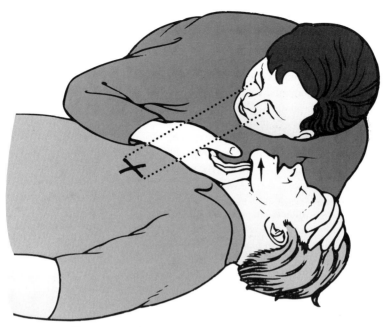

Figure 1. Look, feel, and listen for air movement.

or another dental appliance, remove it. If there is no chance of a cervical spine injury (see page 35) and it appears that the victim may vomit, position him on his side. If you're concerned about a neck injury, use the logrolling maneuver (see page 38).

Near the condition of death, a person may show "agonal respirations," characterized by infrequent mouth openings without any chest rise, sometimes accompanied by head lifting.

Pulse Oximetry

A pulse oximeter is a small device that measures the saturation of oxygen in the blood. The oximeter is usually placed on a fingertip or earlobe. A normal oxygen saturation reading depends on the altitude at which it is obtained, because there is less oxygen in the atmosphere as one ascends in altitude. Ninety-four percent to 100% is normal oxygen saturation in a healthy person at sea level. As one ascends to high altitude, the saturation generally drops, but with acclimatization up to an altitude of approximately 12,000 feet should not fall below 90%. If the oxygen saturation is measured lower than its predicted value, this may represent a problem with oxygen supply or delivery (such as occurs with high-altitude pulmonary edema [see page 310]), a state of dehydration, a false reading resulting from placing the oximeter on a cold finger or a finger with nail polish or pressed-on nail, severe anemia, blood volume deficiency or shock (see page 58), exposure of the oximeter to bright light or a strong electromagnetic field, or other causes. If the patient is short of breath in a way that's a cause for concern (see page 190) and the oximeter reading is low (below 90%), it's wise to administer oxygen (see page 405) if it is available. If carbon monoxide intoxication (see page 306) or dark skin pigmentation is present, the pulse oximeter reading may be falsely elevated, so pulse oximetry should not be relied upon in these situations. Although pulse oximetry determination does not predict who will or won't develop acute mountain sickness, it's a useful adjunct to follow the oxygenation of a person at high altitude.

Feel for a pulse. Current American Heart Association guidelines advise laypersons to begin chest compressions without going through a pulse check on victims who are not breathing and who don't show any sign of life. However, basic life support may also be initiated by checking for a pulse. Place the tips of your index and middle fingers (not your thumb, which can generate a "false" pulse—your own!) gently on the radial artery in the wrist (see Figure 17, C, page 31). If you cannot detect a pulse there (particularly if your fingers are cold), move your fingers quickly to the brachial artery (this is particularly useful for infants) at the midpoint of the inside of the upper arm (see Figure 17, E, page 31), the femoral artery in the groin (see Figure 17, B, page 31), or the carotid artery in the neck (see Figure 17, A, page 31). If no pulse is detected in any of these locations (and the victim is not breathing or verbalizing), begin chest compressions (see page 30). Observe the pulse rate; normal is 55 to 90 per minute for adults, 100 to 110 per minute for small children, and 110 to 140 per minute for infants. The pulse rate is faster with excitement or fear and slower in trained athletes. A rapid and weak ("thready") pulse is a sign of impending shock (see page 58), usually as a result of excessive bleeding, dehydration, or heart problems. An irregular pulse may indicate an abnormal heart rhythm.

Locate brisk bleeding. Quickly survey the victim to locate any obvious sources of brisk bleeding. Quickly apply firm pressure to these areas (see page 50). Take blood and bodily fluid precautions (see page 481).

Once you have dealt with these life-threatening problems, begin a careful, complete examination of the victim. Take a step back and consider the general appearance and condition of your patient. Sometimes you will get a sense that something is seriously wrong. An infant who is lethargic is potentially very ill; a senior citizen who is confused and has slurred speech is in trouble. Trust your instincts.

If an injury may be extensive, examine the whole victim. It's easy to become focused on an obvious injury, such as a deformed broken ankle, and overlook other, possibly more serious, injuries. Whenever possible, perform a complete examination of any patient who has anything more than a minor ailment. Particularly dangerous situations include falls; blows to the head, neck, chest, or abdomen; altered mental status; difficulty breathing or shortness of breath; and injuries to children. In these cases, or whenever the diagnosis is not readily apparent, evaluate the victim from head to toe. Weather and appropriate modesty permitting, be sure to undress the victim sufficiently to perform a proper examination. Look around the neck or on the wrist(s) for a medical alert (such as MedicAlert) tag, and in a wallet, helmet, or pack for an information card.

Because most bodies are bilaterally symmetrical, if you're having difficulty determining if a body part is abnormal or deformed, compare it to the opposite side. Always ask a victim to move a body part before you do it for him; if he resists because of pain or weakness, you need to suspect a broken bone or spinal cord (nerve) injury. Don't "force" a motion.

Take as much time as you can afford to explain to a victim what you are going to do. This is usually reassuring. If the victim is a child, it's important to make eye contact and to be continually supportive. If someone is doing or has done something with which you don't agree, make any argument or criticism out of earshot of the victim. If the examiner is opposite in gender to the victim, try to have a same-gender witness (chaperone). When examining a victim, keep talking to him. Closely observe for indications of discomfort or pain.

1. Check the victim's mental status. If he is awake, determine if he is oriented to time, place, and person. ("What is the date? Where are you? Who are you?") Note if the speech pattern is normal, slurred, or garbled. If the answers are in any way abnormal, suspect a head injury, intoxication, stroke, central nervous system infection (such as meningitis), hyperthermia, hypothermia, severe high-altitude illness, low blood sugar, or hypoxia (insufficient oxygen to the brain). Maintain constant observation of the victim until all of his responses are appropriate.

2. Examine the neck. Without turning the victim's head, feel each cervical vertebra and the first few thoracic vertebrae from behind and note tenderness or muscle spasm. The seventh vertebra will be the most prominent. Check for swelling. Feel the Adam's apple in the front of the neck for tenderness or a "crunching" sensation (noted by both the examiner and victim). If there is a chance of neck injury, immobilize the neck (see page 35).

3. Examine the spinal column. Run your fingers down the length of the spine and press to elicit any tenderness. Check for spinal cord injury by having the victim voluntarily move his arms and legs and report his sense of feeling. Ask the victim to squeeze your hand with each of his, and then to "press down on the gas pedal" with each foot against your hand. Pinch the skin on the back of the hand and top of the foot as a crude measure of sensation. If any response (hand-to-hand or foot-to-foot) is asymmetrical, suspect a spinal cord injury or stroke (see pages 35 and 135).

4. Examine the head—but try not to move it. Feel the entire scalp gently for raised or depressed areas, or cuts. *Observe blood and bodily fluid precautions* (see page 481).

   While being careful to not expose yourself unnecessarily to blood, look carefully through thick scalp hair for sites of bleeding. Look into the ears for drainage (clear [spinal] fluid, blood, or pus). If there is blood, capture some on a white absorbent cloth or gauze pad. If the blood forms a ring, with a faded or yellow area toward the center, this may indicate the presence of leaking cerebrospinal ("spinal") fluid. Feel the nose for obvious malalignment or instability. Look up into the nostrils. If you have a flashlight, shine it into the eyes to see if the pupils constrict and are equal in size. If you don't have a flashlight, cover the eyes and then uncover them to see if the pupils constrict. Pinpoint (constricted) pupils may be a sign of brain injury or drug overdose. Unequal pupils may represent a direct injury to an eye or a brain injury. Nonreactive and bilaterally dilated pupils may represent a severe brain injury. Ask the victim to follow your fingers with his eyes; if this cannot be done, if the eyes don't move together, or if he reports blurred or double vision, there may be a problem. If the eyes are spontaneously jerking or wandering, this may also indicate abnormality. If the victim has contact lenses, he may require assistance with their removal (see page 172).

   Have the victim open and close his mouth to see if the teeth fit properly. Feel the nose to check for pain and deformity. Check the teeth for absence, looseness, or breaks, and the tongue for cuts. Have the victim open and close his mouth, and move his jaw from side to side. Ask him to stick out his tongue and move it from side to side. Ask the victim if he can swallow. Ask him to say "Ahh" and see if you can get a glimpse of the back of his throat. If dentures are loose, remove them. Inspect for missing teeth. Smell the victim's breath to detect any abnormal odor (e.g., alcohol or "fruity" breath associated with severe diabetes).

5. Examine the skin. Look for sweating, skin color (normal may—and pale does—indicate inadequate circulation; dusky blue indicates hypothermia or shock; reddened indicates heat illness or sunburn; yellow indicates liver disease; mottled indicates low blood pressure, hypothermia, shock, or massive infection), bruises, rashes, burns, bites, and cuts. Note the skin temperature. Look inside the lower eyelids for a pale color that might indicate anemia or internal bleeding. If you pinch the skin on a victim's forearm and it remains "tented" and loose, the victim may be dehydrated. One method to determine adequacy of the general circulation is to check "capillary refill." To do this, press down firmly on the victim's fingernail in order to blanch (turns pale white) the tissue underneath the nail. When the pressure is released, if the circulation is adequate, normal (usually red-pink) will return within 2 seconds (Figure 2). If it takes longer than 2 seconds, suspect a circulatory problem, which can be general (e.g., anemia, significant dehydration, low blood pressure) or localized (e.g., very cold temperature).

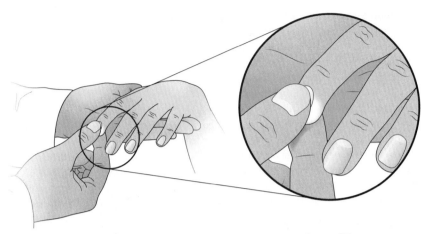

Figure 2. Pressing on a fingernail to check capillary refill.

6. Examine the chest. Observe whether the chest expands fully and equally on both sides with breathing. Feel the chest wall and breastbone for tenderness and inspect for deformation or embedded objects. Run your fingers along the length of the collarbones. Place your ear against each side of the chest to listen for breath sounds.

7. Examine the abdomen. Gently press in all areas to elicit tenderness. See page 116 for a discussion of causes of abdominal pain. Examine the genitals. An uncontrolled penile erection might indicate a spinal cord injury. If you have pressed on the spine and it is not tender, and you otherwise don't suspect a spinal injury, roll the patient (with assistance if possible) and examine the back and buttocks.

8. Examine all bones and joints. Gently press on the chest, pelvis, arms, and legs to elicit any tenderness. As noted earlier, run your fingers down the length of the clavicles (collarbones) and press centrally where they join the sternum. Trace each rib with your fingers. Look for deformation or discoloration. When practical, check circulation, movement, and feeling in all limbs.

9. Take a temperature. Use a digital, mercury, or alcohol thermometer, if possible one that can detect hypothermia or hyperthermia, depending on the circumstance. Rectal temperature measurement is more reliable than oral or axillary (see page 155) measurement, but may be impractical in the field. Always shake down a mercury or oral thermometer, and hold it in place for at least 3 minutes to obtain a reading. Don't rely on skin temperature to accurately reflect changes in the core temperature. Feeling a person's forehead to determine temperature is notoriously inaccurate.

10. Perform a brief mental health evaluation. Notice your patient's speech capability and pattern, ability to reason, and whether or not he makes sense. Ask him if he can recite his name, location, date, and circumstances. Make note of abnormal thoughts, expressions of despair or hostility, and any declaration of auditory or visual hallucinations.

Send for help early. As soon as you have determined that a situation will require extrication, rescue, or advanced life support, initiate your prearranged plan for communication and transportation. Don't assume that someone will call for help; you must assign this task to a specific individual. If you have a medical report form available to send to potential rescuers, do so. If not, try to write down and transmit the following information with a reasonable amount of specificity:

1. Number of victims
2. Location

3. Landing area for helicopter—yes or no; include weather conditions
4. Your name and immediate contact information
5. Communication appliances—mobile phone, radio
6. For each victim:
   a. Age
   b. Gender
   c. Injuries/medical problems
   d. Condition
   e. Therapies (splints, bandages, procedures, medications) undertaken

If you're in a situation in which you can access the emergency medical service (EMS) system (911 or other telephone number), be prepared to provide the following information: the victim's location, your phone number, the nature of the emergency, the number of people needing help, the condition of the victim(s), what is being done to treat the victim(s), and any specific environmental conditions or physical obstacles. Speak slowly and clearly, and don't hang up until the dispatcher tells you he has all the information he needs.

While you are waiting for help to arrive:

1. Complete an adequate history. Listen carefully to the victim; in most cases, he will lead you to the affected organ system. Remember to inquire about allergies, especially to medications.

2. Reassure the victim. Most disorders aren't life-threatening and will allow you plenty of time to formulate a treatment plan. Be sure you have introduced yourself to the victim, and always explain what you are doing in a direct fashion. Avoid making comments such as "Oh my God," "This is a hopeless situation," or "Whoops!" Let the victim know that you are capable and in charge. Accentuate the positive aspects of the situation, to build a climate of hope. Don't argue with other rescuers in the presence of the victim. Be particularly gentle, parental, and reassuring with children. Always warn the victim before you do anything that might cause him pain.

3. Keep the victim comfortable and warm. Don't feed a victim who cannot purposefully swallow. If he can eat and drink, offer water, clear soups, and clear juices. Use oral rehydration salts (ORS; see page 194) or an electrolyte-containing sports beverage to maintain hydration. Avoid coffee, tea, and other caffeinated beverages.

4. Keep a written record of all medications given. If possible, also record symptoms and objective measurements (such as temperature) with times noted.

5. Remove all constrictive clothing or jewelry from any injured areas. If the victim has a hand wound, all watches and rings (see page 447) should be removed before swelling makes doing so impossible. In particular, rings left in place can become inadvertent tourniquets on swollen fingers.

Always reexamine and reevaluate a victim at regular intervals. A person may not experience difficulties until after a time delay, particularly if the problem is related to a head injury or internal bleeding. If you're concerned enough about a person to examine him once, wait a while and then examine him again. The interval between examinations is determined by your level of concern. For instance, someone with possible internal bleeding (see page 57) should be examined every 10 to 15 minutes until you're confident that the severity of the situation has declined sufficiently to warrant less vigilance. *If someone has an altered mental status (particularly after a head injury), he requires your constant attention.*

Try to maintain reasonable hygiene. This includes handwashing with soap and water and/or using an alcohol-based (at least 60%) hand gel. This is particularly important as an interval activity between multiple victims. Be aware that alcohol-based hand gel is not particularly effective against spore-forming bacteria, such as *Clostridium difficile.*

ASSISTING A VICTIM OF STARVATION

In a rare circumstance, you may encounter someone who has been without food and/or water for days or weeks and is in a situation of starvation. If that's the case, the general approach is to:

1. Attend to any life-threatening injuries or medical conditions.
2. Be certain that the person has functioning kidneys. This may be very difficult to determine in the field. If the person can still urinate, for the purpose of immediate care, you should proceed to offer food and drink. If the person is so "dry" that he has not urinated for 24 or more hours, proceed with caution and watch for fluid retention (swelling of the ankles and shortness of breath). Begin with 10 mL (2 teaspoons) of oral fluid per kg (2.2 lb) of body weight consumed every 2 to 3 hours until urination begins. An acceptable fluid is a dilute electrolyte solution (e.g., ORS [see page 194] or half-strength [diluted with water] Gatorade or other sports beverage).
3. Slowly feed the victim small portions of a food that is relatively high in fat (e.g., bacon, eggs, nuts, banana chips).
4. Don't permit the victim to gorge on fluid or food. The sudden sensation of profound fullness may cause nausea and vomiting.

LONG-TERM CARE OF AN UNCONSCIOUS OR GRAVELY DISABLED PERSON

If a person is unconscious or gravely disabled and you need to care for him for more than a day, you may need to attend to the following:

1. Be careful administering oral liquids, food, or medications. The person must be capable of purposeful swallowing.
2. If the eyes are open and the victim cannot blink or protect his eyes, gently tape them shut or provide for regular moisturization/lubrication with "artificial tears."
3. If the victim urinates or defecates and soils himself, he should be cleaned and dry clothing or a diaper applied.
4. To prevent pressure sores, reposition the victim at least every 2 hours to provide full circulation to any compressed soft tissues.

MEDICAL DECISION-MAKING

The art of outdoor medicine absolutely depends on observation, anticipation, and resourcefulness. The cardinal rule is to act conservatively and not take unnecessary risks when making the decision to continue a journey or postpone travel and seek formal medical attention. Similarly, you may need to decide whether to carry out a disabled victim or to stay put and signal or send for help.

Although every situation is unique, all decisions begin with an accurate assessment of the victim's condition. The situation should be categorized as trivial (small cuts, insect sting without allergic reaction, a single episode of diarrhea); minor (sprained ankle, small burn wound, sore throat); moderately disabling (broken wrist, kidney stone, bronchitis); potentially severe (chest pain, severe abdominal pain, high fever); totally disabling (seizure, broken hip, severe high-altitude illness); or life-threatening and limb-threatening (uncontrolled bleeding, extensive frostbite, venomous snakebite with symptoms). In all cases that are other than trivial or minor, it's proper to insist on prompt evacuation or rescue for thorough evaluation. Never overestimate your abilities as a healer or count on good fortune. *The assumption under which you must operate is that a victim's clinical condition will deteriorate, particularly in a harsh environmental setting.* No adventure is worth a lost life or permanent disablement.

If more than one victim is injured, you must set priorities and attend to the most critically injured. Continually evaluate each victim to detect improvement or deterioration over time.

Don't focus on situations that are beyond reasonable hope. For example, if a victim is near death from severe burns, decide if there is really anything you can do to save him, and if not, get busy with the people you can help. These are emotionally charged and extremely difficult decisions, even for those of us who have made them many times for many years.

You may have to decide whether to evacuate a victim or wait for a rescue party. In some instances, this is an easy decision—when a victim must be carried to a lower altitude to treat severe mountain sickness, for instance, or when the transport route is short and easily negotiated. The judgment call is based on weather conditions, the nature and severity of the injury or illness, and the distance that needs to be covered.

Sometimes you may need to care for a person for days, and hand off their care to another person. If you become a caregiver, it's very important that you form the most accurate impression possible of your patient. Here are rules to follow:

1. If the situation permits, ask your new patient to repeat his or her history. If the person is reluctant to engage in a long conversation, at least try to get him to relate current relevant events.

2. Repeat as much of the physical examination as you can. Explain to the patient that you have assumed his care, and that in order to do the best that you can on his behalf, it's important for you to understand his issues and to be able to monitor progress based upon the examination.

3. Assume that until you have talked to the patient or otherwise obtained a comprehensive history, and performed a physical examination with your own hands, eyes, and ears, you don't know as much as you could about your patient.

4. Interview and examine your patient as often as is necessary and practical. If you must be absent from a patient for a longer period than is prudent between examinations, delegate the responsibility to someone else.

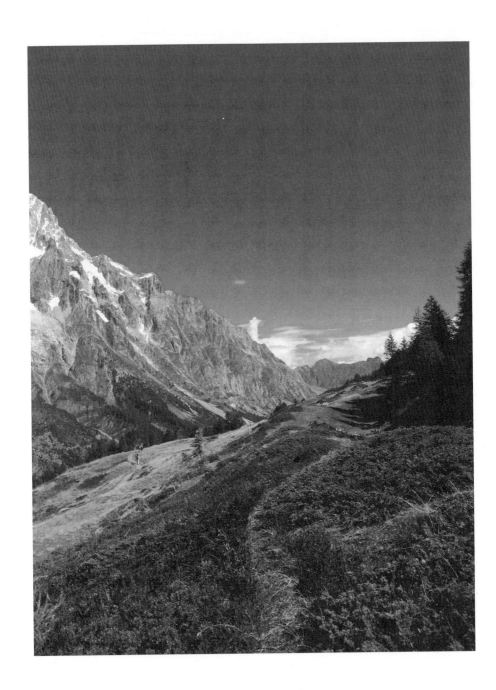

PART TWO

Major Medical Problems

This section describes common disorders that may be life-threatening. The problems are often present in combination and require prompt recognition and management.

AN APPROACH TO THE UNCONSCIOUS VICTIM

Any disorder that decreases the supply of blood, oxygen, or sugar to the brain or that causes brain swelling, bleeding into the brain, or alteration of critical body chemistries can lead to unconsciousness. Thus, virtually every major illness or injury can ultimately render a person unconscious. If you come across someone who cannot be awakened, you must rapidly assess him for any treatable life-threatening conditions, and then try to discover the cause of the altered mental state.

The victim should not be moved until you carefully perform the following examination in sequence. Until you're absolutely certain that the victim does not have a neck injury, don't attempt to arouse him by vigorous shaking methods.

1. Evaluate the airway (see page 22).
2. Evaluate breathing (see page 28).
3. Check for pulses (see page 30).

The "ABC" (airway, breathing, circulation) method as the initial approach to determine whether or not to begin the chest compressions of cardiopulmonary resuscitation (CPR) for cardiac arrest victims has been changed to a "CAB" approach, with initiation of chest compressions first, followed by airway and breathing (see pages 22-34). This does not conflict with the earlier advice. Most of the persons you encounter who are unresponsive are not suffering from cardiac arrest.

1. Protect the cervical spine (see page 35).
2. Control obvious bleeding (see page 50).
3. Examine the victim for chest injury (see page 39), broken bones (see page 67), and burns (see page 108).
4. Consider shock (see page 58), head injury (see page 59), seizure (see page 65), severe allergic reaction (see page 64), low blood sugar (see page 133), stroke (see page 135), fainting spell (see page 154), hypothermia (see page 281), heat illness (see page 296), high-altitude cerebral edema (see page 311), high-altitude pulmonary edema (see page 310), lightning strike (see page 340), poisoning, and alcohol or drug intoxication.
5. Remove contact lenses (see page 172).
6. Transport the victim to medical attention (see page 429).

HELMET REMOVAL

If the victim is wearing a helmet, it may be necessary to rapidly remove it to get to the airway. It is very important to do this in a way that protects the neck from twisting or bending forward or backward. It usually takes two persons to safely remove a helmet:

1. The first rescuer, positioned above the head of the victim, holds the helmeted head steady by grasping it on each side. If necessary to support the airway, the first rescuer can reach down and hold the mandible (lower jaw).
2. The second rescuer, positioned below the head of the victim, prepares the helmet for removal by loosening and removing straps, goggles, and other attachments, so long as this process does not allow for unintended head movement.
3. The second rescuer takes over head stabilization, while the first rescuer continues to hold the helmeted head, by sliding two hands along the sides of the victim's head position; this should be done by either placing one hand behind the base of the head at its junction with the neck and the other hand under the chin or by sliding two hands along the sides of the head and up inside the helmet.
4. The first rescuer completes removal of retaining straps, then slides the helmet off the head using axial (straight up away from the feet, without any twisting) traction.
5. Head positioning and gentle traction are maintained while a cervical collar or other method (see page 35) is used to stabilize the position of the head and neck.

AIRWAY

Airway obstruction is one of the leading causes of death in victims of head injury, and a frequent complication of vomiting in an unconscious person. Adequacy of the airway and breathing must be attained rapidly in every victim. In the absence of hypothermia, an interval of 4 minutes in which there is a failure to oxygenate the brain can lead to irreversible damage.

Figure 3 depicts the anatomy of the respiratory system. Air enters the mouth and nose (where it is humidified), traverses the pharynx (throat), passes through the trachea (windpipe) and bronchi, and normally proceeds into the smallest air sacs of the lungs, known as the alveoli. Within these distal air spaces, inspired oxygen is exchanged for carbon dioxide, one of the end products of human metabolism. During swallowing, the epiglottis and tongue cover the entrance

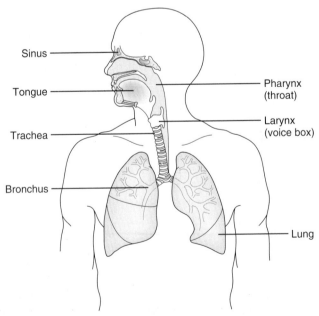

Figure 3. Anatomy of the respiratory system.

(via the vocal cords) to the trachea, so that food and liquid are directed to enter the esophagus and not the airway.

Obstruction of the airway at any level can interfere with the passage of air, delivery of oxygen via the lungs to the blood, and exhalation of carbon dioxide. The mouth and pharynx may fill with blood, vomitus, or secretions. With facial injury, deformation of the jaw or nose may hinder breathing. In a supine (face up) unconscious victim, the tongue may fall back into the pharynx and occlude the opening to the trachea. Inhalation of food can obstruct the opening between the vocal cords and cause rapid suffocation.

Symptoms of airway obstruction include sudden inability to speak, appearance of panic with bulging eyes, blue skin discoloration (cyanosis), choking gestures (hand held to the throat), harsh and raspy or "musical" and high-pitched noise ("stridor") that comes from the throat during breathing, and difficulty with breathing as evidenced by struggling and profound agitation. Any person who collapses suddenly, particularly while eating, or who has been in an accident should be examined rapidly for airway obstruction.

1. *Under no circumstance should the neck be manipulated if there is a possibility of injury to the spine or spinal cord.* If a victim is unconscious and has suffered a fall or multiple injuries, it's safest to assume that his neck is broken. In this situation, keep the airway open by gently but firmly lifting the jaw, either by grasping the lower teeth and jaw and pulling directly forward (away from the face), or by maintaining a forward pull on the angles of the jaw (Figure 4). Don't bend the neck forward or backward. A modified jaw thrust (Figure 5) can be performed by a single rescuer while stabilizing the neck.

2. *If there is no chance of a broken neck,* maintain the airway with the jaw lifts previously described or by tilting the head backward while gently lifting under the neck (Figure 6). The alignment is different for an infant, small child, or older child or adult in terms of

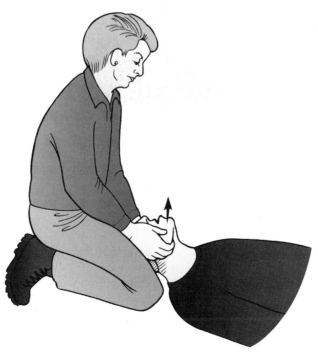

Figure 4. Jaw pull to open the airway.

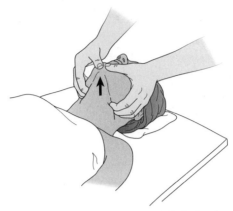

Figure 5. Modified jaw thrust to open the airway while being in a position to minimize motion of the neck. Grasping the angles of the lower jaw firmly, the rescuer pulls forward to lift the tongue out of the throat.

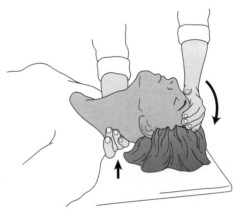

Figure 6. Positioning the head to control the airway. The forehead is gently pushed back while support is maintained under the neck. *Never* manipulate the head or neck if a broken neck is suspected.

where one would position a pad or pillow (Figure 7). A head tilt with chin lift may be used (Figure 8).

3. Keep the airway clear of blood, vomitus, loose dentures, and debris. This can be accomplished by sweeping the mouth with two fingers or by continuous suction with a field suction apparatus powerful enough to extract chunks. Take care not to force objects deeper into the throat. If the tongue appears to be the problem (you may hear a snoring noise when the victim inhales), wrap the end of the tongue in a cloth or gauze bandage, grasp firmly, and pull it out of the mouth (Figure 9). If it cannot be held in this manner, a seemingly brutal, but potentially lifesaving, maneuver may be used. A safety pin or sharp-pointed wire may be passed through the tongue and used to improve the grip (see Figure 9), taking care to avoid the large, visible blood vessels at the base of the tongue. To keep the tongue out of the mouth, a string can be tied to the safety pin and then secured to the victim's shirt button or jacket zipper. Fortunately, in most cases the jaw lift will carry the base of the tongue out of the airway. Another aggressive technique is to use

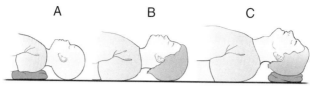

Figure 7. Placement of a pillow to assist airway alignment in an infant **(A)**, small child **(B)** and older child or adult **(C)**.

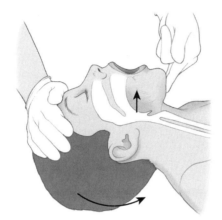

Figure 8. Head tilt with chin lift to bring the base of the tongue forward and open the airway.

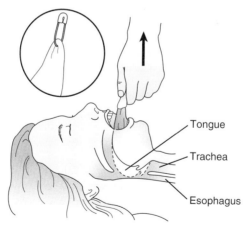

Figure 9. Manual tongue traction. With a cloth or safety pin *(inset)* to secure the grip, the tongue is lifted out of the mouth to clear the airway.

two safety pins to attach the tongue to the face just below the lower lip (Figure 10) or with an extending string to the victim's shirt button or jacket zipper.

4. If the victim is unconscious, and there is no chance of a broken neck or back, don't leave him lying flat on his back. Turn him on his side ("recovery position") so that if vomiting or bleeding occurs, the fluid can drain from his mouth and the victim won't choke or drown (Figure 11). Use a pillow or other paddng as needed for comfort, but don't occlude gravitational drainage from the mouth.

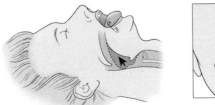
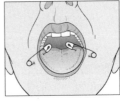

Figure 10. Using two safety pins to attach the tongue to the lower lip to help control the airway.

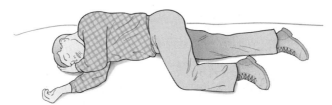

Figure 11. Victim on his side to minimize choking.

5. If the victim is conscious and having airway difficulty, allow him to assume whatever position keeps him most comfortable. This usually protects the airway and allows the victim to handle his secretions (e.g., saliva or bleeding from the mouth and nose).
6. Choking is a life-threatening condition in which the upper airway (above the vocal cords) is obstructed by a foreign object (tongue, broken teeth, dentures, food). The choking person is profoundly agitated (until he becomes unconscious from lack of oxygen), may appear to be panicked with bulging eyes, may grasp at his throat in a choking gesture, cannot breathe, and is unable to speak. You must respond rapidly:

Sweep the mouth with one or two fingers to remove any foreign material. Take care not to force material farther into the throat. Quickly extract loose dentures.

Using an open hand, give the victim two to four rapid, sharp blows on the back between the shoulder blades. This may be more effective if the victim is lying on his side or is bent forward at the waist. If a small child is choking, perform this maneuver while holding him face down or upside down. If the victim is an infant, place him face down on one of your forearms, with his head lower than his body. Support his head. Give five quick back blows, then turn the infant over and give five quick chest thrusts (similar to those given during CPR—see page 30).

Perform the Heimlich maneuver (Figure 12). Position yourself behind the victim and encircle him with your arms, clasping your hands in a fist in the upper abdomen just below his ribs. Squeeze the victim suddenly and firmly ("bear hug") two or three times, in an attempt to produce a brisk exhalation (cough) and ejection of the foreign (choking) material. If your first attempt is unsuccessful, alternate back blows with the Heimlich maneuver. If you are the victim and no one is present to help during a choking episode, you can throw yourself against a log or table edge in an attempt to perform a self-Heimlich maneuver.

If the victim is lying on his back (supine), perform the Heimlich maneuver by sitting astride his thighs, facing his head (Figure 13). Place the heel of one hand on his upper abdomen and cover it with your other hand. Press into the abdomen suddenly and firmly in a direction toward the chest. Do this a few times, and then perform the chin

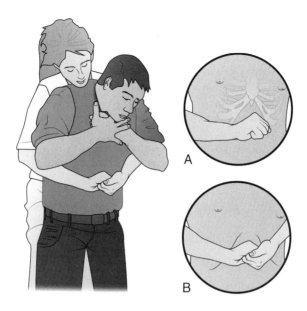

Figure 12. The Heimlich maneuver. **A,** A hand is placed on the upper abdomen. **B,** The second hand interlocks to create a tight grip. A sudden, forceful squeeze ("bear hug") causes the victim to cough.

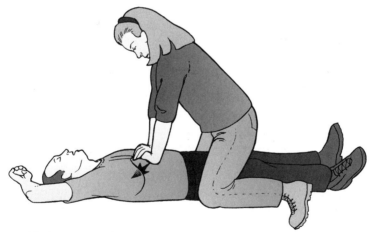

Figure 13. Heimlich maneuver with the victim lying on his back.

lift (see step 1 on page 23) and sweep a finger deeply through the mouth to extract any foreign material forced up by your efforts. Take care not to push anything back into the throat.

For a child older than 1 year of age, keep him supine (because the child is too large to hold face down or upside down) and place the heel of your hand well below his breastbone but above his navel.

If the victim is obese or pregnant, apply the force (with the victim sitting or lying down) to the center of the chest (breastbone), rather than the abdomen.

If necessary, begin mouth-to-mouth breathing (see page 28).

BREATHING

The act of breathing delivers oxygen to the lungs during inhalation, exchanges oxygen for carbon dioxide in the lungs, transfers oxygen into the bloodstream, and removes carbon dioxide during exhalation. The rate and depth of breathing are controlled by the oxygen and carbon dioxide levels in the blood, by the body's oxygen demand, by the ability of the blood to unload oxygen to the tissues, by brain and brainstem regulatory sensory systems, and by emotional factors. If there is a head or spinal cord injury, however, the central nervous system stimulus for breathing may be lost. In many instances, this is only transient (lightning strike is a good example); thus, it's imperative to provide breathing assistance for a period of time before giving up hope. Exhaled air from a human contains 16% oxygen, which is enough to support life (via mouth-to-mouth or mouth-to-[face]mask breathing) at low altitudes.

A direct chest injury (broken ribs, fractured breastbone, bruised or collapsed lung) may render respirations inadequate because of pain or mechanical dysfunction. Accumulation of fluid in the lungs because of inhalation, burns, heart failure, or constriction of the smaller branches of the airway (during an asthma episode or allergic reaction) may make the work of breathing overwhelming for the victim.

How to Assist Breathing (Mouth-to-Mouth)

1. Position the victim's head in the "sniffing position" by placing one hand under his neck and the other on his forehead, to lift behind the neck (gently) and tilt the head backward (see Figure 6). If you suspect a broken neck, don't move the victim's neck; merely lift his jaw (see Figure 5).
2. Quickly sweep two fingers through the victim's mouth to remove any foreign material. Remove loose dentures.
3. Pinch the victim's mouth closed and cover his mouth with your own (Figure 14). If you have a barrier (pocket face mask or mouth shield, such as the NuMask Pocket CPR Kit with one-way valve) to prevent transmission of infectious diseases, use it as directed. An improvised barrier shield for rescue breathing can be created by taking a surgical glove and cutting off the middle finger at the midpoint of its length. The rescuer then stretches the glove across the victim's mouth and nose and blows into the glove (Figure 15). After each breath, uncover the nose to allow the victim to exhale. If you are using the jaw lift technique to open the airway, press your cheek against the victim's nose to occlude it

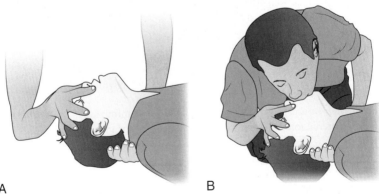

A   B

Figure 14. Mouth-to-mouth breathing. **A,** While the neck is supported with one hand, the nose is pinched closed. **B,** The rescuer covers the victim's mouth with his own and forces air into the victim until the chest rises. This should take approximately 1 to 2 seconds.

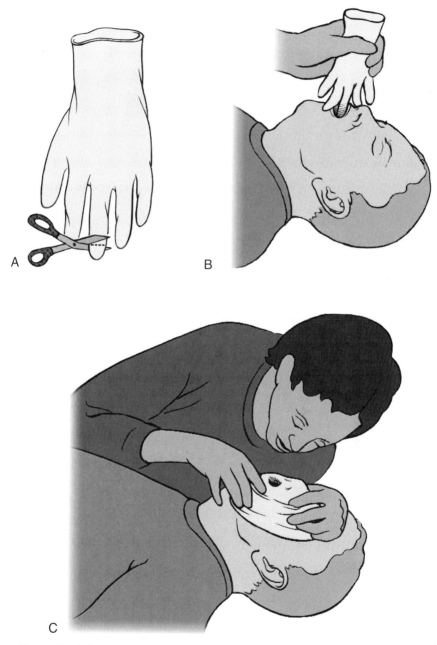

Figure 15. **A-C,** Improvised CPR barrier fashioned from protective surgical glove.

during mouth-to-mouth breathing. For mouth-to-nose breathing, close the victim's mouth and cover his nose with your mouth. For small children and infants, cover both the mouth and nose with your mouth (Figure 16).

4. Blow air into the adult victim until you see his chest rise. This should take approximately 1 to 2 seconds. With small children and infants, don't blow forcefully. Remove your mouth and allow the victim to exhale passively; the chest should fall. The goal is to give two full

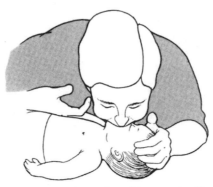

Figure 16. Mouth-to-mouth-and-nose breathing required to resuscitate a child.

breaths, pausing between them to inhale and see if the chest moves properly. If the victim is not spontaneously breathing, coughing, or moving after you have provided the first two breaths, prepare to administer the chest compressions of CPR (see page 32).

5. Repeat the inhale–exhale cycle every 5 seconds for adults, and every 3 seconds for children. If chest compressions are occurring, the ratio is 30 compressions to each 2 rescue breaths for adults and children.

6. If you meet resistance trying to blow air into the victim's lungs and/or the chest does not rise, be certain the airway is open (proper head position, tongue and mouth clear—see pages 23-26). You may need to lift the jaw (see page 23) to pull the base of the tongue up and out of the throat. If the positioning is correct and the chest still does not rise, consider an airway obstruction with a foreign body (see page 26).

7. If it's impossible to blow any air into the victim's lungs, it might be that something is lodged in his airway. Turn the victim on his side and deliver four sharp blows between the shoulder blades, or perform the Heimlich maneuver (see page 27).

8. Mouth-to-mouth breathing usually forces air into the victim's stomach as well as into his lungs. If the stomach fills up with so much air that it becomes tense and you cannot expand the lungs, turn the victim quickly on his side and press on the abdomen. This may make him vomit, so be prepared to clean out the mouth.

CHECK FOR PULSES (CIRCULATION)

Assess the need for CPR. Current American Heart Association guidelines advise laypersons to follow a "Simplified Adult Basic Life Support (BLS) Algorithm." This emphasizes a "Push Hard–Push Fast" approach that specifies that if the victim is unresponsive (without signs of life) and is not breathing (or is gasping only), then the rescuer should activate an emergency response (e.g., call for assistance), obtain an automated external defibrillator (AED), and begin chest compressions. If the AED is applied and the victim is suffering from ventricular fibrillation, a shock may be delivered. Always check with the manufacturer, but be aware that most AEDs, because they are self-grounded, can be used safely in wet environments or on metal surfaces without risk to the rescuer.

　　Determining whether or not BLS has been successful eventually requires checking for a pulse. Check for pulses for 10 seconds at the neck (carotid artery: Figure 17, *A*) or groin (femoral artery: Figure 17, *B*). Use the tips of your index and middle fingers to feel for a pulse. Don't use your thumb, because this finger often has pulsations of its own, which you may confuse with the victim's pulse. Using more than one finger at the same time to locate a pulse may increase your likelihood of feeling it.

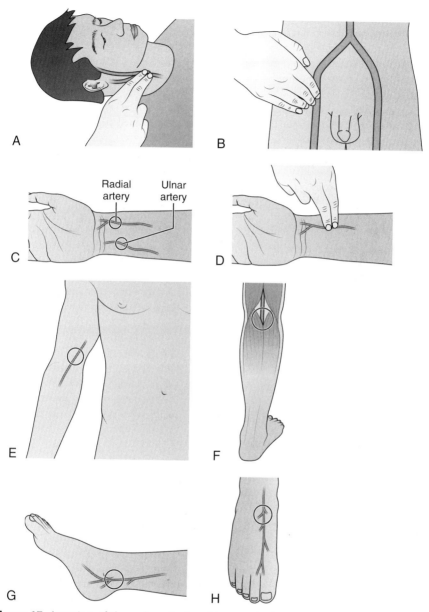

Figure 17. Location of the pulses. **A,** Carotid artery in the neck. **B,** Femoral artery in the groin. **C,** Radial and ulnar arteries in the wrist. **D,** Taking a radial pulse. **E,** Brachial artery in the arm. **F,** Popliteal artery behind the knee. **G,** Posterior tibial artery on the inner aspect of the ankle. **H,** Dorsalis pedis artery on the top of the foot.

Don't rely on the wrist (radial or ulnar artery: Figure 17, C and D) for the determination of heartbeat. The carotid artery is located (see Figure 17, A) at the level of the Adam's apple, between this structure and the large muscle (sternocleidomastoid) that runs from the base of the ear to the collarbone. Pulsations from the femoral artery may be felt (see Figure 17, B) below the abdomen in the groin crease where the front of the leg attaches to the trunk, two fingerbreadths medial (toward the center) to the midpoint in the line from the hipbone (anterior iliac spine) to the bony region directly under the pubic hair (the pubic symphysis). Other locations where the pulse may be felt (often with great difficulty) are on the inner aspect of the elbow (brachial artery: Figure 17, *E*); behind the knee (popliteal artery: Figure 17, *F*); directly behind the bony prominence (malleolus) on the inner side of the ankle (posterior tibial artery: Figure 17, *G*); and centrally on the top of the foot (dorsalis pedis artery: Figure 17, *H*).

A normal resting pulse rate is 55 to 90 per minute for adults, 80 to 110 per minute for small children, and 100 to 130 per minute for infants. A well-conditioned athlete will often have a resting pulse rate of 45 to 50 per minute, because the well-developed vagus nerve's impulses dominate. Failure to feel a pulse means that the heart is not beating (cardiac arrest), the pump (heart) is not squeezing with sufficient force (profound shock or hypothermia), the artery is constricted (hypothermia), there is an injury to the artery (from a fracture or severe cut), or you are feeling in the wrong place.

If no pulse is detected (and the victim is unconscious and not breathing), give 30 chest compressions, then open the airway and deliver 2 breaths, and then continue the CPR sequence of 30 compressions to every 2 breaths. Call or send someone for help.

Chest compressions are performed as follows:

1. Place the victim on his back on a firm surface and position the heel of one of your hands over the center of his breastbone (Figure 18, *A*). The heel of your second hand is placed over the bottom hand. Interlock your fingers (see Figure 18, *B*) and keep them held lightly off the victim's chest.
2. Your shoulders should line up directly over the victim's breastbone, with your arms straightened at the elbows (Figure 19).
3. Using a stiff-arm technique, the adult breastbone is compressed at least 2 inches (5 cm) and then released (Figure 20). Keep your motions smooth. The compression phase should equal the relaxation phase, with a rate of at least 100 compressions per minute for adults and children. Give an initial 30 compressions. With single-rescuer CPR, try to maintain a

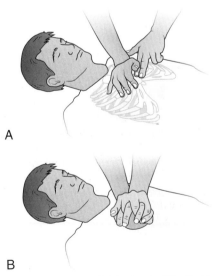

A

B

Figure 18. Positioning the hands for CPR. **A,** The heel of the first hand is placed two finger-breadths above the bottom edge of the breastbone. **B,** The second hand is placed over the first and the fingers are interlocked.

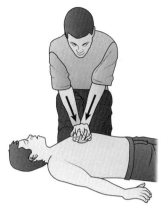

Figure 19. Proper arm and body position for CPR. The rescuer compresses the victim's chest by keeping the arms straight and dropping his upper body weight directly over the victim.

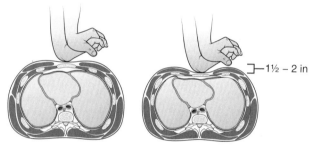

Figure 20. Compression of the chest during CPR. With proper technique, the adult/child breastbone should be compressed 1½ to 2 inches, with 100 compressions per minute.

ratio of 30 compressions interrupted by 2 mouth-to-mouth breaths (see page 28). After the first 4 cycles of compressions and breaths, check for pulses and spontaneous breathing. If both are absent, resume your efforts, checking for signs of life every few minutes.

4. If two rescuers are working together, the second rescuer should give the victim mouth-to-mouth resuscitation, forcing 2 breaths into him with every 30 chest compressions. The artificial breaths should be provided during a brief pause between compressions.

5. Continue CPR until you are relieved by someone, you become exhausted, the victim is revived, or a qualified person pronounces the victim dead. Situations in which CPR is unlikely to revive a victim include cardiac arrest associated with severe injuries, drowning in which the victim has been submerged for more than an hour (with the exception of cold-water immersion—see page 286), the victim having an incompressible chest (extreme cold or prolonged "downtime" with rigor mortis—see page 285), and after 30 minutes of resuscitation effort without any victim response (breathing or pulse).

Chest compressions in infants and small children can be performed by placing a stabilizing hand on the child's back and compressing hand (or fingers) on the chest (Figure 21). With a small child, use one hand to perform the compressions. With an infant, use two fingers. Care should be taken to provide firm compressions without separating the ribs from the breastbone. For a small child or infant, the rate of chest compressions is at least 100 per minute, with 2

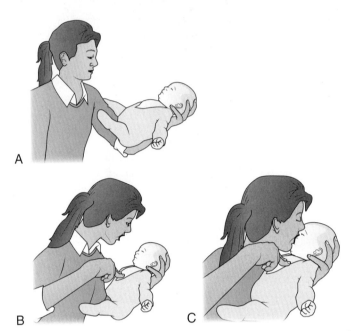

Figure 21. Infant CPR. **A,** Positioning the infant on the forearm. **B,** With the forearm for a back support, two fingers of the opposite hand are used to compress the breastbone. **C,** The mouth and nose of the infant are covered by the rescuer's mouth for rescue breathing.

breaths after each 30 compressions. The compression depth is at least one-third of the anterior–posterior diameter of the chest (approximately 1.5 inch [4 cm] in infants and small children, and 2 inches [5 cm] in large children). Although there are advocates of chest compression-only (i.e., without rescue breathing) CPR in adults, there is emerging information that this approach should not be used in children. Children should receive the full benefits of rescue breathing properly applied during CPR.

Continue to administer rescue breathing and chest compressions until help arrives or you become too tired to continue. Miraculous survivals have been reported in victims of prolonged cardiac arrest from cold-water submersion or lightning strike. During the first 5 to 7 minutes of CPR, if you cannot do both mouth-to-mouth breathing and chest compressions for whatever reason, do the compressions only.

As mentioned previously, if you have access to an AED, attach it to the victim as soon as possible, so that it can determine whether or not a shock (for ventricular fibrillation, in which the heart does not contract, but quivers in such a fashion as to be unable to pump blood) is indicated. If the AED shocks the victim, then check for a pulse and breathing. If the victim continues to require chest compressions because a pulse is not present, continue CPR for 2 minutes and then use the AED again to determine whether or not a shock is indicated. If a shock is successful in terminating ventricular fibrillation, chest compressions may still be necessary for a minute or two to circulate blood (and oxygen) while the heart restores a life-sustaining rhythm and blood pressure. When pulses return and can be felt, discontinue chest compressions.

The Condition of Death

CPR in a wilderness setting is rarely successful. Unfortunately, your best efforts at resuscitation may be to no avail and the victim will die. Signs of death include no detectable pulse; absent breathing; dilated (and often irregularly shaped) pupils that don't contract when exposed to bright light; pale or blue-gray skin, fingernails, and lips; penile erection; uncontrolled urination or bowel movement; cool body temperature; and no movement or response to pain. After a period of an hour or two, the muscles become stiff (rigor mortis), the skin mottles, and blood settles visibly in a dependent fashion due to gravity, causing large discolored blotches on the victim's back, buttocks, and legs (if he is kept supine). *However, it's essential to remember that hypothermic individuals, who are extremely cold, may appear to be dead* (see page 285), when in fact they are alive and might be saved. Severely hypothermic individuals may have fixed and dilated (nonreactive to light) pupils, nondetectable pulses, breathing so shallow that it cannot be detected, skin mottling, stiff muscles, and so forth. Therefore, if severe hypothermia is suspected, "no one is dead until he is warm and dead." In such a case, resuscitative efforts should be carried out until the victim is revived, the rescuers become exhausted or endangered, or a health care professional can pronounce death. This is also true for a victim of lightning strike or cold-water drowning, and for children.

So, for which victim should CPR not be started? Unless the victim is suspected or known to be hypothermic, it's reasonable to not begin CPR if you check for a pulse and breathing for a full minute and cannot detect either; if there is an unsurvivable injury (e.g., decapitation, incineration, or apparent death and decomposition of the body); or if it's unsafe for the rescuer. If a victim is dead, the body should be decently covered and kept in a cool location until extrication is possible. If foul play is suspected, the body should not be moved. If a dangerous communicable infection is suspected as the cause of death, take appropriate precautions and minimize body handling.

If you are in possession of a dead body or bodies and extrication will not be possible, you may need to dispose of the body. Here are some suggestions:

1. Respect local custom and practice, unless it is dangerous. Burial is often the preferred method, but cremation may be advised in certain circumstances of infectious disease.
2. The burial site should be at least 164 ft (50 m) from drinking water sources and 1640 ft (500 m) from the nearest dwelling. Dig the hole at least 5 ft (1.5 m) above the groundwater table, and at least 3.3 ft (1 m) deep.
3. Keep a record of identifying features, including photographs and possessions.
4. If you're able, wrap the victim in a plastic sheet or something similar before burial.
5. Mark the location of the burial.
6. If cremation is done, it should occur at least 1640 feet (500 m) downwind from the nearest dwelling.

PROTECT THE CERVICAL SPINE

If a victim has fallen, is unconscious, or has a face or head injury, he may have a fracture of the cervical spine (neck). High-risk situations include falls from a height greater than 10 feet or any fall that involves an elderly person, motor vehicle accidents at speeds over 35 mph or with a death at the scene, drowning, and diving accidents. If the victim has external evidence of a neck injury; complains of midline neck or back pain; or has a tender neck when examined, broken limb, pelvic pain, altered mentation, head or face injury, chest or back pain, or abnormal sensation or weakness in the hands or feet, be suspicious for an associated cervical spine fracture. In this circumstance, it's prudent to immobilize the victim's head and neck.

Never move the neck to reposition it, except as discussed two paragraphs later. You must immediately immobilize the head and neck. The neck can be immobilized by taping the head to a backboard or stretcher, by applying a rigid collar, or by placing sandbags or their equivalent on either side of the head (Figure 22). Don't use bags of snow to hold the head, because these may melt and allow too much motion; they can also contribute to hypothermia (see page 281).

In general, the most dangerous direction of motion for a neck-injured (spinal cord–injured) person is chin to chest (flexed). Circumferential neck collars that prevent flexion can be purchased preformed or be fashioned from cardboard, Ensolite sleeping pad material, foam-covered

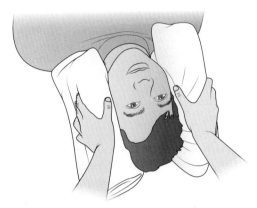

Figure 22. Immobilization of the neck using rolled towels. The rescuer's hands may be replaced with a strap of tape across the forehead to prevent movement.

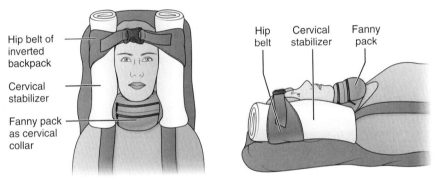

Hip belt of inverted backpack

Cervical stabilizer

Fanny pack as cervical collar

Hip belt   Cervical stabilizer   Fanny pack

Figure 23. Cervical collar fashioned from a padded hip belt on an inverted backpack.

aluminum (the SAM Splint) (see Figure 301), a padded hip belt on an inverted backpack (Figure 23), or other semi-rigid materials. For a neck collar to be effective, it must be rigid or semi-rigid, fit properly, not choke the victim, and allow the victim's mouth to open if he needs to vomit. One way to improvise a splint is to wrap bulky clothing with a wide elastic bandage to compress the material and make it more rigid.

It may be necessary to straighten (align) the victim's head and neck in order to allow extrication or transportation, or to improve the airway (see page 22). If it's absolutely necessary to do this, very slowly (using at least two hands) keep gentle traction on the head and first move it so that the neck is not bent sideways, without performing any head rotation. Stop immediately if any resistance is felt to this maneuver. Then, rotate the head until the head and neck are in a neutral (facing forward) position. Stop immediately if any resistance is felt to this maneuver. *Don't at any point flex the neck forward or extend it backward.* If the victim is awake and can talk to you, instruct him to let you know if moving his head and neck is causing him to have increased pain or to have a worsened neurologic situation (such as numbness in the hand or arm). If that's the case, then don't move the neck if at all possible.

The safest way to move a victim with a suspected neck injury is to apply a protective collar and transport the person on a rigid backboard or vacuum mattress. An improvised spine board can be made by inserting a snow shovel through the centerline attachment points of an internal frame backpack. Pad the shovel, then tape the victim's head to the shovel, which serves as a head bed. The pack suspension system is used to stabilize the shoulders and torso, so that the victim now has his head relatively immobilized. Another possibility is to invert (turn upside down) an internal or external frame backpack and use the padded hip belt as a head bed.

If a rigid collar cannot be applied without forcing the neck into an unnatural (for the victim) position, it may be better to use a soft collar with rigid reinforcements to prevent motion. For instance, if the victim is an elderly person who normally has a forward curvature of the spine, and can inform you of this, it's better to immobilize the neck in a comfortable (for the victim) position with a slight amount of flexion. Applying force to straighten this particular victim's neck might risk worsening a fracture or even causing a spinal cord injury. In any case, the most important thing is to prevent future unintended motion.

If no other equipment is available and if the victim is conscious and cooperative, a thick pad (rolled towel, jacket, or the like) may be placed at the base of his neck. This can be made more rigid by first wrapping (compressing) it with a wide elastic (e.g., ACE) bandage. Secure this by wrapping tape or cloth around the forehead, then crossing it over the pad and bringing it back out under the armpits to be tied across the chest (Figure 24). *Be aware that this technique does not guarantee immobilization in a combative or confused victim, and provides only enough support to remind the victim to not move his head and neck.*

In proportion to the torso, the head of a young child is larger than is the head of an adult. Therefore, when a child is flat on his back, his neck may be flexed instead of in a "neutral" position. To overcome this effect, tilt the head back slightly, or place a blanket or pad under the child's torso.

If the victim becomes uncooperative or agitated, you must hold his head until it can be firmly immobilized and the victim restrained from motion (Figure 25; see Figure 22). All of this is necessary to avoid injury to the spinal cord. If the victim must be moved or turned on his side (most commonly to allow vomiting or to place insulation beneath him), hold his head fixed between your forearms while you hold his shoulders with your hands. In this way the victim can be "logrolled," using as many rescuers as possible to avoid unnecessary motion (Figure 26).

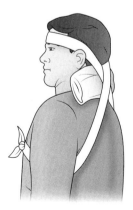

Figure 24. A rolled towel or shirt is secured behind the neck with a firmly wrapped cravat or cloth. This technique should be used solely for an alert and cooperative victim. *It provides only enough support to remind the victim to not move his head and neck.*

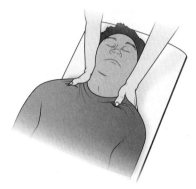

Figure 25. Immobilization of the neck. The rescuer grasps the victim's shoulders and controls the head between his forearms.

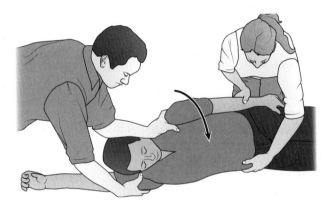

Figure 26. Logrolling the victim. The rescuer at the head immobilizes the neck with his forearms and the victim's extended arm, while an assistant helps turn the body.

Logrolling the Victim (see Figure 26)

The best way to carry and immobilize a person who may have an injured spine is to use a scoop stretcher, or to slide a backboard underneath the victim. However, when these are not available and a spine-injured person must be turned, logrolling is the best alternative.

1. The first rescuer approaches the victim from the head, and keeps the head and shoulders in a fixed position (no neck movement).
2. The second rescuer extends the victim's arm (on the side over which the victim is to be rolled) above the victim's head. The first rescuer takes this arm and uses it to help support the head in proper position.
3. All rescuers work together to turn the victim without moving his neck.

Lifting a Victim

See page 429.

CHEST INJURY

BROKEN RIBS

Direct force applied to the chest wall can break ribs, causing extreme pain with breathing, collapse of a lung (pneumothorax), or both. If the right lower ribs are broken, be alert to the possibility of a bruised or cracked liver, which lies directly below; if the left lower ribs are broken, the underlying spleen may be injured.

FLAIL CHEST

If a number of ribs are broken or detached in series, so that the affected section of the chest wall cannot expand and contract in synchrony with the rest of the chest, then a flail chest (Figure 27) is present. Depending on the size of the flail segment, this can cause severe respiratory compromise. Sometimes the flail segment moves with breathing in a direction opposite to the rest of the chest wall (e.g., it moves inward on inspiration and outward on expiration).

PNEUMOTHORAX

A pneumothorax is a collapsed lung created when there is an air leak (from the lung or from a penetrating wound of the chest wall) into the space between the lung and the inside of the chest wall (pleural space). In the normal situation, the pleural space is undetectable and filled with negative pressure, which allows the lung to expand and contract with chest wall movement (breathing). When air leaks into the pleural space, either from a lung injury or from a hole in the chest wall, the lung collapses. The lung may then be increasingly compressed if air accumulates in the pleural space under pressure (Figure 28). A collapsed lung is recognized by diminished or absent breath sounds (heard through a stethoscope or an ear held against the chest wall) on the affected side, accompanied by chest pain, shortness of breath, and difficulty breathing. If air accumulates under pressure in the affected pleural space, this becomes a "tension" pneumothorax. This is characterized by rapidly progressive difficulty in breathing, cyanosis (blue skin discoloration), distended neck (jugular) veins, and a shift of the windpipe away from the affected side.

Sometimes, the same process that causes air to escape from the lung to create a pneumothorax can direct some of this air to become trapped under the skin, creating a "crackling" sensation when the skin is pressed, sensation of fullness or visible swelling in the neck, change in voice,

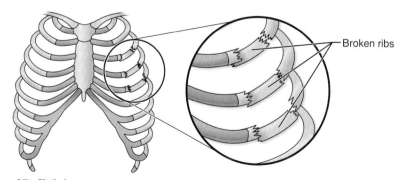

Figure 27. Flail chest. A section of detached (broken) ribs may seriously impede the mechanics of breathing.

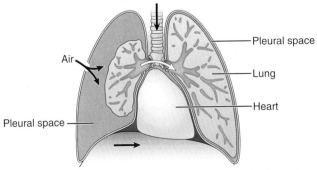

Figure 28. Pneumothorax. Air enters the pleural space lining the lung through the chest wall or from a lung leak, which causes the lung to collapse. A tension pneumothorax occurs when air in the pleural space accumulates under pressure, forcing the lung, heart, and trachea to the opposite side *(white arrow)*.

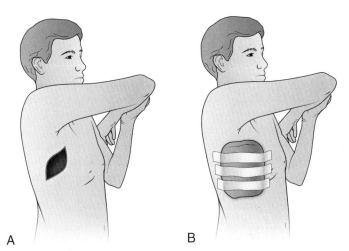

Figure 29. Chest wound dressing. **A,** Open chest wound. **B,** The dressing is held firmly in place with tape or a cloth wrap.

and difficulty swallowing. Although worrisome in appearance, this subcutaneous (under the skin) air absorbs over time and is not nearly as dangerous as a collapsed lung.

BRUISED LUNG

A bruised lung can result when sufficient force is applied to the chest wall. This injury typically causes increased difficulty with breathing after a delay of minutes to hours, as blood and tissue fluid accumulate in the injured lung. In a severe case, the victim will cough up blood clots.

TREATMENT FOR CHEST INJURIES

1. Attend to any chest wounds. All open wounds (particularly those in which air is bubbling) should be rapidly covered, to avoid "sucking" chest wounds that could allow more air to enter the pleural space and thus continue to worsen a collapsed lung (see page 39). For a dressing, a Vaseline-impregnated gauze, heavy cloth, or adhesive tape (Figure 29) can be used. The dressing should be sealed to the chest on at least three sides (Figure 30). If the

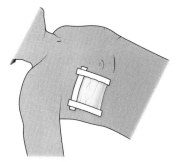

Figure 30. Apply a dressing sealed on three sides to cover a wound over a collapsed lung.

victim develops a tension pneumothorax following a penetrating wound to the chest and his condition deteriorates rapidly (difficulty breathing, cyanosis, distended neck veins, collapse followed by unconsciousness), force a finger through the wound into the chest to allow the air under pressure to escape. If your diagnosis is correct, you will hear a hissing noise as the air rushes out. This allows the lung to partially expand and may save the victim's life. (When a tension pneumothorax occurs and there is no hole in the chest through which the air can escape, a trained rescuer will place a needle or catheter [14 gauge] through the chest wall over the top side of the 2nd to 4th rib in the line directly down from the armpit [axilla] to allow the air to exit.) After the release of air from a tension pneumothorax, cover the wound with a completely occlusive (not permeable to air; so *not* a loosely woven piece of gauze) dressing and seal only three sides (see Figure 30) to create a flutter-valve effect (air can exit, but not enter) and prevent a recurrence—which might come with a complete seal. SAM Chest Seal is an occlusive dressing designed for treating open chest wounds. It comes in forms with or without a one-way valve.

2. Administer oxygen (see page 405). If an oxygen tank is available, oxygen should be administered at a rate of 5 liters per minute by face mask or nasal prongs. Elderly victims who have been heavy cigarette smokers (chronic obstructive pulmonary disease [COPD]: see page 45) should be watched carefully for signs of decreasing consciousness whenever oxygen is administered. If this occurs (in the absence of head trauma or shock), supplemental oxygen should be discontinued.

3. Assess the rate and adequacy of breathing. Watch for chest rise, feel and listen to the chest, place a hand near the nose and mouth to check for air movement, and observe skin color. If necessary, assist breathing. This may be done with mouth-to-mouth breathing (see page 28) or with a face mask device. *If the victim is not breathing, check for pulses and assess the need for CPR (see page 30).*

4. Anyone who has a significant flail chest will be unable to coordinate the muscular act of breathing and will need early assistance. The flail segment should be cushioned firmly with pillows, sandbags, or their equivalent (Figure 31). If necessary, secure the cushion with wide strips of tape or straps, but don't make these circumferential around the chest in such a way that they will restrict chest wall expansion for breathing. Cushioning and strapping limit movement (pain) of the broken bones and ease the act of breathing.

5. Broken ribs are best managed with cushioning in a position of comfort and frequent reevaluation of the ability to breathe. Don't tape or tightly wrap the ribs, because this might prevent complete reexpansion of the chest (lung) with inspiration and therefore predispose the victim to shallow, inadequate breathing and subsequent pneumonia.

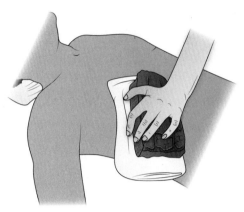

Figure 31. Method of cushioning a flail chest wall segment by applying firm pressure with a blanket and section of tree bark.

However, a moderately snug elastic wrapping of the chest may be necessary to provide sufficient pain relief so that a victim can self-extricate. Encourage the victim to take at least one deep breath or give one good cough each hour. Allow 6 to 8 weeks for the ribs to heal before allowing very strenuous activity.

6. Evacuate the victim as soon as possible. Properly positioning the victim may be helpful. If the chest is injured on one side, transport the victim on his side with the injured side up and the uninjured side down. This may facilitate better oxygenation of the blood. However, take note that a person with a flail segment may occasionally be more comfortable with the injured side down. If that's the case, then facilitate whatever position that allows the greatest amount of pain relief and the victim to be effectively transported.

SERIOUS LUNG DISORDERS

ASTHMA

Asthma is a hyperresponsive disease of the airways and lungs that involves episodes of coughing, shortness of breath, wheezing, and increased secretions in the bronchi. Generally, most people will know that they are prone to asthma attacks; however, a first-time episode may occur during an allergic reaction, on exertion or exposure to cold, or as a result of emotional stress. In most cases, the mechanism is the same: narrowing and spasm of the small airways, with increased mucus production. Asthma is often accompanied by inflammation of the airways. The victim has difficulty breathing, with wheezing during exhalation (most common), during inspiration, or both. Coughing is a major feature. The victim may become quite anxious ("air hunger"). Severe cases lead to rapid respiratory deterioration, cyanosis (blue discoloration of the skin), and the use of accessory muscles of respiration (the victim sits upright and attempts to expand the chest wall by contracting neck muscles and using body movements). When the attack is extreme, wheezing may diminish, because the lungs become so "tight" that there is not enough air movement to create the abnormal breath sounds. The victim may tire out. Worrisome signs that indicate a severe asthma attack are very rapid or very slow breathing rate, and inability to speak or lie down. Diminished or poor feeding in an infant may indicate severe asthma.

Treatment for Severe Asthma

1. Administer oxygen (see page 405) by face mask at a rate of 10 liters per minute. If cold weather precipitated the attack, try to get the victim into a warmer climate.

2. Administer an inhaled (aerosol or "micronized") bronchodilator. Bronchodilators (airway openers) are drugs that carry the advantages of minimal side effects and direct delivery to the site of action. They are available in metered-dose handheld inhalers from which the victim takes therapeutic puffs. An excellent drug for an acute attack is albuterol (Ventolin). The dose for an adult is 200 micrograms (two puffs initially—each puff contains approximately 90 micrograms), followed by two puffs up to 6 times a day. A mild to moderate asthma episode in an adult can frequently be controlled with an inhaled bronchodilator alone, and sometimes even a single puff will be effective. Young children have difficulty using the inhaler, and therefore may require administration of the drug orally in pill or liquid form. The most effective technique for metered-dose inhalation is discharging the contents through a spacer clamped between the lips. The drug should be released (canister pressed down or "triggered") at the beginning of a deep inspiration. After inhalation, the recipient should attempt to hold his breath for 10 seconds. A person with asthma may also be carrying his own long-acting bronchodilator, such as salmeterol or formoterol.

3. Administer epinephrine (adrenaline) if the victim remains in severe distress after inhalation of a bronchodilator. For a severe asthma attack that is not remitting, the drug may be given in a proper dose every 20 minutes for 3 doses. Epinephrine is a powerful bronchodilator that's injected intramuscularly (see page 444) as an aqueous solution of 1:1000 concentration in a dose of 0.3 to 0.5 mL for an adult and 0.01 mL/kg of body weight for a child (not to exceed 0.3 mL). For weight estimation, 1 kg equals 2.2 lb. It should be injected into the lateral thigh. If the thigh is obese, whether in an adult or a child, such that the needle might not reach into muscle, then inject into the lower thigh. If obesity is extreme, consider injecting into the mid-calf. The only reason to administer the drug subcutaneously (see page 446) is if the equipment is not available for an intramuscular injection. The drug is available in preloaded syringes in certain allergy kits, which include the EpiPen autoinjector and EpiPen Jr. autoinjector, the Auvi-Q "talking" autoinjector (0.3 mg or 0.15 mg dose), and the Adrenaclick (0.3 mg or 0.15 mg dose). Other devices worldwide are the Jext, Emerade, Allerject, and Anapen. Instructions for use accompany the kits. For dosing purposes, a 0.3 mg autoinjector should be used for adults and children over 66 lb (30 kg) in weight. Children 66 lb and under should be injected with a 0.15 mg autoinjector.

   Take particular care to handle preloaded syringes properly, to avoid inadvertent injection into an unintended location, such as a finger or toe. Don't intentionally inject epinephrine into the buttocks or a vein. Epinephrine should not be exposed to heat or sun, but does not need to be kept refrigerated. If clear (liquid) epinephrine turns cloudy or discolored, it should be discarded. When administering an injection, *never* share needles between people.

   Epinephrine is not recommended for persons known to have coronary artery heart disease (angina or recent heart attack) or older than 45 years. Epinephrine is the treatment of choice for a severe asthma attack in a child.

4. Administer a corticosteroid. Asthma is often accompanied by inflammation of the airways. The victim should be dosed with prednisone tablets at the earliest possible opportunity, because the onset of their action is delayed by 4 to 6 hours. The dose for an adult is 60 mg, tapered over 8 days (e.g., give 60 mg on days 1 and 2; 40 mg on days 3 and 4; 20 mg on days 5 and 6; and 10 mg on days 7 and 8. The initial dose for a child is 2 mg/kg (1 kg = 2.2 lb) of body weight with a maximum dose of 60 mg; the child is then given

1 mg/kg of body weight (maximum 60 mg) in a single dose each day for the next 4 days. An alternative steroid medication is dexamethasone, beginning with a dose of 10 mg by mouth for an adult and decreasing by 2 mg every 2 days. For children the initial dose is 0.6 mg/kg body weight (maximum dose 10 mg) in a single oral dose, with the dose tapered by one fifth over the next 4 days. If a person with asthma improves greatly (e.g., feels completely normal) after using epinephrine or an inhaled bronchodilator (or both), steroid administration is not absolutely necessary, but in general, it is a highly helpful intervention. If a victim is carrying his own steroid (glucocorticoid) inhaler, such as beclomethasone, budesonide, ciclesonide, or fluticasone, have him use it. Similarly, if he is carrying his own ipratropium (which helps to open the airways), this can be self-administered. Corticosteroids are interchangeable to a certain degree. If you must substitute, here is a rough measure of equivalence: 20 mg prednisone equals 16 mg methylprednisolone equals 3 mg dexamethasone.

5. A person with asthma who is in more than minimal distress or who does not achieve great improvement with these basic pharmacologic maneuvers should be transported rapidly to the nearest medical facility. Great care should be taken to keep him well supplied with oxygen and as exertion-free as possible.

PULMONARY EMBOLISM

A pulmonary embolus is a blood clot that has traveled from a vein somewhere in the body to lodge in the circulation of a lung. Such a clot obstructs the flow of venous blood through a portion of the lung and prevents the normal transfer of oxygen to blood by the affected lung tissue.

The most common sources of the original blood clots are the veins of the pelvis or legs (thrombophlebitis: inflammation of the veins with blood clots). Predisposing factors to thrombophlebitis include dehydration, underlying disease of the veins (such as varicose veins), injuries, cancer, recent surgery, medications (such as birth control pills), injury, obesity, and prolonged immobility (see page 269). There are hereditary genetic factors as well, such as the presence of factor V Leiden thrombophilia, which results in a tendency to form clots in small blood vessels.

If a person has blood clots in the leg(s), symptoms may include leg pain, warmth, or swelling. These clots may be present in the calf or deeper down within the thigh with extension into the pelvis.

Symptoms of pulmonary embolism include sudden onset of sharp chest pain (occasionally worse with deep breathing), cough (occasionally with blood), shortness of breath, increased rate of breathing, light-headedness, and increased or irregular heart rate. The victim may develop a fever. It's often difficult to distinguish pulmonary embolism from pneumonia (see page 45). If the clot is very large, the victim may collapse and die rapidly. This is rare.

If a person develops symptoms that may represent pulmonary embolism, he should be promptly taken to medical attention. If oxygen (see page 405) is available, it should be administered by face mask at a flow rate of 10 liters per minute. If the victim can swallow purposefully, administer an aspirin tablet (325 mg) every 24 hours. If a pulmonary embolism is diagnosed, the patient will be treated with a rapid-acting anticoagulant ("blood thinner"), such as heparin or enoxaparin, while being started on a maintenance anticoagulant such as warfarin (Coumadin), dabigatran (Pradaxa), apixaban (Eliquis), or rivaroxaban (Xarelto).

HEART FAILURE (OFTEN CALLED "CONGESTIVE HEART FAILURE")

Failure of the heart muscle to pump blood effectively may occur suddenly (usually with a large heart attack) or start gradually and worsen with time (after a heart attack; with infections of the heart muscle; from prolonged cocaine, anabolic steroid, or alcohol abuse; from chronic anemia; etc.). The symptoms include shortness of breath (particularly with exertion), swollen feet and ankles (fluid retention), bubbling noises in the lungs (fluid in the lungs), cough, wheezing, and blue skin discoloration (cyanosis) noted under the fingernails, around the lips, and of the earlobes. Frequently, a victim of heart failure cannot lie flat to sleep (because fluid collects in the lungs), so he wakes up at night feeling short of breath.

If a victim with known heart failure rapidly worsens, or if a previously healthy individual develops signs of heart failure (which may represent a new heart attack), he should be kept sitting up, unless he is more comfortable lying on his back. Administer oxygen (see page 405) by face mask at a flow rate of 10 liters per minute, and immediately carry him to medical attention. If the victim must travel under his own power, all exertion should be kept to a minimum. If the victim is awake and alert, you can administer nitroglycerin 0.4 mg by tablet or spray under the tongue. If this makes the person feel better and the blood pressure does not drop dangerously low, the dose may be repeated after 20 minutes. Don't use nonsteroidal antiinflammatory drugs (NSAIDs) in persons with heart failure because of the concern for fluid retention.

If traveling at high altitude, suspect high-altitude pulmonary edema (see page 310).

CHRONIC OBSTRUCTIVE PULMONARY DISEASE

Chronic obstructive pulmonary disease (COPD) refers to a number of diseases suffered by people who have exposed their lungs to long-term insults, particularly cigarette smoke. Chronic bronchitis (infection, inflammation, or bronchospasm—see page 192) or emphysema (scarring that leads to lack of elasticity, overinflation, or lung collapse) are the most common subsets of COPD. People with COPD have poor respiratory reserves and cannot tolerate strenuous exercise or extremes of environment. A victim of COPD suffers attacks of shortness of breath and coughing similar to asthma, but can get into serious trouble much faster because of underlying debilitation. The earliest signs of respiratory fatigue should be heeded, and evacuation to a restful situation and physician evaluation are high priorities.

With the exception of epinephrine, you may treat a victim of COPD with the same drugs used for the management of asthma. Effective bronchodilator drugs include albuterol, ipratropium, formoterol, salmeterol, and tiotropium. After an exacerbation of COPD, the victim may benefit from a 10-day course of oral prednisone (40 mg per day). Corticosteroids are interchangeable to a certain degree. If you must substitute, here is a rough measure of equivalence: 20 mg prednisone equals 16 mg methylprednisolone equals 3 mg dexamethasone.

Administration of high-flow oxygen (greater than 1.5 to 2 liters per minute by nasal cannula, or tube) carries a risk, because correction of the low blood oxygen level (hypoxia) in some individuals with COPD will cause them to stop breathing. This is because they have lost sensitivity to high carbon dioxide levels in the blood as a stimulus for breathing (COPD victims always have a relatively high level of carbon dioxide in the blood), and administration of oxygen removes the remaining stimulus (hypoxia) for breathing. Therefore, any person with COPD who is given oxygen should be watched continuously. If his rate of breathing becomes dangerously slow, or he becomes confused or sleepy, the oxygen flow rate should be lessened. Severe COPD can be catastrophic. If necessary, the person may need to have his breathing assisted.

If a person with COPD shows signs of bronchitis (see page 192) or pneumonia (see next section), the first-line antibiotic should be azithromycin, trimethoprim–sulfamethoxazole, amoxicillin, doxycycline, tetracycline, clarithromycin, levofloxacin, moxifloxacin, or sparfloxacin. Second-line antibiotics include ciprofloxacin, cefixime, cefprozil, ofloxacin, and amoxicillin–clavulanate. There is some evidence that continuing azithromycin 250 mg by mouth once per day over a prolonged period of time may decrease the frequency of acute COPD worsenings.

PNEUMONIA

Pneumonia is an infection of the lung(s) characterized by combinations of fever, shaking chills (often with chattering teeth), cough, painful and difficult breathing, chest pain, weakness, and expectoration of discolored (red, green, yellow, brown) phlegm (sputum). Pneumonia may evolve from bronchitis (see page 192) or arise independently. In toddlers or young children, rapid breathing, abdominal pain, poor appetite, and vomiting may be the presenting complaints.

Treatment for Pneumonia

1. If respiratory difficulty is extreme, administer oxygen (see page 405) at a flow rate of 5 to 10 liters per minute by face mask.
2. Administer an antibiotic for 7 to 10 days, unless otherwise specified. Although many different bacteria, viruses, mycoplasmas, fungi, and other agents can cause pneumonia, the organisms most commonly acquired outside the hospital ("community acquired") respond to the following drugs (for people under 60 years of age): amoxicillin–clavulanate (875 mg twice a day), azithromycin (500 mg the first day, then 250 mg once a day), clarithromycin (500 mg twice a day or 1 g once a day), levofloxacin (500 mg once a day for 5 days), or moxifloxacin (400 mg once a day). If one of these is not available, use cefdinir (300 mg twice a day), cefpodoxime (400 mg twice a day), cefprozil (500 mg twice a day), cefuroxime axetil (500 mg twice a day), or doxycycline (100 mg twice a day for 10 days). A person over 60 years of age or who is debilitated should be treated with levofloxacin or amoxicillin–clavulanate. For a child 4 months to 6 years of age, use amoxicillin, amoxicillin–clavulanate, azithromycin, erythromycin–sulfisoxazole, clarithromycin, or cefuroxime axetil. For an infant 3 weeks to 3 months of age, use erythromycin or azithromycin.
3. Evacuate the victim.

If pneumonia is suspected, it is non-trivial and should be anticipated to worsen. Serious lung problems related to specific environmental conditions are discussed in the sections on high-altitude illnesses (see page 306), drowning (see page 364), and smoke inhalation (see page 113).

CHEST PAIN

Chest pain may be a manifestation of a variety of disorders, ranging from a harmless chest cold or heartburn to a life-threatening heart attack. To try to attain a diagnosis, it's important to ask these questions:

1. Where is the pain?
2. What is the nature of the pain?
3. How severe is the pain?
4. How long have you had the pain?
5. Does the pain extend into the arm, neck, jaw, or abdomen?
6. What relieves the pain?

ANGINA PECTORIS

Angina pectoris ("angina") is caused by narrowing or obstruction (spasm or actual occlusion) of the coronary arteries, which supply the heart muscle. The pain, which lasts from 3 to 15 minutes, is most often described as heavy and pressure-like ("squeezing," like a weight on the chest). It is classically located beneath the breastbone (but may also commonly be present in the left front chest), with occasional radiation to the jaw, back (between the shoulder blades), and left arm. Rarely, it can radiate to the right arm. Associated symptoms include nausea, sweating, shortness of breath, anxiety, and weakness. It is commonly associated with exertion, emotional stress, or both, and may be more frequent at high altitudes (this is debated by doctors), where less oxygen is available. Symptoms are sometimes worse in cold weather or after meals. "Atypical" angina is pain that occurs at rest or that awakens a victim from sleep. Women more commonly have nonclassic symptoms of angina than do men. These include irregular heartbeat, "sharp" or "stabbing" pain, pain that can be reproduced by pressing on the chest, and pain that's localized to underneath the breast. Additional symptoms in elders include shortness of breath with exercise, weakness, or sweating. A first-time angina episode, change in the pattern of existing angina episodes, or increased frequency of episodes may portend a heart attack. Angina may be relieved by rest. Persons with known angina are generally prescribed drugs: nitrates (e.g., isosorbide dinitrate), beta-adrenergic blockers (e.g., metoprolol), or calcium channel blockers (e.g., nifedipine, verapamil, or diltiazem). They also may be taking low-dose aspirin and a "statin" drug to achieve target lipid (e.g., cholesterol) levels. Any person who is taking a nitrate should not be prescribed medication for erectile dysfunction (e.g., sildenafil citrate [Viagra]).

The person who suffers from angina should be kept at absolute rest (sitting or supine) until the pain subsides. If he is carrying his medications, he should place a nitroglycerin tablet (0.4 mg) under his tongue (the tablet dissolves) or use sublingual nitroglycerin spray. If pain persists, this may be repeated after 3 to 4 minutes (not to exceed three tablets or spray applications in 10 minutes). Unless the victim is completely familiar with his angina and declares the episode typical and completely resolved, he should be transported with minimum exertion to an appropriate medical facility. If no relief is obtained, the victim may be suffering a heart attack. Expect a person with chest pain to trivialize his symptoms and deny the possibility of a heart attack.

There is a rare phenomenon, known as myocardial (heart) stunning, which is a severe, reversible abnormality is which a person without coronary artery disease suffers chest pain or decreased heart pump effectiveness (resulting in low blood pressure) when faced with a profound emotional stress, such as death of a parent or extreme fear. The precise mechanism is unknown, but the hypothesis is that this might be caused by an outpouring of "stress hormones." This is one more reason why it's important to try to keep emotions under control in a stressful situation.

HEART ATTACK (ACUTE MYOCARDIAL INFARCTION)

A heart attack is an emergency, because it may rapidly lead to complete cardiac arrest (standstill). A person suffering a heart attack will usually show some or all of the following symptoms: aching (sometimes "crushing") substernal (under the breastbone) chest pain that may extend into the back, left arm or both arms, or neck; shortness of breath; profound weakness; nausea or vomiting; pale, moist, and cool skin; sweating; agitation; abnormal heart rate and rhythm—slow, fast, or irregular; and collapse. Typically, the chest pain does not subside with administration of nitroglycerin. When cardiac arrest occurs, the victim stops breathing and has no heartbeat. Any elderly person with chest pain requires prompt physician evaluation.

Risk for a heart attack is greater in persons over the age of 65 years, with high cholesterol, a prior heart attack or family history of heart attacks, high blood pressure, diabetes, cigarette smoking, or frequent angina. Women, particularly under the age of 54 years, are more likely than men to have heart attacks without typical chest pain. The implication is that a young woman with risk factors (e.g., diabetes, obesity, tobacco use, unsatisfactory lipid profile, high blood pressure, and/or family history of heart attacks) might be well advised to see a physician for a thorough evaluation before strenuous outdoor activities.

A "silent" heart attack, in which there is a paucity of symptoms, more commonly occurs during sleep or in a diabetic victim.

Aortic Dissection

Aortic dissection refers to a tear in the aorta, commonly associated with a prior history of high blood pressure. The classic symptoms include sudden "tearing" (sharp) chest pain, which can be unbearably intense. It reaches maximal intensity almost immediately, and may be described by the victim as if a knife was being stuck in the chest. The pain may spread to the jaw, neck, arms, between the shoulder blades, or into the back. This is a true emergency, so if suspected should lead to prompt evacuation.

Treatment for a Suspected Heart Attack

1. Send someone for help.
2. If the victim has a pulse and is breathing, he should be kept at absolute rest and arrangements should be made for immediate transport to a medical facility. Administer one non–enteric-coated aspirin tablet (325 mg) by mouth. Have the victim chew and swallow it to hasten absorption from the stomach into the bloodstream. If oxygen is available, it should be administered by face mask at a flow rate of 5 to 10 liters per minute.
3. If the victim collapses, *assess the need for CPR* by feeling for a pulse (see page 31) and checking for breathing (see page 12). If these are absent, begin CPR (see page 30).

VERY RAPID HEART RATE

Supraventricular tachycardia (SVT), sometimes called paroxysmal atrial tachycardia (PAT), is a disorder that causes a person's heart to beat very rapidly, sometimes up to 250 beats per minute. This can make the victim extremely uncomfortable, with a sensation of pounding or fluttering in the chest, palpitations, chest discomfort or tightness, anxiety, light-headedness, shortness of breath, nausea, or weakness. If he is not carrying appropriate medications to treat this condition, you might try having the victim bear down and hold his breath as if straining to lift a heavy weight, or immerse his face in a pool of ice water. Another technique is to have him close his eyes, then have him press firmly on both eyeballs for 15 seconds to the point of moderate discomfort. Don't suggest this if the victim has glaucoma or recent eye surgery. Rubbing and pressing ("massaging") one of the carotid arteries (see page 31) in the victim's neck can sometimes send a reflex signal through the nervous system to the heart to cause it to slow to a normal rate ("break" the SVT). Carotid artery massage must be done in elders with extreme caution, because on rare occasion it has been noted to precipitate a stroke (see page 135). SVT is definitively treated by a physician with an intravenous injection of a specific medication (often adenosine), or in a dire emergency with a controlled (synchronized) electrical shock ("cardioversion") to the heart. Persons may carry medications to control or treat SVT. These include diltiazem (or another calcium channel blocker), metoprolol (or another beta-blocker), and many others.

NONCARDIAC CAUSES OF CHEST PAIN

Infection

Chest pain may be caused by a lung infection, such as pneumonia, bronchitis, or pleuritis. Typically, infection is characterized by pain that's sharp in nature and associated with fever, cough, weakness, and production of colored (nonwhite) sputum. Deep breathing usually makes the pain worse. The treatment of these disorders is discussed in other sections. Consult the index.

Pulmonary Embolism

Chest pain may be caused by a blood clot that has traveled to a lung(s); this is called pulmonary embolism (see page 44).

Heartburn

The pain of gastrointestinal upset (in particular, reflux of food and acid from the stomach into the esophagus) may closely mimic angina. Typically, heartburn (reflux esophagitis, or "reflux") occurs after a large meal, especially when the victim immediately lies down. Foods that are often troublesome include alcoholic and carbonated beverages, coffee, chocolate, and fats. The discomfort radiates sharply from the stomach through the breastbone and into the throat. Pain, belching, and a sour taste in the mouth may indicate a hiatal hernia, which allows reflux of

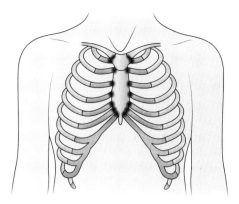

Figure 32. Costochondritis. The attachments of the ribs to the breastbone are inflamed and exquisitely tender to pressure.

stomach acid back up into the esophagus. Treatment for heartburn is discussed on page 208. If there is any suggestion that angina (see page 46) is present, seek medical attention. Because the symptoms of a heart attack can be easily confused with those of heartburn, any elderly person with chest or abdominal pain requires prompt physician evaluation.

Muscle Injuries

Heavy physical exertion can lead to overuse syndromes. The pain is related to muscle motion and is accompanied by pain with motion and soreness to the touch. Treatment for these injuries is discussed on page 262.

Costochondritis

Costochondritis is an irritation of the cartilaginous ends of the ribs where they attach to the sternum (Figure 32). The pain is sharp and well localized to the breastbone and adjacent rib ends. It is worsened considerably by pressing on the area or by deep breathing. Occasionally, slight painful swellings of the rib ends can be felt. The treatment is administration of aspirin or a NSAID.

BLEEDING

For a discussion of wound management (cleaning, closing, and dressing), see page 240.

Whenever you are going to be exposed to blood or other potentially infectious bodily fluids, wear nonpermeable nitrile gloves from your first-aid kit. If you are allergic to latex rubber, don't use sterile latex rubber gloves. If you have eyeglasses, put them on.

While it's occasionally visually distressing, bleeding can be one of the easiest problems to manage, because the treatment options are so straightforward. The severity of the injury determines the rate of blood loss and what measures you must take to control the bleeding. Evaluate the following considerations:

1. Where is the bleeding? It's important to consider and identify internal bleeding as well as external bleeding. Considerable blood loss can be associated with blunt (nonpenetrating) abdominal injury (liver, spleen), as well as long bone or pelvic fracture (2 quarts, or liters, of blood can rapidly accumulate in the thigh following a broken femur). *Examine the entire victim!*

2. Is the bleeding from an artery or from a vein? Because arterial blood is under higher pressure, blood loss tends to be more rapid from a severed artery than from a vein. Arterial bleeding can be recognized by its spurting or pulsatile nature and rapid outflow. All blood exposed to air, in the absence of unusual drug intoxications, turns red fairly quickly, so you cannot rely on color to indicate origin.
3. A victim who has lost 25% to 30% of his blood volume may suffer from shock. Treatment is discussed on page 58.
4. Prolonged uncontrollable bleeding is rare unless a major blood vessel or more than one vessel is disrupted, the victim is taking an anticoagulant (blood thinner) medication, or the victim suffers from hemophilia. In such a case, heroic intervention may be lifesaving.

TREATMENT FOR BLEEDING

First, remove all clothing covering the wound so that you can see precisely where the bleeding is coming from. *Almost all external bleeding stops with firm, direct pressure.* This should be applied directly to the wound with the heel of your hand, using the cleanest available thick (four or five thicknesses of a 4 inch by 4 inch—or 10 cm by 10 cm—sterile gauze pad, for instance) bandage or cloth compress (Figure 33). Army battle dressing (ABD) pads are excellent for this purpose and don't take up much space in your pack. Maintain pressure for a minimum of 10 minutes, to allow severed vessels to close by spasm (an artery contains small amounts of muscle tissue in its walls) and to allow early blood clot formation. Peeking at the wound under the compress interrupts the process and prolongs active bleeding. The application of cold packs or ice packs over the compress (*not* under it) may hasten the process by initiating spasm and closure of disrupted blood vessels. It's also useful to have the victim lie down and to elevate the bleeding part above the level of his heart. A scalp wound tends to bleed freely and may require prolonged pressure or wound closure for control (see page 63).

If direct pressure to the wound does not stop the bleeding, you must make certain that you're applying the pressure in the correct spot. Check quickly to see that you're pressing precisely over the bleeding point. If you are a fraction of an inch off, you can miss the best compression spot for a torn blood vessel; in this case, simply piling on more bandages may not solve the problem. Once you have repositioned your pressure, wait again for 5 to 10 minutes. If the pressure appears to be working, once the bleeding has substantially subsided you can apply a pressure dressing. Do this by covering the wound with a thick wad of sterile gauze pads, ABD pads, or the cleanest dressing available, and wrapping the area firmly with a rolled gauze or elastic bandage. Don't apply the dressing so tightly that circulation beyond it is compromised (as indicated by blue fingertips or toes, or by numbness and tingling). Watch the dressing closely for blood soaking and dripping, which indicate continuous bleeding.

Pressure points are external body locations that can be compressed in order to diminish or stop bleeding. This is accomplished by impeding blood flow through the underlying artery.

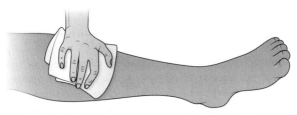

Figure 33. Firm pressure applied to a bleeding wound.

Pressure point compression can be used to attempt to control bleeding that cannot be controlled by direct pressure to the wound, and as a bridge to application of a tourniquet (see later discussion). The pressure point for locations on the arm beyond the pressure point is on its inside to occlude the brachial artery, accomplished between the biceps and triceps muscles (see Figure 17, E). For the leg, it is directly over the femoral artery (see Figure 17, B). The pressure point should be compressed for approximately 10 to 15 minutes, to allow the severed blood vessel(s) to constrict and for the bleeding to be controlled by direct pressure on the wound. If pressure point constriction is not successful at halting life-threatening bleeding, it may be necessary to apply a tourniquet. In the case of torrential bleeding, most rescuers will go directly from pressure over the wound to the application of a tourniquet.

There are "blood stopper" (hemostatic) products that can be used to assist in controlling bleeding. Whenever one of these products is used, it's still necessary to apply direct pressure to the wound for at least 3 minutes. For profound bleeding from a large leg wound near the femoral artery and vein (see page 31), it might even be necessary to apply pressure by kneeling on the bandages. In any case of a bleeding wound, if the bleeding only partially ceases, repeat the application of the hemostatic product. Some of these products are:

1. Nonmedicated "Blood Stopper"—type bandage designed for compression that consists of an absorbent dressing attached to an elastic gauze wrap.
2. QuikClot adsorbent hemostatic gauze (Z-Medica Corporation), which delivers a zeolite-based clotting agent. This product is also available in a mesh 3.5 inch by 3.5 inch "sponge" configuration as QuikClot Sport (with or without silver as an antibacterial agent).
3. Combat Gauze (Z-Medica Corporation), which is 50% rayon and 50% polyester blended gauze impregnated with mineral kaolin powder. In a popular package, it is vacuum packed and Z-folded for ease of use.
4. BleedArrest (Hemostasis, LLC) over-the-counter powder and foam are advertised to be useful for minor to moderate bleeding wounds.
5. HemCon dressings containing chitosan. Chitosan is manufactured by chemical modification of chitin, which is the structural element in the exoskeleton ("external" skeleton) of crustaceans (crabs, shrimp, and so forth). Chitosan is not known to commonly invoke an allergic reaction ("shellfish allergy" is not a contraindication to use), and can be sterilized.
6. Celox (hemostatic granules) is a high-performance hemostatic material that has been created to control high-volume arterial bleeding. Composed of a proprietary marine biopolymer (including chitosan), it is poured as a granular mixture into a bleeding wound, where it helps to facilitate blood clot formation without causing any tissue damage. It is thought to do this by aggregating negatively charged red blood cells, which are attracted to the positively charged granules. According to promotional material distributed by Sam Medical Products, the granules assist a clot to form within minutes without generating any heat, burning sensation, or rigid structure formation within the wound. A gelled mass formed by excess granules protects the clot and is easy to remove. Celox works in cold conditions and also on blood that has been heparinized (e.g., a person being treated with this category of "blood thinner" or, presumably, with enoxaparin [Lovenox]). There is no mention of whether or not it has been or would be expected to be effective if a victim is currently taking warfarin (Coumadin), clopidogrel (Plavix), dabigatran (Pradaxa), apixaban (Eliquis), or rivaroxaban (Xarelto), which are prescribed medications intended to inhibit blood clotting. To apply Celox, pour the granules from a sterilized, sealed packet (15 g or 35 g) into the wound and then hold them in place with a gauze bandage for 5 minutes. A compression bandage, such as an elasticized wrap, is then wrapped over the gauze-covered wound and the victim is brought to medical care.

Applying a Tourniquet

A tourniquet is indicated in a life-threatening situation and is best applied by an experienced person. In the case of torrential bleeding, a tourniquet is more advantageous than continuous pressure. The decision to apply a tourniquet is one in which a limb is possibly sacrificed to save a life. Massive bleeding from an arm or leg may require application of a tourniquet.

A tourniquet should be applied to the limb between the bleeding site and the heart, as close to the injury as is effective (usually 2 to 3 inches [5.1 to 7.6 cm] above the wound), and tightened to the point at which the bleeding can be controlled with direct pressure over the wound. The reason for placing it close to the bleeding is to preserve as much living tissue (which is "above" the tourniquet) as possible.

The combat application tourniquet (e.g., CAT) is used by the military and available for purchase to laypersons. It is applied to a bleeding victim as follows:

1. Place the wounded limb through the loop of the band. Position the tourniquet 2 to 3 inches above the wound (Figure 34). Before tightening any tourniquet, be sure to first take out the slack.
2. If the leg is the limb involved, direct the self-adhering band through both sides of the friction adapter buckle (Figure 35). If the arm is involved, this is not necessary.
3. Feed the self-adhering band tightly around the limb and securely fasten it back on itself (Figure 36).
4. Adhere it completely along the band until it reaches the clip (Figure 37).

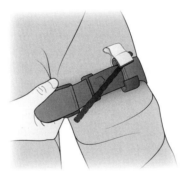

Figure 34. Initial positioning of a combat application tourniquet (CAT).

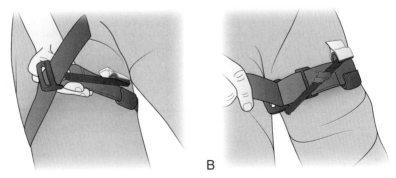

A   B

Figure 35. Positioning the self-adhering band of a CAT through the friction adapter buckle. **A,** On a leg. **B,** On an arm.

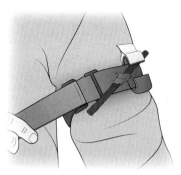

Figure 36. Secure the self-adhering band of the CAT tightly back upon itself.

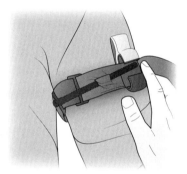

Figure 37. Adhere the band of the CAT until it reaches the clip.

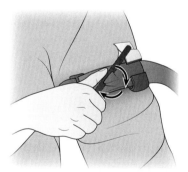

Figure 38. Twist the windlass rod of the CAT until the bleeding stops.

5. Twist the windlass rod until the bleeding stops (Figure 38).
6. Lock the windlass rod in place with the windlass clip (Figure 39).
7. Grasp the windlass tip, pull it tight, and adhere it to the windlass clip (Figure 40).
8. Observe for cessation of bleeding. If needed, apply a second tourniquet above and side-by-side to the first tourniquet.

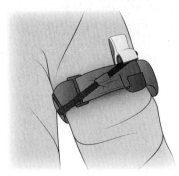

Figure 39. Lock the windlass rod of the CAT in place.

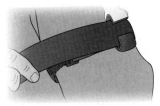

Figure 40. Adhere the windlass tip of the CAT to the windlass clip.

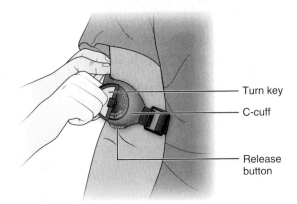

— Turn key

— C-cuff

— Release
button

Figure 41. Application of the E-MAT Emergency Tourniquet.

The CAT can be carried in its one-handed configuration, with the free-running end of the self-adhering band passed through the buckle, forming a loop for the arm to pass through. Then, one pulls the self-adhering band tightly and securely fastens it back upon itself. The windlass rod is twisted until the bleeding has stopped. To maintain the tightness, the windlass rod is locked in place with the windlass clip. Then, the self-adhering band is wrapped over the windlass rod. To complete the application, the windlass rod and self-adhering band are secured with the windlass strap. A person should be practiced in this technique before having to deploy it in the field.

Another commercially available tourniquet is the E-MAT Emergency Tourniquet (Pyng Medical). This is applied as follows (Figure 41):

1. Place the E-MAT on an arm or leg with the housing facing upward.
2. Click the strap buckle into place.

3. Pull the strap tight.
4. Turn the key further to tighten the strap.
5. To reapply the tourniquet, push in and hold the release tab, then pull the strap all the way out. Reposition the tourniquet, then follow instructions 1 through 4.

To construct an improvised tourniquet, use a 2 to 4 inch (5 to 10 cm) bandage—not something thin (such as a string, wire, or cord) that will cut through the skin. Wrap the bandage around the limb several times, and then tie a half or an entire square knot, leaving loose ends long enough to tie another knot (Figure 42, A). Place a stick or stiff rod over the knot, and then tie it in place with the loose ends. Before tightening the tourniquet, be sure that you have taken out the slack. Twist the stick (windlass) until the bandage is tight enough to stop the bleeding, and then secure it (see Figure 42, B) in place with another cloth, tape, or circular bandage. If the tourniquet is applied correctly, it should only take approximately 3 turns of the windlass to stop blood flow. If you must leave the victim after applying a tourniquet, and therefore can no longer apply direct pressure to the wound, be certain to check that the tourniquet is still effective after you have released pressure.

After placing any tourniquet, write the initial time of placement on the device or nearby skin with an indelible marker. The goal is to not need the tourniquet to control bleeding by 2 hours after its application. However, loosening the tourniquet should not be attempted if the bleeding was torrential or additional bleeding of any amount would cause the victim to become seriously compromised. That having been said, some authorities recommend loosening the tourniquet an hour after its initial placement under physical and visual control, which might be all right if the bleeding is not brisk. If the bleeding can now be controlled with direct pressure, don't retighten the tourniquet, but keep a very close watch on the situation. If the original wounding damaged or severed a very large blood vessel, it's likely that you will need to keep the tourniquet

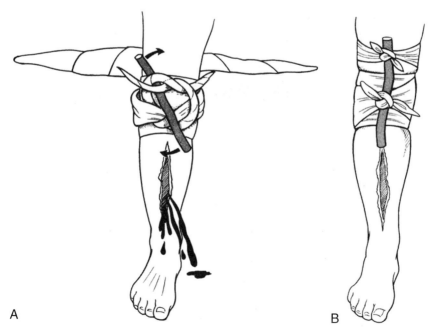

A   B

Figure 42. Application of an improvised tourniquet. **A,** Wrap the bandage around the limb, then tie a square knot. Tie a stick in place over the knot. Twist the stick to tighten the tourniquet just until the bleeding stops. **B,** Secure the stick.

in place for more than an hour. Always keep a tourniquet in plain view, so that it doesn't get left in place longer than necessary just because someone didn't know or forgot it was there. After a tourniquet has been in place continuously for 2 or more hours, don't remove it until you reach advanced medical care.

If a single tourniquet has been placed and bleeding continues, attempt first to tighten the tourniquet. If this is not successful in staunching the bleeding, then apply a second tourniquet side-by-side to the first tourniquet, between the first tourniquet and the heart.

1. If the victim has suffered a large wound through which internal organs (such as loops of bowel) (Figure 43, *A*) or bones (see page 67) are protruding, *don't attempt to push these back inside the body or under the skin unless they slide back in easily (essentially without your assistance).* Moving organs (i.e., gently returning extruded bowel to within the abdominal cavity) or realigning bones to stop bleeding and/or apply traction to allow a prolonged evacuation may be necessary. Before exposed bowel or bones are moved, irrigate away any gross dirt or other debris. If the bowel or bones remain external to the skin, cover them with continually moistened bandages (pads of gauze or cloth) held in place without excess pressure (see Figure 43, *B*). Seek immediate medical attention.

2. If the victim has suffered a severe cut in his neck, take special care to not disturb the wound, because such disturbance might remove a blood clot that's controlling the bleeding from a large blood vessel. Apply a firm pressure dressing (don't choke the victim with the bandage) and seek immediate medical attention. Continually assess the airway (see page 22), because an expanding blood clot within the neck can compress the throat and windpipe. If the victim begins to have raspy breathing or a changed voice, evacuation is maximally urgent.

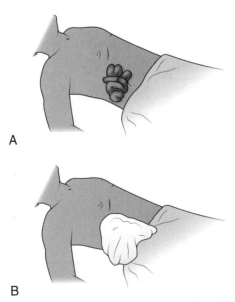

A

B

Figure 43. A, Loops of bowel protrude from a laceration in the abdomen. **B,** These should be covered gently with a moistened bandage or cloth. Do not try to push them back into the abdomen unless necessary for evacuation (e.g., if the victim must walk out under his own power and such activity is forcing more bowel to extrude from the wound).

3. Bleeding can be quite brisk from a ruptured or torn varicose (dilated) vein in the leg. This can usually be managed with direct pressure, while elevating the leg. Follow this with a pressure dressing.

4. If a foreign object (such as a knife, tree limb, or arrow) becomes deeply embedded (impaled) in the body, don't attempt to remove it, because the internal portion may be occluding a blood vessel that will hemorrhage without this "plug." Any attempt at removal may create more damage than already exists, which includes increasing the bleeding. This is particularly true with a hunting (broadhead) arrow. Pad and bandage the wound around the object, which should be fixed in place with tape if possible (Figure 44). The external portion of the object may be cut to a shorter length (cut off the shaft of the arrow a few inches above the skin, for example), if necessary, to facilitate splinting and transport of the victim. Another way to protect the impaled object from being jostled is to use a splint (see Figure 310).

5. A gunshot wound may cause severe internal damage that's not readily visible from the surface wound. Any victim who has suffered a gunshot wound should be brought to immediate medical attention, no matter how minor the external appearance. If bleeding cannot be controlled such that it is welling up from the wound, try packing the wound with a bloodstopper gauze, such as Z-Fold QuikClot Combat Gauze (see page 51) and apply pressure. Always disarm the victim. A head-injured or otherwise confused victim carrying a loaded weapon could accidentally create an additional victim. If you don't know how to handle a gun, move the weapon at least several feet away and point it in the direction where accidental discharge will do the least harm.

6. After the bleeding has stopped, immobilize the injury. Check all dressings regularly to be certain that swelling has not made them too tight. Signs that a bandage is too tight are blue discoloration of the fingernails/fingertips/toenails/toes, cool and pale skin color, tingling or loss of feeling beyond the bandage, difficulty moving the fingers or toes, and pain underneath or beyond the bandage.

INTERNAL BLEEDING

If bleeding is internal, such as from a bleeding ulcer, broken bone, injured spleen or liver, leaking abdominal aneurysm, or lung cancer, the victim may suffer from shock. Symptoms of internal (undetected) bleeding are the same as those of external bleeding, except that you don't see the blood. They include rapid heartbeat, shortness of breath, general weakness, thirst, dizziness or fainting when arising from a supine position, pale skin color (particularly in the fingernail beds and conjunctivae), and cool, clammy skin. Other signs include increasing pain and firmness of the abdomen after an injury, vomiting blood or "coffee grounds" (blood darkened by stomach

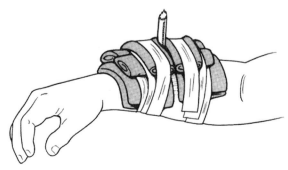

Figure 44. Padding and bandages to prevent motion of a penetrating object.

acid), blood in the urine or feces, or large bruises over the flank or abdomen. Because it's difficult to predict the rate of internal blood loss and because the only effective treatment for many causes of severe internal bleeding is surgery, medical help should be sought immediately.

SHOCK

Shock is a condition in which the blood supply that carries oxygen and nutrients to various organs of the body is insufficient to meet metabolic demands. In simple language, the shock state is the beginning of cell death. The signs and symptoms are restlessness, low blood pressure, weak and rapid (thready) pulse, altered mental status (restlessness, anxiety, confusion), moist and cool (clammy) skin, rapid shallow breathing, inability to control urination and bowel movements, nausea, and profound weakness. It is a life-threatening condition and may follow a large number of inciting events. Causes of shock include severe internal or external bleeding (25% to 30% acute loss of an adult's total blood volume, equivalent to 1.5 to 2 liters out of 6 liters), overwhelming infection, burns, dehydration, heart attack or disease, hormonal insufficiency, hypoglycemia, hypothermia, hyperthermia, allergic reaction, drug overdose, and spinal cord injury (loss of sympathetic nervous system support allows blood vessels to dilate because they lose tone). If shock is caused by blood loss (hemorrhage), the following rough estimates apply:

1. Blood loss of 750 mL to 1 liter corresponds to heart rate ("pulse") of up to 100 beats per minute and respiratory rate of approximately 14 to 20 breaths per minute. Blood pressure may remain normal.
2. Blood loss of 1 to 1.5 liters corresponds to heart rate greater than 100 and respiratory rate of 20 to 30. Blood pressure is decreased.
3. Blood loss of 1.5 to 2 liters corresponds to heart rate greater than 120 and respiratory rate of 30 to 40. Blood pressure is decreased.
4. Blood loss of greater than 2 liters corresponds to heart rate greater than 130 and respiratory rate greater than 35. Blood pressure is decreased.

Shock is a true emergency. Unfortunately, there is little that the rescuer can do in the field. The management of shock includes the following:

1. Position the victim on his back, with the legs elevated about 30 degrees (8 to 12 in or 20 to 30 cm), to encourage blood in the leg veins to return to the central circulation (heart) and head (brain) (Figure 45). Don't elevate the legs if the victim has a severe head injury (see page 59), difficulty breathing, a broken leg, or a neck or back injury, or if such a maneuver causes any pain. If the victim is short of breath because of heart failure (see page 44), he may be more comfortable in the sitting position.
2. Keep the victim covered and warm. Remove him from harsh weather conditions. Remember to insulate him from below. If insufficient bundling is available, lie next to the victim to share body heat. Take special care to keep his head, neck, and hands covered.
3. Administer oxygen (see page 405) at a flow rate of 10 liters per minute by face mask.
4. Control any obvious sources of external bleeding (see page 50). Splint all broken bones.
5. If the victim is diabetic, consider a hypoglycemic reaction (see page 133). If the victim is conscious and can purposefully swallow, administer Glucose paste (see page 133) or a sugar-sweetened liquid or gel by mouth in small sips. Otherwise, don't give the victim anything to eat or drink unless he is alert and thirsty or hungry. If the victim is in shock because of diarrhea and dehydration, attempt to initiate oral fluid intake (see page 194).
6. If the victim has been stung by an insect or appears to be suffering an allergic reaction (see page 64), treat the allergic reaction.
7. Transport the victim to a hospital as rapidly as possible.

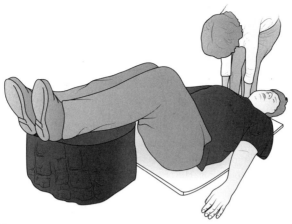

Figure 45. Positioning a victim who is in shock. Elevate the legs, cushion the back, protect the airway, and keep the victim warm.

HEAD INJURY

Victims of head injury (when it involves the brain, commonly referred to as "traumatic brain injury" or TBI) can be roughly divided into two groups, according to whether or not they have lost consciousness. Always be aware that the dazed or unconscious victim cannot protect his airway; you must be vigilant in your observation. The most common immediate serious complication of head injury is obstruction of the airway with the tongue, blood, or vomitus. The most common associated serious injury is a broken neck.

Persons who are taking medications ("blood thinners") that inhibit blood clotting, such as warfarin (Coumadin), dabigatran (Pradaxa), clopidogrel (Plavix), apixaban (Eliquis), or rivaroxaban (Xarelto) are at increased risk for bleeding inside the skull (either within the brain or in the space between the brain and the inside of the skull) following an injury, so they must be watched particularly closely after any blow to the head or sudden deceleration event. The most common indication that such bleeding is happening is persistent or increasing headache.

CONCUSSION, WITH OR WITHOUT LOSS OF CONSCIOUSNESS

Concussion is a form of traumatic brain injury (TBI). If a person struck in the head has lost consciousness, he has suffered at least a concussion. However, a person does not need to have gone unconscious to have suffered a concussion. The working definition of a concussion is an immediate and temporary impairment of brain function, sometimes accompanied by a brief period of amnesia after a blow to the head. The following signs and symptoms are commonly associated with a concussion: unaware of what happened; confusion; cannot recognize people or surroundings; loss of memory (not typically including, however, one's name and address); loss of consciousness; headache or sensation of pressure in the head; dizziness; balance problems; nausea; vomiting; feeling "foggy," "dazed," or "stunned"; visual problems (e.g., seeing stars or flashing lights, or seeing double); hearing problems (e.g., ringing in the ears); irritability or emotional changes; slowness or fatigue; inability to follow directions or slow to answer questions; easily distracted or poor concentration; inappropriate emotional behavior; glassy-eyed or vacant staring; slurred speech; seizure. With regard to the latter, a single brief seizure immediately following a concussion is not necessarily an ominous sign. Headache, dizziness, and difficulty concentrating may persist for weeks after a concussion, so the victim should not be in a position, such as lead climber, to put others at risk.

1. *Protect the airway (see page 22) and cervical spine (see page 35).*

2. If the victim wakes up after no more than a minute or two and quickly regains his normal mental status and physical abilities, he has probably suffered a minor injury—so long as there is no relapse into unconsciousness or persistent lethargy, nausea or vomiting, or severe headache. If the victim is far from help, he should undertake no vigorous activity and be kept under close observation for at least 24 hours. It is commonly taught that after someone has sustained a head injury with loss of consciousness (implying a concussion), he or she should be kept awake. It is also taught that if the victim falls asleep, he should be awakened regularly, presumably to demonstrate that he can be awakened and has not worsened or lapsed into a coma. However, be aware that sleeping in and of itself has no influence on the progression of the head injury. Furthermore, some persons who have suffered a concussion (or worse) become sleepy. If they fall asleep, they will not worsen because they fall asleep. If they worsen, it is part of the progression of the head injury, not related in any way to sleep. You cannot keep someone awake forever, because they need sleep in order to rest. So, if you're in a situation in which you are assessing someone who has suffered a head injury to determine his neurologic status, you need to set reasonable intervals at which to perform the examinations. There is no magic number, but if you're concerned that someone is worsening, at least once an hour seems reasonable. Signs of worsening following a blow to the head include nausea and vomiting, blurred vision, increasing headache, and any change in mental status (e.g., declining alertness, ability to converse, or ability to follow commands; increasing confusion; or decreasing level of consciousness). If someone seems more sleepy than usual after a head injury, particularly if he is a child, perhaps difficult to assess and compounded with exhaustion, it's better to be safe than sorry. Bring that person to medical attention as soon as possible.

3. Confusion or amnesia for the event that caused the blackout is not uncommon and not necessarily serious, so long as the confusion does not persist for more than 30 to 45 minutes. Because a serious brain injury may not become immediately apparent, the wilderness traveler who has been knocked out should not venture farther from civilization for 24 hours. If headache or nausea persists beyond 2 to 3 hours, the victim should begin to make his way (assisted by rescuers) to medical care. If the injury is minor and evacuation is not undertaken, advance the victim's activity as follows: no physical activity and complete rest until without symptoms; next, light walking without any heavy lifting or resistance activity; next, mild exercise with slight resistance; finally, full activity. Don't progress beyond one "level" each 24-hour period. It may be helpful to not only avoid physical exertion for the first day, but also to avoid mental exertion.

4. If the victim wakes up and is at first completely normal, only to become drowsy or disoriented, or to lapse back into unconsciousness (typically, after 30 to 60 minutes of normal behavior), he should be evacuated and rushed to a hospital. This may indicate bleeding from an artery inside the skull, causing an expanding blood clot (epidural hematoma) that compresses the brain. Frequently, the unconscious victim with an epidural hematoma will be noted to have one pupil significantly larger than the other (Figure 46).

5. If the victim awakens but has a severe headache, bleeding from the ears or nose with no obvious external injury to those organs, clear fluid draining from the ear or nose, unequal-sized or poorly reactive (don't constrict promptly on exposure to bright light) pupils, weakness, bruising behind the ears or under the eyes, vomiting, or persistent drowsiness, he might have a skull fracture. Such signs mandate immediate evacuation to a medical facility.

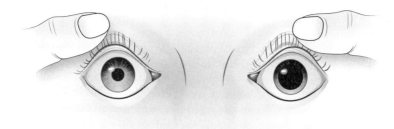

Figure 46. Unequal pupils.

6. If the victim suffers a seizure (see page 65) after a head injury, no matter how brief, he should be transported to a medical facility.

7. If the victim does not wake up promptly after a head injury (unconscious for more than 10 minutes), has bleeding from an ear, has unequal or nonreactive (don't constrict to bright light) pupils, has clear fluid from the nose, has a profound headache, is weak in an arm or leg, is disoriented, or has a fluctuating level of consciousness (normal one minute, drowsy the next), he may have suffered a significant brain injury and should be immediately rushed to a medical facility. Because there is a high incidence of associated neck injuries, any person with a serious head injury should have his cervical spine immobilized (see page 35). Head injuries often cause vomiting. Therefore, be prepared to turn the victim on his side so that he doesn't choke (see page 25).

8. Glasgow Coma Scale (GCS). This scale is used by medical professionals as a guide to the presence of head injury and to follow the progress of a head-injured victim. However, because the GCS was never intended as a tool to sequentially follow someone with a head injury, its use for this purpose is somewhat falling out of favor. However, for the time being, it is the most commonly used scale, so you should be familiar with it and prepared to report your findings.

Eye Opening	Spontaneous	4
	To voice	3
	To pain	2
	None	1
Best Verbal Response	Oriented	5
	Confused	4
	Inappropriate	3
	Incomprehensible	2
	None	1
Best Motor Response	Obeys commands	6
	Localizes pain	5
	Withdraws from pain	4
	Flexes the limbs in response to pain	3
	Extends the limbs in response to pain	2
	None	
Total Score		3 to 15

- 15 is normal (no brain injury)
- 13 to 14 is mild brain injury
- 9 to 12 is moderate brain injury
- 3 to 8 is severe brain injury

Persons with a GCS score of 15 can deteriorate even if they have suffered apparently minor head injuries. Warning signs for persons who might have a serious problem include increasing headache; persistent vomiting; restlessness; increased confusion or sleepiness; observed decrease in GCS score; uncontrolled urination or bowel movement; clear or blood-tinged fluid coming from an ear or the nose without an injury to these areas; raccoon eyes or Battle's sign (see page 74); a convulsion; weakness or numbness of a body part; and a focal blow to the side of the head. So, if a person appears normal, but has suffered any one of these, he is perhaps at a greater risk for having a serious brain injury. This person therefore should be watched very closely. If you are far from medical attention, you should make plans for a prompt evacuation.

9. Simpler neurologic assessment scales. As mentioned earlier, the GCS was developed as a scoring system not for acute care, but rather for repeated bedside assessment of persons with changing states of consciousness and to measure duration of coma. So, it may not be sufficiently reliable, in part because it is subjective (relative to the examiner's ability to apply it) and difficult to remember. Therefore, one may also use one of three other more simple neurologic assessment scales:
   - Simplified Motor Scale
     - Obeys commands
     - Localizes pain
     - Withdrawal or a lesser response to pain
   - AVPU
     - A—Alert
     - V—Responds to verbal stimuli
     - P—Responds to painful stimuli
     - U—Unresponsive to all stimuli
   - ACDU
     - A—Alert
     - C—Confused
     - D—Drowsy
     - U—Unresponsive

   The purpose of using any score is to be able to get a handle on the patient's initial condition and then to be able to "follow" the patient over time in a consistent fashion, in order to know if the patient is improving, staying the same, or deteriorating. This can be very important for treatment and rescue decisions, including selection of a method of evacuation.

10. Pain control. For the purpose of treating a post–mild TBI headache, avoid using aspirin, ibuprofen, or naproxen in order to lessen a potentially increased risk of bleeding. However, if the victim appears to be doing well, ibuprofen may be used. If possible, don't use drugs, such as diphenhydramine or narcotics, that might alter the victim's state of consciousness.

NO LOSS OF CONSCIOUSNESS

If a person has been struck on the head but was never knocked out, he will rarely have incurred a serious injury to the brain. The scalp should be inspected for cuts, which generally bleed freely; it may require considerable pressure to stop the bleeding (see later discussion). If the victim seems normal (answers questions appropriately; knows his name, the location, and the date; walks normally; appears coordinated; has normal muscle strength), there is probably no need to perform a hurried evacuation. If the victim is in any way abnormal, however, he should be rapidly transported to a medical facility. A person with minor head injury who displays any of the following should be watched very closely: vomiting, persistent headache, age over 60 years, intoxication with drugs or alcohol, problem(s) with short-term memory, and any physical evidence of injury above the collarbone. A small child who has been struck on the head and begins to vomit, refuses to eat, becomes drowsy, seems apathetic, or generally appears abnormal should be examined by a physician as soon as possible.

LACERATIONS OF THE SCALP

Cuts of the scalp tend to bleed freely, because the blood vessels are positioned in the thick skin in such a way that they cannot go into spasm and seal off after they are severed. For this reason, it's important to apply prolonged firm pressure to any head wound and to seek care as soon as possible. If possible, any closure method should be preceded by a quick, vigorous rinse of the wound to remove any large pieces of dirt, gravel, or other debris. After that, control bleeding by applying pressure to the wound with the cleanest cloth available. Next, attempt to close the wound. One way to keep the edges of the wound together is to dry the hair as best possible, then twirl hair (if it is at least 1.2 inches [3 cm] in length) on directly opposite sides of the wound to form strands, and then pull these strands toward each other to pull the skin together, then twirl them around each other. Then put a drop of rapid-cure cyanoacrylate glue (such as Super Glue) at the lowest junction of the strands while you're holding them together, and allow the glue to set up, which will occur very quickly. If a cyanoacrylate glue is not available, another way to do

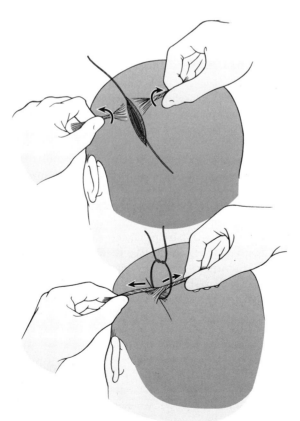

Figure 47. String and hair-tying method for closing a scalp wound.

this is to first lay a long piece of string or dental floss along and beyond the length of the wound. Then, twirl the hair to form the strands, and twirl the strands together as described above. Next, use the string to tie the hair strands together (Figure 47). Repeat the gluing or tying process as necessary to account for the entire open length of the wound. If the wound is large and you don't have a cyanoacrylate glue or any string, you may be able to bring the edges together by directly tying the twirled hair taken from opposite sides of the wound, but this is usually quite difficult.

For information regarding wound repair and bandaging, see pages 240 and 255.

ALLERGIC REACTION

A severe allergic reaction (anaphylaxis) can be life-threatening. It is caused by exposure to insect and animal venoms (such as wasp or jellyfish stings), plant products, medications, or any other agent to which the victim's immune system has been previously sensitized. The foods that most commonly cause allergic reactions are eggs, milk, fish, shellfish, nuts, soy, and wheat.

Symptoms include low blood pressure (shock); difficulty breathing (severe asthma) with wheezing; swelling of the lips, tongue, throat, and vocal cords (leading to airway obstruction); itching; hives (red, raised skin welts that may occur singly or in large patches); nausea and vomiting; diarrhea; abdominal pain; seizures; and abnormal heart rhythms. Any or all of these symptoms may be present in varying severity. The most common life-threatening problem is respiratory distress. Facial swelling indicates that the airway may soon become involved. *Be ready at all times to protect and support the airway.*

TREATMENT FOR AN ALLERGIC REACTION

1. Administer epinephrine (adrenaline) if the victim remains in severe distress after inhalation of a bronchodilator. Epinephrine is a powerful bronchodilator that is injected intramuscularly (see page 444) as an aqueous solution of 1:1000 concentration in a dose of 0.3 to 0.5 mL for an adult and 0.01 mL/kg of body weight for a child (not to exceed 0.3 mL). For weight estimation, 1 kg equals 2.2 lb. It should be injected into the lateral thigh. If the thigh is obese, whether in an adult or a child, such that the needle might not reach into muscle, then inject into the lower thigh. If obesity is extreme, consider injecting into the mid-calf. The only reason to administer the drug subcutaneously (see page 446) is if the equipment is not available for an intramuscular injection. The drug is available in preloaded syringes in certain allergy kits, which include the EpiPen autoinjector and EpiPen Jr. autoinjector, the Auvi-Q "talking" autoinjector (0.3 mg or 0.15 mg dose), and the Adrenaclick (0.3 mg or 0.15 mg dose). Other devices worldwide are the Jext, Emerade, Allerject, and Anapen. Instructions for use accompany the kits. For dosing purposes, a 0.3 mg autoinjector should be used for adults and children over 66 lb (30 kg) in weight. Children 66 lb and under should be injected with a 0.15 mg autoinjector.

   Take particular care to handle preloaded syringes properly, to avoid inadvertent injection into an unintended location, such as a finger or toe. Don't intentionally inject epinephrine into the buttocks or a vein. Epinephrine should not be exposed to heat or sun, but does not need to be kept refrigerated. If clear (liquid) epinephrine turns cloudy or discolored, it should be discarded. When administering an injection, *never* share needles between people.

2. Administer diphenhydramine (Benadryl) by mouth. This is a histamine-1 receptor antagonist drug. A milder reaction that does not require epinephrine or corticosteroids may be managed with diphenhydramine alone. The adult dose is 50 to 75 mg every 4 to 6 hours; the pediatric dose is 1 mg/kg (2.2 lb) of body weight, also every 4 to 6 hours. The

major side effect of this medication is drowsiness. A nonsedating antihistamine suitable for this purpose is fexofenadine (Allegra) 60 mg capsule for adults.

3. In case of a severe reaction, administer corticosteroids. Prednisone tablets in a dose of 50 to 80 mg should be given to an adult; the pediatric dose is 1 mg/kg (2.2 lb) of body weight. The onset of action of steroids is delayed for 4 to 6 hours; therefore, this drug should be given early in the course of therapy. Corticosteroids are interchangeable to a certain degree. If you must substitute, here is a rough measure of equivalence: 20 mg prednisone equals 16 mg methylprednisolone equals 3 mg dexamethasone.

4. Administer an inhaled (aerosol or "micronized") bronchodilator. Bronchodilators (airway openers) are drugs that have the advantages of minimal side effects and direct delivery to the site of action. They are available in metered-dose handheld inhalers from which the victim inhales therapeutic puffs. An excellent drug for an acute attack is albuterol (Ventolin). The dose for an adult is 2 to 6 puffs initially, followed by 2 to 4 puffs every 3 to 6 hours. A child over age 12 who can manage the device may use a handheld inhaler; younger children often require oral (liquid) medication in the appropriate dose.

5. Administer a histamine-2 receptor antagonist drug. This can be ranitidine (Zantac) 150 or 300 mg for an adult or famotidine (Pepcid) 10 or 20 mg for an adult.

6. Transport the victim for medical evaluation.

Reactions to specific agents (such as bee stings, plant contact, hay fever, etc.) are discussed elsewhere. Consult the index.

SEIZURE

A seizure ("fit"; epilepsy) represents vigorous involuntary muscle activity and altered consciousness associated with abnormal electrical discharges within the brain. It may be caused by a number of underlying disorders, which include structural abnormalities of the brain (scars, birth defects), injury, tumor, infection, bleeding (stroke), uncontrolled hypertension, lack of oxygen, abnormal blood chemistries (calcium, sodium, glucose), and "recreational" drug abuse (including drug or alcohol withdrawal).

Most seizures have been grouped into various classifications, which include the following types:

Partial. This seizure is initiated in a focal, or "restricted," part of the outermost layer (cortex) of the brain. Consciousness may (complex seizure) or may not (simple seizure) be impaired.

Generalized. This seizure involves the cortex of the brain in a symmetrical and synchronous manner, and may lead to "automatic," "absent," or profoundly agitated behavior patterns.

Grand mal ("big illness"). In this type of generalized seizure disorder, the victim classically becomes unconscious and has violent repetitive muscle activity with tongue biting, grunting, eye deviation to one side, difficulty breathing, and occasional loss of bladder or bowel control. Following the seizure, the victim will be confused or combative for a time (10 to 60 minutes) as he slowly returns to normal. He may sleep for a while after a seizure.

Status epilepticus. This is defined as prolonged seizure activity for a period that exceeds 1 to 2 minutes, or as multiple seizures without a return of normal consciousness between fits. Status epilepticus is a true medical emergency.

Petit mal ("little illness"). This is an "absence" attack generally seen in a child; in it, he seems to be daydreaming, distracted, or confused. It is not associated with violent abnormal physical behavior.

Psychomotor (temporal lobe). This is an episode of patterned abnormal behavior, such as lip smacking, olfactory hallucinations, vulgar speech, or repetitive movements such as arm waving. The origin of the electrical activity is thought to reside in the temporal lobe of the brain.

TREATMENT FOR SEIZURE

1. Protect the airway (see page 22). If the victim vomits, do your best to clear the mouth and nose of debris. Turn the victim on his side. He may suddenly bite down and hold his teeth clenched, so take care not to get your fingers caught in the mouth. A padded object that cannot be bitten through (such as a leather wallet edge) may be used as a bite block to keep the teeth apart and prevent tongue biting, but take extreme care not to obstruct the airway. Don't place a hard object in the mouth that might break the teeth. Take care not to force the tongue backward into the throat. *Never try to pour liquids into the mouth of a seizing victim.*
2. Protect the cervical spine (see page 35).
3. Protect the victim from injuring himself during the seizure. This may be done with cushions, sleeping bag, or constant repositioning of the victim. If he needs to be physically restrained, keep him on his side. Loosen all clothing around the neck.
4. In most cases, a grand mal seizure will only last 30 seconds to 2 minutes and will be self-limited. The victim will be confused for a few minutes to an hour after the seizure and should be watched closely for recurrence or difficulty in breathing. If the victim continues to seize or does not wake up between seizures (status epilepticus), he must be transported to a medical facility as soon as possible for drug administration. Any victim who does not fully awaken, who awakens but has never previously had a seizure, or who appears weak or feverish after a seizure should be rapidly evacuated.
5. When the victim awakens, determine if he has ever had a seizure before and whether he is supposed to be taking anticonvulsants. The most common cause of a seizure is failure to take prescribed antiseizure medication(s). If the victim has been delinquent, he should take his medicine as soon as possible. For an adult, common medications are phenytoin sodium (Dilantin) 300 to 400 mg per day, phenobarbital 30 to 60 mg three times a day, or diazepam (Valium) 5 to 10 mg three to four times a day. Other common antiseizure medications include levetiracetam (Keppra), lamotrigine (Lamictal), pregabalin (Lyrica), valproic acid (Depakote), clonazepam (Klonopin), gabapentin (Neurontin), trimethadione (Tridione), primidone (Mysoline), and ethosuximide (Zarontin). Never administer an oral medication to anyone unless he is awake and capable of purposeful swallowing.
6. A possible cause of unconsciousness or seizure in a person who suffers from diabetes is low blood sugar (hypoglycemia). If a diabetic suffers a seizure, he should be given sugar as soon as possible. This may be difficult to do away from the hospital, because intravenous injection will be required if the victim cannot swallow. If a diabetic feels weak, sweaty, dizzy, or nauseated, he should immediately ingest a sugar-containing beverage, food (see page 133), or concentrated liquid glucose (Glutose: one tube contains 15 g). If the victim is unconscious, sugar granules or small squirts of Glutose can be placed under the tongue, from where they can be passively swallowed. Once a diabetic suffering from hypoglycemia perks up from ingesting something containing sugar, be certain that the total amount of carbohydrate ingested is 15 to 20 g. This can be accomplished with 4 ounces of carbohydrate-containing juice or non-diet (sweetened) soda, 8 ounces of milk, sugar tablets or 4 teaspoons of table sugar, a tube of Glutose, 5 hard candies, 2 tablespoons of raisins, 5 soda crackers, or a tablespoon of honey. If a glucose meter is handy, check to see that the blood sugar is at least 70 mg/deciliter, and preferably above 100 mg/deciliter. If not, repeat the feeding. Instructions for administering glucagon by injection to a diabetic suffering from severe hypoglycemia are found on page 134.

7. If a woman in her final (third) trimester of pregnancy suffers a seizure, she should be assumed to be suffering from a disorder known as eclampsia, which can be life-threatening. Eclampsia includes high blood pressure, kidney dysfunction, and perhaps central nervous system hypersensitivity. The woman should immediately be rushed to a medical facility, where she will likely be treated with intravenous magnesium and perhaps induction of labor to deliver her child.

8. A person, particularly when emotionally distressed, may have a "pseudoseizure" (false seizure; not a real seizure). In such cases, the patient may be thrashing, turning the head briskly from side-to-side, have normal color and breathing, flutter the eyelids, and awaken rapidly (nearly immediately) to a normal conscious state. He may or may not be tearful, and will not have suffered tongue biting or loss of bladder/bowels. When in doubt, always treat the victim as having suffered a true seizure and take appropriate safety and medical precautions and actions.

FRACTURES AND DISLOCATIONS

A bone fracture (break) may be simple (one clean break) or comminuted (multiple breaks or shattered) (Figure 48). Furthermore, it may be closed (skin intact) or open ("compound," with the skin broken, often with the bone visible in the wound). An open fracture is highly prone to infection. A fracture may be associated with injuries to adjacent nerves and blood vessels.

A broken bone or dislocation (displacement of a bone at the joint) should be suspected whenever there has been sufficient force to cause such an injury, if a snap or crack was heard, if

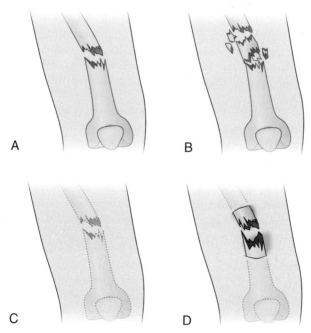

A   B

C   D

Figure 48. Fractured bones. **A,** Simple fracture (one break). **B,** Comminuted fracture (multiple breaks). **C,** Closed fracture (skin unbroken). **D,** Open, or compound, fracture (skin broken).

the victim cannot move or bear weight on the body part, or if an injured body part is painful, swollen, discolored, or deformed.

It's helpful to use a standardized approach to examining an injured limb with a certain routine, to be certain that the examination is complete and nothing significant overlooked:

1. When examining an injury, always begin with an uninjured area and work toward the injury, so that the victim's response to pain doesn't interfere with your exam.

2. Otherwise, begin your examination at the furthest point of the limb and work your way back to the origin. For instance, for the upper extremity, examine the fingers, hand, wrist, forearm, elbow, upper arm, and shoulder, in that order. Pain with a broken bone tends to be instantaneous, constant, and worsened considerably with motion, which may also create a grating sensation and noise. If something is deformed or "grates" with movement, apply a splint. A broken or dislocated bone should be compared with the normal opposite limb; asymmetry is a key sign of a significant injury.

3. A small child with a fracture or dislocation will not use the affected body part and will cry vigorously with the slightest manipulation. Pain and swelling in the vicinity of a joint of a child should be assumed to be a fracture or dislocation.

4. Ask the victim to move the limb through a full voluntary range of motion in order to identify any painful area.

5. If the victim cannot cooperate, then take the limb through a range of motion. If there is resistance, grating, or deformity, stop and apply a splint.

6. If necessary, manage a dislocation (described in various sections later) and then apply a splint. Take care during application of the splint to not reproduce the dislocation.

If you think that a bone may be broken, it's best to treat it as a break until an x-ray can be obtained or the situation shows obvious marked improvement (which usually requires 4 to 6 days).

Because of the force necessary to break or displace a bone, any person with a fracture or dislocation should be examined carefully for other injuries. All fractures and some dislocations cause a certain amount of bleeding, which can be significant with the larger bones (femur, pelvis). For instance, it's possible to lose 250 to 500 mL of blood at the site of a humerus fracture, 350 to 650 mL from a tibia fracture, and 800 to 1200 mL from a femur fracture. Be prepared to treat the victim for shock (see page 58). Don't manipulate a broken limb unnecessarily, even if circulation to the limb seems normal; excess motion increases the risk of damage to the bones, nerves, and blood vessels.

If the skin has been disrupted in the vicinity of the broken bone, the fracture is open. The bone end may or may not be visible through the wound, and bleeding may be minor or major. If a victim has sustained an open fracture, is alert enough to swallow liquids, and is more than 6 hours distant from a medical facility, administer penicillin, erythromycin, amoxicillin, or cephalexin 500 mg by mouth every 4 hours. Rinse the wound with tap water or disinfected drinking water to remove any obvious dirt (and thus, bacteria), and then cover it with a sterile dressing. Don't vigorously scrub or irrigate the wound. Unless there are signs of loss of circulation (coldness, blue color or paleness, numbness) or it's necessary to realign the limb to allow splinting and evacuation, don't try to reposition the injury or to push the bone back under the skin. If you must manipulate the limb, rinse any visible bone with water or disinfectant (such as povidone–iodine 10% solution), and then allow the bone to slide under the skin without touching it. While holding traction (pulling on the end portion of a limb in a longitudinal axis to achieve correct anatomic alignment), immediately apply a splint (see page 70) to prevent further motion and damage.

In general, it's unwise to manipulate an injured limb. If the extremity is deformed, but the circulation is intact (normal pulses, sensation, temperature, and color), don't attempt to straighten it; instead, splint it in the position in which you found it ("splint 'em as they lie"). On the other hand, if the circulation to an extremity is obviously absent (the extremity is numb, cold, and blue or pale), if the victim is in extreme discomfort, or if gross deformity prevents moving the victim out of a dangerous situation or prevents the application of a splint, then an attempt to restore the part to a normal position is justified. Early realignment is easier than delayed realignment, may alleviate a major amount of pain, helps control blood loss into the surrounding soft tissues, may decrease the incidence of fat emboli (fat from the bone marrow entering the bloodstream and causing severe illness), and often allows easier splinting and transport. Be advised, however, that the relocation of a fracture or dislocation may be difficult and transiently very painful for the victim. If you're going to make an attempt to realign a limb, it should be done as soon as possible after the injury (preferably, within 3 hours), before swelling and increasing pain and muscle spasm make the maneuver impossible. If there is no deformity, splint the injured body part in the "position of function" (the position it would assume if it were at rest) (Figure 49).

To attempt to reposition a displaced body part, apply steadily increasing traction (pulling force) to the injury along the normal axis of alignment while applying countertraction above the injury. Don't forcefully lever the bone or snap a bone back into position with a quick, forceful motion. To gain mobility in a deformed area, it's sometimes necessary to gently rock the body parts or slightly accentuate the deformity ("distract" the joint to create maneuvering space between the bones) while applying continuous traction away from the body. This allows the dislocated part to clear any obstruction and slip back into position. If the part is repositioned, it should be held in place while you splint it. After such maneuvers, check to see that circulation has been restored. *In no circumstance should you try to reposition a suspected cervical spine injury unless it is absolutely necessary to establish an airway in order to allow the victim to breathe (see pages 23-24).*

COMPARTMENT SYNDROME

Within the limbs (legs, arms, forearms, feet, hands, and fingers), there are "compartments" defined by inelastic boundaries of tough connective tissue, or fascia. These compartments contain bones, groups of muscles, blood vessels, and nerves. If swelling occurs within a compartment—typically caused by bleeding, continuous excessive external pressure, or a crush injury—the

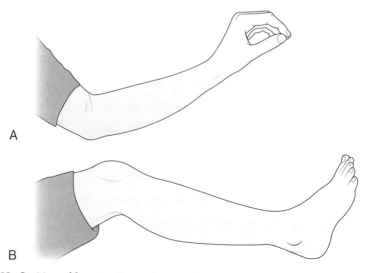

A

B

Figure 49. Position of function (normal anatomic resting position). Unless otherwise specified, the upper and lower limbs should be bandaged and/or splinted in these positions. **A,** Upper extremity. **B,** Lower extremity.

pressure can exceed 30 mm of mercury, which is the pressure at which blood travels through microscopic blood vessels, such as capillaries. This effectively squeezes the tiniest blood vessels and occludes flow through them, cutting off circulation to the compartment and rapidly causing tissue death. The most common cause of compartment syndrome in a wilderness enthusiast is swelling surrounding a broken bone or associated with a severe blunt injury, such as occurs after a fall. The lower leg and forearm are the most common sites. Compartment syndrome is rare following snakebite (see page 315), because most of the swelling following a bite is confined to superficial soft tissues.

Signs and symptoms include the "5 Ps": pain, pallor (pale color of the skin), pulselessness (although pulses may be present), paresthesia (numbness and tingling), and paralysis of the affected body part. Severe pain seems out of proportion to the injury. The underlying tissue feels extremely tight, and pain is increased markedly with external pressure. Stretching the muscles that run through the compartment causes worsened pain. There may be decreased sensation or tingling in those skin areas supplied by the nerves that run through the compartment—for example, decreased sensation to pinprick or light touch on the top of the foot in the web space between the great and second toes because of pressure on the deep peroneal nerve, which runs through the anterior leg compartment. The limb may become pale or show a bluish tinge. When pulses become diminished or lost, the situation has become severe, and the limb will be weak or become useless (paralyzed).

Field treatment involves elevation of the affected limb, splinting, padding to protect against further injury, and rapid evacuation. A true compartment syndrome must be treated with surgery to open the compartment and allow the pressure to be reduced. Severe damage can occur within 6 hours of the onset of the syndrome or may be delayed by hours or days as the limb swells, so it's important to frequently reexamine (every 30 minutes for the first 2 hours; every hour for the next 12 hours; every 2 hours for the next 24 hours, then every 4 hours for the next 48 hours) the person who has suffered an injury that makes him vulnerable to a compartment syndrome. Don't administer aspirin to the victim. Cold packs are of limited, if any, benefit; never immerse a limb in ice water.

SPLINTS AND SLINGS

A splint should be applied to any broken bone, bad sprain, or severely lacerated body part after gross deformity is corrected, to maintain proper position and immobilize the injured part (or parts) so that it cannot be displaced. This prevents further nerve, blood vessel, and muscle damage, and keeps broken bone ends from grating against each other or from poking through the skin. A sling-and-swathe combination (see Figure 61) helps to further immobilize a limb. Pain may be lessened or relieved by eliminating unnecessary motion, allowing more rapid transport.

These general guidelines should be followed in the application of splints:

1. Examine every suspected fracture to see if it is open or closed (see page 67). Check the circulation below the fracture site by inspecting pulses, skin color, sensation, and movement of fingers and toes. In the arm, check the radial and brachial pulses; in the leg, check the popliteal, dorsalis pedis, and posterior tibial pulses (see Figure 17).
2. Control bleeding (see page 50) and apply a dressing if necessary.
3. Splint the joint above and below the injury. For instance, to keep the knee from moving, you often need to prevent motion at the ankle, knee, and hip. There will be times when this is difficult, but do the best you can.
4. If possible, fashion the splint first on an uninjured body part or on a bystander, and then transfer it to the injured area. This lessens manipulation of the injured part and minimizes pain associated with splinting.

5. Splints can be fashioned from sticks, cardboard, foam pads, rolled newspapers, pack frames, ski poles, or other similar objects (Figure 50). Foldable or rollable wire splints can be constructed by cutting 6 inch by 30 inch (15 cm by 76 cm) and 18 inch by 36 inch (46 cm by 91 cm) pieces of ⅛ inch or ¼ inch (3 mm or 6 mm) wire mesh and covering the sharp edges with adhesive or duct tape. Fasteners can include belts, triangular bandages, tape, elastic wraps, shirtsleeves, and blankets. Slings can be fashioned from triangular bandages, cravats, sheets, ropes, and vines.

6. An inflatable air splint is sometimes less desirable, in that it can attain only one shape and may create circulation problems by exerting too much pressure on injured tissues. If you use an air splint, be sure that it has a mechanism to adjust for volume expansion (heat and high altitude). When stored at freezing temperatures, it should be kept partially inflated so that any frozen moisture (from inflating breaths) within the air bladder doesn't cause the walls to adhere.

7. The SAM Splint has become a standard item for the outdoor first aid kit. The core of the SAM Splint is a long rectangle of "O" temper, ultrathin aluminum alloy. The covering layers are made of dermatologically safe closed-pore foam. The splint is available in a standard size of 4¼ inches by 36 inches, which rolls easily to become a 3 inch by 4¼ inch cylinder. It can be shaped to splint a great number of body parts. The splints also comes in a 5½ inch wide XL version, in prepackaged lengths of 18 inches and 9 inches, and as a finger splint that measures 3¾ by 1¾ inches. Appendix Four shows all of the common applications of the SAM Splint.

8. When applying a splint, try not to move or displace the injured area. Use clothing pulled tightly against the skin for a grip, or place hands above and below the estimated break in a bone in order to apply traction and maintain alignment while handling the limb. Take care to apply the splint in a way that it doesn't cut off the circulation. Watch what you're doing at all times so that you can observe the position of the bone(s).

9. The specific positioning of splints is discussed with each injury, but in general, attempt to apply splints so that the body part is in a "position of function." For the hand, this would be like holding a soda can; for the wrist, straight or slightly bent upward; for the elbow, bent at a right angle; for the hip, slightly flexed; for the knee, straight or slightly bent; and for the ankle, bent at close to 90 degrees.

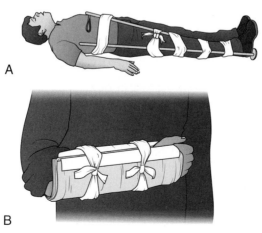

A

B

Figure 50. Splints may be fashioned from items such as (A) ski poles and (B) rolled newspaper.

10. Pad the splint properly by filling empty space to allow even pressure and stability, protect all bony prominences, alleviate pressure points, and immobilize injuries as best as possible. This may be done with foam, a sleeping pad, pack material, or clothing.

11. If the injury is closed (skin unbroken) and there are no signs of decreased circulation, apply ice or snow packs intermittently (10 minutes "on" alternated with 10 minutes "off") to the swollen area. Don't apply snow or ice directly to the skin; protect the skin with cloth.

12. Remove all constrictive jewelry (watches, bracelets, rings, and so forth). Left in place, these can become inadvertent tourniquets on swollen limbs and fingers (see page 447).

13. Administer appropriate pain medication.

14. After a splint is applied, check the limb periodically to make certain that swelling inside the splint has not cut off the circulation. This is particularly important in cold weather, in which numbness can be a confusing factor.

15. Elevate the injured part as much as possible, to minimize swelling.

16. Insist that all victims seek medical evaluation when they return home, to be certain that all bones are properly aligned and that no further intervention is needed.

To learn more about specific splints and slings, read about the specific injuries (in following sections).

TAPING

Taping techniques are usually mastered by athletic trainers. It's not likely that outdoor adventurers will be carrying the padding, foam prewrap, benzoin spray, and athletic tape necessary to complete a comprehensive taping of large joint injuries or to tape for injury prevention. However, just in case the supplies are handy, instructions for taping appear with a few specific injuries. In general, taping does not supply the same amount of support as does splinting. The most common tape is white athletic tape; a very useful product is self-adherent elastic wrap, such as Coban. Adhesive tape can be applied directly to skin, but it will lose adhesion if the skin is not shaved first. If you shave, do so very carefully to avoid nicks and the possibility of creating a site(s) for infection. Plus, when tape is removed from hairy skin, it can be quite painful. Be very careful when applying tape to an acutely injured body part, because swelling underneath the constricting tape can cause circulation problems. Avoid leaving gaps in the tape because this leads to blisters. Try to apply the tape in a way that follows the skin contours and avoids wrinkles, and try to overlap the tape a half-width on successive wraps or strips. If there are any small cuts, skin nicks, or abrasions, always cover these with antiseptic ointment and a bandage before taping. Avoid tension over bony prominences.

SPECIFIC INJURIES

The major bones of the skeleton are illustrated in Figure 51. Check Appendix Four for instructions on how to use the SAM Splint for specific injuries.

Neck

If a fracture of the cervical spine is suspected because of neck pain, weakness or loss of feeling in an arm or leg, tingling in an arm or leg, or mechanism of injury (e.g., a victim who has fallen, is unconscious, and has a face or head injury), you must immediately immobilize the head and neck. This can be done by taping the head to a backboard or stretcher, by applying a rigid collar (which may be fashioned from a SAM Splint, as in Figure 301), or by placing sandbags or their equivalent on either side of the head (see Figure 22). Another technique is to use the padded hip belt of an inverted backpack (see Figure 23). *Don't move the neck to reposition it unless this is absolutely necessary to allow the victim to breathe or be transported (see page 35).*

For the ambulatory, cooperative victim with minor neck discomfort, a thick pad (rolled towel, jacket) can be placed posteriorly at the base of the neck. Secure this by wrapping

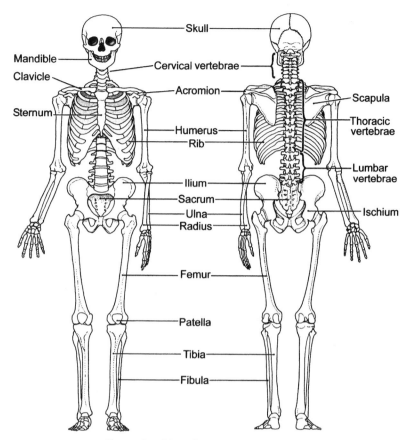

Figure 51. Major bones of the skeleton.

tape or cloth around the forehead, and then cross it over the pad and bring it back out under the armpits to be tied across the chest (see Figure 24). Alternatively, use a thick removable waistband from a backpack or a rolled Ensolite pad in a horse-collar configuration. *Soft-collar techniques should not be relied on to hold the neck immobile; they merely offer gentle support.*

If the victim is uncooperative or agitated, hold his head until you can firmly immobilize it and restrain the victim from motion (see Figure 25). All of this is necessary to avoid injury to the spinal cord. If the victim must be moved or turned on his side (most commonly to allow vomiting or to place insulation beneath him), hold his head fixed between your forearms while you hold his shoulders with your hands. In this way the victim can be "logrolled," using as many rescuers as possible to avoid unnecessary head, neck, and spine motion.

Logrolling the Victim (see Figure 26)

1. The first rescuer approaches the victim from the head, and keeps the head and shoulders in a fixed position so that the neck doesn't move.
2. The second rescuer extends the victim's arm (on the side over which the victim is to be rolled) above the victim's head. The first rescuer uses this arm to help hold the victim's head in proper position.
3. All rescuers work together to roll the victim without moving the neck.

In no circumstance except for life-saving airway management or critical transport should you try to reposition a suspected cervical spine injury. An alert victim with a broken neck or severely torn ligament will usually have enough discomfort from the injury and muscle spasm to force him to hold his neck still. However, someone with a head injury or who is under the influence of alcohol or drugs may feel no pain and can have an undetected serious injury that will be worsened by motion.

Any victim with a suspected neck fracture should be transported on a firm board or in a scoop stretcher, if possible.

"Clearing" a Cervical Spine

It's sometimes as important to know when an injury is not present as it is to recognize when it is present. This is true in the case of a broken neck. "Clearing" the spine means determining that there is likely not a broken neck. Steps to take to determine the presence or absence of a broken neck may be done only if the victim is awake and alert, not intoxicated or otherwise with an altered mental status, is cooperative, and is not distracted (in particular, by pain from another area of the body). To decide that such a person does not have a broken neck, trained medical professionals are taught to do the following actions in *precisely* the order listed:

1. Ask if there is any numbness, tingling, or other abnormal sensation in any arm or leg (which could be attributed to a spinal cord injury). If there is, then you may not "clear" the cervical spine.
2. Ask if the victim has any pain in his neck. If there is pain, then you may not "clear" the cervical spine.
3. Feel each bone (vertebra) in the neck beginning from just below the skull to the first few bones in the upper back (thoracic spine). If there is pain or neck muscle stiffness, then you may not "clear" the cervical spine.
4. Have the victim voluntarily turn his head to the right to a distance of 45 degrees. Instruct him to stop if he feels any pain. If there is pain, then you may not "clear" the cervical spine.
5. Have the victim voluntarily turn his head to the left to a distance of 45 degrees. Instruct him to stop if he feels any pain. If there is pain, then you may not "clear" the cervical spine.
6. Have the victim tilt his head backward, extending the neck. Instruct him to stop if he feels any pain. If there is pain, then you may not "clear" the cervical spine.
7. Have the victim touch his chin to his chest. Instruct him to stop if he feels any pain. If there is pain, then you may not "clear" the cervical spine.

If you complete this evaluation without the victim complaining of neck pain or stiffness, then you can be reasonably certain that he does not have a broken neck.

The "Canadian C-Spine Rule" may assist with determining who may have suffered a significant cervical spine injury. Persons with a high risk for a broken neck are greater than or equal to 65 years of age; fall from a height greater than or equal to 3 feet; fall down 5 or more stairs; receive a direct blow to the top of the head; are in a motor vehicle accident characterized by high speed, rollover, or passenger ejection; are in a motorized recreational vehicle accident; or have numbness/tingling in an arm or leg.

Skull and Face

See page 59. If there is a fracture of the skull, the victim may demonstrate black eyes ("raccoon eyes"), bruising behind the ears ("Battle's sign"), or cerebrospinal (clear or watery blood-tinged) fluid (CSF) leaking from the nose or ears. If CSF is seen to be leaking from the nose or ears, then elevate the head 30 to 60 degrees from the flat position if there is no reason to not do so (such as a suspected spine fracture). If there are fractures of bones in the face, there will usually be swelling and pain of the overlying soft tissues. If the swelling is severe around the nose, breathing may be impaired. If the bones around the eye socket are broken, there may be double vision or inability of the affected eye (or eyes) to traverse its full range of motion.

Nose

See page 180.

Jaw

A fractured jaw is usually caused by a fall or a blow from a closed fist. The lower bone (mandible) may be broken in one or more places. The victim will complain of pain, swelling, inability to close his mouth, improper fit of the teeth, perhaps missing or broken teeth, and difficulty talking. If the fracture extends into the oral cavity, there may be bleeding from the mouth. Treatment is to wrap a bandage over the top of the head and under the jaw for support (Figure 52). *It should be easily removable in case the victim needs to vomit.* A liquid diet should be maintained until the victim can reach the hospital. If a person has a significant facial injury, particularly if there is bleeding or vomiting, allow him to sit in order to lean forward and drain these fluids without choking. If he needs to be recumbent, don't place him on his back. Rather, put him in the recovery position (see page 25).

A dislocated jaw can occur from a blow, from a wide-mouthed yawn, or even during sleep. The mandible slips loose from one or both of its two bony sockets below the ears and slides forward (Figure 53). To reposition the mandible, approach the seated victim from behind and grasp the jaw by placing your thumbs (with cloth or gauze padding for traction) inside the mouth against the lower molars (rear teeth), holding the bone firmly with your remaining fingers. Exert steady pressure straight down until you feel the mandible "pop" back into place, and the victim says his teeth fit properly (see Figure 53, *B*). It's sometimes possible to reposition the jaw by

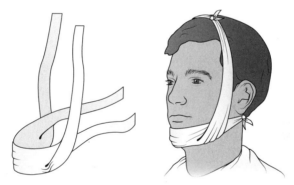

Figure 52. Bandage for a fractured or dislocated jaw. The bandage must be easy to remove, in case the victim needs to vomit.

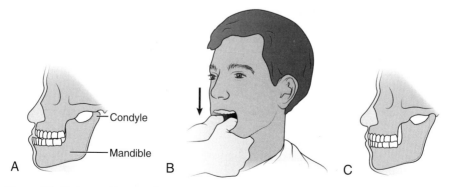

Figure 53. Dislocated jaw. **A,** The condyle of the mandible slips forward out of the joint. The teeth do not fit together properly. **B,** The rescuer applies firm downward pressure to relocate the jaw. **C,** Normal position is restored, and the teeth fit properly.

pushing down and back from the outside on the prominent bones in front of the ears. If both sides of the jaw are dislocated, attempt to reposition one side at a time. After the jaw is repositioned, tie a bandage under the chin and over the top of the head to keep the jaw from easily dislocating again (see Figure 52). *The bandage should be easily removable in case the victim needs to vomit. Another way to keep the mouth from opening widely is to wrap a rolled towel around the neck in such a way as to limit vertical jaw motion.*

Wrist, Hand, and Finger

A fracture or dislocation of the hand, wrist, or finger should be positioned and splinted in the normal resting position (position of function; see Figure 49, *A*). For a wrist or hand injury, this may be accomplished by allowing the victim's fingers to rest around a padded object in his palm (such as a rolled pair of socks, rolled elastic bandage, or wadded cloth; Figure 54), with a circumferential wrap to maintain position (Figure 55). Every attempt should be made to allow the fingertips to remain uncovered, to assess circulation. If the wrist is involved, place a rigid splint on the underside of the hand, wrist, and forearm to prevent motion (Figure 56; see Figures 294

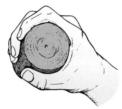

Figure 54. A rolled elastic bandage is gripped gently to maintain the hand in the "position of function."

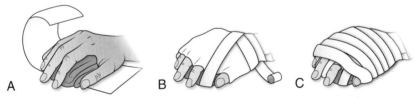

A   B   C

Figure 55. Hand dressing in the "position of function." **A,** The fingers hold a pad of cloth in the palm. **B,** A circumferential wrap is applied, taking care to pad between the fingers. **C,** The completed wrap leaves the fingertips exposed, so that they can be checked for adequate circulation.

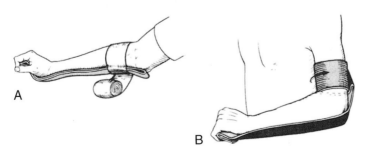

A

B

Figure 56. A SAM Splint fashioned to stabilize the wrist and forearm. **A,** In this method, the elbow is free to bend. **B,** The splint can be extended to immobilize the elbow.

and 297). Another way to splint a wrist fracture and at the same time provide immobilization of the elbow is to use a "sugar tong" type of splint (see Figure 299). Fingers may be splinted independently or taped together (with padding in between) for support (Figures 57 and 58).

A commonly missed fracture of the wrist is that of the scaphoid (navicular) bone (Figure 59). This occurs commonly from a fall on an outstretched hand. Pain and swelling are common, and the examiner notes tenderness when pressing directly on the scaphoid bone via the "anatomical snuffbox" (Figure 60). Even if swelling is not present, if there is "snuffbox tenderness," then the wrist should be splinted in a position of function (see page 69) and the victim brought to a physician for evaluation.

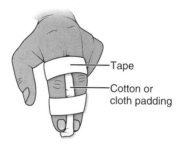

Figure 57. Buddy-taping method to immobilize a finger.

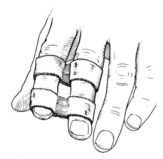

Figure 58. A variation of the buddy-taping method to immobilize a finger. If the fingers are taped together tightly, cotton or cloth should be placed between them for padding.

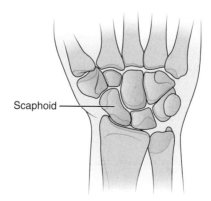

Figure 59. Scaphoid (navicular) bone of the wrist.

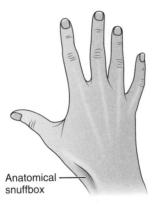

Figure 60. "Anatomical snuffbox" used to determine possibility of scaphoid fracture by applying direct external pressure.

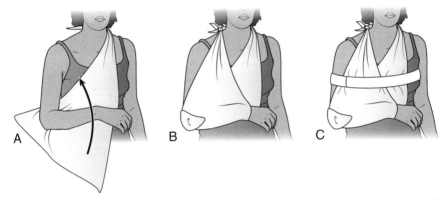

Figure 61. Sling and swathe. **A,** A triangular bandage is draped under the arm and over the opposite shoulder. **B,** Two corners are tied behind the neck, and the third is pinned at the elbow. **C,** A cravat swathe holds the arm against the chest.

A sling can be applied to the forearm for support and pain relief. A swathe may be added for further immobilization. To make a classic arm sling out of a triangular bandage, lay the bandage under the arm as shown in Figure 61. Tie two corners together with a square knot at the opposite shoulder—which creates the arm cradle—and then pin the remaining elbow corner up onto the body of the sling. If the corner cannot be pinned, it can be twisted into a "tail" and then tied into a knot (Figure 62). If the injury is to the upper arm, the victim may be more comfortable if the bandage is brought under the arm to be tied off on top (Figure 63). A rolled or folded triangular bandage becomes a cravat (see page 255), which is wrapped around the sling-encased arm and chest (as a swathe) to hold the arm snug against the body wall (see Figure 61, C). If materials to fashion a sling aren't available, the victim's shirt can be pulled up and pinned to create a crude hammock for the arm (Figure 64), or the shirt sleeve can be pinned to the body of the shirt after the elbow is flexed to the proper position (Figure 65).

If a finger is dislocated at the middle or distal joint (Figure 66, A), make a gentle attempt at relocation by applying steady, firm traction to the fingertip (see Figure 66, B). Don't try to reposition the joint with a sudden forceful snap. It's often easiest to relocate a finger if you hold

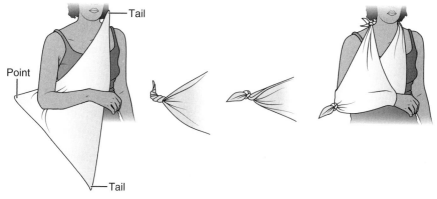

Point

Tail

Tail

Figure 62. Tying off the tail of a sling instead of using a pin.

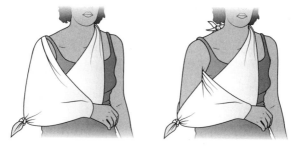

Figure 63. Alternative route for more comfortable bandage placement for a sling.

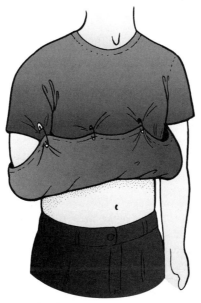

Figure 64. Pinning the shirt to make a hammock sling for the arm.

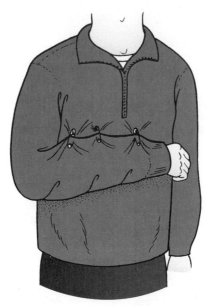

Figure 65. Pinning a shirt sleeve to the chest.

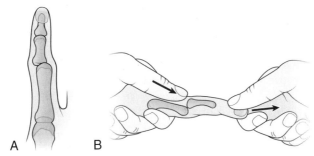

A   B

Figure 66. A, Dislocation of a finger joint. **B,** Relocation of the bones with firm steady traction.

the joint slightly bent and push the distal (overriding) bone back into position with your thumb while you're pulling the bones back into their proper position. It's nearly impossible to reduce a dislocation at the knuckle of the index finger without an operation. After a finger is realigned, it should be taped to one or two adjacent fingers for splinting (see Figures 57 and 58).

A "mallet finger" (Figure 67, *A*) results from disruption of the extensor tendon, which normally pulls the tip of the finger into a straight position. The finger should be splinted with a slight amount of hyperextension (see Figure 67, *B*). A different injury at this joint is disruption of the flexor tendon ("rugby jersey finger"), which normally pulls the tip of the finger down into a bent position. In this case, the end of the finger will often be swollen, bruised, and tender and will be observed to be held straight at the most distant joint, unable to be voluntarily bent toward the palm. This finger should be splinted slightly bent and the victim referred promptly to a hand surgeon for repair.

If the thumb is dislocated or fractured, it can be taped to prevent further injury, by fixing it with an anchor to the index finger (Figure 68, *A*) or directly against the hand (see Figure 68, *B*). You can use the anchor technique to hold any two fingers together.

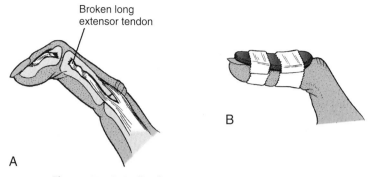

Broken long
extensor tendon

A

B

Figure 67. A, Mallet finger. **B,** Splinting a mallet finger.

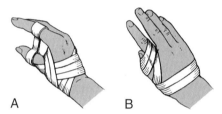

A   B

Figure 68. Taping the thumb for immobilization. **A,** The buddy-taping method. **B,** A thumb-lock. If possible, padding should be placed between the thumb and the forefinger.

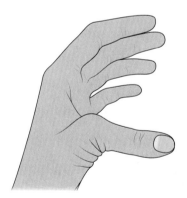

Figure 69. "Gamekeeper's thumb."

A "gamekeeper's thumb" is a disruption of the ulnar collateral ligament, often associated with a tiny avulsion fracture where the ligament attaches, at the base of the thumb (Figure 69). This is a ligament on the inner aspect of the thumb that keeps it from being pulled out away from the hand into an exaggerated hitchhiking gesture. It typically occurs when someone falls onto a ski pole or hiking pole, forcing the thumb outward and rupturing the tendon. The thumb should be taped to limit motion and the victim brought promptly to medical attention for consideration for surgical repair.

Forearm

A fracture of the forearm should be splinted to immobilize the wrist and bent elbow (see Figure 56, B). This may also be done in a "sugar tong" fashion (see Figure 299). Fashion a sling and attach it to the trunk with a swathe (see Figure 61).

Elbow

A fracture of the elbow should be splinted to include the wrist and shoulder, if possible, and at an angle of 60 to 90 degrees. However, if it's painful for the victim to move his elbow, splint it in the position in which you found it. A sling should be fashioned and attached to the trunk with a swathe. A dislocated elbow should be realigned if necessary to restore circulation to the hand. Hold the arm bent 45 to 90 degrees at the elbow and use a lever motion to pull the bones of the forearm back into position, while holding the upper arm fixed in countertraction (Figure 70). This may require a fair amount of force to accomplish and is usually difficult if the victim cannot relax.

"Nursemaid's Elbow"

The radius and ulna are the long bones of the forearm, and join with the humerus (the long bone of the upper arm) at the elbow joint. In young children, if a sudden straight pulling force is applied to the arm, such as when a child's hand is tugged to pull him along, or he is swung in a circle vigorously by the arms, the ligament that holds the radius in place may slip off the head of the radius within the elbow. There may be an audible snapping sound and immediate pain, but the pain may subside rapidly, after which the child will not use the arm. If this occurs and you're close to medical care, splint the arm as for a fracture. However, if you are far from care and wish to see if you can remedy the situation (that is, return the ligament to its proper position), take the child's arm and do the following. First, rotate the hand and forearm such that the thumb moves away from the body (accentuated hitchhiker's gesture) (Figure 71). Next, bend the arm at the elbow to 90 degrees while maintaining the external rotation. If no "pop" is felt or heard, keep the thumb pointed away from the body and move the forearm toward the upper arm (that is, "flex" the arm) until you have moved it as far as you can (Figure 72). If the

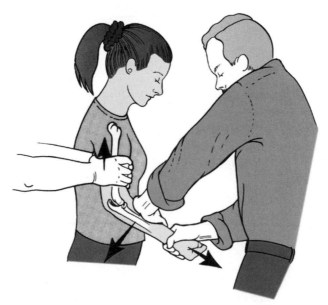

Figure 70. Repositioning a dislocated elbow.

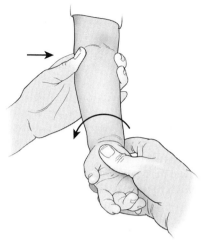

Figure 71. To reduce a nursemaid's elbow, rotate the hand and forearm as shown, then flex the forearm up toward the shoulder.

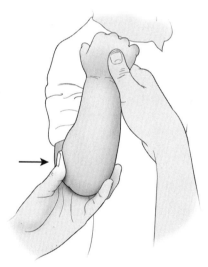

Figure 72. If no pop is felt after rotating the elbow and flexing the forearm toward the shoulder, then maintain the rotation and flexion and push the hand more firmly toward the upper arm.

ligament moves back to its proper position, the child will begin to use his arm again within 10 minutes. After that, there is no need for a sling or splint. If the child still will not use his arm, seek medical attention.

Upper Arm

The entire length of the bone of the upper arm (humerus) can be palpated for tenderness or deformity from the arm's inner aspect. A fracture of the humerus can be differentiated from a dislocated shoulder by observing how the victim holds his arm. With a humeral fracture, the arm is often held close to the chest, whereas a dislocation of the head of the humerus from the shoulder socket (shoulder dislocation—see page 85) prevents the victim from pulling his arm into his body. Also, if a "crunching" or grating sensation is felt when the arm is manipulated, or it rotates freely as if disrupted, a broken bone may be present. Because the radial nerve runs around the back of the humerus, if a fracture is present, there may be numbness of the top of the hand as well as weakness/inability to raise (extend) the wrist and fingers.

A fracture of the upper arm, particularly if it's close to the shoulder, is often quite difficult to splint. A "sugar tong" splint can be fashioned using a SAM Splint, by laying the splint along the inner and outer surfaces of the arm, with the U of the "tong" at the elbow (Figure 299). If possible, the elbow should be kept bent at 90 degrees and the arm placed in a sling. Attach the sling to the body by using a circumferential (around the chest) swathe fashioned from a belt, rope, or long piece of cloth to prevent motion of the arm at the shoulder (see Figure 61). Another method is to use a cravat to hold the upper arm against the body (Figure 73).

Two padded board splints can be used to stabilize an arm fracture above the elbow (Figure 74). The splints cross the upper part of the arm and the midforearm to create a triangle with the elbow. A sling is added for support.

Collarbone (Clavicle)
A fracture of the collarbone is best managed with a sling and swathe (see Figure 61), simple sling, or a modified figure-of-eight bandage (or both). The latter is created by draping a rope, cloth,

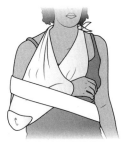

Figure 73. Using a cravat to hold the upper arm against the body.

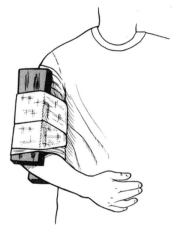

Figure 74. Padded boards to splint the upper arm.

or cravat behind the neck across the shoulders, then forward over the shoulders and under the arms (pad the armpits, if possible), to be tied in the back (Figure 75). This will pull the shoulders back into the military position. To provide a tighter fit, tie the cross-shoulder section to the lower knot (giving a figure-of-eight appearance). After the figure-of-eight bandage is pulled snug, the affected arm may be fixed to the chest using a sling and swathe. Another technique is to weave a figure-of-eight bandage with a long, rolled elastic bandage (Figure 76). *If any figure-of-eight bandage increases the victim's discomfort or if the collarbone is felt to be broken very close to the shoulder, you can use just a sling, with or without a swathe.* A collarbone fracture appears to heal equally well with any of these methods, so the major goal is sufficient support and immobilization for comfort.

Another alternative is to have the victim wear a properly fitted backpack with shoulder straps and carry approximately 15 lb of weight in the pack. The most comfortable sleeping position may be in a reclining chair or propped semi-upright.

Shoulder Dislocation

The long bone (humerus) of the upper arm fits into the shoulder joint with a ball-and-socket mechanism, held in place by muscles and tendons (Figure 77, *A*). When a person falls onto his shoulder or an outstretched arm, or has his arm twisted or pulled forcefully, the head of the

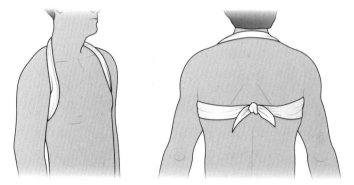

Figure 75. Modified figure-of-eight bandage for a broken collarbone.

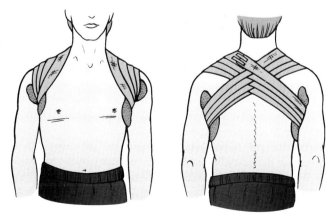

Figure 76. Woven figure-of-eight bandage for a broken collarbone.

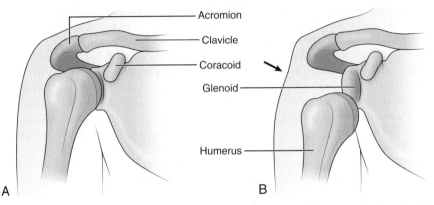

Figure 77. Dislocated shoulder. **A,** Normal anatomy. **B,** With dislocation, the head of the humerus slips out of the glenoid (socket), and a depression *(arrow)* is noted in the external appearance of the shoulder.

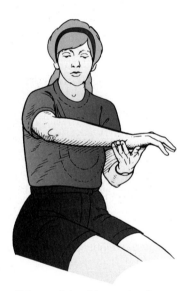

Figure 78. The victim with a dislocated shoulder carries the arm up and away from the body.

humerus can dislocate out of the shoulder joint (see Figure 77, *B*). This is usually quite painful and may be associated with a fracture of the humerus or the lip of the shoulder socket. The diagnosis of shoulder dislocation is made by observing and feeling a depression in the shoulder where the upper arm bone should be located (see Figure 77, *B*), noting that the victim holds the arm up and away from the body (Figure 78), and feeling the head of the humerus as a firm ball 2 to 3 inches (5 to 7.5 cm) below its normal position. There is reduced range of motion of the joint and absence of a "grating sensation" (indicating absence of a broken bone). Those who have previously suffered shoulder dislocations are often prone to recurrent episodes with lesser forces applied to the joint than are needed to cause a first-time dislocation.

If the injured victim can be transported to a medical facility within 2 hours, there is no absolute need to attempt relocation of the arm unless he is in extreme pain. If you decide to not attempt to relocate the humerus by any of the techniques described later, place the arm in a sling, position some padding underneath the arm and against the chest, and secure the sling to the victim's chest with a swathe to minimize motion and discomfort (see Figure 61). Alternatively, you can support the arm using a splint manufactured from a SAM Splint (see Figure 302).

It's usually easiest to relocate the arm ("reduce" the dislocation) if this is done soon after the injury, to avoid the effects of worsening muscle spasm and sometimes internal bleeding, both of which contribute to soft tissue swelling and difficulty with the reduction. So, if more than 2 hours will elapse before medical help is obtained, if the dislocation is recurrent (has happened to the same shoulder before), or if the victim is suffering severe pain, you can make an attempt to reposition the arm bone in its socket. Don't attempt relocation if the upper arm or elbow is deformed in a manner that would suggest a broken bone. Elders who fall are more likely to have broken their arm than are younger persons with more sturdy bones.

The "Cunningham technique" is simple to attempt (Figure 79). The victim should be calm and cooperative. Have him sit upright in a chair or on a rock or log, in a comfortable position. Sit or kneel directly opposite the victim and have the victim rest the hand of his affected arm on your shoulder in order to slightly bend at the elbow. You should be close enough to the victim so that he doesn't need to reach for you. If the left arm is involved, rest your left wrist across the victim's forearm so that you can exert slight downward pressure by holding the arm at the elbow. With your right hand, massage the victim's biceps muscle and then trapezius muscle to eliminate spasm and promote relaxation. Ask the victim to sit up straight and pull his shoulders back while you continue to massage. Ask the victim to shrug his shoulders. If the technique works, the head of the humerus will move back into its socket. Warn the victim that it may feel odd when bone is moving, but to try to remain relaxed. For a dislocation on the opposite side, reverse your hands.

Another simple technique for relocation is to pull with steady, forceful traction on the injured arm, directed at a 45- to 90-degree angle away from the body. At the same time, someone should provide countertraction by holding a sheet or blanket that's wrapped across the victim's chest and under the affected armpit (Figure 80). The easiest technique is to tie a sheet, belt, webbed strapping, or avalanche cord around the rescuer's waist and the victim's bent forearm, so that the rescuer (standing or kneeling) can lean back to apply traction, keeping his hands free to guide the head of the humerus back into position (Figure 81). In all cases, place padding in the armpit and bend of the elbow to prevent a pressure injury to sensitive nerves beneath the skin. A single rescuer can provide countertraction by placing his foot against the victim's chest just below the

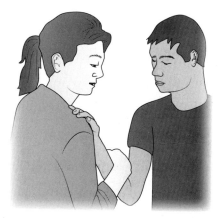

Figure 79. Proper position for using the Cunningham technique for reducing a shoulder dislocation.

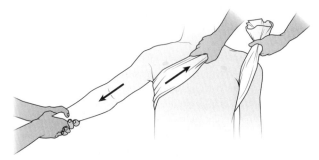

Figure 80. Technique for relocating a shoulder dislocation. One rescuer applies traction at the forearm while another applies countertraction at the chest.

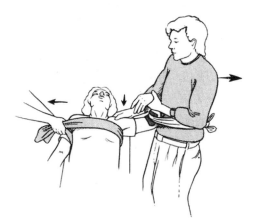

Figure 81. Repositioning a dislocated shoulder. Attached to the victim's forearm with a strap, rope, or sheet, the rescuer uses his body weight to apply traction, leaving his hands free to manipulate the victim's arm. A second rescuer applies countertraction, or the victim can be held motionless by fixing the chest sheet to a tree or ground stake.

armpit or fixing the countertraction sheet or rope to a tree or ice ax buried in the ground; he can also use a life jacket as a foot brace (Figure 82). *Don't jerk the arm, attempt to twist or lever it into position, or pull with a tugging motion.*

Another technique is to have the victim lie prone so that his injured arm can dangle free. Place a thick pad under the injured shoulder. Attach a 10- to 20-lb (4.5 to 9 kg) weight to the wrist or forearm (don't have the victim attempt to hold the weight) and allow it to exert steady traction on the arm, using gravity to relocate the humeral head (Figure 83). Alternatively, have the standing victim bend forward at the waist as you pull steadily downward on his arm to simulate the gravity effect, with gentle side-to-side (at the wrist) rotation (Figure 84).

In the scapular manipulation technique, the victim is placed in a prone position so that his injured arm can dangle free. Apply traction for 5 to 10 minutes. Then, while maintaining traction, push the tip (lower edge) of the scapula ("wingbone") in toward the spine while pulling the upper portion (toward the shoulder) of the scapula away from the midline. This can also be done with the victim in a standing position (Figure 85, *A*). If the victim is standing, it may help to pull the arm forward as well as down (see Figure 85, *B*). This can also be done with the victim lying on his back. Have one rescuer hold the victim flat by pressing on his chest while another

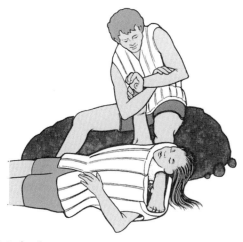

Figure 82. Life jacket brace to assist in the relocation of a dislocated humerus.

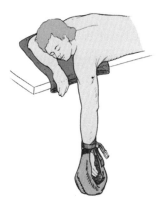

Figure 83. A fanny pack filled with rocks can be used for a weight in the "dangle" method of shoulder relocation.

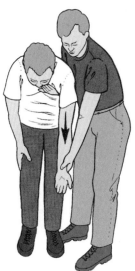

Figure 84. Pulling on the hanging arm to relocate a dislocated humerus.

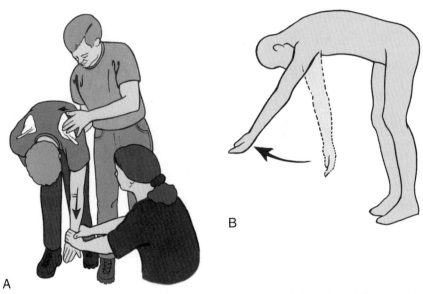

Figure 85. A, Pushing the lower edge of the scapula toward the spine while an assistant pulls downward on the hanging arm to assist in the relocation of a dislocated humerus. **B,** The downward pull on the arm may be slightly forward to help put the arm bone back in the shoulder socket.

pulls the arm upward at a 90-degree angle (Figure 86). The third rescuer reaches underneath the victim to manipulate the scapula. *The scapular manipulation technique can be combined with any other technique,* such as the Cunningham technique. There needs to be enough rescuer hands to combine techniques.

In the Spaso technique, the victim lies on his back. The rescuer slowly lifts the affected arm while applying traction. When the arm is fully lifted and pointing toward the sky, the rescuer applies external rotation (rotate the thumb out to the hitch-hiking position) (Figure 87).

In the Eskimo technique, the victim lies on the ground with the uninjured shoulder down and the injured shoulder up. It usually takes two persons to lift the victim by the wrist and forearm of the injured arm, so he is hanging by the injured arm (Figure 88). If this technique is successful, the head of the humerus pops back into position within a few minutes.

In the Milch technique, the victim attempts self-reduction of the dislocation. He should sit, stand, or lie on his back and slowly reach, using the hand of the injured shoulder, behind the head in order to touch the opposite shoulder (Figure 89). Another way to describe this technique is to have the victim reach up and backward with the injured arm as if going into a windup to throw a baseball. If the technique works, the victim will feel a "pop" as the dislocation is corrected. If you wish to assist the victim, use one hand to gently cup his elbow and assist him with this procedure, while using your other hand to steady the affected shoulder.

If you are the victim, you can attempt the Milch technique. Alternatively, you can get in a sitting position with knees bent up to your chest, wrap your arms around your knees, lock hands by grasping the wrist of the injured arm with your good hand, and then spread your knees.

If pain medicine is available, the victim should be medicated before relocation is attempted, to allow the greatest possible shoulder and chest muscle relaxation. As the arm bone moves back into proper position (this may require 15 minutes of steady traction), it will sometimes "give" in little movements, with a final "pop" back into the socket. Once the bone is back in place, the victim will be able to bring his arm across the chest. If the victim cannot relax his muscles

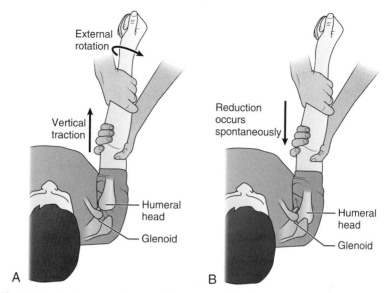

Figure 86. Reducing a dislocated humerus while the victim is lying on his back.

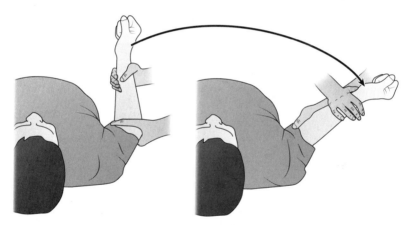

Figure 87. Spaso technique for reducing a dislocated humerus.

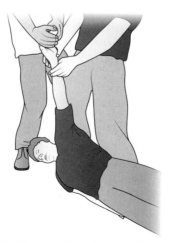

Figure 88. Eskimo technique for reducing a dislocated humerus.

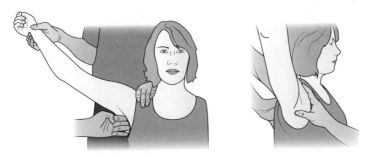

Figure 89. Milch technique for reducing a dislocated humerus.

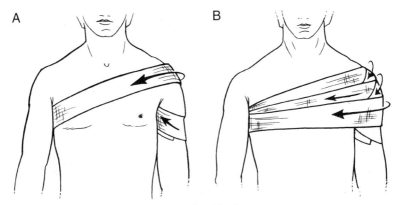

Figure 90. Shoulder harness.

sufficiently to allow relocation, if your attempts cause excruciating pain, or if you're otherwise unsuccessful after 30 minutes, leave well enough alone (no one ever died of a dislocated shoulder). Place padding in the armpit and fix the arm near the body in as comfortable a position as possible with swathe bandages, and then go for help. A shoulder harness (Figure 90) may be useful. The victim who cannot walk should be transported in a sitting (for comfort) position, if possible. If the shoulder relocates, it should be placed in a sling and swathe, to prevent a repeat dislocation (see Figure 61). A first-time shoulder dislocation that is relocated should be immobilized for 3 weeks. A recurrent dislocation that is relocated can be exercised gently after 3 to 5 days.

Shoulder Separation

A shoulder separation, as contrasted with a dislocation, occurs when the collarbone's ligamentous attachments to the acromion and coracoid structures of the triangular scapula are weakened or disrupted (Figure 91). This can range from small tears in the ligaments, which don't result in a visible deformity, to full disruption of the ligaments, leading to a "free-floating" collarbone. The injury usually follows a direct blow to the shoulder, such as occurs when you fall onto your side and cannot break the fall with an outstretched arm.

If tenderness is elicited when pressing directly over the acromioclavicular (AC) joint, particularly with swelling and a spongy sensation over the end of the collarbone, suspect a shoulder separation. Treat as for a broken collarbone (see page 84).

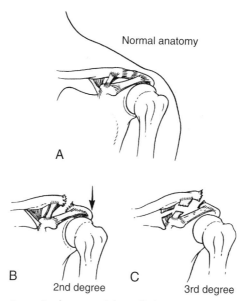

Normal anatomy

A

B
2nd degree

C
3rd degree

Figure 91. A, Ligamentous attachments of the collarbone at the shoulder. **B,** Second-degree shoulder separation. **C,** Third-degree shoulder separation.

Rib

A broken rib can be very painful, but there is little that the rescuer can do to improve the situation. Pad the chest wall with blankets or clothing (if the victim needs to be carried out on a stretcher) to restrict unnecessary motion and contact. Never bind the chest tightly; this inhibits deep breathing and prevents full expansion of the lungs, which predisposes the victim to partial lung collapse and pneumonia. Encourage the victim to breathe deeply (sigh) or cough a few times an hour. If there is a segment of detached (flail) ribs (see page 39), attempt to stabilize its position with padding (see Figures 27 and 31). Because of the force necessary to break a rib, anticipate internal bleeding (lungs, liver, and spleen) (see page 57). A rib will sometimes break during forceful coughing. In this case, internal injury is not a concern.

Spine (Chest and Lower Back)

A victim who falls a great distance and lands on his feet may fracture his heel(s), ankle(s), and lumbar vertebrae (lower bones of the spine—see Figure 51). Symptoms of spinal cord injury include back pain, particularly in the midline; weakness, numbness or tingling below the injury; loss of bladder or bowel control; numbness in a "saddle" distribution (where a person's skin would contact a saddle when sitting on a horse); and low blood pressure ("spinal shock"). If a fractured spine is suspected, the victim must be completely immobilized to avoid damage to the spinal cord. Position him on a firm litter or backboard, and secure him so that no motion of the back is possible (see page 35). If a scoop stretcher or backboard is not available and the victim must be moved, he should be logrolled (see page 38). If a patient has a suspected spine injury, but must be repositioned to allow placement on a backboard or other conveyance, use as many assistants as you need to try to avoid unnecessary twisting and bending of the spine. Pay particular attention to the neck and lower back.

Pelvis

If pressing inward on the victim's hips or downward on the pubic bone causes pain, suspect a fracture of the pelvis and immobilize the victim from his waist down. A pelvic fracture is frequently associated with severe internal injuries and bleeding, so rapid evacuation is a high priority. Be prepared to treat the victim for shock (see page 58). Don't allow a victim with a suspected pelvic fracture to walk. A SAM Pelvic Sling is a force-controlled circumferential pelvic sling belt for effective reduction and stabilization of pelvic fractures. Another device is the Pelvic Binder (www.pelvicbinder.com). If this type of device is not available, the pelvis can be wrapped tightly with a sheet, sleeping pad (held in place with tape), blanket, or jacket to attempt to keep the bone fragments from moving, which hopefully diminishes instability, internal bleeding, and pain (Figure 92). A windlass (see Figure 106) applied to the material wrapped around the pelvis can be used to achieve tightness. Another method is to wrap an inflatable sleeping pad snugly around the pelvis and secure it with tape. After it is secured, it can be inflated to snug it up and apply pressure (Figure 93). Before applying any pelvic sling, be sure to empty the patient's pockets and remove his belt so that the external pressure doesn't press any items against the pelvis. For transport, place padding between the victim's legs and gently tie his legs together to minimize motion and improve comfort.

Tailbone (Coccyx)

If someone slips and falls directly into a sitting position on a very hard surface, such as a boulder or rock slab, he may break his tailbone. This causes pain at the tip of the spine, felt at the top end of the crease between the buttocks, and almost always with sitting. It may also cause pain with bowel movements. Treatment consists of positioning to avoid pressure on the area. This includes leaning forward when sitting to rest the weight anywhere other than on the tailbone, improvising a doughnut-shaped sitting cushion, and avoiding constipation.

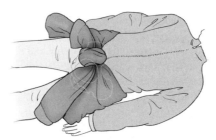

Figure 92. Pelvic sling improvised with a jacket provides compression to the pelvis to control bleeding.

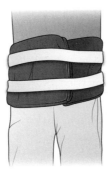

Figure 93. Using an inflatable sleeping pad to stabilize a fractured pelvis.

Femur

A fracture of the femur (the large bone of the upper leg—the longest and strongest bone in the body) can be diagnosed by severe pain, inability to bear weight, deformity, and rapid swelling (from bleeding). Often, the affected leg is shortened and the foot is rotated away from the other leg. Sometimes a fracture of the neck of the femur can be subtle, as the victim complains only of minor pain on the inside of the groin or knee and may continue to walk. On close inspection, the affected leg may be seen to be slightly shortened, and there may be some swelling and pain in the anterior hip area. Any disabling femur fracture requires splinting from the hip to the ankle. Because the muscles of the thigh are quite powerful and will tend to force the broken bone ends to overlap (Figure 94, *A*), traction is often necessary to control bleeding, maintain position, decrease pain, and prevent further internal muscle and blood vessel damage (see Figure 94, *B*). The recommended amount of traction is the equivalent of 10% of body weight, not to exceed 15 lb (6.8 kg). If sufficient rescuers are available, one person should maintain firm traction on the leg at the ankle to oppose the strong muscle contractions of the thigh (Figure 95). A broken

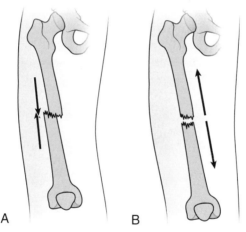

A   B

Figure 94. Fracture of the femur. **A,** Without traction, strong muscles of the thigh pull the broken bone ends together, causing pain and deformity. **B,** Traction straightens the leg and helps control bleeding and pain.

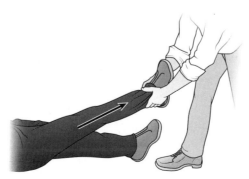

Figure 95. Technique for applying traction to the lower leg to stabilize a broken femur.

femur can bleed 2 quarts (liters) of blood into the thigh rapidly, so evacuation is a high priority. Be prepared to treat the victim for shock (see page 58).

The standard Thomas ("half ring") splint allows traction to be applied to the femur. A Hare splint has a ratchet mechanism at the end to provide mechanical traction. A Sager splint allows traction by facilitating lengthening of its long, rigid axis rod. The Kendrick Traction Device is a lightweight, portable field traction apparatus that operates on the same principle and can easily be carried and applied in a wilderness setting. The Slishman Traction Splint, available in ski pole and EMS versions, is an excellent, lightweight device. The ski pole version is similar to a single ski pole system (Figure 96). Practice using any commercial splint before you have to use it "for real."

You can also prepare an improvised traction splint that replicates the features of a Thomas splint: a half ring to anchor up against the pelvic bone (ischial tuberosity) underneath the lower crease of the buttock, two longitudinal rigid rods to run the length of the leg, a fixed spacer at the lower (foot) end between the two rods, and a traction mechanism to pull on the leg to align the fracture. The half ring can comprise a SAM Splint (see Figure 309). See later for details.

The ankle should be padded with foam or cloth pads, or a boot should be worn. If the latter is done, you can cut away the toe section to assess the circulation (skin color, sensation) (Figure 97).

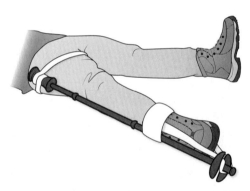

Figure 96. Single ski pole system for applying traction to stabilize a broken femur.

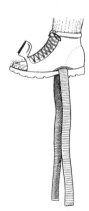

Figure 97. The toe section of a boot can be cut away to allow inspection for adequate circulation. A cravat or piece of webbing can be passed through a boot as the first step in creating a traction harness.

A traction harness must be created to pull the leg straight down away from the head. One method is to cut two slits through the victim's sturdy boot, above the sole just in front of the heel and directly below the leg bones. Pass a cravat or nylon webbing (such as a pack strap) through the opening (see Figure 97); the ends of the strap will be secured to the rigid object that will form the spacer at the foot end of the leg splint. The paired-loop ("double runner") method of creating an ankle hitch uses paired lengths of cravat, nylon webbing, or rope (Figure 98, *A*). Fold each in half, creating a single turn at one end. Lay one cravat over the top of the ankle and one behind the ankle (behind the Achilles tendon), with the curved ends pointed in opposite directions. Pass the free ends of each cravat through the loop in the other cravat, and tighten the cravats so that they fit snugly and flat against the ankle. The free ends should now hang down (see Figure 98, *B*) and will be secured to the spacer, directly or with an interposed pulley system, that connects the long, rigid rods of the splint. Another method to apply traction is "Buck's traction," in which a pad is secured firmly around the lower leg in such a way that the pad can get enough purchase to allow it to anchor tape stirrups (Figure 99). If the ankle is injured, a suitable traction harness would be the S-configuration hitch, which is applied to the leg just above the ankle (Figure 100).

The traction splint rods can be fashioned from two ski poles, rigid tree limbs or saplings, tent poles, or anything else that's approximately a foot (30 cm) longer than the distance from the top of the thigh to the bottom of the foot. To measure the proper length, lay the rods next to the victim on either side of the thigh, with the top of the inner rod tucked up against the groin crease and the top of the outer at the top of the thigh. Cut the lengths to be even at a distance of approximately 8 to 12 inches (20 to 30 cm) below the foot (Figure 101).

Construct the splint away from the victim. Using a cravat, ski pole straps, webbing, or rope, attach the tops of the two poles with a length that approximates half the circumference of the thigh at this point, to create the half ring that will be snugged up underneath the victim into the lower buttock crease (Figure 102). This splint may also be accomplished using a SAM Splint (see Figure 309) to create the half ring. At the lower (foot) ends of the rods, attach a perpendicular rigid spacer about 8 in (20 cm) in length (Figure 103). This could be a piece of ski pole, a wrench, a piece of tree limb, or the like. Then lay four cravats (two for above the knee, two for below) or straps (that can be fastened) over the rods and wind them to be configured as cradle hitches (Figure 104). These will fix the rods to the leg after traction has been applied. Velcro straps are nice, if you have them.

Holding traction on the leg, lift it enough to slide the splint underneath. Snug the half ring up into the buttock crease, remembering to keep the shorter rod on the inside of the leg. Attach the

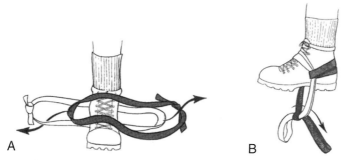

Figure 98. Paired-looped webbing to create an ankle hitch. **A,** Position the webbing around the ankle. **B,** Pull the harness tight with the ends pointed down for fixation to the splint.

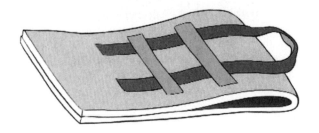

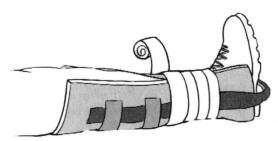

Figure 99. Buck's traction.

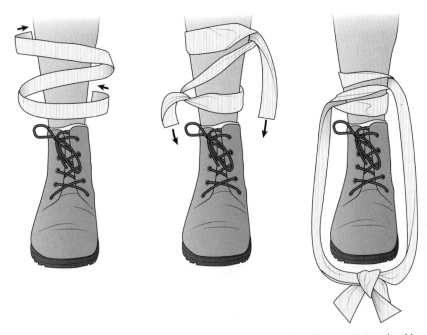

Figure 100. S-configuration hitch traction harness applied above an injured ankle.

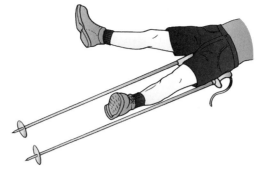

Figure 101. Proper length of traction splint rods.

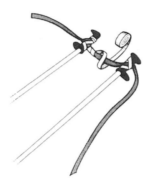

Figure 102. Creation of the half ring, which snugs up into the buttock crease.

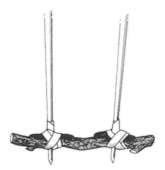

Figure 103. Attachment of the spacer at the foot end between the splint rods.

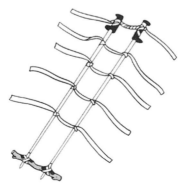

Figure 104. Configuration of cravats for cradle hitches.

splint firmly to the leg with tape or a cravat around the front of the thigh (over thick padding, if available) at the top of the splint above the suspected point of the fracture (Figure 105).

Tie the free ends from the traction harness (which you created through the boot or around the ankle) to the spacer at the end of the long splint. Create a "Spanish windlass" by inserting a short, rigid stick or rod between the tied-down free ends and twisting to produce the desired amount of traction (Figure 106). Fix the twister rod in place by tying it to the adjacent long splint rods (Figure 107). Another way to apply traction is to use a webbing belt and sliding buckle (Figure 108).

Finally, secure the splint to the leg with the cradle hitches, two above the knee and two below (Figure 109). Pad everything. The victim may be more comfortable if you apply traction while his knee is very slightly bent.

With a broken femur, the rescuer would ideally remove the victim's shoe or boot to be able to assess whether or not the circulation is intact, by checking the dorsalis pedis artery pulse on the top of the foot (see page 30) and observing for normal skin color and sensation. This should be done only if it will not interfere with splinting and if the foot can be protected from the elements (e.g., to avoid frostbite). If the footwear is removed, tent up the sock and cut a hole just large enough to allow a finger to enter to find the pulse and to get a peek at the skin color.

After applying any femur traction splint, remember to check at 30-minute intervals to be sure that the traction has not lessened beyond where you desire it to be. It's not uncommon for professional and improvised traction splints alike to slip or otherwise lose tension.

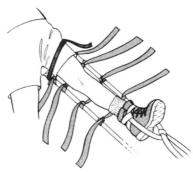

Figure 105. Attaching the splint to the leg above the suspected point of the fracture.

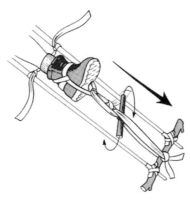

Figure 106. Tie the free ends of the foot harness to the spacer. Then twist the Spanish windlass to create downward traction on the leg.

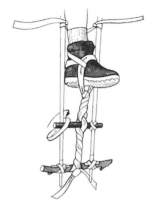

Figure 107. After the windlass is twisted to achieve the desired traction, tie the windlass rod to the long struts of the splint to maintain the traction.

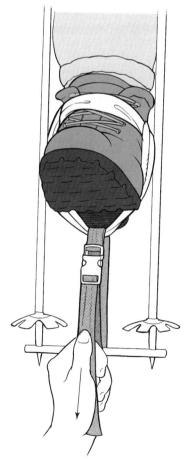

Figure 108. Applying traction to a long leg splint using a webbing belt and sliding buckle.

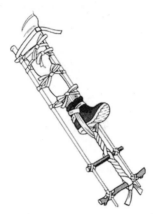

Figure 109. Secure the splint in place by tying off the cradle hitches.

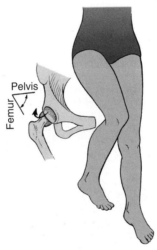

Pelvis

Femur

Figure 110. Position of the leg with posterior hip dislocation.

Hip

If a person (usually elderly) falls with great force directly onto his knee, the large leg bone may be forced backward out of the hip socket and create a posterior hip dislocation. In such a case, the affected leg appears shorter and is bent at the knee; the foot and knee are also turned inward (toward the other leg) (Figure 110). With an anterior hip dislocation, the ball of the femur slips forward out of the hip socket, and the leg is shorter and externally rotated (knee and foot face outward) (Figure 111). Either dislocation is a serious condition, because the blood supply to the head of the femur (the "ball" of this ball-and-socket joint) is disrupted. If medical attention cannot be reached within 1 hour, make an attempt at relocation—*unless there is a deformity of the upper leg or knee (indicating a fracture)*. Hold the leg and knee of the victim firmly, and exert forceful traction pulling on the thigh directly down toward the victim's feet, in an attempt to slide the head of the femur back into the hip socket. If this is successful, you will feel a "give," and the leg, knee, and foot will regain proper alignment.

Because of the force required to perform this maneuver, it's generally necessary to have a second rescuer provide countertraction to the victim's upper body. The two-rescuer method

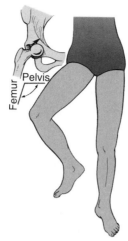

Figure 111. Position of the leg with anterior hip dislocation.

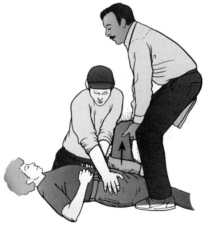

Figure 112. Two-rescuer method for repositioning a dislocated hip.

involves the first rescuer straddling the supine victim directly over his hips, facing toward the victim's head and holding the victim's bent leg between his knees. The second rescuer holds the victim's pelvis to the ground while the first lifts upward on the dislocated femur (Figure 112).

The "Captain Morgan technique" (named for the pose of the pirate on a bottle of Captain Morgan rum) is performed as follows: Have the victim lie on his back on a backboard, stretcher, or other surface to which the victim can be secured by a strap across the pelvis. Bend the joints of both the leg (at the hip) and the knee on the affected side to 90 degrees (right angle). The rescuer then places one of his feet on the backboard directly underneath the victim's leg such that the rescuer's knee is positioned underneath the victim's calf as close as possible to the knee. The rescuer holds the victim's ankle to keep the knee bent and applies an upward force to the hip by lifting his calf, while gently rotating the lower leg back and forth to see if this helps slide the femur back within the pelvis (Figure 113). This technique can be done with a single rescuer, but it's always helpful to have someone assist by holding the victim's pelvis firmly on the ground.

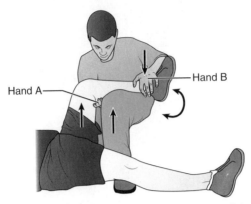

Figure 113. Captain Morgan technique for reducing a dislocated hip.

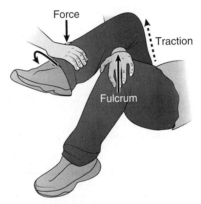

Figure 114. Whistler technique for reducing a dislocated hip.

Another single-rescuer technique is the "Whistler technique." In this case, the rescuer's forearm is used as a fulcrum against which to apply the necessary force to put the dislocated femur back into place (Figure 114). Have the victim lie on his back on a backboard, stretcher, or other surface to which the victim can be secured by a strap across the pelvis. The uninjured leg is put up into a bent flexed position. The rescuer slides his forearm under the injured leg behind the knee and uses his hand to hold onto the flexed knee of the uninjured leg. With his other hand, the rescuer holds firmly onto the ankle of the injured leg, which should be put into a position of approximately 90 degrees flexed (at the hip). Now, the rescuer uses his forearm (underneath the dislocated leg) as a fulcrum and the lower leg as a lever. Putting downward force on the leg should now flex the knee and put traction on the femur, pulling its head back into the hip socket. It may help to rotate the leg back and forth to get the hip to go back into position.

If relocation is successful, firmly splint the hip by securing the victim's legs together, slightly bent at the hips and knees with padding in between; he should be promptly evacuated, and should not attempt to walk.

Knee and Kneecap

A suspected fracture of the knee or kneecap should be splinted from hip to ankle. If there is such great deformity that the foot becomes numb and turns blue or pale and cold (usually with severe dislocation of the knee joint) and pulses cannot be felt, then dislocation of the knee joint should be suspected and the rescuer should use traction to attempt to realign the leg in a position of function (with the knee bent at a 15- to 30-degree angle; see Figure 49, *B*) to reestablish circulation. It's very difficult to correct a knee dislocation in this manner, so it's likely that the attempt will be unsuccessful. If pulses don't return even after the knee has been repositioned, the major artery that traverses the knee joint may have been torn or crushed and occluded. A knee fracture or dislocation is a surgical emergency. Even if the relocation attempt is successful, the victim still must be evacuated promptly for a full evaluation.

The kneecap can be dislocated to the outside (lateral dislocation—more common) or to the inside (medial dislocation). If the kneecap becomes dislocated, gently straighten the leg, then push the kneecap back into place. It may be necessary to slightly hyperextend ("overstraighten") the knee to accomplish this. To relax the quadriceps muscle, it may help to slightly flex the hip. Another technique is to have the victim lie face down, then hold the patella firmly while lifting the affected leg slowly off the ground to relax the hamstring muscles. Then, release your grip on the patella and slowly straighten the leg to see if the kneecap will move back into proper position. Occasionally, the kneecap will not move back into position. If any maneuver is painful or not easily accomplished, don't apply force. After the kneecap is repositioned, splint the leg straight or at a 15-degree bend (knee) using an Ensolite or foam pad and elastic bandage(s). If the leg is in this position and splinted, the victim may gently bear weight. If the splint slips, duct tape can be used to fashion suspenders (Figure 115). To prevent the kneecap from becoming dislocated, a person with a history of frequent (patellar) dislocation may choose to wear an Aircast patellar brace or similar support. This stabilizes the kneecap and compresses the surrounding soft tissue with a circular cushion of air.

If the knee has been dislocated or fractured, the victim must be carried. If a kneecap dislocation is the only injury, however, successful treatment will allow the victim to walk, using an ice ax, ski pole, or other object as a crutch.

The knee can be sprained (or strained) when it twists or withstands impact. The supporting ligaments that bind the joint on the outside and inside (lateral and medial collateral ligaments) and those that cross front to back through the interior of the knee joint (cruciate ligaments) can be stretched, slightly torn, or completely disrupted. This causes immediate pain with weight bearing (walking), motion (trying to bend the knee or extend the leg), or touch (pressing against

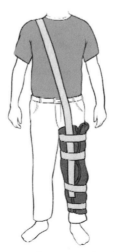

Figure 115. Duct tape suspenders support an improvised knee splint.

the injured side of the knee). Often, there is swelling and a spongy feel to the knee. As swelling increases, the knee becomes less flexible and more difficult to bend. If you suspect more than a minor sprain, immobilize the knee as if for a fracture; the victim should avoid weight bearing.

Sometimes the mechanism of injury can suggest what has been damaged:

- Striking the bent knee from the outside commonly injures the medial collateral ligament.
- Striking the straight knee from the inside commonly injures the lateral collateral ligament.
- Striking the front of the knee commonly injures the posterior cruciate ligament.
- A knee being severely twisted or completely giving out on impact or pivot commonly is caused by anterior cruciate ligament disruption.
- The medial and lateral menisci are cartilaginous cushions within the knee joint. Pain with knee rotation or clicking/locking of the knee may indicate a meniscal tear. A "bucket-handle" tear of a meniscus can cause the attached torn fragment to become lodged in the knee joint, which is very painful, and results in a "locked" knee, which cannot be bent (flexed) or straightened (extended) without sharp excruciating pain (because the fragment is being pinched). If this happens, it's sometimes possible to release the trapped fragment. First, position the affected side down to take advantage of gravity. Next, gently and slowly bend the knee to an angle of about 30 degrees, and then apply pressure to the lower leg in an attempt to slightly open the affected side of the joint. For instance, if the pain is on the outer side of the knee, the pressure is applied to the lower leg and ankle in an inward fashion, with slight inward rotation of the ankle, with a hand pressing on the inside of the knee in a direction toward the ground. If the pain is on the inner side of the knee, pressure is applied to the lower leg in an outward fashion, with slight outward rotation of the ankle, with a hand pressing on the outside of the knee in a direction toward the ground. If the maneuver is successful, the pain will be relieved immediately, and the knee will "unlock" (be able to bend and straighten without pain).
- Inability to step up ("climb stairs") after a "pop" is felt or heard may indicate injury to the quadricep/patellar tendon. Sometimes this tendon is irritated from overuse, which causes pain underneath and just below the kneecap. The treatment is rest, ice, and an NSAID, as for any other sprain or strain. Some persons report pain relief if they apply a patellar tendon strap around the leg just below the knee. This can be improvised from a rolled cravat or bandanna.

Lower Leg

A fracture of the lower leg should be splinted from knee to ankle. If necessary, the legs can be attached side by side with padding in between. If the knee is not involved, keep it bent at 15 to 30 degrees.

If the head of the fibula (smaller bone of the lower leg) is dislocated from its position adjacent to the head of the tibia (larger bone of the lower leg), there will be pain and a bulge at the site of the dislocation. This injury commonly occurs when the knee is bent (flexed) while the foot is rotated inward with forefoot and toes forced downward. If this happens and pain prohibits the victim from walking, then an attempt may be made to relocate the fibular head by pressing over it while simultaneously bending the knee and rotating the foot outward while lifting the forefoot toward the knee, to cause a "pop."

Ankle

A fracture of the ankle can be stirrup-splinted or wrapped to prevent movement. This can be accomplished using a SAM Splint, parka, or piece of rolled foam taped or wrapped into place (Figure 116; see Figures 303 to 305). Remove or loosen the boot or shoe to avoid entrapment due to swelling, which could impair circulation. However, if the victim must walk out under his own power, replace footwear as soon as possible, before swelling makes this impossible.

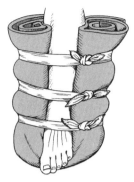

Figure 116. A piece of rolled foam can be used as a "stirrup" to hold the foot and ankle motionless.

Toe

A fractured toe may be splinted by buddy-taping. This is performed by placing some padding (cloth or cotton) between the toes and taping the injured toe to a healthy adjacent toe for support.

AMPUTATION

Amputation is detachment of a body part, such as an ear, finger, or foot. It is usually associated with a serious force or crushing injury, such as an animal bite. The immediate threats to life are bleeding and shock (see page 58).

If a body part is detached, apply firm pressure to the site of the bleeding where the tissue loss has occurred. Manage any serious bleeding (see page 50). Cover the wound with the cleanest available bandage, and then wrap firmly. *Don't attempt to reattach the detached body part.* If a digit is hanging on by a small "bridge" of skin or muscle, attempt to bandage it without completing the separation.

If the body part can be easily recovered and the victim can be brought to a hospital within 18 hours of the injury, do the following:

1. Gently rinse the body part if the cut end is contaminated with dirt.
2. Wrap the body part in clean cloth or gauze and keep the covering moist. The ideal solution is saline (*not* ocean water, because of infection risk), if that is available; if not, fresh water will do. Don't immerse the part in a bag of water; merely keep the covering moist. Keep the body part cool by placing it on ice after wrapping it securely in a bandage, cloth, or towel. Don't freeze the amputated tissues. To avoid a freezing injury, *don't apply ice directly to the body part or immerse it in ice water.*
3. Bring the body part with the victim to the hospital.

The application of a tourniquet to stop bleeding is essentially a decision to possibly sacrifice the limb in order to preserve life. If any salvageable part of the limb is still attached and bleeding is not so severe that a tourniquet is needed, don't apply a tourniquet to stop bleeding until you have exhausted all pressure techniques (see page 50). If the limb is completely severed and the bleeding is torrential, a tourniquet may be applied until the muscular walls of the arteries constrict and bleeding can be controlled by direct pressure (see page 52).

After 5 to 10 minutes, loosen the tourniquet briefly to see if the bleeding can be controlled with pressure techniques alone.

BURNS

DEFINITIONS (Figure 117)

First-degree burn. This is a burn that involves the outermost layer of skin, the epidermis. It is often quite painful. The skin is reddened, but there is no blister formation. When a large surface area is involved, as with an extensive sunburn, the victim may become quite ill, with fever, weakness, chills, and vomiting.

Second-degree burn. This is a burn that involves the epidermis and portions of the next-deeper layer of the skin, called the dermis, which contains the sweat glands, hair follicles, and small blood vessels. It is usually more painful than a first-degree burn, and blisters are present. Large areas of second-degree injury impair the body's ability to control temperature and retain moisture. Thus, a severely burned victim loses large amounts of fluid and can rapidly become hypothermic in a cold environment.

Third-degree burn. This is a burn that has penetrated the entire thickness of the skin, and may involve muscle and bone. It is typically painless because of nerve destruction. The appearance is dry, hard, leathery, and charred. Occasionally, the skin will appear waxy and white with small clotted blood vessels visible as purple or maroon lines below the surface. Because a third-degree burn is usually surrounded by an area of second-degree injury, the edges of the wound may be quite painful. Third-degree burns almost always require a skin graft for coverage.

Partial-thickness burn. First-degree or second-degree burn.

Full-thickness burn. Third-degree burn.

Inhalation injury. This is a burn that involves any portion of the airway. Inhalation injury occurs when a victim is trapped in a fire and inhales smoke, steam, or superheated air (see page 112).

TREATMENT FOR BURNS

1. Remove the victim from the source of the burn. If his clothing is on fire, roll him on the ground or smother him in a blanket to extinguish the flames. If clothing is soaked with

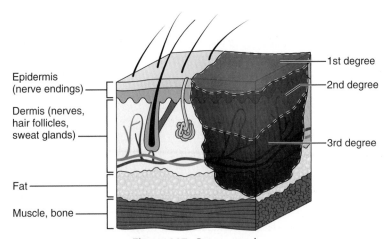

Figure 117. Burn wound.

hot liquid, quickly remove the clothing. Remove all materials that are hot or burned. If the victim has been burned with chemicals, *gallons* of water should be used to wash off the harmful agents. If chemicals may be present in an article of clothing, remove it. If the eyes are involved, they should be irrigated copiously. Phosphorus ignites on contact with air, so any phosphorus in contact with the skin must be kept covered with water. Don't attempt to neutralize acid burns with alkaline solutions or vice versa; the resultant chemical reaction may liberate heat and worsen the injury. Stick to irrigation with water. If clothing remains stuck to the skin and does not fall away with irrigation, don't tear the clothing away. Cut around it.

2. Evaluate the airway. Look for evidence of an inhalation injury: burns of the face and mouth, singed nasal hairs, soot in the mouth, swollen tongue, drooling and difficulty in swallowing saliva, muffled voice, coarse or difficult breathing, coughing, and wheezing. If it appears that an inhalation injury has occurred, administer oxygen (see page 405) by face mask at a flow rate of 5 to 10 liters per minute, and transport the victim to a hospital as quickly as possible.

3. Examine the victim for other injuries. Unless the airway is involved or the victim is horribly burned, the burn injury will not be immediately life-threatening. In your eagerness to treat the burn, don't overlook a serious injury such as a broken neck. Control all bleeding and attend to broken bones before applying burn dressings.

4. Treat the burn. Cool the burned area. This is usually done with cool or cold, wet compresses. Don't apply ice directly to skin to avoid creating a frostbite injury. If the burn is acquired suddenly (as when a child grabs a hot rock), prompt application of cold can limit the extent of the tissue damage.

   First-degree: A first-degree burn, such as a mild to moderate sunburn, may be treated with cool, wet compresses for 10 to 20 minutes. Oral administration of an antiinflammatory drug, such as aspirin or an NSAID, may provide considerable relief for sunburn. Because sunburn may cause itching, topical remedies that may be effective include pramoxine (Prax) lotion, menthol plus camphor (Sarna) lotion, pramoxine plus camphor plus calamine (Aveeno anti-itch) lotion, and lidocaine plus camphor (Neutrogena Norwegian Formula moisturizer). For severe sunburn ("cooked lobster") when no blisters are present, administration of oral prednisone in a rapid taper (80 mg the first day, 60 mg the second, 40 mg the third, 20 mg the fourth, 10 mg the fifth) may be helpful. Corticosteroids should always be taken with the understanding that a rare side effect is serious deterioration of the head ("ball" of the ball-and-socket joint) of the femur, the long bone of the thigh. Corticosteroids are interchangeable to a certain degree. If you must substitute, here is a rough measure of equivalence: 20 mg prednisone equals 16 mg methylprednisolone equals 3 mg dexamethasone.

   Topical corticosteroid creams or ointments are of no benefit in treating a burn wound. Anesthetic sprays that contain benzocaine work for a few hours, but may induce allergic reactions. They should be used sparingly. If no blisters are present, a moisturizing cream (such as Vaseline Intensive Care) will help soothe the skin. Aloe vera gel or lotion of at least 60% concentration seems to promote resolution of extensive first-degree burns. Burnaid first-aid burn gel (Rye Pharmaceuticals), which also comes in an impregnated dressing, contains 2% to 4% melaleuca oil and is advertised to provide relief from the pain of minor burns and scalds.

   Second-degree: A second-degree burn should be irrigated gently to remove all loose dirt and skin. This should be done with the cleanest cool water available. *Never apply ice directly to a burn;* this may cause more extensive tissue damage. Cool compresses may be used for pain relief for 10 to 20 minutes. Mild soap and water may be used to clean the burn.

After the wound is clean and dry, cover it with a hydrocolloid dressing (e.g., DuoDERM), polyurethane film dressing, hydrogel wound dressing (e.g., Spenco 2nd Skin), or silver-impregnated wound dressing. These appear to promote more rapid healing with less discomfort than application of silver sulfadiazine antiseptic cream. However, if silver sulfadiazine (Silvadene) is available, it may be used. An alternative is mupirocin ointment or cream, or bacitracin ointment. A nonadherent dressing layer directly over the antiseptic is easier to change than coarse gauze. Regardless of what is applied directly to the burn wound, it may be helpful (to keep the burn wound area clean) to apply a somewhat bulky dressing made of gauze or cloth bandages, taking care to keep the dressing snug but not tight. Silver sulfadiazine should not be used on the face or in victims who are pregnant, infants, or nursing mothers with children younger than 2 months.

Spenco 2nd Skin is an inert hydrogel composed of water and polyethylene oxide. It absorbs fluids (so long as it doesn't dry out), which "wicks" serum and secretions away from the wound and promotes wound healing. Other occlusive hydrogel-type dressings are NU-GEL (preserved polyvinyl pyrrolidone in water) and Hydrogel, which can absorb up to $2\frac{1}{2}$ times its weight in exuded (from the wound) fluids. Yet another covering for a burn is a layer of petrolatum-impregnated Aquaphor gauze under a dry (absorbent) gauze dressing.

Don't apply butter, lanolin, vitamin E cream, or any steroid preparation to a burn. These can all inhibit wound healing and may facilitate infections with increased scarring.

Dressings should be changed each day to readjust for swelling and to check for signs of infection. Be certain to keep burned arms and legs elevated as best possible, to minimize swelling and pain.

Blisters should not be opened, unless they are obviously infected and contain pus (this will generally not occur until 24 to 48 hours after the burn injury). If a blister remains filled with clear fluid, it's an excellent covering for the wound and will minimize fluid loss and infection. There is no rush to remove charred skin from a burn wound. As the wound matures and dressings are changed, gentle scrubbing will lift off dead tissue.

A victim with large areas of second-degree burns may need to be treated for shock (see page 58).

Third-degree: A third-degree burn should be irrigated gently and may be cleansed with mild soap and water. It should then be covered with antiseptic cream or ointment or a hydrogel-type dressing, and then with a dry sterile dressing.

If a first-degree burn involves more than 20% of the body surface area and the victim suffers from fever, chills, or vomiting, a physician evaluation is required. If a second-degree burn involves a significant portion of the face, eyes, hands, feet, genitals, or an area greater than 5% of the total body surface area, a physician evaluation is required. Body surface area can be estimated using the "rule of nines" (Figure 118). For an adult, each upper limb equals 9% of total body surface area (TBSA), each lower limb equals 18%, the anterior and posterior trunk equal 18% each, the head and neck combined equal 9%, and the genital/groin area (perineum) equals 1%. For a small child, each upper limb equals 9% of TBSA, each lower limb equals 14%, the anterior and posterior trunk equal 18% each, the head and neck combined equal 18%, and the perineum equals 1%. Another method to estimate involved body surface area is the "palm of hand" rule, which is that the surface area of the victim's palm with the fingers represents approximately 1% to 1.5% of his TBSA. All third-degree burns are serious and should be seen by a physician. A physician's care should

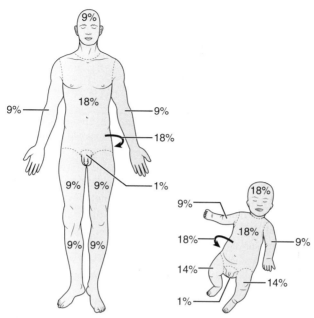

Figure 118. Rule of nines for body surface area estimate.

also be sought if the burn covers more than 5% of TBSA; is severe and involves the face, hands, or genitals; or the victim becomes ill with fever, vomiting, or general deterioration.

Wet versus Dry Dressings

If the burn surface area is small (less than 10% of total body surface area), cool, moist dressings (*not ice*) may be used to initially cover the burn wound. These often provide greater pain relief than do dry dressings. If the surface area involved is large, however, dry, nonadherent dressings should be used, to avoid overcooling the victim and introducing hypothermia (see page 281). Because the skin is the major thermoregulatory organ of the body, it's difficult for an extensively burned victim to control his body temperature, so great care must be taken when wetting down such a person. If the victim begins to shiver, the cooling is too extreme.

Fluid Replacement

A person who has suffered an extensive burn will rapidly become dehydrated. Because water quickly shifts from the blood volume into the tissues of the body, the injured skin cannot retain moisture, and associated immune suppression leads to overwhelming infection and shock. Oral rehydration with balanced salt solutions is little help, but in the wilderness, it's usually the only option. Try to get the victim to drink—in sips, if necessary—enough liquid to keep the urine copious and light-colored (see page 195). If a burned victim cannot drink because his airway is injured, consciousness is altered, weakness prevails, or vomiting is persistent, immediately call for an evacuation.

Antibiotics

Antibiotics aren't necessary for burns unless they become infected. This is indicated by the presence of pus, foul odor, cloudy blisters, increased redness, and swelling in the normal skin that surrounds the burn, and fever greater than 101°F (38.3°C). If a burn becomes infected, administer dicloxacillin, cephalexin, or erythromycin, and be certain to change all dressings daily. If a person sustains a serious burn that becomes infected after exposure to ocean water, administer ciprofloxacin, doxycycline, or trimethoprim–sulfamethoxazole in addition to the other antibiotic chosen. Blisters that appear to be infected should be "unroofed" and drained, then covered with a proper dressing.

Tar Burn
If a victim is splashed with hot roofing tar or paving asphalt, immediately immerse the affected area in cool water to solidify the tar and limit the burn. If a small area is covered with tar and you cannot reach a physician, you can remove the tar by gently massaging it with repeated coatings of bacitracin or mupirocin ointment, or mayonnaise, which will turn brown as the tar dissolves into it. Don't injure the skin by attempting to roughly peel off the tar. After the tar is removed, treat the burn as described previously. If you cannot dissolve the tar, cover the wound with bacitracin ointment or mupirocin ointment or cream, and a clean dressing.

Beach Tar Removal
These same tar-dissolving substances will work to remove the sticky tar sometimes found washed up on the beach. Other substances that are effective for this purpose include olive oil, 50/50 ointment (50% liquid paraffin and 50% soft paraffin), baby oil, cooking oil, mineral oil, or tanning oil. Goo Gone is a product containing naphtha, petroleum, heavy aliphatic terpenes and terpenoids, and citrus oil. It should not be applied to a burn. If it is used to remove beach tar, then wash the skin very carefully with soap and water after you have finished with the tar removal.

BURN PREVENTION
1. Obey all posted warnings regarding campfires.
2. Use flame-resistant tents and sleeping bags.
3. Keep all campfires a sufficient distance (minimum 20 ft) from tents and other flammable materials. Create a clear, fuel-free perimeter of at least 3 feet around any campfire or grill. Don't sit too close to a campfire, particularly in windy conditions. Don't allow children to play near a campfire.
4. Don't add lighter fluid, gasoline, kerosene, or any other flammable liquid to a flaming fire or hot coals/embers.
5. Store flammable liquids in approved metal containers that are tightly sealed. Don't fill lamps and stoves with fuel anywhere near intense heat or open flames. Use a funnel to pour flammable liquids, and clean up any spills immediately.
6. Keep a bucket of water within easy reach of a campfire.
7. Thoroughly extinguish the campfire before going to sleep or leaving the campsite.
8. Don't handle camp sauna hot rocks or cook pots without wearing proper hand protection.
9. Don't allow children to handle containers with hot water.
10. Don't set containers of hot water or food on unstable or uneven surfaces.
11. Use battery-operated lights in or near tents or campers.

INHALATION INJURIES

Inhalation injuries include thermal (heat) and chemical (smoke, noxious gas) inhalations. A third type of inhalation injury is aspiration (inhalation) of stomach contents; blood; or ocean, river, lake, or pool water into the lungs. The severity of the injury is determined by the chemical nature of the substance, temperature, volume of inhaled material, and underlying health of the victim. In a likely scenario, such as a boating accident or a seizure that occurred in the water, you must have a high index of suspicion for an inhalation injury. Drowning is discussed on page 364.

THERMAL INJURY

In thermal inhalation, the airway is injured by the introduction of superheated air or steam. Such injuries almost always occur in an enclosed environment, although occasional mishaps occur in association with wildland fires (see page 303). Because water conducts heat approximately 30 times as efficiently as air, the risk of injury is far greater with steam than with dry superheated air.

The heat injures the inside of the mouth and nose, throat, vocal cords, trachea, bronchi, and occasionally lungs. External signs of an inhalation injury include burns of the face and mouth, singed nasal hairs, and soot in the mouth and nose. Symptoms include shortness of breath; wheezing; coughing (particularly of carbonaceous black sputum); raspy, coarse breathing (stridor) noted most often during inspiration, with a barking quality that seems to originate in the neck; muffled voice; drooling; difficulty swallowing; swollen tongue; and agitation.

Once the burn injury has occurred, there is no effective way to limit its progress, so *the victim should be transported as rapidly as possible to an emergency facility.* If oxygen (see page 405) is available, it should be administered at a flow rate of 5 to 10 liters per minute by face mask. If the victim's condition deteriorates rapidly because the airway becomes swollen and obstructed, the only hope for survival is the placement of a tube directly through the vocal cords and into the trachea, or the creation of an air passage through the neck (tracheotomy).

SMOKE (CHEMICAL) INJURY

Most smoke is composed of soot and various chemicals. Although each specific substance causes its own variation on the basic lung injury, the immediate first-aid approach is the same. Remove the victim from the offending agent and *immediately administer oxygen* at a flow rate of 5 to 10 liters per minute (see page 405) by face mask. If the victim is having difficulty breathing or is without respirations, he should be supported with mouth-to-mouth breathing (see page 28). Difficulty in breathing may be delayed for a few hours after smoke inhalation, so a victim should seek immediate medical attention even if he feels fine initially.

The utmost caution must be exercised when removing a victim from the source of suspected toxic gases, so as not to create additional victims. Rescuers should wear gas masks if they are available. Carbon monoxide intoxication is discussed on page 306.

Smoke from wildland fires can affect your health. A person does not acclimate to smoke in any way, and repeated exposures can diminish lung function. So, avoidance is very important.

Intense exposure to heat and smoke when in the immediate proximity of a raging forest fire causes burns, asphyxiation from lack of oxygen, carbon monoxide poisoning, and injury by other severe, acute causations.

Smoke exposure of a degree to create a hazy horizon, where you can see, smell, and taste the smoke, may also cause health problems. Healthy persons are usually not at a major risk from such smoke. But of course, it's always a good idea to avoid breathing smoke if you can help it. Smoke is not good for you.

Smoke is a mixture of gases and fine particles produced when wood and other organic matter burn. It reflects the fuel, so can contain products of combustion from rubber, plastics, and any other material consumed in the blaze. Firefighters have the greatest exposures to smoke, and they are often affected. It has been estimated that nearly 40% to 50% of medical encounters by wildland firefighters are for respiratory problems. Whether or not this statistic can be perfectly extrapolated to a non-firefighter population passively exposed to wildfire-generated smoke is not known, but it's highly likely that respiratory ailments and diminished lung function would be a logical result of exposure to smoke.

What's in the smoke? Some of the combustion products of concern include these classes of materials: particulate matter (organic and inorganic), carbon monoxide, ozone, organic acids, polynuclear aromatic hydrocarbons, volatile and semi-volatile organic compounds, and free radicals. These are present or absent in varying degrees depending on the fuel burned, temperature of the fire, suppression method(s) used, and other factors. Therefore, the toxicity of the smoke may vary, but for the purposes of this discussion, all smoke from wildland fires should be considered comparable.

Because particulate matter dominates in proportion within wildland fire smoke, the greatest health threat from smoke comes from the fine particles, which are often microscopic. The particles easily get into the eyes and respiratory system, where they can cause health problems such as burning eyes (conjunctivitis), irritated throat, runny nose (sometimes associated with an allergic response), and illnesses such as bronchitis (cough). Fine particles also can worsen chronic heart and lung diseases. Because death rates from these conditions have been noted to rise in a smoky environment, the smoke has been linked to premature deaths in people with these conditions, in a fashion analogous to increased mortality rates during heat waves.

Persons who are more susceptible to ill effects at lower smoke levels are those with heart disease (congestive heart failure, symptomatic angina, cardiomyopathy), lung disease (asthma, reactive airway disease, chronic obstructive pulmonary disease [COPD]), and any medical condition in which oxygen delivery and heart and lung function are essential for health and wellness.

Older adults appear to be at increased risk of being affected by smoke, as are children with high activity levels. Firefighters, athletes, soldiers, and others who exercise in smoky conditions often report feeling poorly, sometimes to the point of incapacitation.

If you develop symptoms, it's not difficult to know if smoke is affecting you. Obvious symptoms are burns around the mouth and nose; singed nostrils; irritated and reddened eyes; painful throat; fatigue; decreased exercise tolerance; palpitations; chest pain; shortness of breath or inability to draw a deep breath; coughing; wheezing; sinus irritation; headache; or worsening of preexisting conditions that manifest any of these symptoms.

Prevention is key. One must know how to limit exposure to smoke:

1. Pay attention to local air quality reports and to the Environmental Protection Agency's Air Quality Index (AQI—see later discussion). Stay alert for any news coverage or health warnings related to smoke. Use visibility guides, if they're available. Not every community has a monitor that measures particle levels in the air. In the western United States, some areas without air quality monitors have developed guidelines to help people estimate the AQI based on how far they can see.

2. Common sense is the cornerstone of wilderness medicine. If it's smoky outside, don't plan to exert yourself or run the race, and consider keeping your children indoors. If you develop smoke-related symptoms, curtail any contributing activities and seek an environment away from the smoke. Ordinary dust masks are designed to filter out large particles, so don't count on them to diminish exposure to small particulate matter found in smoke.

3. The air indoors is also important during times of high smoke levels outdoors. So, you should keep indoor air as clean as possible. Unless it's extremely hot outside and you need to open windows and doors for air circulation, you should keep them closed. If you have an air conditioner, allow it to run, with the fresh air intake closed and the filter clean. Certain air cleaners might decrease particulate matter indoors, but be certain that the device does not emit ozone. Don't smoke tobacco products, and don't burn anything that will emit smoke. If it becomes too hot inside a building or enclosure, find a cooler shelter, so that you aren't overcome by the heat. When driving a car in smoky areas, keep the windows and vents closed.

AIR QUALITY INDEX FOR PARTICLES

The AQI, which is often depicted as a color-coded chart, is an index for reporting daily air quality that indicates how clean or polluted the air is, and what associated health effects might be of concern. The Environmental Protection Agency (EPA) calculates the AQI for five major air pollutants regulated by the *Clean Air Act:* ground-level ozone, particle pollution (also known as particulate matter), carbon monoxide, sulfur dioxide, and nitrogen dioxide. Ground-level ozone and airborne particles are the two pollutants that pose the greatest threat to human health in the United States. In the setting of smoke from a wildland fire, it is the particulate matter that is of greatest concern.

The AQI is reported as a numerical rating that runs from 0 to 500. The higher the AQI value, the greater the level of air pollution and the greater the health concern. For example, an AQI value of 50 represents good air quality with little potential to affect public health, whereas an AQI value over 300 represents hazardous air quality. When AQI values are above 100, air quality is considered to be unhealthy, at first for sensitive (to the harmful components) groups of people, and then for everyone as AQI values get higher.

The AQI categories are:

- *0 to 50 (Green): Good.* Air quality is considered satisfactory, and air pollution poses little or no risk.
- *51 to 100 (Yellow): Moderate.* Air quality is acceptable; however, for some pollutants there may be a moderate health concern for a small number of people.
- *101 to 150 (Orange): Unhealthy for Sensitive Groups.* Members of sensitive groups may experience health effects. The general public is not likely to be affected when the AQI is in this range.
- *151 to 200 (Red): Unhealthy.* Everyone may begin to experience health effects. Members of sensitive groups may experience more serious health effects.
- *201 to 300 (Purple): Very Unhealthy.* This triggers a health alert, because everyone may experience more serious health effects.
- *301 to 500 (Maroon): Hazardous.* This triggers health warnings of an emergency nature. The entire population is more likely to be affected.

People living in close proximity to the fire-stricken areas should remain indoors and avoid inhalation of smoke, ashes, and particulate matter in the area. Ordinary dust masks, designed to filter out large particles, will not help because they allow the more dangerous smaller particles to pass through. High-efficiency particulate air (HEPA) filter masks can remove nearly all airborne particles 0.3 micrometers (microns) in diameter, but are more expensive and may be difficult to use for people with lung disease, because it can be hard to draw air through them.

If outdoor trips in smoky areas are necessary, breathing through a damp cloth may help filter out some of the particles that are floating in the air, but this is a temporizing measure only and should not be counted on to significantly diminish smoke exposure for more than a few minutes.

ASPIRATION INJURY

Vomiting and inhalation of stomach contents is a common complication of severe hypothermia or drug overdose, and often follows head injury. The key factor is altered mental status, because a person who has a depressed level of consciousness does not protect his airway. In any situation in which a victim is unconscious and prone to vomit, *and the neck is highly suspected or known to be uninjured,* place the victim on his side so that vomitus and blood will drain from his mouth to the ground, rather than into his lungs. If you suspect a neck injury, and the victim must be kept on his back with the neck immobilized, keep constant watch for vomiting. If the victim vomits, he must be quickly turned on a stretcher or backboard or logrolled (see page 38), and his mouth manually cleared of debris.

ABDOMINAL PAIN

The causes of abdominal pain are myriad. There are serious causes and minor disturbances. As with most disorders, the purpose of taking a history and performing a physical examination is to determine the urgency of the situation, in order to plan for evacuation if necessary. Because differentiation between various causes is often difficult, the recommendations that follow are ultraconservative. Any person with severe abdominal pain should be seen by a physician as soon as possible. Signs and symptoms indicative of a serious cause for abdominal pain are persistent, severe, or worsening abdominal pain; a "rigid" abdomen (stomach muscles tightened involuntarily in response to the examiner pressing on the abdomen); "rebound" tenderness (see pages 117-118); fever; persistent vomiting; blood (red or "coffee grounds") in the vomit or bowel movement; and/or black tar-like bowel movement.

A special word of caution—when an elder person complains of severe abdominal pain, extra caution applies. Sudden, severe, diffuse, and relentless central abdominal pain, particularly if associated with bloody stools, can be a sign of decreased blood flow and lack of oxygen (ischemia) to the bowel, caused either by obstruction of an essential blood vessel or by the bowel kinking or telescoping back upon itself. This situation is a surgical emergency. Ripping pain in the lower abdomen or back (often with an expanding girth) may be from an abdominal aortic aneurysm (see later discussion).

GENERAL EVALUATION

Obtain the history:

1. *Nature of the pain.* Is the pain sharp (knife-like), aching (constant), colicky (intermittent and severe), or cramping (squeezing)? Has the victim ever suffered a similar episode? Been given a specific diagnosis? Is it minor or severe? Have the victim characterize it on a scale of 1 to 10, with 10 being the worst, so that you can track the victim's progress.
2. *Location of the pain.* Is the pain well localized to one particular area, or does it radiate to another region (from the back to the groin, for example)? Did the pain begin in one region and move to another?
3. *Mode of onset of the pain.* Did the pain occur suddenly, or has it gradually increased in intensity? How long has the victim been in pain?
4. *Associated symptoms.* Is the victim short of breath, nauseated, vomiting, suffering from diarrhea or constipation, or dizzy? Is the victim vomiting blood, bile (green liquid produced by the gallbladder), or "coffee grounds" (blood darkened by stomach acid)? Does the vomit smell like feces (indicative of a bowel obstruction)? Does the victim have a fever (indicative of an infection)? Does he have blackened, tarry bowel movements (indicative of bleeding in the gastrointestinal tract)?
5. *Relief of pain.* Is there a position that the victim can assume that will lessen the pain? Does the victim feel better in a quiet position, or is he agitated and constantly moving around?
6. *Menstrual history.* In the female victim, it's important to determine if there is any chance that the abdominal pain is related to a disorder of pregnancy.

PHYSICAL EXAMINATION

Perform the physical examination:

1. Observe the victim. Note whether he is active or avoids movement. If possible, note the severity of distress when the victim has his attention diverted (and so is not focusing all of his attention on your examination).

2. Note the victim's skin color, pulse rate and strength, rate of respirations, effort of breathing, mental status, and temperature. Abnormalities of any of these heighten the possibility of a serious problem.

3. Examine the abdomen. This is best done by having the victim lie quietly on his back, with his knees drawn up. Gently press on the abdomen, *proceeding from the area of least discomfort to the area of greatest discomfort.* For the purposes of examination, the abdomen can be divided by perpendicular lines through the navel into four quadrants: right upper, left upper, right lower, and left lower (Figure 119). The epigastrium is the area of the abdomen directly below (not underneath) the breastbone in the midline. Note

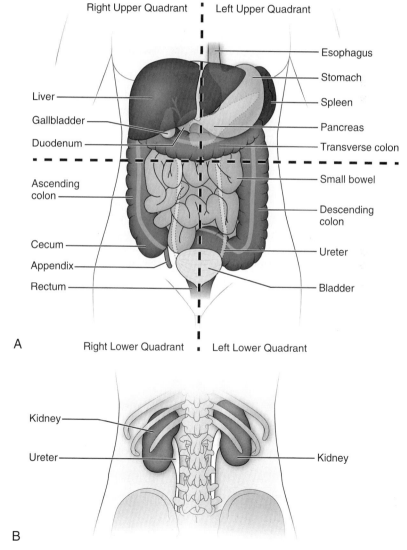

Figure 119. Location of the abdominal organs. **A,** View from the front, with the abdomen divided into four quadrants. **B,** The kidneys are located posteriorly and may be the cause of flank or back pain.

where the victim complains of pain and whether the pain is affected by your examination. If the victim has increased sharp pain when you suddenly release your hands from his abdomen after a pressing maneuver, this may indicate "rebound" pain associated with general inflammation of the lining of the abdominal cavity (peritonitis). Rebound pain may be caused by severe infection or leakage of blood or stomach/bowel contents into the abdominal (peritoneal) cavity, or by other problems that are generally quite severe.

When a specific area of the abdomen is tender, there are certain disorders to consider:

Epigastrium. Heart attack, ulcer, gastroenteritis, heartburn, pancreatitis.

Right upper quadrant. Injured liver, hepatitis, gallstones, pneumonia.

Left upper quadrant. Injured spleen, gastroenteritis, pancreatitis, pneumonia.

Right lower quadrant. Appendicitis, kidney stone, ovarian infection (pelvic inflammatory disease), ectopic (fallopian tube ["tubal"]) pregnancy, colitis, bowel obstruction, hernia, miscarriage, kidney stone, painful menses.

Left lower quadrant. Diverticulitis, colitis, kidney stone, ovarian infection, ectopic (fallopian tube ["tubal"]) pregnancy, bowel obstruction, hernia, miscarriage, kidney stone, painful menses.

Lower abdomen (central). Abdominal aortic aneurysm, ovarian infection, ovulation disorder, twisted or telescoped bowel, ischemic (dying) bowel, ectopic (fallopian tube ["tubal"]) pregnancy, bladder infection, colitis, bowel obstruction, inflammatory bowel disease ("irritable bowel").

Flank. Abdominal aortic aneurysm, kidney stone, kidney infection, pneumonia.

By quadrant, brief descriptions of and treatments for these disorders follow.

EPIGASTRIUM

Heart Attack (see page 47)

The symptoms of a heart attack can include pain that's located in the epigastrium, rather than in the chest. If the victim has a history of heart disease and complains of dull epigastric pain, nausea, shortness of breath, and weakness, consider the possibility of a heart attack. If you suspect a heart attack, even minimally, plan for immediate rescue or evacuation.

Ulcer (see also page 209)

An ulcer is an erosion in the lining of the stomach (gastric ulcer) or duodenum (peptic ulcer) that penetrates the protective mucous layer and allows acid and digestive juices to erode deeper into the tissues (Figure 120). This causes extreme pain and can lead to

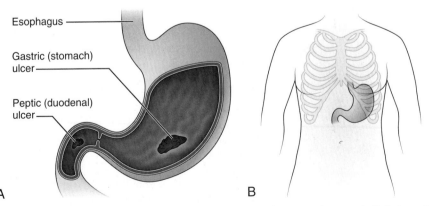

Figure 120. Ulcers. **A,** Location of ulcer craters in the duodenum and stomach. **B,** Epigastric region of the abdomen, where ulcer pain is often noted.

bleeding from leaking blood vessels in the ulcer crater. Symptoms include constant burning pain in the epigastrium that's made worse by pressing and is often associated with nausea and/or belching. In a minor case, the pain may be relieved by a meal. In a severe case, when the ulcer has eroded into a blood vessel or has perforated the wall of the stomach or bowel, the victim will vomit red blood or dark brown clotted blood ("coffee grounds") and complain of pain that may radiate to his back. Rebound tenderness and peritonitis may be present. Dark black tarry bowel movements (melena) are caused by blood that has made its transit through the bowel. Bright red blood or blood clots with a bowel movement can be caused by brisk bleeding from an ulcer, but more commonly originate from bleeding that's occurring within the large intestine (colon) or rectum, or from hemorrhoids (see page 206). Mild bleeding from an ulcer may actually transiently decrease the pain, because blood acts as an antacid. Some ulcers are caused by bacterial (usually, *Helicobacter pylori*) infection. To eradicate the bacteria and allow the ulcer to heal, a physician must prescribe specific, intense antibiotic therapy.

Gastroenteritis

Gastroenteritis is often called the "stomach flu" (see the discussion of diarrhea on page 193). Symptoms include waves of crampy upper and/or lower abdominal pain, followed by loose bowel movements. Nausea and vomiting may be present. Occasionally, the victim has symptoms of an upper respiratory infection, with cough, runny nose, sore throat, headache, and fever. The treatment for viral gastroenteritis consists of an adequate liquid diet (hydration is the key to recovery—see page 194), which can sometimes only be accomplished by first administering medicine for persistent vomiting (see page 208). When a victim vomits green bile, this should be taken as a sign that the problem is more serious than straightforward gastroenteritis, although bilious vomiting can occur with repetitive retching, when the stomach has been emptied and duodenal contents are all that is left for regurgitation.

Heartburn

See page 208.

Pancreatitis

The pancreas is an organ situated in the posterior upper abdomen that secretes a number of enzymes used to digest food. The pancreas also secretes insulin, the hormone that allows us to use and store glucose. The digestive enzymes travel from the pancreas through a duct, from which they are released through a small opening into the duodenum (the first portion of the bowel after the stomach). If the pancreas becomes inflamed, either by alcohol abuse (heavy drinking is far and away the most common cause), viral infection, or blockage of the main secretory duct by a gallstone, severe epigastric pain is the rule. Sometimes the victim will have diffuse abdominal pain with radiation to the back. Pain is accompanied by nausea and vomiting (which may contain bile). The victim may be restless and prefer to sit and lean forward for pain relief. A person with pancreatitis needs to be hospitalized, because the most effective treatment is to eliminate oral intake for a time (to decrease stimulation of the pancreas). Out of the hospital, allow the victim clear liquids and antacids only, and pain medicine if pills can be kept down. Seek immediate physician care. If a person with severe abdominal pain has blue discoloration around the umbilicus or of the flanks, this may indicate internal bleeding, known as hemorrhagic pancreatitis.

RIGHT UPPER QUADRANT

Injured Liver

If a fall or blow to the abdomen, right flank, or right lower chest is followed by abdominal pain that's worsened by pressing on the right upper quadrant, a torn or bruised liver should be considered. The victim is at risk for severe internal bleeding and should be observed for signs of shock (see page 58). Evacuate him as soon as possible.

Hepatitis

See page 210.

Gallstones (Cholelithiasis)

Gallstones are formed in the gallbladder, which lies under the liver in the right upper quadrant of the abdomen. The gallbladder stores bile (manufactured in the liver), which is released into the duodenum to aid in digestion following each meal (Figure 121). An attack of gallbladder inflammation (cholecystitis) occurs when the outlet from the gallbladder or the main bile duct into the duodenum becomes obstructed (usually by a gallstone) and the gallbladder cannot empty. This causes stretching of the gallbladder, inflammation, and painful contraction against an impenetrable passage. There is often an element of infection.

A typical attack occurs immediately after a meal and is sudden in onset. The pain is colicky and located in the right upper quadrant or epigastrium. It may be associated with nausea, vomiting, and fever. Occasionally, it radiates to the back or right shoulder. Examination of the

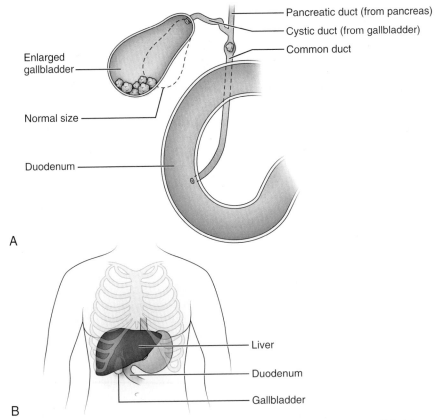

Figure 121. Gallbladder with gallstones. **A,** The stones are formed in the gallbladder and travel through a narrow passageway (cystic and common ducts), which is easily blocked. **B,** Location of the gallbladder adjacent to the liver in the right upper quadrant of the abdomen.

abdomen demonstrates tenderness in the right upper quadrant. Occasionally, you can feel a tennis ball–sized tender mass—the swollen gallbladder.

The definitive treatment for cholecystitis is removal of the gallbladder, although many surgeons prefer to "quiet down" the situation first with antibiotics, pain medicine, and intravenous fluids. The victim of a gallbladder attack should be transported to a hospital for evaluation. Pain medicines can be given safely, although certain narcotics may increase spasm of the bile passage and, paradoxically, briefly worsen pain. Solid foods (particularly fats) are prohibited during an attack. Maintain the victim on clear liquids and begin antibiotic therapy with ciprofloxacin, ampicillin, amoxicillin, or amoxicillin–clavulanate, any of these combined with metronidazole, if pills can be kept down.

Pneumonia
See page 45.

LEFT UPPER QUADRANT
Injured Spleen
If a fall or blow to the abdomen, left flank, or left lower chest is followed by abdominal pain that's worsened by pressing on the left upper quadrant, consider a torn or bruised spleen. The victim is at risk for severe internal bleeding and should be observed for signs of shock (see page 58). Evacuate the victim as soon as possible.

Gastroenteritis
See page 119.

Pancreatitis
See page 119.

Pneumonia
See page 45.

RIGHT LOWER QUADRANT
Appendicitis
The appendix is a small (average length 3.5 inch [9 cm]) sausage-shaped outpouching of the cecum (which is a part of the small bowel), with no modern physiologic function, that is located near the transition point where the small bowel becomes the large bowel (colon) (Figure 122). When it becomes obstructed or infected/inflamed (acute appendicitis), the victim typically has a history of crampy pain that begins in the central abdomen (often around the umbilicus), and then moves, over the course of a few hours, to become constant in the right lower quadrant. He may also suffer loss of appetite, constipation or diarrhea, vomiting, fever, and weakness. Pain nearly always precedes any other symptoms. There may be burning on urination if the appendix rests against a ureter carrying urine from the kidney to the bladder. Sometimes, if one presses on the left lower quadrant of a victim of appendicitis, there is pain noted in the right lower quadrant. If an inflamed appendix lies close to the obturator or psoas muscles, there may be pain when the right leg is internally rotated (obturator) or pulled away from the midline (psoas) of the body.

Examination of the abdomen demonstrates tenderness in the right lower quadrant. Frequently, the victim will resist any movement of the body or legs, because such movement causes abdominal pain. Rebound tenderness is associated with a swollen appendix that's ready to burst or has already ruptured. After the appendix ruptures, the pain may diminish considerably for a few days while an abscess forms. Untreated appendicitis may cause the victim to develop peritonitis, rapid breathing and heart rate, and low blood pressure. If you suspect appendicitis,

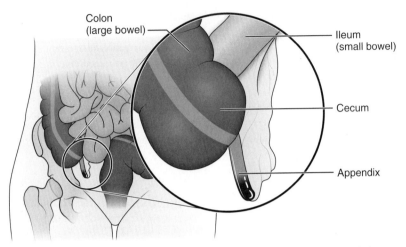

Figure 122. Appendicitis. Pain is felt in the right lower quadrant of the abdomen.

transport the victim to a hospital for surgical evaluation. If transport will take more than 24 hours and the victim can tolerate oral fluids (is not actively vomiting), allow clear liquid intake to prevent dehydration. An antibiotic (cephalexin, amoxicillin–clavulanate, cefixime, or cefpodoxime) should be administered if more than 24 hours will elapse before arrival at a hospital. If the victim is allergic to these agents, a combination of ciprofloxacin and metronidazole can be substituted.

If a woman of childbearing age develops right lower quadrant pain, the diagnosis of ectopic pregnancy (see page 126) should always be considered. It's useful to carry a urine pregnancy test kit in the first-aid kit.

Kidney Stone
See page 128.

Ovarian Infection (and Other Disorders of the Female Reproductive System)
See page 125.

Colitis
See page 204.

Bowel Obstruction
If the intestine becomes obstructed by scar tissue, cancer, injury, or feces, the victim rapidly becomes quite ill. Symptoms include nausea and vomiting, frequently of green bile or feculent (feces-like) material. The victim has waves of cramping pain that coincide with bowel motion (contractions) that may be visible through the abdominal wall, which is often distended by the dilated loops of bowel. Occasionally, the victim will have small, squirting bowel movements, as a little liquid slips past the obstruction. If a bowel obstruction is suspected, the victim should be immediately evacuated to a hospital.

An ileus is functional inactivity (no food or fluid absorption, lack of normal peristalsis) of the bowel that leads to intestinal dilation, vomiting, and abdominal pain. It commonly follows an intraabdominal injury or physiologic catastrophe (such as extensive burns, disseminated infection, or shock).

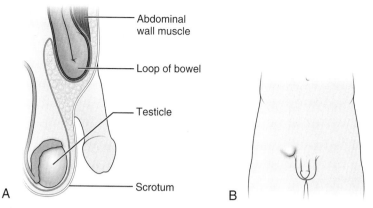

Figure 123. Inguinal (groin) hernia. **A,** A loop of bowel bulges through a defect in the lower abdominal wall. **B,** Location of external bulge. In some cases, the swelling extends into the scrotum.

Hernia

If the intestine slips through the muscles of the abdominal wall, usually in the groin or around the umbilicus (navel), a hernia is formed (Figure 123). Symptoms include a visible bulge, abdominal pain, and pain at the site of the hernia. The victim should be made to lie quietly on his back with his knees drawn up; place cold packs directly on the bulge. Give pain medicine to control the discomfort. If sufficient relaxation is obtained, the hernia may slip back through the wall, and the bulge will disappear. Afterward, the victim should wear a support (truss or belt) to prevent recurrence until the problem can be corrected surgically. Straining and heavy lifting should be avoided.

If a victim has a painless hernia (bulge) that cannot be corrected, he should avoid straining, particularly when holding his breath, and seek the advice of a physician.

If the intestine will not slip back through, the hernia is trapped (incarcerated). This is an emergency, because if the blood supply to the bowel is pinched off, the tissue can be severely damaged or die, and/or a bowel obstruction (see page 122) can be created. An incarcerated hernia is extremely painful, and if the bowel is injured, the overlying skin frequently becomes reddened or dusky in appearance. Because the aforementioned maneuvers for reduction of a hernia will not be successful and pain will increase, the victim should be rapidly evacuated to a hospital.

LEFT LOWER QUADRANT
Diverticulitis

Diverticula are small outpouchings that develop at weak points along the wall of the colon (large bowel), probably because of high pressures associated with muscle contractions during the passage of stool. When these sacs become obstructed and/or inflamed (most frequently in middle-aged or elderly individuals), they enlarge and create pain and fever. Usually, the left lower quadrant is involved, because diverticula tend to form in the left-side portion of the colon (descending colon) more frequently than in the right-side portion (ascending colon) or horizontal connecting section (transverse colon). A ruptured diverticulum can cause a clinical picture much like that of a ruptured appendix (see page 121), with pain in the left side of the abdomen instead of the right side. The victim should generally seek medical attention, and his diet should be limited to clear fluids. Physical activity should be minimized. Antibiotics (metronidazole, metronidazole combined with doxycycline, amoxicillin–clavulanate, trimethoprim–sulfamethoxazole, cefixime, ciprofloxacin, or cefpodoxime) should be administered if help is more than 24 hours away.

Doctors have historically advised persons with known diverticular disease to avoid eating nuts, seeds, popcorn, corn, and other high-residue foods. This is on the presumption that these food products pass through the bowel partially or complete nondigested, so they may be prone to cause trauma to the diverticuli or to lodge in them. This has never been proved true, so one may eat a "backpackers" diet without fear of inducing diverticulitis.

Colitis
See page 204.

Kidney Stone
See page 128.

Ovarian Infection (and Other Disorders of the Female Reproductive System)
See page 125.

Bowel Obstruction
See page 122.

Hernia
See page 123.

LOWER ABDOMEN (CENTRAL)
Abdominal Aortic Aneurysm
An aneurysm is a dilated blood vessel that has been weakened by the ravages of age, high blood pressure, and atherosclerosis (Figure 124). At a certain point, the wear and tear become too much and the blood vessel rips, causing either a slow leak or rapid, massive bleeding that leads to sudden collapse and death. This generally occurs spontaneously most commonly in the elderly, unless there is a congenital defect; traumatic tears of the aorta occur in all age groups.

The aorta is the large artery that carries blood from the left ventricle of the heart to the body. The symptoms of a ruptured abdominal aortic aneurysm are intense, unrelenting, ripping pain

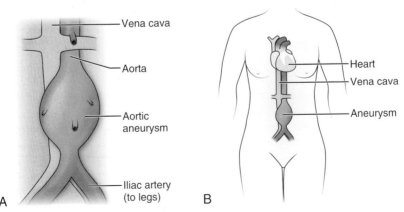

Figure 124. Abdominal aortic aneurysm. **A,** Age, high blood pressure, and disease ravage the dilated aorta. **B,** Location of the aorta in the abdomen. Leaking or rupture causes pain in the abdomen, back, and flank.

in the abdomen that may radiate to the back or chest; weakness; discoloration of the legs with mottling; and rapid collapse. Gentle examination of the abdomen may demonstrate a pulsating, expanding mass. Abdominal rigidity is due to rapid accumulation of blood.

Any elderly person who suddenly develops abdominal pain or back pain associated with weakness, a fainting spell, decreased sensation and/or abnormal color in the legs or feet (even if transient), or shortness of breath should be immediately rushed to a hospital. In the best of circumstances, this is a highly critical situation. Be prepared to treat the victim for shock (see page 58).

Ovarian Infection

The ovaries and fallopian tubes (Figures 125 and 126), which carry eggs from the ovaries to the uterus, may become infected, commonly with the bacteria that cause gonorrhea (a form of venereal disease) or by other infectious agents, such as *Chlamydia trachomatis*. Symptoms include abdominal pain in the lower quadrants (greatest on the side of the affected ovary), fever, shaking chills, nausea, vomiting, and weakness. Occasionally, the victim will complain of a yellow-greenish vaginal discharge. If you suspect an infection, take the victim to a hospital immediately. If more than 24 hours will pass before a doctor can be reached, the victim should be treated with azithromycin 1 g by mouth single dose or doxycycline 100 mg two

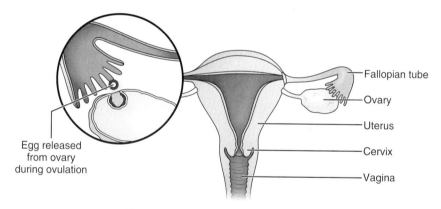

Figure 125. Female reproductive tract.

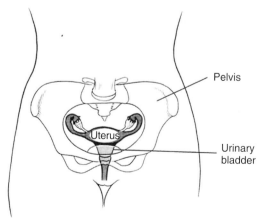

Figure 126. Location of female reproductive tract within the pelvis.

times a day for 7 days. If these are not available, then use tetracycline 500 mg four times a day or amoxicillin–clavulanate 500 mg two to three times per day for 7 days (doxycycline and tetracycline are effective against *Chlamydia*). If you suspect gonorrhea, bring the victim to a health care professional for an injection of ceftriaxone while administering the medications for chlamydia infection. Away from professional medical care, if more than 24 hours will pass before a doctor can be reached, to treat the gonorrhea, administer cefixime 400 mg orally as a single dose. Alternative single-dose therapies for gonorrhea are cefpodoxime 200 mg, cefuroxime 1 g, ciprofloxacin 500 mg, ofloxacin 400 mg, azithromycin 2 g, and norfloxacin 800 mg. To attempt to treat gonorrhea and chlamydial infection with one medication at the same time, you can use the single-dose 2 g azithromycin therapy (see page 276). If the victim is pregnant or allergic to penicillin and gonorrhea is suspected, administer azithromycin 2 g in a single dose or erythromycin base 250 mg four times a day for 14 days.

Ovulation, Ovarian Cyst, and Torsed (Twisted) Ovary

Some women suffer sudden, intense abdominal pain at the time of ovulation (when the egg is released from the ovary) (see Figure 125). This is caused by a small amount of blood and ovarian fluid, which irritates the lining of the abdomen. Symptoms include pain that suddenly develops in the right or left lower quadrant and is worsened by movement or deep palpation of the area. Treatment is pain medicine and rest. A ruptured ovarian cyst (which releases tissue fluid or blood) or torsed (twisted) ovary causes similar but much more severe symptoms, which may include excruciating pain, nausea and vomiting, and a rigid (to the pressing hand) abdomen. Any of these conditions may be difficult to distinguish from appendicitis (see page 121) if the right ovary is involved. Treatment for a torsed ovary may require surgery. *Any sudden abdominal discomfort in a woman of childbearing age should be promptly evaluated by a physician.*

Bleeding from the Vagina

If bleeding from the vagina accompanied by abdominal pain is not clearly part of a normal menstrual period, a woman should seek prompt medical attention. Possible causes include fibroids, uterine polyps, cancer, "dysfunctional uterine bleeding" (having a menstrual period without ovulation), and pregnancy-related bleeding. If the bleeding is clearly part of a normal menstrual period, and the pain is unquestionably due to menstrual cramps, the victim may benefit from administration of an NSAID.

If abnormal (in amount or character) pain and/or bleeding occur during or between menstrual periods, the cause should be determined by a physician. Until the evaluation is performed, exertion should be kept to a minimum. If periods have been missed (or if the victim is known to be pregnant) and copious vaginal bleeding develops, place the victim at rest and transport her rapidly—by litter, if possible—to a physician. If the bleeding is spotty, the victim may walk with assistance. A ruptured tubal (ectopic) pregnancy can rapidly become life-threatening. In this situation, a pregnancy situated in a fallopian tube (rather than in the uterus) causes the tube to rupture. The symptoms include vaginal bleeding, lower abdominal pain (which can become severe), and signs of shock (see page 58). This is a true medical emergency.

Vaginitis, Vaginal Discharge, and Vaginal Infections

The most common causes of female genital tract discharge are infection, reaction to a foreign object, injury, or allergic reaction. In the healthy vagina, bacteria (lactobacilli) produce lactic acid and promote an environment (pH of 3.8 to 4.5) that resists infection, although there are other microorganisms (such as *Staphylococcus, Ureaplasma,* and *Mycoplasma*) present.

Vaginitis is a condition of irritation and inflammation of the vagina, commonly noted as a secondary condition that follows administration of an antibiotic, such as ampicillin, to a woman.

The antibiotic alters the normal bacterial population of the vagina and allows overgrowth of the causative (for vaginitis) agent, which is often yeast. With a *Candida albicans* yeast (candidiasis or moniliasis) infection, the victim notes a thick, white, and creamy or curdy ("cottage cheese") discharge, vulvar and vaginal itching and redness, and burning pain on urination. She should use clotrimazole (Gyne-Lotrimin). Administer vaginal 100 mg tablets once a day for 7 days, or twice a day for 3 days; a vaginal 500 mg tablet for 1 day (single dose); or 1% cream in a 5 g dose for 7 to 14 days. An alternative drug is miconazole nitrate (Monistat); administer 100 mg vaginal suppositories once a day for 7 days, 200 mg vaginal suppositories once a day for 3 days, 1200 mg vaginal suppository in one dose, or 2% cream in a 5 g dose for 7 days. Other acceptable treatments are a single fluconazole (Diflucan) 150 mg tablet by mouth; tioconazole 6.5% (Vagistat-1) ointment in a single 5 g application; butoconazole nitrate 2% (Femstat) cream in a 5 g dose for 3 days; or terconazole (Terazol) vaginal cream 0.8% in a 5 g dose once a day for 3 days, vaginal cream 0.4% in a 5 g dose once a day for 7 days, or vaginal suppositories 80 mg once a day for 3 days.

Bacterial vaginosis is caused by a shift in vaginal bacterial flora from lactobacilli-dominant to mixed flora, and is characterized by a milky (yellowish or gray), sticky, homogeneous, and sometimes thin discharge with an abnormal ("fishy," particularly after intercourse) odor, as well as occasional itching and pain. It is definitively diagnosed by measuring the vaginal pH at a value greater than 4.5 and noting a specific type of cell ("clue cell") when the discharge is examined with a microscope. Treatment is either metronidazole 500 mg by mouth twice a day for 7 days or 0.5% or 0.75% metronidazole vaginal gel (such as MetroGel Vaginal) once a day for 5 days; or clindamycin phosphate 300 mg by mouth twice a day or 1 applicator (5 g) of 2% vaginal cream at bedtime for 7 consecutive nights; or 2% extended-release clindamycin cream, one application intravaginally.

If the infection is due to trichomoniasis (caused by *Trichomonas vaginalis*), the victim will suffer a copious, occasionally frothy, and white-gray or yellowish (sometimes foul-smelling) discharge and may also have abdominal pain and fever. The vulva may be irritated. In such a case, the antibiotic of choice is tinidazole or metronidazole 2 g in a single dose. Don't drink alcohol while taking tinidazole or metronidazole or for 3 days thereafter. The male sex partner should be treated with the same treatment.

On return to civilization, an appropriate gynecologic exam should be sought to exclude other causes of vaginal infection, which include herpes simplex virus, *Neisseria gonorrhoeae* (the causative agent of gonorrhea), and *Chlamydia trachomatis*.

Genital herpes is caused by herpes simplex virus type 1 (HSV-1) or type 2 (HSV-2). HSV-1 is transmitted predominantly by oral–genital sexual contact and HSV-2 by genital–genital contact. After exposure, the incubation period is 2 to 12 days, with an average of 4 days. Early symptoms include a red rash and small bumps, followed by a blistering rash with ulcers. Other symptoms may include pain at the site of the rash, tender local lymph nodes, fever, headache, fatigue, and muscle aching. If the blisters and ulcers occur on external skin, they heal in 9 to 12 days after a crusting phase; if they occur on mucous membranes (e.g., inside the vagina or the mouth), they heal without first crusting. After the first episode of genital herpes has resolved, recurrent episodes may be preceded by tingling or sharp pain in the buttocks, legs, or hips from a half hour to 5 days before the rash erupts. Antiviral treatment can shorten the first episode or a recurrent episode, or can be used to suppress the onset of an eruption. The following are recommended doses of medications:

For first episode of genital herpes (take medication by mouth for 10 days): Acyclovir 400 mg three times a day; or valacyclovir 1 g twice a day; or famciclovir 250 mg three times a day.

For recurrent episode of genital herpes: Acyclovir 800 mg twice a day for 5 days or three times a day for 2 days; famciclovir 125 mg twice a day for 5 days or 1 g twice a day for 1 day; or valacyclovir 500 mg twice a day for 3 days or 1 g once a day for 5 days.

For suppressive therapy against genital herpes (take medication twice a day for as long as suppression is desired): Acyclovir 400 mg, valacyclovir 500 mg, or famciclovir 250 mg. It's possible that taking any of these medications once a day, rather than twice a day, may be effective.

The herpes sufferer should be advised to adhere to excellent handwashing and avoid touching the sores, because the affliction can be mechanically spread.

In the event that emergency contraception is desired (e.g., for unprotected sexual intercourse or contraceptive failure), levonorgestrel tablets 0.75 mg (Plan B) are available over the counter. This medication does not protect against infection with human immunodeficiency virus (HIV) and other sexually transmitted diseases. The medication provides a short burst of hormones that affects the lining of the uterus and alters sperm transport, which prevents sperm from meeting the egg to achieve fertilization. Levonorgestrel is most effective if given within 3 days (72 hours) of intercourse, but is particularly effective if given within the first 24 hours after intercourse, and may be effective up to 5 days after intercourse. The dose is one pill by mouth, followed by a second pill 12 hours after the initial pill. Plan B One-Step is a single 1.5 mg dose of levonorgestrel taken orally as soon as possible within 72 hours after unprotected intercourse. Another approach is ulipristal acetate 30 mg (Ella), a prescription progestin drug that may be taken by mouth as soon as possible within 5 days after unprotected sexual intercourse. It works by preventing or delaying the release of an egg from the ovary and perhaps by altering the lining of the uterus.

Bladder Infection
See page 272.

Colitis
See page 204.

Bowel Obstruction
See page 122.

FLANK
Abdominal Aortic Aneurysm
See page 124.

Kidney Stone
A "kidney stone" originates in the urine-collecting system of the kidney, and most commonly causes pain when it travels down the ureter (ureteral stone) to the bladder (Figure 127). After traversing the bladder, it may enter the urethra and continue to wreak havoc. The most common compositions of stones are calcium-derived (80%), struvite (15% to 20%; magnesium ammonium phosphate), uric acid (5% to 10%), and cystine (less than 1%).

The pain of a kidney stone is usually sudden in onset and often becomes intolerable. The location of the pain is related to the location of the stone. If the stone is high in the ureter, the pain localizes to the victim's back (on the affected side), with some radiation to the abdomen. Lightly tapping over the flank and lower ribs on the back of a victim with a kidney stone will often cause extreme pain. If the stone is passing through the lower ureter, the victim will have extreme pain in the back, abdomen, and genitals. When the stone is not moving, the pain (renal "colic") may disappear as quickly as it began. A small (less than or equal to 2 mm in diameter) stone may take 7 to 10 days to pass; a 2 to 4 mm stone may take up to 2 weeks; and a stone larger than 4 mm may take up to 3 weeks.

A victim who is passing a kidney stone finds no relief from remaining motionless, and will appear quite agitated, constantly changing positions. Associated symptoms include nausea, vomiting, bloody urine, an urge to urinate, pain on urination, and sweating.

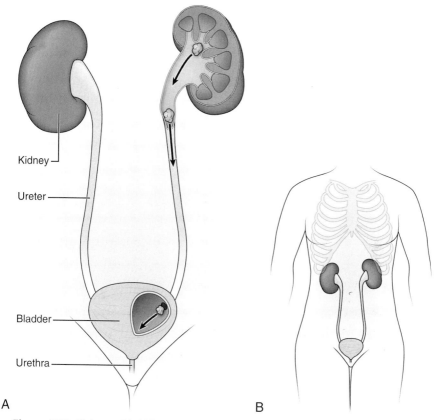

Figure 127. Kidney with kidney stones. **A,** The stones are formed in the kidney and travel through the ureter, bladder, and urethra before they are passed in the urine. **B,** Location of the genitourinary (urogenital) system.

If the diagnosis of a kidney stone appears relatively certain, give the victim the strongest pain medicine that's necessary and available, and encourage him to drink copious amounts of fluid. Ketorolac (10 mg by mouth every 4 to 6 hours, not to exceed 5 days) has been recommended as a pain medication for kidney stone because it may decrease spasm in the ureter; it may be given along with a narcotic drug, such as hydrocodone, to enhance the analgesic effect. Another useful drug if ketorolac is not available is diclofenac (50 mg by mouth two or three times a day). Some urologists recommend adding tamsulosin (Flomax) 0.4 mg by mouth once a day for a few days after the onset of pain associated with passing a kidney (ureteral) stone. It should be noted that this particular therapy may cause low blood pressure as a side effect. Seek physician evaluation as soon as possible. *If the victim is elderly, consider the diagnosis of ruptured aortic aneurysm* (see page 124). If you have any suspicion that the victim might have an aneurysm, evacuate him immediately.

Kidney Infection
See page 273.

Pneumonia
See page 45.

EMERGENCY CHILDBIRTH

When a woman is ready to give birth, the contractions of labor are usually intense and uninterrupted, or separated by intervals of less than 3 to 5 minutes. If the child to be born is not the woman's first, labor can progress very quickly, so don't wait until the last minute to set up. On the other hand, don't deliver a baby in the woods if it isn't necessary. If the child is the mother's first, if the contractions are more than 5 minutes apart, if the waters have not "broken" (a gush of fluid from the ruptured amniotic sac) and there has been no passage of bloody mucus, and if no bulging is present in the vaginal area, consider whether you have time to make it to the hospital. If the waters have broken and labor has not begun, it's best to evacuate the mother, because delivery must occur or be induced within 24 hours to avoid the onset of an infection that could jeopardize the infant and mother. *If the umbilical cord or any other part of the infant other than the head is showing at the vagina, the delivery will be difficult and should be performed if at all possible by a skilled obstetrician.*

If delivery is imminent (the mother wishes to push) and you're outdoors, spread a towel or blanket. The birthing process is fairly messy, so don't expect to salvage the ground cloth. Wear sterile surgical gloves from your first-aid kit. If you don't have gloves, wash your hands with soap and water. Have the following supplies ready: four towels for drapes; two sturdy strings to tie the umbilical cord; a sharp pair of scissors, scalpel, or knife to cut the umbilical cord; a towel to dry the baby; a blanket to wrap the baby; a rubber suction bulb for the baby's mouth and nose; and a large plastic bag to carry the placenta.

Have the mother undress below the waist and cover her with a blanket or sheet. She should lie on her side between contractions until she feels that she is ready to push. When she wants to push, have her lie on her back with her legs spread as far apart as possible. Place a towel (drape) over each thigh, across the abdomen, and under the buttocks to "frame" the vagina.

It's extremely helpful to elevate the buttocks with a folded blanket or pile of towels. This is because the most difficult part of a normal birth is delivery of the upper shoulder, which is facilitated by pushing the infant downward at the proper time.

When the mother is undergoing a contraction, and you see some wrinkled skin and a wisp of hair from the infant's head showing in her vagina, have the mother grab behind her legs and pull them up toward her head, or plant her feet firmly, while she bears down (like having a bowel movement) and pushes. This may go on while the vaginal entrance stretches to accommodate the infant's head. If the fluid-filled, transparent amniotic sac is bulging out in front of the infant's head, it can be nicked with a sharp blade or scissors to allow the fluid to be released and the delivery to proceed. Don't do this unless you're absolutely certain that the childbirth will occur away from a hospital. A mother may prefer to squat during delivery, but this makes assisting her more awkward.

During a push, put one hand gently on the infant's head and another underneath his head, providing countertraction against the woman's perineum (the area between the anus and the vaginal opening) to allow gradual stretching of the opening and to then assist delivery of the head and control the speed of delivery. You don't want the head to "pop out," to avoid a large tear in the vagina.

A baby is delivered in (ideally) two stages. First, the head and face appear, usually with the face down (Figure 128). Once the infant has appeared to the level of his eyebrows, instruct the mother to stop pushing. The baby will be extremely slippery. When his face appears, run your fingers around the infant's neck to see if the umbilical cord is wrapped around it. If it is, see if you can slip it over the head. If not, tie (clamp) it off tightly twice, with about 1½ inch (3.8 cm)

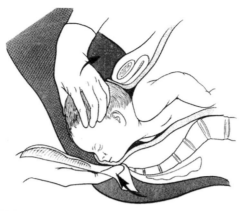

Figure 128. Appearance of the head and face during childbirth.

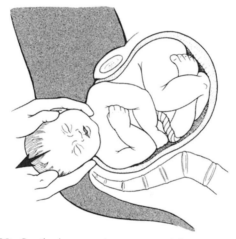

Figure 129. Gentle downward pressure to deliver upper shoulder.

between ties, and cut carefully between the ties. The ties must be tight and not slip off, or the baby could suffer severe bleeding.

In the moment between the delivery of the head and the beginning of the shoulders' emergence, support the head with one hand and gently wipe the face with a clean cloth. Although some authorities believe that suctioning a newborn is not necessary, it's alright to gently suction the mouth (first) and nose, using the bulb syringe, by squeezing the air out, placing the tip in the mouth and each nostril, and letting the bulb inflate. Squirt out any extracted material before each reinsertion of the tip. Suction each nostril at least twice.

The baby's head and body will spontaneously rotate 90 degrees (don't twist them) to one side as the body starts to emerge. Have the mother resume pushing. While supporting the head, grasp the uppermost (with respect to the ground) shoulder and apply gentle downward pressure until the upper shoulder is delivered from the vagina (Figure 129). Don't tug on the head or pull from underneath the infant's armpits. After the upper shoulder is out, exert gentle upward pressure to free the lower shoulder (Figure 130). At this point, hang on to the baby tightly, because the rest of the baby will shoot out, usually with a big gush of amniotic fluid and some blood.

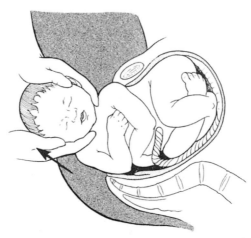

Figure 130. Gentle upward pressure to deliver lower shoulder.

Hold the baby in a towel or blanket and dry him. Hold him firmly by the ankles, but don't dangle him upside down. If you have not already done so, tie (clamp) the umbilical cord with two ties (preferably sterile—dipped in boiling water, for example), one at 6 inches (15 cm) and one at 8 inches (20 cm) from the child. Use cord that won't slip a knot, shoelace material, or cotton tape. Cut carefully between the ties. Although some authorities believe that suctioning is only necessary on occasion as a stimulus for a newborn to breathe, you may suction the baby's mouth (first) and nose (newborns are obligate nose breathers), and stimulate him by rubbing with a towel until he begins to cry. Gently wipe off all slimy material. Wrap the child in a blanket and hand him to the mother to hold. The mother may begin to breastfeed at this point.

The long end of the umbilical cord, which is still attached to the placenta that is attached to the inside wall of the uterus, will be hanging from the mother's vagina. The placenta will deliver spontaneously, so don't pull on the umbilical cord. *Don't massage the mother's abdomen (uterus) until after the placenta is delivered.* Place the placenta in a plastic bag and bring it to civilization for inspection. After the placenta is delivered, gently massage the mother's abdomen for 30 minutes. This stimulates the uterus to contract and helps control bleeding. It will feel like a firm, rounded, grapefruit-sized mass in the middle of the lower abdomen just above the pubic bone. If bleeding starts again, massage more vigorously. You may have to repeat this a few times during the hours immediately following childbirth. It may be uncomfortable for the mother.

If bleeding seems profuse after the placenta is delivered, or if the placenta does not spontaneously deliver after 60 minutes, be prepared to treat for shock (see page 58).

If the vagina is torn, apply pressure with a sterile compress. After the bleeding slows, the vaginal area can be gently washed, with the mother on her back, so that rinse water flows away from the vagina toward the anus. Take care to keep any contaminating material or solutions out of the vagina. Lay a sterile compress or clean sanitary napkin over the vagina.

After a wilderness birth, administer an antibiotic (cephalexin, amoxicillin–clavulanate, or erythromycin) to the mother for 48 hours.

COMPLICATED DELIVERIES

Breech Delivery

In a breech delivery, the infant's buttocks and legs come out first. Let him deliver spontaneously (don't pull) until the level of his umbilicus (where the umbilical cord attaches) appears. At this point, take a firm hold on the baby's pelvis and apply gentle traction. Don't pull on his legs or back.

Determine which shoulder is lower, and try to swing the baby's body to the other side to allow that shoulder to exit the vagina. Gently move him to the opposite side to deliver the other shoulder. Don't let go of the baby. If the first shoulder won't deliver, you may need to reach inside the vagina with two fingers to locate one of the infant's arms and swing it down across his anterior chest, so that the hand and forearm are delivered. Repeat this procedure for the second arm.

Position the baby so that his face is down. With one hand tightly holding the baby by his ankles, slide your other hand underneath him and slip your middle finger into the vagina, then into the baby's mouth for a grip. During a contraction, when the mother is pushing, extract the baby. If the extraction takes a few minutes, let the baby rest on your forearm with your finger in his mouth and his arms and legs dangling on either side, and use your other hand to push the vaginal tissues away from his face.

Prolapsed Umbilical Cord; Single Arm or Foot

A prolapsed umbilical cord occurs when the cord falls out of the vagina and becomes trapped between the baby and the opening. This can be a catastrophe, because if the cord is pinched and obstructed, the blood supply to the baby will be interrupted.

Turn the mother on her side or have her kneel in the knee-to-chest position and try to interrupt labor. Don't encourage pushing. Place a moistened (with disinfected saline, preferably) towel over the cord and vagina and expedite an emergency evacuation of the mother from the wilderness. If the delivery continues, try to have it occur without undue delay. Do your best to keep the head from compressing the cord.

If a single arm or foot hangs out of the vagina, have the mother kneel in the knee-to-chest position and try to get her to a hospital as quickly as possible.

Cellulitis of the Breast (Mastitis)

A nursing mother may develop infection of the soft tissue of the breast. Risk factors for mastitis include plugging of the milk ducts due to delayed infant feeding (causes breast engorgement), cracked nipples, fatigue, and poorly fitted (rubbing) clothing. The affected part of the breast becomes reddened, warm, and painful. The mother may suffer from fever, chills, body aches, and nausea and vomiting. Unresolved, mastitis may develop into a breast abscess. The mother should continue to breastfeed the child, because the infection will not be transmitted to the child. Nurse first on the unaffected side, then on the affected side. If the breast remains engorged, attempt to pump after feeding. Encourage frequent breastfeeding. Administer dicloxacillin or cephalexin 500 mg by mouth four times a day for 10 days. If the patient is allergic to penicillin, administer clindamycin 300 mg or erythromycin 500 mg by mouth four times a day for 10 days. Warm packs applied to the breast may encourage drainage and hasten resolution. The woman should stay well hydrated and wear a supportive bra.

DIABETES

Diabetes is a disorder in which the pancreas cannot create sufficient insulin (type 1 or insulin-dependent diabetes) or in which insulin is not effective (type 2 or non–insulin-dependent diabetes). Insulin allows the body to use and store sugar; in the diabetic state, the victim suffers from high blood sugar and an array of physiologic derangements (kidney failure, skin ulcers, bleeding into the vitreous of the eye) associated with deterioration of small blood vessels. Many diabetics need to take insulin by injection or inhalation to manage the disease; others can control their blood sugar by diet, oral medications (hypoglycemic agents), or both. Oral medications include drugs that stimulate pancreatic cells to produce more insulin (e.g., glipizide [Glucotrol]), reduce sugar production in the liver (e.g., metformin [Glucophage]), reduce carbohydrate absorption and sugar "peaks" after eating (e.g., acarbose [Precose]), inhibit glucose reabsorption through the kidneys (e.g., canagliflozin [Invokana]), or reduce insulin resistance in the body. Exenatide (Byetta) injection is used as a supplemental drug for certain patients with type 2 diabetes. Insulin analogs, such as insulin lispro, are rapidly acting and when used in conjunction with standard insulins, which have longer onset and duration of action, can allow the outdoor enthusiast who suffers from diabetes to have greater flexibility in the timing of meals, snacks, and exercise. One product is the Humalog KwikPen.

The most common dangerous acute situation incurred by a diabetic is a hypoglycemic reaction (low blood sugar) induced by an inadvertent overdose of insulin, or after a normal dose of insulin or glucose-lowering agent accompanied by extraordinary exercise or insufficient food intake. The manifestations of an insulin reaction are weakness, sweating, hunger, abdominal pain, and altered mental status (which may include confusion, belligerent behavior, fainting, seizures, or coma). The solution is to administer sugar as rapidly as possible. If the victim is unconscious, it's generally prohibited to administer anything by mouth, because of the danger of choking and aspiration of food or fluid into the lungs. However, sugar granules or concentrated liquid glucose (Glutose: one tube contains 15 g) can be inserted under the tongue, to dissolve and be passively swallowed. Otherwise, sterile glucose solution must be injected intravenously, which obviously requires a trained individual. If the victim is awake and capable of swallowing, a naturally sweetened solution (apple or orange juice, sugar-containing soft drink), banana, or candy bar (chocolate, sugar cube) should be eaten. Once a diabetic suffering from hypoglycemia perks up from ingesting something containing sugar, be certain that the total amount of carbohydrate ingested is 15 to 20 g. This can be accomplished with 4 ounces of carbohydrate-containing juice or non-diet (sweetened) soda, 8 ounces of milk, sugar tablets or 4 teaspoons of table sugar, a tube of Glutose, 5 hard candies, 2 tablespoons of raisins, 5 soda crackers, or a tablespoon of honey. If a glucose meter is handy, check to see that the blood sugar is at least 70 mg/deciliter. If not, repeat the feeding. As soon as the victim feels better, he should eat a meal, to avoid a recurrence.

Glucagon is a hormone that causes the liver to release glucose. In a hypoglycemic emergency, it can be administered into a muscle of the victim to raise the blood glucose level. Here are the steps for administration:

1. Find the diabetic person's glucagon injection kit (GlucaGen HypoKit), most likely stored in a small zippered case. There will be a vial of powder and a syringe containing liquid with an attached needle.
2. Remove the plastic cap from the vial. Pull the needle cover off the syringe. Insert the needle through the rubber stopper (within the marked circle) of the vial containing the GlucaGen powder and inject all the liquid from the syringe into the vial.
3. Without taking the needle out of the vial, gently shake or roll the vial back and forth until the powder has completely dissolved and the solution appears clear.
4. Make sure that the plunger on the syringe is completely down. While keeping the needle in the liquid within the vial, withdraw all the liquid into the syringe. Take care to not pull the plunger out of the syringe. Pull the syringe and needle out of the vial or leave it within the vial for the next step.
5. Point the needle and syringe up so that the air floats to the top of the syringe just under where the needle attaches to the syringe (see page 444). Push the plunger gently until a few drops of liquid drip out to be sure that there is no air in the syringe and needle. Continue to push the plunger until you have the correct dose for the injection. If you haven't yet removed the needle from the vial, do so now.
6. Stab the needle all the way into a muscular area such as the curve of the calf or into a muscular thigh. Try not to push it into fatty tissue, such as a buttock. While holding the needle and syringe motionless, pull back on the plunger to be sure that

the needle is not positioned in an artery or vein, in which case blood would freely enter the barrel of the syringe. If no blood is returned, then push the plunger all the way down without any hesitation. For a child weighing less than 44 lb (20 kg), administer only half of the contents of the syringe. Don't administer the glucagon injection directly into a vein. After the injection, remove the needle and apply light pressure at the injection site. A person injected with glucagon may suffer momentary sweating and nausea.

7. When the person revives, give him some kind of fast-acting simple sugar (Glutose paste, glucose tablets, fruit juice, or hard candy), as long as he is capable of purposeful swallowing. Because the blood glucose level will remain adequate only for an hour or so because of the injection, it's important to observe the person closely and be sure that he continues to ingest food and liquid. If you have a glucose meter, try to keep the glucose level above 100 mg/deciliter.

Anyone who suffers from diabetes should wear appropriate identification, in case he requires assistance. No one who is insulin dependent should attempt physical exertion in a dangerous environment without adequate glucose intake. Even a person taking only an oral hypoglycemic drug, such as micronized glyburide or glipizide, should be cautious.

If the blood sugar gets dangerously high, the diabetic may become very ill, because the blood becomes acidotic with the by-products of metabolism (known as ketones), dehydration increases, and body chemistries become unbalanced. Such a patient is confused, combative, or comatose. His breathing rate increases, breathing becomes shallow, and exhaled breaths have a fruity or acetone (like fingernail polish remover) odor. He may be vomiting, complain of abdominal pain, and be intensely thirsty. Because of dehydration, the pulse is rapid and weak, skin is very dry, eyes may appear "sunken," and there is little sweating (dry armpits). Such a clinical picture calls for immediate transport of the victim to the hospital. If he can drink, he should be encouraged to ingest unsweetened fluids. The definitive treatment for ketoacidosis is intravenous fluids and insulin injections, which must be carefully dosed according to the measured blood sugar level.

If you cannot differentiate between an insulin reaction (low blood sugar) and altered mental status caused by excessively high blood sugar, you should err on the side of predicting a hypoglycemic episode and give the victim something sweet to eat or drink. If you have guessed correctly, the improvement will be dramatic; if your diagnosis was wrong, the extra sugar will not cause any significant harm. If a diabetic person is carrying a blood glucose meter (such as FreeStyle Lite, FastTake, Accu-Chek, or SureStep), be sure you're instructed in its proper use before you need to use it. At high altitudes, the Accu-Check Compact Plus blood glucose meter is a good choice because it relies on a chemical reaction that doesn't depend on the presence of oxygen.

If a person with diabetes develops a skin infection, particularly if it is on the foot, an appropriate antibiotic choice is dicloxacillin, amoxicillin–clavulanate, or ciprofloxacin.

If a person with diabetes develops gastroenteritis (see page 119) with vomiting, it's wise to administer an antiemetic drug early, to try to prevent dehydration and to allow adequate eating and drinking, thereby making it somewhat easier to manage blood sugar swings.

STROKE

A stroke is caused by a blood clot that blocks an artery supplying part of the brain, or by bleeding from a leaking vessel into the brain. It occurs suddenly and can be minor or major, depending on the area and amount of the brain involved. If a stroke involves the brainstem, it may affect the breathing center and cause rapid death. A stroke may be caused by rupture of a cerebral artery aneurysm; when this occurs, the victim may suffer from a form of bleeding known as subarachnoid hemorrhage, in which case the victim typically complains of the "worst headache of my life."

Symptoms include sudden headache without another cause; numbness of the face, arm, or leg; nausea and vomiting; blurred or double vision; weakness or paralysis of the arm(s) and/or leg(s) (particularly if it occurs on one side); difficulty speaking or understanding speech; difficulty walking; dizziness, confusion, and/or loss of balance or coordination; loss of consciousness; coma; seizure; and collapse. If someone has stroke symptoms that last for a few minutes to an hour and then gradually resolve, he has suffered a transient ischemic attack (TIA), which is a warning that he may soon suffer a full-blown stroke. So, even if stroke symptoms are fleeting, the victim should see a physician as soon as possible. If a person is believed to have suffered a TIA, he should begin to take aspirin, 50 to 325 mg by mouth once a day, until he is evaluated by a neurologist. If a stroke occurs, aspirin should not be administered.

A rapid simple neurologic examination may reveal subtle changes indicative of a stroke. This exam consists of the following:

Mental status. Ask the victim his name, age, and location, as well as time, day, and year.

Vision. Have the victim count fingers that you display. Check each eye by itself and then both eyes together. Check that the pupils are equal. Ask the victim to follow a moving object with his eyes.

Facial muscles. Ask the victim to pucker his lips and then to whistle. Check the cheeks and mouth for symmetry. Have the victim clench his jaw while you feel the jaw muscles on each side. Have the victim tightly close his eyes. Have him relax with his eyes closed; lightly touch his face to locate any numb spots.

Hearing. Make a soft noise (yet loud enough that you can hear it) in each of the victim's ears.

Swallowing and speech. Ask the victim to swallow. Ask him to stick his tongue out and move it from side to side voluntarily. Listen carefully to note if his speech is clear or slurred.

Muscle strength. Have the victim squeeze one of your fingers with each hand, straighten each leg against resistance, bend each leg against resistance, bend and straighten each elbow and wrist against resistance, extend and flex each ankle against resistance, and shrug both shoulders against resistance.

Sensation. Using a light touch, move your fingers over the entire body and try to identify any areas of decreased sensation.

Coordination. Ask the victim to stand perfectly still in an upright position with his eyes closed and his arms at his sides. Be prepared to catch him if he begins to fall. Have him open his eyes, and then clap one hand into the palm of the other as fast as possible. Ask him to move an index finger back and forth between the tip of his nose and your finger, held 18 inches (46 cm) away. Have him walk heel-to-toe and on tiptoes.

If someone displays the symptoms of a stroke, he should be placed at absolute rest with his upper body and head elevated by an angle of at least 30 degrees. If his level of consciousness declines, pay attention to his airway (see page 22) so that he does not vomit and choke. Seek immediate medical attention. Low blood sugar may cause symptoms that mimic a stroke. If the victim can swallow purposefully without choking, sugar granules or concentrated liquid glucose (Glutose: one tube contains 15 g) can be inserted under the tongue, to dissolve and be passively swallowed (see page 133).

If stroke symptoms are associated with scuba diving, they might indicate an air embolism (see page 360). In this case, the victim needs to be transported in a head-up and/or left-side-down position and delivered to a hyperbaric chamber as soon as possible.

INFECTIOUS DISEASES

Foreign travel is increasingly a component of the wilderness experience, and thus American travelers are exposed to numerous diseases that are not indigenous to the United States. In addition, domestic outdoor activities expose us to the vectors (carriers, such as mosquitoes or ticks) and microorganisms that generate diseases such as malaria, Rocky Mountain spotted fever, and Lyme disease. People who handle wild animals or ingest animal products are at increased risk. This section addresses some of the more common and worrisome infectious diseases associated with outdoor activities. Immunizations are discussed on page 420.

Recommendations for drugs to treat these diseases are based on current literature. These recommendations may change—and some undoubtedly will, because new and better treatments are being discovered, organisms can acquire resistance to certain chemical agents, and toxic side effects to certain drugs will be revealed. It's important for physicians and laypeople who will assume responsibility for treating others to remain informed about current therapies.

MALARIA

Malaria is caused by infection with one of four microscopic protozoan parasites: *Plasmodium falciparum, P. vivax, P. malariae,* or *P. ovale.* These are transmitted in the wild by the bite of an infected *Anopheles* mosquito. Of the nearly 430 species of *Anopheles* mosquitoes, only 30 to 40 transmit malaria. Most cases of malaria acquired by U.S. citizens are contracted in sub-Saharan Africa; most of the remainder are linked to travel in Southeast Asia, Central and South America, the Indian subcontinent, the Middle East, and Oceania (Papua New Guinea, Vanuatu, and the Solomon Islands).

Mosquitoes bite humans to obtain a blood meal in order to produce eggs. When a female mosquito bites a human infected with malaria, it ingests an immature form of the parasite. In approximately 2 weeks, the parasite matures within the mosquito. When the infected mosquito bites a noninfected human, it releases malaria sporozoites (an immature form of the parasite), which mature in the human liver to become merozoites, and which then invade red blood cells. From these locations, the organisms can penetrate the vital organs, such as the brain, lungs, liver, and kidneys. Within a few days, the infected red blood cells burst and the parasites infect more red blood cells.

The incubation period between acquisition of the parasites and the onset of symptoms is 8 to 40 days, depending on the species. Up to a third of victims may not show the disease until after 60 days from the time of the initial mosquito bite. Malaria should be considered in any person with a fever who is in or has recently been in a malarious location. Typical symptoms include a flu-like illness, with any or all of the following: headache, chills, sweats, fatigue, backache, pale skin, loss of appetite, muscle aches, nausea, diarrhea, and vomiting. These are soon followed by episodes of headache, intense chills (rigors), high fever, and sweating. Jaundice and anemia may occur. The episodes last 1 to 8 hours and are separated by 2 to 3 days, depending on the species. Onset of fever may be delayed by a few days.

Persons infected with falciparum malaria may be significantly more ill, with episodes of fever and chills at closer intervals (sometimes seemingly constant) and lasting for more than 30 hours. In addition, there may be alteration in mental status, abdominal pain, seizures, difficulty breathing, blood in the urine, severe anemia, and shock. Severe malaria can be fatal or lead to anemia, heart and kidney failure, and/or coma; untreated infections can cause recurrent illness for years.

Identification of the specific plasmodium is accomplished by observing the parasites under the microscope in blood smears. Three "negative" (no parasites seen) blood smears interpreted by a trained examiner and spaced 12 to 24 hours apart are necessary to rule out malaria. Rapid diagnostic tests, such as BinaxNOW, are sometimes used to diagnose malaria when a trained microscopist is not available.

Unfortunately, there is not yet a useful vaccine against malaria. Avoidance of mosquito bites is key to prevention. Because the *Anopheles* mosquito tends to feed during the evening and nighttime, it's particularly important to wear adequate skin-covering clothing; sleep under nets or screens; spray living quarters (with, for instance, a pyrethrin-containing product) and clothing (with, for example, permethrin 0.5%, Duranon, or Repel Permanone; or concentrated Perma-Kill 4-Week Tick Killer, diluted and applied to clothing); and use insect repellent (N,N-diethyl-3-methylbenzamide, called DEET) at these times (see page 336). Insect Shield Repellent Apparel and Insect Shield Repellent Gear are impregnated with a proprietary permethrin formula. The clothing is claimed to withstand 70 launderings and retain repellency.

If you travel to a region where *P. falciparum* is resistant to chloroquine and pyrimethamine–sulfadoxine, prophylaxis (prevention) can be accomplished with mefloquine. The adult dose is 250 mg (salt) weekly. The pediatric dose varies according to the weight of the child: weight 15 to 19 kg, 63 mg; weight 20 to 30 kg, 125 mg; weight 31 to 45 kg, 188 mg; and over 45 kg, 250 mg. (For estimating purposes, 1 kg equals 2.2 lb.) Mefloquine should be started 1 to 2 weeks before travel, and then administered once a week during travel in malarious areas and for 4 weeks after you leave such areas. Mefloquine should not be taken during pregnancy. This drug should not be used by persons with psychiatric disease or history of depression or seizures. Side effects include nausea and vomiting, dizziness, mood changes, difficulty sleeping and nightmares, headache, and diarrhea.

An alternative drug for travelers who cannot take mefloquine is doxycycline (the adult dose is 100 mg a day beginning 1 to 2 days before travel and continuing for 5 to 6 weeks after; the pediatric dose for those more than 8 years of age is 2 mg/kg of body weight a day, up to the adult dose). Doxycycline is not advised for pregnant women or children under age 8 years, and it may cause increased skin sensitivity to sunlight.

A final drug prophylaxis regimen against malaria is chloroquine phosphate (the adult dose is 300 mg of the base once a week; the pediatric dose is 5 mg/kg of the base, up to the adult dose, once a week), which should be taken 1 to 2 weeks before you enter a malarious region and continued until 1 month after your journey. Chloroquine is recommended for travelers, particularly pregnant women and children who weigh less than 33 lb (15 kg), who cannot take mefloquine or doxycycline. If you use chloroquine for prophylaxis, you should also carry three tablets of Fansidar to be taken in the event of a flu-like illness or other unexplained fever, assuming the absence of an allergy to sulfonamide antibiotics. Chloroquine should not be used by persons with retinal problems and has side effects of headache and itching.

Proguanil (Paludrine) is a drug that may be used for antimalarial prophylaxis in areas where *P. falciparum* is resistant to chloroquine. The drug is available without prescription in parts of Europe, Scandinavia, and Africa, but is as yet unavailable in the United States. It is administered in an adult dose of 200 mg daily (pediatric dose: under 2 years, 50 mg; age 2 to 6 years, 100 mg; age 7 to 10 years, 150 mg; over 10 years, 200 mg), along with weekly chloroquine (the latter to protect against other forms of malaria). It can be used by those who will spend more than 3 weeks in rural areas of East Africa (particularly Kenya and Tanzania), but does not appear to be useful in Papua New Guinea, West Africa, or Thailand.

Atovaquone in combination with proguanil hydrochloride is available as the drug Malarone. The drug is taken at the same time each day with food or a milky drink. Treatment should be started 2 days before entering a malaria-endemic area and continued for 7 days after return. The adult dose is one tablet (250 mg atovaquone/100 mg proguanil) per day. Each pediatric tablet of Malarone contains atovaquone 62.5 mg/proguanil 25 mg. The pediatric dose is based on weight: 11 to 20 kg, one pediatric tablet per day; 21 to 30 kg, 2 tablets; 31 to 40 kg, 3 tablets; greater than

40 kg, one adult tablet. It should be noted that if Malarone is taken with tetracycline, metoclopramide, rifampin, or rifabutin, it may be less bioavailable and thus potentially less effective. It should not be used by persons with significant kidney disease.

Pyrimethamine plus dapsone (drug combination: Maloprim) is prescribed in many malaria-endemic regions outside the United States. This drug cannot be used by pregnant women; it can also cause bone marrow suppression.

If you are stricken with malaria in an area where the malaria organism(s) is believed to be sensitive to chloroquine, but you have not been taking prophylaxis, begin treatment with chloroquine (adult dose, 600 mg of the base immediately, followed with 300 mg at 6 hours and once a day on days 2 and 3; pediatric dose, 10 mg/kg of body weight [up to 600 mg] of the base immediately, followed by 5 mg/kg at 6 hours and once a day on days 2 and 3). In a region where *P. falciparum* is resistant to chloroquine, administer quinine sulfate (adult dose, 650 mg every 8 hours for 3 days; pediatric dose, 8 mg/kg [up to 650 mg] every 8 hours for 3 days) *plus* tetracycline (adult dose, 250 mg four times a day for 7 days; pediatric dose, 5 mg/kg [up to 250 mg] four times a day for 7 days) or Fansidar (adult dose, 3 tablets; pediatric dose: weight 5 to 10 kg, ½ tablet; weight 11 to 20 kg, 1 tablet; weight 21 to 30 kg, 1½ tablets; weight 31 to 45 kg, 2 tablets; weight over 45 kg, 3 tablets). (For purposes of estimation, 1 kg equals 2.2 lb.) Malarone is sometimes used to treat acute malaria caused by *P. falciparum*. For dosage, see the first recommendation in the following list for "stand-by treatment."

In addition to the treatment recommendations above, there are two "stand-by treatment regimens" offered by the Centers for Disease Control and Prevention (CDC):

1. Atovaquone-proguanil (Malarone): The dosage for each of 3 consecutive days of treatment is based on body weight: 5 to 8 kg, 2 pediatric tablets; 9 to 10 kg, 3 pediatric tablets; 11 to 20 kg, 1 adult tablet; 21 to 30 kg, 2 adult tablets; 31 to 40 kg, 3 adult tablets; greater than 40 kg, 4 adult tablets. This treatment regimen is not recommended for someone who has been taking this medication for prophylaxis against malaria.

2. Artemether-lumefantrine (Coartem): The 3-day regimen is based on body weight: 5 to less than 15 kg, 1 tablet per dose; 15 to less than 25 kg, 2 tablets per dose; 25 to less than 35 kg, 3 tablets per dose; 35 or greater kg, 4 tablets per dose. The person should receive the first dose, then the second dose 8 hours later, then one dose twice per day for the next 2 days. This treatment regimen is not recommended for someone who has been taking mefloquine for prophylaxis against malaria.

Persons who have taken prophylaxis may contract malaria. In any case of suspected malaria, seek the advice of a physician as soon as possible. Anticipate that a stricken individual, particularly a child, may develop extremely low blood glucose (sugar).

To determine the malaria risk within a specific country and to learn of the most recent recommendations for prophylaxis and drug therapy, you can seek information from one of many sources on the Internet, such as www.cdc.gov/malaria/.

YELLOW FEVER

Yellow fever is a viral disease transmitted in the jungle by mosquitoes of the genus *Haemagogus* and in urban areas of the species *Aedes aegypti*. "Jungle" yellow fever is seen in forest-savanna zones of tropical Africa, parts of Central America, forested areas of South America, and Trinidad. The "urban" variety is seen in South America and West Africa. The disease has not yet been noted in Asia.

The illness begins 3 to 6 days after the culprit mosquito bite(s). Symptoms include sudden onset of fever, headache, chills, red eyes, muscle aching, no appetite, nausea, and vomiting. These symptoms last for 3 to 4 days, after which there may be 12 to 24 hours of remission. Soon thereafter comes a "toxic phase," in which the seriously stricken victim develops fever, skin rashes, altered mental status, severe abdominal pain, vomiting, low blood pressure, profound hepatitis, and liver and kidney failure. In such cases, the victim becomes jaundiced (hence, "yellow" fever) and bleeds easily. The disease can be fatal in up to half of persons who enter the toxic phase. Treatment is supportive and based on symptoms. Because of the bleeding problems, don't use aspirin to control fever.

Since yellow fever is so difficult to treat, it's essential to use yellow fever vaccine and mosquito control measures (see page 336). A live-virus vaccine is available. A single injection induces immunity after 10 days that is adequate for 10 years (see page 424).

DENGUE

Dengue (sometimes called dengue fever) is a viral (flavivirus) infection transmitted by *Aedes aegypti* and *A. albopictus* mosquitoes. It is estimated that 50 million people in more than 100 countries are infected each year with dengue viruses. There are four different serotypes of dengue virus (DEN-1, DEN-2, DEN-3, and DEN-4), and there appears to be little cross-immunity, so a person may be stricken with dengue four times in his life, with each subsequent infection generally being worse than the preceding ones. The current thinking is that while a first infection with DEN-1 may provide a slight boost in short-term (6 months to 1 year) overall immunity to dengue, it may also increase the possibility of severe disease after this period from the other serotypes. The most active feeding times for dengue vector mosquitoes is for a few hours after daybreak and in the afternoon for a few hours just after dark (dusk). As opposed to the night-feeding mosquitoes that transmit malaria, these species tend to be "urban," may also feed during daylight hours (also indoors, in the shade, and during an overcast), and are known to bite below the waist. Dengue is seen chiefly in the Caribbean and South America, as well as other tropical and semi-tropical areas, such as Southeast Asia, Africa, and Mexico. In the United States, cases have been noted in Texas, Hawaii, and Florida. The larvae flourish in artificial water containers (e.g., vases, tires), often in a domestic environment.

The incubation period following a mosquito bite is 3 to 7 days. The disease is self-limited (5 to 7 days) and characterized in older children and adults by a sudden onset of severe headache (with or without pain behind the eyes), sore throat, fatigue, cough, high fever (greater than 101.3° F or 38.5° C), chills, muscle aches, sore throat, reddened eyes, enlarged lymph nodes, nausea and vomiting, bone and joint pain ("breakbone fever"), bruising, and a fine, red, itchy skin rash that typically appears (as the fever subsides) on the proximal arms, legs, and trunk (it spares the face, palms, and soles). It may then spread to the face, and farther out on the arms and legs, becoming slightly darker and more solid. The rash usually lasts for up to 4 days. Although the fever usually remits spontaneously, an occasional victim will relapse. Some victims have a cycle of a few days of fever, then 1 to 3 days without fever, then fever again. It's not uncommon to suffer central nervous system manifestations, such as irritability, depression, seizures, or severe altered mental status. Children and young adults appear to be particularly vulnerable to especially severe forms of dengue virus infection (formerly called "dengue hemorrhagic fever"), associated with severe abdominal pain, persistent vomiting, fever transitioning to low body temperature (hypothermia), and bleeding problems: nosebleed, bleeding gums, bloody vomiting, darkened stool, restlessness, weakness, etc. This may progress to include breathing difficulties and circulatory problems that can lead to extremely low blood pressure (shock—see page 58). When this occurs (generally 3 to 6 days after the first onset of symptoms of dengue), the victim may develop a diffuse, dark purple, blotchy rash caused by bleeding into the skin.

Treatment is supportive and based on symptoms. Fever should be treated with acetaminophen, and not with aspirin or NSAIDs. There is no commercial vaccine available yet against dengue, but researchers are working diligently on this aspect of prevention. Insect repellents (particularly those containing DEET; see page 336) are critical for prevention.

CHIKUNGUNYA ILLNESS

Chikungunya illness is similar to dengue. It is indigenous to tropical Africa and Asia, and should be particularly suspected in persons returning from the Caribbean. Caused by transmission of an alphavirus from a bite by the mosquito *Aedes aegypti* or *A. albopictus*, Chikungunya disease carries an incubation period of 1 to 12 (usually 2 to 4) days, followed by sudden onset of fever greater than 101.3° F (38.5° C), and pain and stiffness of multiple joints, particularly fingers, toes, wrists, ankles, and knees. The joint symptoms are often in the hands and feet. Other symptoms may include headache, backache, sore muscles, pain on looking at the light, pain behind the eyes, sore throat, nausea, vomiting, and weakness. On days 2 to 5 after the onset of fever, there may appear a red rash on the trunk, arms, and legs (less commonly on the face, palms, and soles). The arthritis may last for months to years, or it may disappear and then return 2 to 3 months after the initial illness. There are blood tests to confirm the diagnosis. Therapy is symptomatic. Aspirin should be avoided. Proper use of insect repellents is critical for prevention.

WEST NILE VIRAL DISEASE

West Nile (named from the West Nile province of Uganda) viral disease (West Nile virus [WNV]) is caused by a flavivirus (similar to those that cause St. Louis encephalitis, Japanese encephalitis, and Murray Valley encephalitis) carried predominantly by mosquitoes (*Culex pipiens* in the eastern United States, *C. pipiens quinquefasciatus* in the southern United States, and *Culex tarsalis* in the western United States, *Aedes*, *Anopheles*, and many other species) and at least 160 species of birds, although it has been found in small mammals and to an alarming degree in horses. The mosquitoes become infected by feeding on birds and many animals (e.g., bats, horses, chipmunks, dogs, rabbits, reindeer, squirrels, and even alligators). It appears to be transmitted to humans by mosquito bite and has been presumed to have arrived in the United States from the Middle East. In rapid fashion, it appears to have spread across the country. The four top species of wild birds affected by WNV are American crows, Western scrub-jays, yellow-billed magpies, and Steller's jays. Mosquitoes bite the birds and thus acquire the virus. West Nile viral disease is endemic in Africa, the Middle East, and West Asia. The virus has been spread to the recipient of an organ transplant from an infected donor, from a pregnant mother to a fetus, by blood transfusion, and possibly through breast milk. Otherwise, it does not appear to spread from human to human. While much of the clinical WNV activity is noted in summer and autumn, it's certainly possible to acquire the disease in winter from the bite of an infected mosquito.

The incubation period after a bite from an infected mosquito until the onset of illness is 3 to 14 days. The victim usually suffers a flu-like illness lasting for 3 to 6 days, characterized by fever, headache, neck stiffness and pain, swollen lymph glands, muscle aches and weakness, loss of appetite, fatigue, diarrhea, vomiting, red (smooth, bumpy, or lace-patterned) rash (commonly on the chest, abdomen, and back; sometimes on the arms and/or legs), and aversion to light (sometimes interpreted by victims as eye "pain"). Fatigue may be a residual symptom for up to a month. In 1 in every 100 to 300 cases, the victim suffers severe encephalitis (inflammation of the brain) with stiff neck and severe altered mental status (including coma or double vision), as well as paralysis. Convulsions are rare. Elders are more prone to suffer severe or fatal illness. Death is uncommon.

Most (80%) people infected with WNV never realize that they have had the disease, because they remain without symptoms. Twenty percent of infected people develop West Nile fever, and less than 1% of people infected develop severe medical illness, including meningitis and/or encephalitis (characterized by seizures, loss of vision, and disorientation) or paralysis. There are blood tests for WNV that measure antibodies to the virus and show positive in most infected people within 8 days of the onset of symptoms. However, they may initially be "negative" and need to be repeated at a later date. There is no specific treatment other than supportive therapy. Recovery is generally complete for survivors, although persistent neuropsychological problems (fatigue, memory problems, weakness, tremor, word-finding difficulties, headaches, and depression) may occur, even if the acute disease was mild.

Prevention is essential. First and foremost, that means preventing mosquito bites. Here are some recommendations:

1. Don't maintain standing water that serves as a breeding ground for mosquitoes, which lay eggs in the water. Drain or dump all standing water on a weekly basis. This includes water as shallow as 1 inch deep, as may be found in flower pots, planter bases, old tires, child pools, and so on.
2. Be sure that all doors and windows have tight-fitting screens. Repair any holes or rips, and if possible, treat screens and door jambs with mosquito control products.
3. Most bites occur at dawn and dusk, so limit outdoor activities during these times.
4. Use effective insect repellents, such as those containing DEET (N,N-diethyl-m-toluamide) or picaridin (KBR 3023). Use repellents according to the manufacturer's labeled instructions, and reapply frequently, particularly if you swim or become sweaty.
5. Wear clothing designed to cover your arms and legs, including long sleeves and pants.

EASTERN EQUINE ENCEPHALITIS

Eastern equine encephalitis (EEE) is caused by the EEE virus, which is transmitted by mosquito bites, most commonly from the species *Culiseta melanura*. This is a potentially fatal disease that's endemic to the eastern United States, particularly the forested swamp areas of the mid-Atlantic and New England states. It is also found in Latin America.

After an incubation period of 4 to 10 days from the time of the mosquito bite, EEE virus infection can lead to two different types of illness. The first is "systemic" and involves the rapid onset of fever, chills, fatigue, and muscle and joint pains, all lasting up to 2 weeks. Vomiting and diarrhea may occur. The second type of illness, which is much more severe, is encephalitis, which results in swelling of the brain. This occurs after a few days of the systemic illness. Symptoms include severe headache, altered mental status, weak breathing efforts, blue or pale skin color, seizures, and unconsciousness leading to coma. Up to a third of persons who become seriously ill with EEE will die, and survivors often have long-term neurologic problems.

There is no effective vaccine or treatment for humans, which emphasizes the importance of prevention. Outbreaks of infections with EEE virus occur in horses and humans following amplification of virus populations in a song bird–mosquito cycle. The prime time of risk is summer to early autumn. Mild winters and warmer summers attributable to global climate change may contribute to the risk.

RELAPSING FEVER

The sporadic (in occurrence) form of relapsing fever is caused by various borrelial organisms transmitted by argasid (soft) ticks of multiple *Ornithodoros* species. For instance, tick-borne relapsing fever in the western United States and Canada is caused by *Borrelia hermsii*, transmitted by the *Ornithodoros hermsii* tick. The epidemic form of relapsing fever is transmitted by the human body louse. In the United States, relapsing fever is largely confined to the western portion of the country, where the ticks inhabit coniferous forests in the remains of dead trees and burrows occupied by mice, rats, and chipmunks.

The disease is more common in men, who may occupy the poorly maintained cabins and huts that rodents like to visit. The classic case involves a tick bite and a 7-day incubation period, followed by the abrupt onset of high fever, shaking chills, severe headache, muscle and joint aches, abdominal pain, nausea, and vomiting. This lasts for about 3 (but may be 1 to 17) days, until there is a crisis wherein the fever drops while the victim undergoes drenching sweats and intense thirst. For a subsequent period that averages 7 days, there is no fever and minimal symptoms, and then a relapse into illness. This cycle recurs an average of three times, with each episode of illness generally less severe. The sporadic (tick-borne) variation tends to be less severe; mortality rates of up to 40% have occurred in louse-borne epidemics.

A physician can make the diagnosis by examining a smear of the victim's blood under the lens of a microscope and observing the causative organisms. Treatment is doxycycline 100 mg twice a day, or tetracycline or erythromycin 500 mg by mouth four times a day for 10 days. When the victim ingests the antibiotics, he may suffer a high fever and low blood pressure (shock—see page 58) as a reaction to the death of the organisms within his bloodstream. Therefore, if you suspect relapsing fever, unless the victim is extremely ill, it's best to have him treated in a hospital, where this reaction can be anticipated and managed. If you are forced to treat in the field, be certain that the victim is well hydrated (see page 194), and administer a lower dose (250 mg) of antibiotic for the first four doses.

TYPHOID AND PARATYPHOID FEVERS

Typhoid and paratyphoid fevers are caused by the bacteria *Salmonella typhi* and *S. paratyphi,* respectively, which are transmitted among humans through ingestion of contaminated food or water. Most cases are acquired abroad under conditions of poor hygiene.

After an incubation period of 10 to 14 days, victims suffer fever with or without diarrhea and abdominal pain. Most victims also complain of headache, fatigue, and loss of appetite. "Rose spots," which are 2 to 4 mm red spots on the trunk that blanch (lose their color) when pressed, are seen in some cases. The liver may become inflamed.

Most cases resolve in 3 to 4 weeks (paratyphoid infection typically resolves in a shorter time period). The seriously stricken individual may suffer a severely inflamed bowel, distended abdomen, bleeding from the gastrointestinal tract, pneumonia, heart failure, severe fever, and death.

A physician who diagnoses typhoid or paratyphoid fever (the latter is also known as enteric fever) will treat the victim with an intravenous antibiotic. The layperson can use ciprofloxacin or azithromycin 10 mg/kg (2.2 lb) of body weight by mouth twice a day for 7 days. The pediatric dose (up to the adult dose) is calculated by the same formula. An alternative is trimethoprim–sulfamethoxazole; administer one double-strength tablet twice a day. You can also use ampicillin 100 mg/kg (2.2 lb) of body weight in four divided doses. It's important to keep the victim from becoming dehydrated (see page 194).

Injectable and oral vaccines (see page 426) to prevent typhoid fever are available to people traveling to areas of high risk.

EBOLA, LASSA, AND OTHER VIRUSES THAT CAUSE "HEMORRHAGIC FEVERS"

The viral hemorrhagic (bleeding) fevers (Ebola, Lassa, Marburg, and Crimean-Congo) can all be spread among humans by transfer of secretions (blood and bodily fluids: vomit, urine, feces, sweat, feces, saliva, semen, other fluids). Therefore, it's important to isolate suspected victims as best as possible from other humans during their care. Personal protective equipment (PPE; breathing masks, along with liquid-impermeable gloves, face shields/goggles, and protective clothing or gowns with leg/foot components) that covers all skin should be worn by caregivers. Transfer to a medical facility for therapy may be critical to survival. Field care is supportive and similar to that for yellow fever (see page 139).

At the time of this writing, Ebola virus disease is pandemic in West Africa. Because of international travel, it has appeared on other continents. It is highly infectious and spreads in people by human-to-human transmission, from contact with blood and body fluids. It can also be contracted by handling infected animals, such as fruit bats and chimpanzees found in Africa. "Bush meat" should be avoided as a dietary item. The incubation period is 2 to 21 days after exposure, prior to the onset of symptoms. The infected victim typically has onset of fever, severe headache, sore throat, abdominal pain, vomiting, diarrhea, joint and/or muscle pain, and weakness. If the disease worsens, there is profound vomiting and diarrhea, leading to dehydration and collapse. In some cases, there can be diffuse bleeding and essential organ failure. To date, therapy is supportive and there is not yet a vaccine. Anyone suspected of being infected with Ebola virus should be strictly isolated, and all available precautions, such as proper PPE, should be used to avoid contact with his blood or body secretions. The current thinking is that Ebola virus only spreads when people are sick (e.g., have symptoms), and that after 21 days, if an exposed person does not develop symptoms, he will not become ill with Ebola virus disease.

Lassa fever is a viral disease transmitted to humans principally through the body secretions of the *Mastomys natalensis* rat. It occurs primarily in sub-Saharan West Africa. The infected victim suffers a gradual onset of headache, fever, and fatigue. There is often a severe sore throat, and there may be diarrhea and/or reddened eyes. Victims often complain of chest pain behind the breastbone, which may be caused by inflammation of the throat and esophagus. Roughly a quarter of victims develop bleeding complications. If the case is nonfatal, resolution begins in 8 to 10 days. In a fatal case, the victim progresses to develop altered mental status, shock, and severe breathing disorders.

SCHISTOSOMIASIS

Schistosomiasis is a term that describes a variety of diseases caused by different species of parasitic flatworms of the genus *Schistosoma*. The intermediate hosts are freshwater snails, which release the immature infective stages into the water; thus, the infections are acquired by people who bathe or swim in contaminated water. It is not acquired in saltwater. The early symptoms caused by all of the species of worms are similar. When the fork-tailed cercariae (early stages of the immature worm) penetrate the skin, they cause itching and a rash at the site of entry that may begin within a few hours to a week after exposure and last for 1 to 2 days. Two to eight weeks later, the victim shows loss of appetite, fatigue, night sweating, headache, muscle aches, diarrhea, hives, and late-afternoon fever lasting 5 to 10 days ("snail," "safari," "Katayama," or "Yangtze River" fever).

After a few months, the different species cause specific organ damage. *Schistosoma haematobium* is prevalent in Africa, the Middle East, the islands of Madagascar and Mauritius, and India. The worms take residence in the blood vessels of the bladder and genitalia and induce bloody, painful, and frequent urination. The other four species of worms cause scarring in the intestines and liver. *S. mansoni* is prevalent in Africa, the Arabian Peninsula, Madagascar, Brazil, Suriname, Venezuela, and some Caribbean islands. The worms take residence in the blood vessels surrounding the large bowel and induce bloody and mucus-laden diarrhea. In late stages of the disease, the liver can be severely damaged. *S. japonicum* is prevalent in China, the Philippines, Japan, and the island of Sulawesi. The worms take residence in the blood vessels supplying the small bowel and induce severe, bloody, and mucus-laden diarrhea. *Schistosoma intercalatum* infections occur in sub-Saharan Africa and *Schistosoma mekongi* infections along the Mekong River in Cambodia and Laos. "Katayama fever" consists of fever, headache, muscle aches, abdominal pain in the right upper quadrant (liver), and bloody diarrhea. This occurs 2 to 6 weeks after the onset of schistosomiasis.

The diagnosis is usually made by identification of schistosome eggs in feces or urine. Treatment for schistosomiasis includes the prescription anthelminthic (antiparasitic) drug praziquantel.

To prevent schistosomiasis, it's necessary to prevent the entry of cercariae into the body. In a region of high risk, it's unwise to bathe or swim in an untreated pond or stream. Shallow, stagnant water is more contaminated than that in swift-moving currents. Always wear hip boots or waders when passing through streams or swamps. If contact with water occurs, apply rubbing alcohol to your skin and briskly towel off, but understand that these methods may not be effective. Applying

DEET (see page 336) to the skin before water immersion may block some of the penetrating cercariae, but this is not a reliable preventive measure. Boil or disinfect all bathing water, or store it for 3 days (the life span of the cercariae) before using it; also be certain that it is free of snails. Heating bathing water to 122° F (50° C) for 5 minutes is also an effective method. Artemether is a drug that can be given alone or in combination with praziquantel to prevent schistosomiasis in high-risk situations. There is not yet an effective repellent or vaccine against schistosomiasis.

ROCKY MOUNTAIN SPOTTED FEVER

Rocky Mountain spotted fever is caused by *Rickettsia rickettsii,* a tick-borne parasite. The disease is most commonly noted in late spring and early summer, when people are more likely to be outside and become hosts for the dog tick *(Dermacentor variabilis)* or western wood tick *(Dermacentor andersoni).* Other ticks can carry the parasite. Most infections are reported in the southeastern states: North Carolina, South Carolina, Texas, Tennessee, Virginia, Maryland, and Georgia.

The incubation period is 2 to 14 (average 7) days after the tick bite, at which time a high fever abruptly begins. At 2 to 6 days after the onset of fever, the red-spotted rash typically begins on the wrists and ankles, then spreads toward the trunk, and may spread to involve the hands (including the palms) and feet (including the soles). The face is less often involved. At first, the rash is composed of pink spots that blanch with pressure; these later become darker red or purplish. As the disease advances, the spots coalesce to form purple blotches. However, some victims never develop a rash (Rocky Mountain "spotless" fever).

Other symptoms that begin before the onset of the rash include headache (common), chills, joint and muscle aching, cough, puffy eyelids and face, swollen hands and feet, reddened eyes, abdominal pain, nausea, and vomiting. Severe cases can affect multiple organ systems and cause death.

If you suspect that someone is suffering from Rocky Mountain spotted fever, seek a physician's help immediately. Doxycycline (adult dose, 100 mg twice a day) or tetracycline (adult dose, 500 mg four times a day; pediatric dose, 10 mg/kg four times a day) should be given for 6 days, or continued until the victim is without fever for 3 days. Although it's generally not recommended that you administer doxycycline or tetracycline to a pregnant woman or to a child younger than 6 years of age, because of the risk of tooth discoloration or abnormal bone development (the latter in a fetus during pregnancy), in a case of suspected Rocky Mountain spotted fever when a physician is not available to administer an alternative antibiotic, doxycycline or tetracycline should be given.

COLORADO TICK FEVER

Colorado tick fever is caused by a virus transmitted to humans by the wood tick *Dermacentor andersoni,* and perhaps by other species. It is a seasonal illness that occurs from late March to early October, with peak incidence in May and June, usually in people who recreate outdoors.

The usual incubation period—from tick bite to symptoms—is 3 to 6 days. The victim complains of sudden onset of fever, severe headache, muscle aches, and fatigue. Other symptoms may include aversion to light, eye pain, loss of appetite, abdominal pain, and nausea and vomiting. Only 5% to 10% of victims develop a skin rash. The hallmark feature, which is observed in only half of victims, is a distinctive fever pattern. There is a fever for 2 to 3 days, a 1- to 2-day remission, and then an additional 2 to 3 days of fever. Permanent effects and serious complications are rare, but do occur, more commonly in children under 10 years of age.

A victim of Colorado tick fever may require 3 weeks or longer to recover fully; the most common persistent symptoms are fatigue and weakness. However, infection appears to confer lifelong immunity to subsequent exposures to the virus. Treatment is supportive.

LYME DISEASE

Lyme disease, caused by infection with the spirochete *Borrelia burgdorferi,* is the most common tick-borne illness in the United States. Occurrence is most frequently in summer and early autumn, during peak outdoor activities. The two hard ticks implicated in transmission of the spirochete from mammal to mammal (e.g., from white-footed mouse *Peromyscus leucopus* to the white-tailed deer *Odocoileus virginianus* in the South; from the dusky-footed wood rat *Neotoma fuscipes* and the California kangaroo rat *Dipodomys californicus* to larger mammals in northern California) are *Ixodes scapularis* (deer tick) in the Northeast, South, and Midwest, and *I. pacificus* (western black-legged tick) in the West.

The adult ticks of these species are extremely small—about the size of a sesame seed. Worse yet, the disease can be transmitted by the nymphal forms, which may appear only as minuscule black spots on the skin. Other potential carriers of *B. burgdorferi* in the United States include the dog tick, wood tick, rabbit tick, and Lone Star tick *(Amblyomma americanum);* however, these ticks may not transmit the disease. Lyme disease has been reported in Canada, the Soviet Union, Australia, Europe (linked to the sheep tick *I. ricinus*), Scandinavia, Japan, and China. In Asia, the culprit tick is *I. persulcatus.* The Lone Star tick may also transmit the Heartland virus, which has been identified thus far in Missouri and Tennessee, causing a flu-like illness for which there is only symptomatic treatment.

The distinctive skin lesion of Lyme disease, erythema migrans, appears 3 to 32 days (usually, about a week) after the tick bite, most commonly at the bite site. It is attributed to *B. burgdorferi* that are spreading locally in the skin and is usually found on the trunk, upper arm (or armpit), or thigh as a small red spot that expands into a large (average 7 in or 18 cm, but up to 30 in or 76 cm, in diameter) and irregular circle or oval with a red, raised, or flat outer border surrounding paler ("fading," but slightly red) skin in the center. The rash may itch or burn and is warm to the touch. The initial central spot may turn into a blister or small ulcer, or it may turn blue in color. In some cases, multiple similar red areas appear simultaneously, occasionally within the larger primary lesion, but never on the palms or soles. These areas clear spontaneously over 1 to 14 (average 4) weeks. Variations of the rash include diffuse hives or a more measles-like eruption. An untreated victim may develop recurrent rashes 1 to 14 months after the initial rash disappears.

Within days to weeks of infecting a human, the *B. burgdorferi* organisms spread from the skin through the bloodstream and lymphatic system to affect other organs. Therefore, appearing just before, or coincident with, the skin rash(es) are flu-like symptoms that include muscle aching (particularly of the calves, thighs, and back), stiff neck, fatigue, low-grade fever, chills, painful joints, loss of appetite, nausea, cough, sore throat, swollen lymph glands, enlarged spleen, headache, abdominal pain (particularly in the right upper quadrant), irritated eyes (conjunctivitis), swelling around the eyes, and aversion to light. Most of the symptoms disappear in 2 to 3 weeks (along with the rash), but fatigue and muscle aching may last for months.

More serious symptoms include severe headaches and a stiff neck suggestive of meningitis (see page 162), confusion, profound sleepiness or insomnia, memory disturbances, emotional changes, and poor balance. Pain in the joints and symptoms of hepatitis may also occur.

Pets can also contract this disease, suffering lameness, swollen joints, lethargy, and loss of appetite.

If Lyme disease is not treated with an antibiotic, the disease can progress to facial paralysis and severe heart and nervous system disorders weeks to months after the initial rash disappears. Months or years later, up to 60% of untreated victims will suffer arthritis. If a person is successfully treated for Lyme disease with an antibiotic and has a subsequent episode of the erythema migrans rash, it's quite possible that he has been reinfected with a different strain of *B. burgdorferi.*

Antibiotic therapy for Lyme disease at the time of the initial rash or symptoms should be given for 14 to 21 days. For an adult, use doxycycline 100 mg twice a day. An alternative is amoxicillin 500 mg orally three times a day. If the victim is allergic to doxycycline/tetracycline and amoxicillin, he may take cefuroxime axetil 500 mg orally twice a day or erythromycin 250 mg orally four times a day. A child should be treated with amoxicillin 17 mg/kg (2.2 lb) of body weight (up to 250 mg) three times a day. If the child is allergic to penicillin, administer cefuroxime axetil 125 mg or 15 mg/kg (2.2 lb) of body weight or erythromycin 250 mg or 10 mg/kg (2.2. lb) of body weight three times a day. Nearly 15% of persons treated with antibiotics for Lyme disease in this fashion may develop fever, flushed skin, and low blood pressure within 24 hours of treatment. This may require physician intervention for intravenous fluids.

A physician may elect to treat certain Lyme disease victims with a daily injection of ceftriaxone for 2 weeks. There are occasional treatment failures; these people may require hospitalization for another intravenous antibiotic.

Prevention is key. Avoid tick bites by wearing proper clothing (light colored for spotting ticks, tightly woven collared shirts, closed boots, long sleeves and pant legs, hats) impregnated with 0.5% permethrin (Permanone) insecticide or N,N-diethyl-3-methylbenzamide (DEET) repellent (see page 336). Insect Shield Repellent Apparel and Insect Shield Repellent Gear are impregnated with a proprietary permethrin formula. The clothing is claimed to withstand 70 launderings and retain repellency. When traveling in tick country, keep shirts and pant cuffs tucked in. All hair-covered areas and warm, moist locations on the skin should be inspected carefully. Any tick found on the skin should be removed promptly and properly (see page 332). Following a tick bite, watch for the characteristic rash and symptoms. Some authorities believe that a tick must be attached to a human for at least 36 to 48 hours to transmit Lyme disease, but this has not yet been proved. Most authorities agree that the risk of transmission increases with the duration of tick attachment.

It has not yet been proved that administration of an antibiotic to every person bitten by an *Ixodes* tick is a cost-effective method to prevent this disease. However, in an area where carrier ticks and the disease are frequent, it's not unreasonable to administer an appropriate antibiotic within 72 hours following removal of an embedded or blood-engorged tick. This should be considered only if the attached tick is identified as an adult or nymphal deer tick; the tick is felt to have been attached for 36 hours or longer; the drug can be given within 72 hours of tick removal; there is a high rate of infection (greater than or equal to 20%) within local ticks; and doxycycline is not contraindicated. For the currently recommended single dose therapy, use 200 mg of doxycycline for adults, and for children 8 years of age or older doxycycline 4 mg/kg (2.2 lb) of body weight (up to a total dose of 200 mg).

EHRLICHIOSIS

Human ehrlichiosis (there is also a canine form) is present in two forms, one caused by a rickettsial organism known as *Ehrlichia chaffeensis,* which is spread by *Amblyomma americanum* tick bites, and the other caused by the rickettsial organisms *E. phagocytophila* and *E. equi,* spread by *Ixodes* tick bites. Infection is usually acquired by a person who inhabits a rural environment. The average incubation period after a bite is approximately 7 to 10 days. The victims, who are more commonly middle-aged adults than children and young adults, complain of a flu-like syndrome with high fever, chills, fatigue, headache, muscle aches, vomiting, and a variety of skin rashes, which can be punctate, bumpy, like tiny bruises, or broad and reddened. A victim often has decreased counts of various types of blood cells, as well as liver dysfunction. The treatment is doxycycline 100 mg twice a day or tetracycline 500 mg four times a day for 10 days. The few children who have been diagnosed with ehrlichiosis have been treated with doxycycline 3 mg/kg of body weight in two divided doses per day. Untreated or treated after a delay in diagnosis, up to 15% of victims can develop severe infections, kidney failure, bleeding disorders, seizures, and/or coma.

ANAPLASMOSIS

Human anaplasmosis, also called human granulocytic anaplasmosis, is caused by infection of white blood cells by a bacterium named *Anaplasma phagocytophilum*. Like ehrlichiosis, anaplasmosis is disseminated by bites of *Ixodes* ticks, the blacklegged tick *(I. scapularis)* in the Northeast and upper Midwest, and the western blacklegged tick *(I. pacificus)* on the West Coast. Infected persons have the onset of illness 5 to 21 days after a bite, with symptoms of fever, headache, fatigue, and muscle aches, which may progress to more serious illness affecting the kidneys, central nervous system, lungs, and blood system. A rash is rarely present. The treatment is the same as for ehrlichiosis.

AFRICAN TICK-BITE FEVER

African tick-bite fever (also known as South African tick typhus) is caused by a bite from the tick *Rickettsia africae*. It is a common cause of fever in returned (to the United States) travelers who have been to sub-Saharan Africa or the West Indies. Symptoms include fever, fatigue, headache, chills, sweats, muscle and joint aching, and a bumpy or blistering rash on the limbs that may also appear on the palms and soles, with swollen lymph nodes in the bitten limb. A hallmark sign is a slightly painful bite site with a blackened center and red surrounding tissue. This may be hidden underneath scalp hair if that is where the tick attached. The onset of illness is within 2 weeks after the tick bite. Treatment is with doxycycline 100 mg by mouth twice a day for 5 to 7 days. This usually causes symptoms to improve within 48 hours. On occasion, African tick-bite fever can cause severe illness with overwhelming infection, pneumonia, kidney failure, heart problems, and diffuse bleeding, so it is important to administer the doxycycline, even to children under the age of 8 years. In such a case, the doxycycline can be given for 2 days, followed by azithromycin for an additional 5 days.

BABESIOSIS

Babesiosis is caused by protozoan parasites that invade human red blood cells. They are transmitted from mammals and rodents to humans by the bite of certain hard ticks. For instance, *Babesia microti* in New England is transmitted by the northern deer tick *Ixodes scapularis,* which can also transmit the spirochete agent of Lyme disease.

An infection manifests itself in a human with symptoms of fatigue, loss of appetite, and weakness, followed within a few days to a week by fever, sweats, and muscle aches. Less common symptoms include headache, nausea, vomiting, and chills. There is rarely a rash. The victim may suffer anemia and an enlarged spleen. A person who no longer has a spleen, either because it is not present or not functioning properly (e.g., persons with sickle cell anemia) may suffer a more serious or prolonged illness.

A physician can make the diagnosis by observing the parasites in a smear of human blood under the lens of a microscope. Most victims recover without treatment. In severe cases, a physician may administer drugs, such as atovaquone (750 mg by mouth twice a day) plus azithromycin (500 or 1000 mg by mouth on day one, then 250 mg per day) for 7 to 10 days; if the bacteria are stubborn, antibiotic therapy may be necessary for 6 weeks or longer. Babesiosis should be suspected in persons if they have been diagnosed with Lyme disease or anaplasmosis and they develop severe disease or a poor response to usual antibiotic therapy.

TRICHINELLOSIS (TRICHINOSIS)

Trichinellosis (trichinosis) is a disease that occurs in humans who consume the larvae of *Trichinella* species (such as *spiralis* and *nativa*) that have encysted in animal muscle tissue (meat). Most of us are familiar with the risk associated with eating undercooked pork, but be aware that cases have resulted from consumption of horse meat, wild boar, bear, walrus, and cougar, the latter in jerky form (which was brined and smoked, but never heated during preparation). Squirrels, woodchucks, capybaras, mice, and rats are infected in nature.

Victims of trichinellosis first develop gastrointestinal distress (nausea, vomiting, diarrhea, and abdominal pain) during the week following ingestion of infested meat. This may continue for 4 to 6 weeks. During the second week, when the larvae are invading human muscle tissue, high fever, muscle aches, swelling (edema, puffiness) of the soft tissues around the eyes, weakness, skin rash, and joint aches develop. There may be tiny red hemorrhages under the fingernails or visible within the skin. In addition, analysis of human blood shows an unusually high count of eosinophils, which are a cell type associated with allergies and certain parasite infestations.

The migrating larvae can cause damage to the lungs (cough, bloody sputum, shortness of breath, pain with breathing), heart, and brain.

The larvae encyst in the muscle tissues, beginning the second or third week of infection, which causes muscle aches and stiffness. Then the larvae die; they become calcified 6 to 18 months after the infection first occurred.

The definitive diagnosis is made in humans by a blood test or muscle biopsy (examining a small piece of muscle harvested from the patient for *Trichinella* cysts and muscle inflammation with a concentration of eosinophils). Treatment for a person with trichinellosis is not yet totally satisfactory; it involves administration of the drug mebendazole.

Although most species of *Trichinella* are killed by freezing, there are freeze-resistant strains, so all meat that is at a high risk for carrying the parasite should be cooked thoroughly to a temperature of at least 150° F to 170° F (65.6° C to 77° C), which generally occurs when the meat turns from pink or red to gray. Certain brining solutions may kill *Trichinella;* however, the curing temperature must be sufficiently high.

LEPTOSPIROSIS

Leptospirosis is caused by spirochetes of genus *Leptospira*. The organisms are shed in the urine of wild and domestic animals, including cows, dogs, and pigs. Humans acquire the disease by contacting contaminated soil or water, which includes freshwater ponds and streams. The spirochetes can enter through nicked or abraded skin, through the mucous membranes of the eye and mouth, or by being ingested.

After an incubation period of 2 to 21 days, many victims display fever, chills, fatigue, muscle aches, headache, swollen lymph glands, and red eyes without a discharge. Nausea, vomiting, abdominal pain, and cough are common symptoms as well. This presentation lasts for about a week, and then is followed by a few days of improvement, after which a second stage of the disease begins. This is characterized by more muscle aches, nausea and vomiting, and a diffuse skin rash (red or purplish patches of skin). A sore throat, enlarged spleen, abnormal heart rhythms, low platelet count, and enlarged liver with jaundice may develop. In very severe cases, the victim may suffer from kidney and liver dysfunction, and even bleeding from the lungs.

Antibiotic treatment lessens symptoms and the duration of illness. Severe leptospirosis is treated with intravenously administered penicillin. If hospitalization is not needed, the treatment is doxycycline 100 mg by mouth twice a day, or tetracycline 500 mg four times a day, for 7 days. Other oral antibiotics that can be used are amoxicillin, cefuroxime axetil, azithromycin, penicillin, and erythromycin.

To avoid infection, it's best not to swim in freshwater ponds and streams likely to be heavily contaminated by urine from livestock or wildlife.

TULAREMIA

Tularemia is caused by the bacterium *Francisella tularensis,* which can be transmitted to humans by tick bites or by handling, skinning, or eating improperly cooked infected rabbit meat. Rarely, it can be transmitted (e.g., from a bite or handling sick or dead animals) from a cat, bear, deer, beaver, or muskrat. Even more rarely, it can be inhaled (associated with gardening and lawn care) and cause pneumonia. The incubation period after exposure to the bacteria is usually 3 to 6 days, but ranges from 1 to 21 days.

There are multiple clinical presentations of the disease, with combinations of the following signs and symptoms: painful and tender ulcers on the hand (from handling an infected animal) with associated swollen lymph glands behind the elbow and in the armpit; swollen lymph glands in the groin, associated with insect bites of the legs; sore throat; conjunctivitis in one eye with a swollen lymph gland in front of the ear on the same side; fever; headache; chills; weakness; pneumonia; and weight loss. In some cases, the victim suffers from nausea and vomiting, diarrhea, and abdominal pain.

A physician will use blood tests to confirm the diagnosis. Treatment is best rendered with intramuscular injections of streptomycin. If the victim cannot be brought to medical attention promptly, therapy may be initiated with oral doxycycline 100 mg twice a day, tetracycline 500 mg four times a day, or ciprofloxacin 750 mg twice a day for 2 to 3 weeks.

MENINGOCOCCAL DISEASE (INCLUDING MENINGITIS)

One of the most feared infectious diseases is meningitis caused by the bacterium *Neisseria meningitidis (meningococcus)*. The infection can appear in outbreaks, most commonly abroad, particularly in sub-Saharan Africa and China. The infection is spread in the respiratory secretions of humans.

The disease appears in many forms, the most common of which are meningitis, pneumonia, and disseminated bacterial infection. The typical presentation of meningitis is fever, headache, and a stiff neck (see page 162). If the cause is meningococcus, the victim may develop a skin rash, which consists of red dots or bumps, or a flat, more patchy dark red discoloration. If the dark red dots begin to enlarge and coalesce into large purplish bruise-like discolorations, this is a bad sign. In the worst cases, the victim develops shock, respiratory failure, diffuse bleeding, and death. Approximately 1 in 10 victims of meningococcal meningitis dies.

This is a true emergency. The victim needs large doses of intravenous antibiotics, such as ceftriaxone. If these aren't available, administer a high oral dose of penicillin, cephalexin, cefixime, cefpodoxime, or amoxicillin–clavulanate acid for 10 days. If the victim is allergic to penicillin, use trimethoprim–sulfamethoxazole or ciprofloxacin. Ciprofloxacin may also be administered for prophylaxis to all close ("household") contact adults in a single dose of 500 mg. Azithromycin in a single dose of 500 mg by mouth may also be effective for prophylaxis. Rifampin may also be used for this purpose in adults (600 mg a day by mouth for 2 days) and children (younger than 1 month: 5 mg/kg by mouth every 12 hours for 2 days; older than 1 month: 10 mg/kg by mouth every 12 hours for 2 days). A physician may elect to prescribe an injection of ceftriaxone for this purpose.

An effective meningococcal vaccine is available (see page 424).

RABIES

Rabies is discussed on page 369.

DEALING WITH DEATH

Despite best efforts to do the right thing, sometimes people die. They may have died of "natural causes," been severely injured, or expired because of an acute or chronic illness. The physical condition of death is described on page 34.

If you encounter a dead person in the wilderness, you must do the best you can to deal with the situation. This involves both caring for the dead person(s) and caring for the living.

HANDLING A DEAD BODY

If the body is to be recovered and transported, then do your best to handle it with dignity and respect. If there is any consideration of a communicable disease, then be particularly cautious when handling the remains. Whenever possible, use blood and bodily fluid precautions (see page 481). This is mandatory when a person has died because of Ebola virus disease, for which full PPE is essential. If possible, keep the body covered and in a cool or cold location, to attempt to limit decomposition and the accompanying difficult-to-handle sight and smells. Try to limit your and other's exposure to the body. If there is any question of foul play, try not to move or otherwise disturb what might become a crime scene. If a person is obviously dead, don't put yourself at risk trying to recover the body. Examples would include someone trapped underwater in the midst of swift water or a person who has expired after a long fall on a glacier and requires a technical approach to be retrieved. Coordinate with local authorities to obtain assistance for body recovery and transportation. If you must leave the scene without taking the body, so long as you do not suspect an infection as the cause of death, bring along whatever personal effects you can reasonably gather without compromising your ability to safely travel. These may be important to family members and friends. See page 35 for information about burial of bodies.

EMOTIONAL CONSIDERATIONS

It's natural to be sad and perhaps remorseful, frightened, or repelled by the situation. Talk to others and allow yourself to express your emotions, so long as you can function as a problem-solver. Allow others to speak to you and work through what they are feeling. Don't impose your cultural or religious beliefs on others unless they request this assistance. Be strong, be consistent, and above all, show compassion.

OBTAINING ASSISTANCE

If an American citizen dies away from the United States, try to notify a U.S. embassy or consulate.

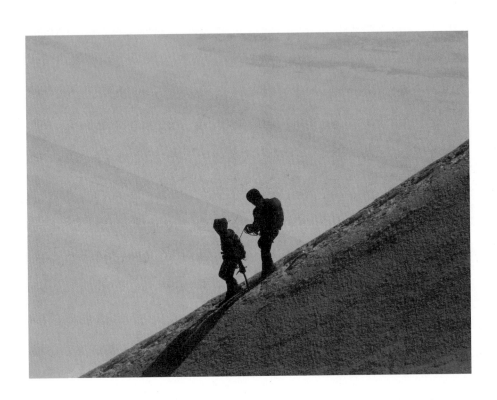

PART THREE

Minor Medical Problems

Although the afflictions discussed in this section are rarely life threatening, they account for the majority of health care problems encountered in a recreational or wilderness setting. For the sake of simplicity, this section is organized by body organ system. Specific disorders can be rapidly located by using the index.

Whenever a person becomes ill, it's wise to consider how the disorder can become worse. For instance, bronchitis can progress to pneumonia in situations of stress and suboptimal environmental conditions. Therefore, if someone develops severe bronchitis, he should not continue to travel farther from civilization until it's clear that medical management is going to halt progression of the illness.

I have not included all of the problems that originate from substance abuse or indiscriminate sexual encounters. However, it's critical to observe that drinking alcohol or using mind-altering drugs impairs judgment and is a major contributor to injuries. It is inexcusable to dull your senses when such activity places you and others at risk.

GENERAL SYMPTOMS

UNCONSCIOUS (OR SEMICONSCIOUS) VICTIM

As discussed in detail in the section "Major Medical Problems" (see page 21), a proper approach to the unconscious (comatose) victim may make the difference between life and death. You must evaluate the behaviorally changed or semiconscious (stuporous, dazed, confused, or combative) individual with the same degree of concern. To discover the cause of an altered mental status, you must be a bit of a detective, while also performing the tasks that prevent the victim from hurting himself. Always assume that an unconscious person may be seriously injured.

1. Open and maintain the airway (see page 22). Check for adequacy of the pulse (see page 30).
2. Protect the cervical spine (see page 35). *Every injured person has a broken neck until proven otherwise.*
3. Carefully examine the victim for evidence of an obvious injury and treat accordingly. Consider traumatic brain injury (see page 59).
4. Consider low blood sugar, and treat the victim with glucose if he is alert enough to cooperate (see page 133). If not, and glucagon for injection is available, consider its use (see page 134).
5. Consider that the victim may have suffered a seizure (see page 65).
6. Consider infection, in particular of the central nervous system (see page 14) or generalized and severe (see pages 137-150).
7. Consider hypothermia (see page 281).

Don't:

1. Don't shake a victim vigorously to awaken him without first protecting the neck. *Never shake a victim to awaken him if you suspect that hypothermia (see page 281) is present.*

If you think that the victim is merely intoxicated, you may snap an ammonia inhalant or hold "smelling salts" under his nose and allow him a few whiffs to stimulate awakening. If there is any chance of a neck injury, don't perform this maneuver without maintaining the head and neck in a stable position.

2. Don't attempt to carry an unconscious victim or manage a belligerent person if this might exhaust you. Send someone for help and stay with the victim until help arrives.

3. Unless there is no other way to get lifesaving help, never leave an unconscious or dazed person unattended.

FAINTING

Fainting is defined as sudden brief loss of consciousness not associated with a head injury. There are innumerable causes of fainting, but most episodes are associated with decreased blood flow (oxygen and/or glucose) to the brain. This may be caused by low blood sugar (hypoglycemia—see page 133), slow heart rate (vasovagal or "vagal" reaction, in which the vagus nerve, which slows the heart rate, is overstimulated: fright, anxiety, stomach irritation, bowel dilation, drugs, fatigue, prolonged standing in one position), rhythm disturbances of the heart, dehydration, heat exhaustion, anemia, or bleeding.

If you witness a fainting episode, or are with someone who is becoming lightheaded (sweating, weak, ashen colored, dizzy), quickly help the person lie down and elevate his legs 8 to 12 inches (20 to 30 cm). This position increases venous blood flow back to the heart, which in turn pumps more blood to the brain. If the victim begins to vomit, turn him on his side. If he has fallen, examine him for injuries. A cool, moistened cloth wiped on his forehead, on his face, and behind his neck may make the victim feel better. Don't splash or pour water on his face. Don't slap the victim's face.

After a victim suffers a fainting episode, he should be examined for any sign of serious illness or injury. If you don't suspect anything serious, have him lie still for a few minutes, and then sit for a few minutes. If the victim is alert and capable of purposeful swallowing, offer him cool sweetened liquids to drink—preferably one that contains electrolytes (see page 194)—to correct dehydration. When the victim feels normal, he may slowly regain an upright posture. If the victim is elderly, and particularly if his pulse is irregular or he has chest discomfort, seek immediate medical assistance. Anticipate a heart attack (see page 47) or stroke (see page 135).

A vagal reaction, as described earlier, is often preceded by warning signs of lightheadedness, a sensation of warmth, nausea, sweating, and "tunnel vision." It most commonly occurs in persons who are standing. If a person suddenly loses consciousness, wakes up, and does not recall any of the warning signs of a vagal reaction, particularly if it occurred during exercise or when the person was sitting or supine, then suspicion is heightened for an abnormal heart rhythm that requires formal medical evaluation.

FATIGUE

Fatigue (lethargy, tiredness, exhaustion, generalized weakness, decreasing exercise tolerance) can be a sign of any disorder or dysfunction that diminishes a person's energy level. Accompanied by fever, it can be indicative of an infection; accompanied by certain associated symptoms, it may indicate a hypoactive thyroid. In the outdoors, anyone who began the trip in good condition but is now fatigued should be examined carefully for signs and symptoms of hypothermia (see page 281), hyperthermia (see page 296), high-altitude illness (see page 306), infection, emotional depression (see page 278), anemia (pale membranes inside the eyelid, pale fingernail beds, sallow skin complexion), dehydration (see page 194), or starvation. A diabetic who becomes fatigued may suffer from high or low blood sugar (see page 133). If fatigue is accompanied by shortness of breath, don't travel any farther from civilization until you determine a treatable cause or the victim clearly improves. Sudden onset of fatigue can be indicative of a heart attack (see page 47).

If a person is suffering physical exhaustion, allow him at least 12 hours of rest, encourage adequate food intake, and take particular care to correct dehydration.

In a situation of extreme exercise within a particular muscle group—the legs during forced or military-style marching, or long-distance or marathon running; the arms during repetitive, relentless exertion such as weight lifting—muscle tissue can be broken down. This is more common under conditions of environmental heat (see page 296). Substances (particularly myoglobin, a pigment that carries oxygen) are released into the bloodstream, which in large concentrations can cause the kidneys to fail. The victim has very darkened (brown) urine (myoglobinuria), sore muscles, and extreme fatigue. In this situation, remove the victim from environmental heat, place him at as near complete rest as possible, and encourage him to drink as much liquid as he can to correct dehydration and flush the pigment from his system (see page 194).

FEVER AND CHILLS

Fever is an elevation in body temperature sometimes caused by infection. The causative organism (most commonly a bacterium or virus) releases substances into the bloodstream; these quickly reach the part of the brain that acts as the body's thermostat. Thus, body temperature is "reset" at a higher level. This probably helps fight infection, but the temperature may need to be lowered if the elevation is extreme or prolonged.

Normal body temperature is 98.6°F (37°C) measured orally, and 99.6°F (37.5°C) measured rectally. To convert degrees Fahrenheit (F) into degrees Centigrade (C, or Celsius), subtract 32, then multiply by 5, then divide by 9. To convert degrees C into degrees F, multiply by 9, then divide by 5, then add 32. A temperature conversion chart is found on page 476.

Temperature should be measured with a thermometer. Electric (digital) thermometers are easiest to use and require the least time to record a temperature. If you use a mercury or alcohol thermometer, first shake it to pool the mercury or alcohol below the 94°F (35°C) marking. If you suspect the victim to be hypothermic, a special thermometer is necessary (see page 281). To take a temperature by mouth, place the thermometer under the tongue, close the mouth, and take a reading after 3 to 4 minutes. To take a temperature rectally (the more reliable method, and necessary in a case of suspected hypothermia, so long as it can be done in a location where the patient will not be exposed to the elements and become colder), the thermometer is *gently* placed—ideally lubricated with oil or petroleum jelly—1 inch (2.5 cm) into the rectum. It is held for at least 2 minutes and then extracted and read. Never leave a child or confused adult unattended with a thermometer in the mouth or rectum. *Don't rely on skin temperature to vary consistently with changes in core body temperature.*

Armpit (axillary) temperatures are far less reliable, because they may underestimate the temperature elevation. However, a high temperature recorded from the armpit may be interpreted to mean that there is some elevation in body temperature. An armpit temperature may be the only one you get in an uncooperative child less than 2 years of age. Since such a temperature tends to read on the low side, add 1.4°F (0.8°C) to obtain the equivalent rectal temperature.

Generally, infection will not elevate the core (rectal) body temperature higher than 105°F (40.5°C). Anyone with a temperature measured above that level should be examined for heat illness (see page 296), stroke (see page 135), or drug overdose. Vigorous prolonged muscular activity (seizure or marathon running) can raise the core temperature above 107°F (41.7°C).

A child is considered to have a fever if his rectal temperature is greater than 100.4°F (38°C), oral temperature is greater than 100°F (37.8°C), or armpit temperature is greater than 99°F (37.2°C). You should be concerned about a fever greater than 100.4°F (38°C) in an infant less than 3 months of age or greater than 104°F (40°C) in any small child, because this can indicate a severe infection. If a child greater than 2 years of age has a fever greater than or equal to 106°F (41.1°C), and if there is no clear diagnosis of a viral infection, he should be treated with a broad-spectrum antibiotic (e.g., amoxicillin–clavulanate), on the rationale that there is a significant likelihood of a bacterial infection. Prolonged fever in a child should be investigated by a physician. Signs of a serious infection in an infant include lethargy ("floppy baby"), pain (persistent crying), labored breathing, purple skin rash, excessive drooling, a bulging "soft spot" (fontanel) on the top of the head, or a stiff neck.

If a person has a temperature higher than 100.5° F (38° C) that's thought to be due to an infection, he will be made more comfortable (fever lowered) by administration of aspirin, a nonsteroidal antiinflammatory drug (NSAID), or acetaminophen (Tylenol). *To avoid Reye syndrome (postviral encephalopathy and liver failure), don't use aspirin to control a fever in a child under age 17.* The traditional teaching is that infants and small children with fevers (usually due to ear infections or viral illnesses) should be treated as soon as any elevation of temperature is noted, in order to prevent febrile seizures, although this may not actually be effective. An infant (younger than 6 months) with a fever should be seen as soon as possible by a physician. Sponging a child with cold water doesn't help much to reduce fever and can even be counterproductive if the child struggles or begins to shiver, both of which generate heat. If the fever is greater than 104° F (40° C), however, sponging can be attempted using lukewarm water. Never sponge a child with alcohol, because it can be absorbed through the skin and act as a poison.

If the victim suffers from environmental heat-induced illness (see page 296), he will not benefit from and should not be given aspirin or acetaminophen. An NSAID is not as dangerous but is also *not* helpful.

Whether to use an antibiotic for a "fever of unknown origin" (a fever that cannot be definitively linked to a specific site of infection) is a judgment call. If a person has an altered immune system (acquired immunodeficiency syndrome [AIDS], cancer, diabetes, chronic corticosteroid administration) and a high or persistent fever not associated with symptoms suggestive of a particular infection, it's probably wise to administer a "broad-spectrum" antibiotic, such as ciprofloxacin or azithromycin. If there are symptoms that lead you to a specific site of infection (such as cough—pneumonia; burning on urination and flank pain—kidney infection), the appropriate antibiotic should be started. Finally, any feverish small child can become rapidly debilitated; he will rarely suffer from being given a common antibiotic, such as amoxicillin or trimethoprim–sulfamethoxazole.

Chills are caused by the release of bacteria or viruses (or their toxins) into the bloodstream. The victim will suddenly feel very cold and begin to shiver, with teeth chattering, goose bumps (piloerection), and weakness. The "chill" may actually occur during a temperature spike within a fever.

FEVER IN A RETURNED TRAVELER

It's not uncommon to acquire an infectious disease during outdoor travel, particularly to foreign (non-U.S.) countries. These illnesses are often accompanied by fever. As a general rule, infectious diseases follow periods of incubation. The incubation periods of travel-related infectious diseases, some of which may have fever as a component, are (with overlap, often because diseases may have different presentations during different stages) as follows:

- *Less than 10 days:* Influenza, dengue, yellow fever, gonorrhea, plague, ehrlichiosis, hantavirus, paratyphoid fever, Chikungunya virus, Japanese encephalitis, leptospirosis, Mediterranean spotted fever, African tick-bite fever, Rocky Mountain spotted fever, Colorado tick fever, trichinosis, tularemia, anthrax, tick-borne diseases
- *10 to 21 days:* Malaria, viral hemorrhagic fevers (such as Ebola, Rift Valley, and Marburg), typhoid fever, scrub typhus, Q fever, relapsing fever caused by *Borrelia* organisms, African trypanosomiasis, Epstein-Barr virus, hepatitis, Lyme disease
- *More than 21 days:* Malaria, filariasis, brucellosis, hepatitis (A, B, C, E), rabies, schistosomiasis, leishmaniasis, amoebic liver abscess, tuberculosis

The location of travel provides clues to the possible cause of fever. For instance, if a person has traveled to the Caribbean, then dengue and malaria are high on the list, with rare clusters of cases of histoplasmosis and leptospirosis. In sub-Saharan Africa, it would be more common to suspect malaria, tick-borne rickettsial infection, schistosomiasis, or filariasis, with less common cases of African trypanosomiasis. The Centers for Disease Control and Prevention (CDC) Health Information for International Travel *(The Yellow Book)* is an excellent resource to help guide the patient and clinician (www.cdc.gov/travel).

COUGH

Cough is a common symptom. Often associated with an upper respiratory infection, cough can also be due to throat irritation, postnasal drip, nasal irritation or inflammation, overuse of nasal spray decongestants, sinusitis, bronchitis (see page 192), serious infectious disease (e.g., pneumonia—see page 45), whooping cough (pertussis—see below), asthma (see page 42), heart failure (fluid in the lungs—see page 44), reflux esophagitis ("heartburn"—see page 208), allergy, blood clot in the lungs (see page 44), high-altitude pulmonary edema (see page 310), or drug side effect.

Treatment of cough depends on the cause. For instance, the cough associated with asthma requires that the asthma be properly treated. For the cough associated with a minor upper respiratory infection, usually viral, cough medicine may be helpful. Some suggested remedies are listed on page 470. One favored by experts is dexbrompheniramine 6 mg plus pseudoephedrine 120 mg twice daily for 1 week. An alternative is ipratropium 0.06% nasal spray, two sprays per nostril 3 to 4 times daily for 2 weeks. *A U.S. FOOD AND DRUG ADMINISTRATION ADVISORY PANEL IN 2007 RECOMMENDED THAT THERE IS NO EVIDENCE THAT OVER-THE-COUNTER COLD AND COUGH MEDICINES WORK IN CHILDREN AND THAT THE PRODUCTS SHOULD NOT BE GIVEN TO CHILDREN YOUNGER THAN 6 YEARS OF AGE.* Children ages 2 to 18 years may benefit from 2 teaspoons of buckwheat honey (buckwheat, eucalyptus, citrus, and labiatae honey have been tested; other varieties might work) for treatment of nocturnal (nighttime) coughing. *It is not advised to feed honey to infants or children under age 12 months because of the risk for infant botulism.*

Whooping cough (pertussis) is a highly communicable infectious disease of the upper respiratory system caused by the bacterium *Bordetella pertussis* or *B. parapertussis.* Other species of *Bordetella* may cause disease in humans. It is transmitted by respiratory secretions or large droplets from the respiratory tract of an infected person. In children, whooping cough is typified by coughing episodes that are sudden, intense, and sometimes accompanied by vomiting and inspiratory "whoops," indicating throat spasms on inhalation. Most deaths from whooping cough occur in children younger than 12 months of age. It's not uncommon for the victim to cough in severe spells and to have gagging or vomiting after a coughing spell. The incubation period after exposure is usually 7 to 10 days. In adults, whooping cough most commonly presents like a common cold (nasal congestion, sore throat, red eyes, mild cough, slight fever) for a week or two (this is the most infectious period). The cough then becomes progressively severe. The cough in both children and adults is described as fits of repeated coughing during a single exhalation, followed by a "whooping" inspiration. After coughing, the victim may be exhausted or vomit. It may involve difficulty breathing. Persons with whooping cough usually appear well between coughing fits, which may be so severe as to cause nosebleeds, severe chest wall muscle strain, or even broken ribs. Untreated, the cough may last for 6 to 10 weeks in children and for more than 100 days in adults, as the illness gradually subsides. If this diagnosis is made, the victim should be treated with azithromycin (10 mg/kg of body weight [not to exceed 250 mg] by mouth once a day on day 1, then 5 mg/kg on days 2 through 5 for children; 500 mg day 1, then 250 mg days 2 through 5 for adults); erythromycin (40 to 50 mg/kg per day in four divided doses [not to exceed 2 g per day] for 14 days for children; 500 mg four times a day for 14 days for adults); clarithromycin (15 mg/kg per day in two divided does [not to exceed 1 g per day] for 7 days for children; 500 mg twice a day for 7 days for adults); or trimethoprim–sulfamethoxazole (8 mg/40 mg/kg per day in two divided doses for 14 days for children; 160 mg/800 mg twice daily for 14 days for adults). All of the aforementioned doses for children are for ages 6 months or older. For infants ages 1 to 5 months, the doses are azithromycin 10 mg/kg once a day for 5 days, erythromycin 40 to 50 mg/kg per day in four divided doses for 14 days, or clarithromycin 15 mg/kg/day in two divided doses for 7 days. Antibiotic administration shortens the course of the disease if started within 3 weeks of the onset of cough symptoms. After that time, antibiotics don't shorten the course of the disease, but may help prevent disease spread. The protective effect of diphtheria-tetanus-pertussis (DTaP) vaccine wanes 5 to 10 years after the last dose, so adults remain vulnerable to the disease if they don't receive booster immunizations of Tdap vaccine. This is recommended for persons ages 11 to 64 years.

   Croup is a disease of children, rarely seen in adults, in which there is hoarseness, raspy breathing on inhalation, and a seal-like, barking cough associated with narrowing of the soft tissues of the larynx. If croup is suspected, the victim should be given a single oral dose of a corticosteroid, such as dexamethasone (0.6 mg/kg [2.2 lb] body weight for a child, up to 4 mg total dose; 4 mg for an adult). While some support the home remedy of breathing cool air, there is no evidence that breathing cool air, warm air, or humidified air makes any difference in resolving the illness. If croup is very severe, a health care practitioner may administer inhaled epinephrine.

COUGHING BLOOD

The blood coughed up by a victim may have originated anywhere from the mouth to the lungs. Causes of coughing blood include the following.

Sore Throat

The victim will complain of an irritated throat and difficulty swallowing, and will cough up whitish phlegm streaked with blood. If the victim is not short of breath or in distress, rapid medical attention is not necessary (see page 44). If a person has a nosebleed, he may cough and spit a lot of blood (see page 179).

Pneumonia

The victim will complain of fever, chills, chest pain, and shortness of breath. He may cough up green or rust-colored thick sputum (see page 45).

Pulmonary Embolism

The victim will complain of difficult and painful breathing, shortness of breath, agitation, and weakness. Generally, only severely ill persons will cough up small clots of blood (see page 44).

Lung Cancer

The victim will suddenly cough up small pieces of spongy lung tissue or tumor, along with blood clots. Attend to the airway (see page 22) and seek medical attention.

Lung Injury

If a victim is struck in the chest, and particularly if his ribs are broken, the underlying lung can be bruised or torn. The victim will cough up small clots of blood or, if the injury is major, mouthfuls of blood. This is extremely serious and requires constant attention to the airway (see pages 22 and 40).

HICCUPS (HICCOUGHS)

Hiccups are sudden inhalations (caused by involuntary rhythmic contractions of the diaphragm and breathing muscles) immediately followed by rapid closure of the opening between the vocal cords. There is no known physiologic purpose for hiccups. Usually they last a moment or two and are a mere annoyance. However, they sometimes persist and become fatiguing or painful. There are many anecdotal remedies, which include biting into a lemon or lime, taking repetitive small sips of liquid for at least 30 seconds, causing a fright, gargling with or immersing the face into ice water, breath-holding or hyperventilating for 30 seconds, eating a teaspoon of granulated sugar (with or without peanut butter), or pulling on the tongue. One method is to gently stimulate the back of the throat with a spoon, just to the point of causing the victim to gag. If all else fails, a more aggressive technique is to gently stimulate the back of the inside of the nose by carefully passing a thick fishing line (e.g., leader) up into one nostril until it is just felt to tickle the back of the throat (without gagging the person). Leave the line in that position and slightly jiggle it until the hiccups (hopefully) cease, then remove it by pulling it back out the way it entered. Take care to use a long enough length of line so that there is no chance of losing your grip and having the line lost inside the nose or throat, and don't force it up into the nose—it should slide easily without pain, scraping, or causing a nosebleed. An alternative to fishing line is a well-greased length of very thin, flexible rubber tubing.

DIZZINESS

Dizziness is a feeling of lightheadedness, with or without a sensation of spinning (vertigo). It often precedes a fainting episode (see page 154) or may accompany a stroke (see page 135), heart attack (see page 47), low blood sugar (see page 133), heat illness (see page 296), ear infection (see page 163), the bends (see page 362), plant poisoning (see page 374), motion sickness (see page 411), and many other disorders. Frequently, dizziness is caused by an infection or disorder of the middle ear, which controls balance. Indeed, if the external ear canals are blocked by wax, this alone can cause dizziness.

If a victim is dizzy, he should lie on his back and attempt to regain orientation to his surroundings. Examine him for obvious causes and treat accordingly. If the dizziness does not resolve, and particularly if the victim is elderly (in which case it might indicate a stroke), he should be taken to a physician. True vertigo is very distressing to the victim and described by him as "the room spinning around," with nausea and/or vomiting, weakness, ringing in the ears (tinnitus), and occasional slow jerking or fluttering movements of the eyeballs (nystagmus). Benign paroxysmal (sudden) positional vertigo (BPPV) may be caused by free-floating calcium carbonate crystals in the inner ear. It is typified by episodes of a spinning sensation lasting for a minute or less, usually caused by a change in head position, accompanied sometimes by nausea and vomiting. It usually resolves spontaneously or can be remedied by head repositioning maneuvers performed by someone properly trained in these techniques.

Inflammation of the inner ear (often associated with a recent cold) is known as vestibular neuronitis ("labyrinthitis"). It is treated with the same medications used for motion sickness (see page 411). In addition, a 3-week taper of a corticosteroid (such as methylprednisolone) in a starting dose similar to that for a severe poison oak rash (see page 218) may hasten recovery. Antiviral agents have not been proved effective for this condition. The benzodiazepine class of drugs (including lorazepam or clonazepam 0.5 mg by mouth twice a day, or diazepam 2 to 5 mg by mouth every 6 hours as needed) may be useful to suppress vertigo, but carry the side effect of sedation. If dizziness is accompanied by nausea and vomiting, it may be helpful to give the patient ondansetron (4 mg dissolving tablet) or another anti-vomiting medication (see page 467). Vestibular neuronitis is a diagnosis to be reached by a physician after more serious problems are excluded.

If BPPV is suspected, it's worth attempting to reposition the particles within the inner ear that might be irritating the hair cells that affect balance. This is done by having the patient lie at a slight head-down incline with one ear down until the vertigo is gone or nearly gone. Then, have the patient turn his head to have the other ear down. From this point forward, assist the patient (with patient's chin tucked to chest) to a sitting position and see if the symptoms are gone. If the vertigo recurs, move the patient sequentially through the following two positions for a minute or two, allowing symptoms to subside: lying on one side with nose turned to the ground, and lying on the opposite side with nose turned to the ground. Then, check the sitting position to see if these maneuvers have been successful.

HEAD (ALSO EYE, EAR, NOSE, THROAT, AND MOUTH)

HEADACHE

Worrisome headaches (some of which are described later) include those that are made worse by holding one's breath and straining; associated with fever and/or chills; progressive in frequency or severity; of sudden onset; associated with "focal" and persistent neurologic findings (such as weakness in an arm or leg); associated with a stiff neck; where the pupils of the eyes are unequal; where there is a rash of herpes infection; when accompanied by a dental abscess; with head injury; or accompanied by any new diffuse body rash. In these cases, one should seek prompt medical attention.

Tension or fatigue headache is characterized by throbbing pain in the temples, over the eyes, and in the posterior neck and shoulder muscles. It can be treated with rest, sunglasses, and moderate pain medication, such as aspirin or acetaminophen every 3 to 4 hours. Sometimes, applying warm packs or massage to tense muscles relaxes them and helps relieve the pain.

Migraine headache is generally more severe. It is defined as episodic attacks of headache lasting 4 to 72 hours and characterized by at least two of the following: moderate to severe intensity, one-sided pain, throbbing or "pulsating," and worsening with movement. In addition, there is nausea or vomiting, which may be treated with promethazine (Phenergan) or metoclopramide (Reglan). Ondansetron (Zofran) may not be as effective, and may worsen the headache. There may be aversion to light (photophobia) or sound (phonophobia). Migraine headaches have many variations, which may include stuffy or runny nose and weakness of an arm or a leg, difficulty with balance, speech impairment, diminished hearing, or double vision. Some people experience an "aura" before the "classic" migraine headache, in which they may smell strange odors or see flashing lights. Others develop tunnel vision—diminished peripheral vision. The headaches are characterized as excruciating, pounding, or explosive. They commonly awaken people from sleep. Occasionally they will respond to NSAIDs, but often require stronger pain medications. A person suffering from a migraine should be placed in a quiet, dark area to minimize external stimuli. He should be encouraged to drink enough liquid to treat or prevent dehydration and offered an NSAID, ketorolac, acetaminophen, or aspirin. Caffeine may be helpful (or make the situation worse—see later).

Specific antimigraine medications include the "triptans," such as sumatriptan (Imitrex), naratriptan (Amerge), rizatriptan (Maxalt), and zolmitriptan (Zomig). These medications should be given as early as possible in the course of the headache to achieve maximal effectiveness. Other medicines that are effective include propranolol or metoprolol, amitriptyline, methysergide, flunarizine, and prochlorperazine (Compazine) given with diphenhydramine (Benadryl). Ergotamine drugs (such as dihydroergotamine mesylate [Migranal] nasal spray) directly constrict arteries; these should only be used under the direct supervision of a physician, since they may worsen the effects of certain types of migraines. If other drugs aren't effective, dexamethasone in an adult dose of 8 mg by mouth may be effective. If an oxygen (see page 405) tank is available, the victim may get some relief by breathing 10 liters per minute by face mask. An elderly person with a severe migraine, which may be confused with a stroke (see page 135), should seek immediate medical attention. A migraine headache may be precipitated by lack of sleep, high altitude, emotional stress, fatigue, dehydration, bright lights, loud noises, types of weather, missing meals, excessive exercise, cyclical hormone changes, noxious odors, and certain ingested substances (such as caffeine and monosodium glutamate). Therefore, the migraine sufferer should seek to obtain regular sleep (go to bed and wake up at the same times every day), rest, and meals (don't skip or delay); limit caffeine consumption to the equivalent of two cups of coffee or two 12-ounce sodas per day; avoid tobacco products; avoid known personal triggers (e.g., red wine); practice relaxation techniques; and strive to maintain fitness through regular exercise and dietary discretion. For certain sufferers, a neurologist may prescribe topiramate (Topamax) to be taken between episodes of migraine to reduce the frequency of headaches.

The Cerena Transcranial Magnetic Stimulator is a device for treatment of migraine headache that's preceded by an aura (see earlier). It works by releasing a pulse of magnetic energy to stimulate the occipital cortex in the brain, which may stop or lessen the pain of the headache. The Cefaly device is a small, portable, battery-powered unit that is worn like a headband across the forehead. It applies an electric current to the skin and underlying tissues to simulate branches of the trigeminal nerve.

Cluster headache is on one side of the head, is severe and lasts from 30 to 90 minutes, and is associated with eye redness and tearing, runny or congested nose, and sometimes eyelid swelling. The headaches may occur many times in a day and are not usually associated with nausea and vomiting. The same treatments for migraine, particularly inhalation of oxygen, are sometimes effective for cluster headaches. Prevention techniques are likewise similar.

Paroxysmal hemicrania is somewhat similar to cluster headache in that it is an adult headache that involves severe throbbing pain on one side of the face, in-around-and-behind the eye, and perhaps all the way to the back of the head and neck. It also has similar eye and nose symptoms. The headache comes in "attack" form, lasting 2 to 3 minutes up to 40 times per day. It is debilitating. This type of headache shows amazing relief after administration of the NSAID indomethacin (Indocin) 25 mg by mouth two or three times per day.

Sinus headache is associated with sinus infection (see page 181) and is typified by fever, nasal congestion, production of a foul nasal discharge, and pain produced by tapping over the affected sinus(es). It should be treated with an oral decongestant (pseudoephedrine), nasal spray (Neo-Synephrine 0.25% or Afrin 0.05%), an antibiotic (azithromycin, amoxicillin–clavulanate, erythromycin, or ampicillin), and warm packs applied over the affected sinus(es).

Occipital neuralgia is pain in the back of the head, upper neck, and sometimes up over the top of the head, and less commonly behind the eyes. It is attributed to damage to the occipital nerves. The pain becomes chronic, and the sufferer describes it as sharp, shocking, or stabbing. In addition to the medications used to treat migraine headaches, there may be relief from rest and local application of heat, and in the hands of a skilled medical practitioner, nerve blocks with anesthetic drugs or even surgery to cut or decompress the nerves.

Subarachnoid hemorrhage is bleeding that occurs, usually suddenly, from a leaking blood vessel (commonly an aneurysm) underneath the thin tissue layer that surrounds the brain and spinal cord. The headache is usually sudden in onset, described as "the worst headache of my life," and may be associated with a fainting spell, altered mental status, seizure, and collapse. If a person suffers a subarachnoid hemorrhage and remains awake, he may complain of a stiff or painful neck with or without back pain about 2 to 4 hours after the bleed. Anyone who complains of a severe headache after extreme physical straining (such as lifting a heavy weight or having a difficult bowel movement) or who collapses suddenly after reporting a headache should be suspected to have suffered a subarachnoid hemorrhage and be brought rapidly to a hospital.

Meningitis, an infection that involves the lining of the brain and spinal cord, is a true emergency. The headache of meningitis is severe and often accompanied by nausea, vomiting, photophobia, fever, altered mental status, and weakness. A purplish skin rash indicates infection with the bacteria *Neisseria meningitidis,* a particularly fulminant and contagious form ("meningococcal") of infectious meningitis. The classic signs of meningitis are a stiff neck with a fever. The victim demonstrates extreme discomfort when the chin is flexed downward against the chest, and may complain that the pain also occurs in the back (along the course of the spinal cord). It's important to note that an infant can suffer meningitis without a stiff neck and may present only with poor feeding, fever, vomiting, seizures, and extreme lethargy ("floppy baby"). If meningitis is suspected, the victim must be evacuated rapidly. If antibiotics are available, the recommendations currently given to doctors for antibiotics are as follows: age 16 to 50 years, vancomycin plus either cefotaxime or ceftriaxone; age greater than 50 years, vancomycin plus either cefotaxime or ceftriaxone, as well as ampicillin.

Giant cell arteritis is a type of inflammation that occurs in elders (it is rare in persons younger than 50 years of age) that can affect the temporal artery, which travels in a path along the sides of the scalp over the ears (temples). The associated headache may be quite severe and accompanied by thickened and tender arteries that may be noticeably enlarged with or without overlying reddened skin. Pulses may or may not be appreciated in these arteries, and the victim may have pain radiating down the side of the face as low as into the jaw. Permanent partial or complete loss of vision may occur in one or both eyes, which makes this condition an emergency. The immediate treatment is administration of a high dose of a corticosteroid, such as prednisone 80 to 100 mg by mouth each day until a physician can evaluate the patient. Hopefully, symptoms will improve within a few days of beginning the corticosteroid medication. Corticosteroids are interchangeable to a certain degree. If you must substitute, here is a rough measure of equivalence: 20 mg prednisone equals 16 mg methylprednisolone equals 3 mg dexamethasone.

A headache that is atypically severe or prolonged may represent a serious problem, such as accelerated (out of control) high blood pressure (hypertension), brain tumor, infection, glaucoma, blood clot within the brain, carbon monoxide poisoning, inflammation of the temporal artery, or hemorrhage. The victim should be evaluated by a physician at the earliest opportunity. If a person develops a severe headache associated with a fainting spell or stiff neck, or is known to suffer from high blood pressure, keep him as calm as possible and urgently seek assistance. If high blood pressure is known to be the problem, and the victim is taking antihypertensive drugs, he should be advised to avoid using medications or other substances that might counteract the effects of his antihypertensives. These include ephedra, phenylephrine, certain herbal supplements (such as ginseng and yohimbine), appetite suppressants, anabolic steroids, and certain NSAIDs.

In general, *particularly worrisome headaches* include a single headache that is the "first" or "worst" of a person's life; headache with a fever that is not explained by an obvious illness; headache with vomiting that is not explained by an obvious illness; headache associated with a neurologic sign, such as weakness or altered speech; headache associated with altered mental status; headache associated with neck pain when the chin is flexed to the chest; progressively worsening headache; sudden headache in an elder; headache in someone suffering from cancer; headache after a blow to the head; headache following an episode of loss of consciousness; or headache in someone suffering from immunosuppression.

When at high altitude (see page 306), always first assume that a headache is a high-altitude headache, a manifestation of acute mountain sickness, or part of evolving high-altitude cerebral edema. It's important to differentiate these problems from other causes of headache, because prompt descent from high altitude may effectively treat the headache, or more important, save a person's life.

BELL'S PALSY

Bell's palsy is a form of facial paralysis caused by a problem with the seventh (facial) cranial nerve that supplies the face. The palsy is rapid in onset and can cause the muscles of one side of the face to be completely paralyzed less than 72 hours after the first weakness is noted. There is usually no pain except perhaps a slight discomfort behind the ear on the affected side. This pain may appear a day or two before the weakness. Bell's palsy may mimic a stroke. With Bell's palsy, the muscles of the forehead are affected. If they are not, the victim should be immediately evacuated for a full medical evaluation. The cause of Bell's palsy may be involvement of the nerve with herpes virus. Another cause is Lyme disease, for which the victim may need to be treated (see page 146). The current recommendation is to treat with prednisone 1 mg/kg (2.2 lb) of body weight by mouth per day for 7 to 10 days. It's often recommended to also treat with the antiviral drug acyclovir (800 mg by mouth five times a day for 7 days) or valacyclovir (1000 mg by mouth twice a day for 7 days). Antiviral therapy alone without prednisone (or another oral steroid) is not advised. It's also important to protect the eye if the victim cannot close his eye or blink. The eye can be patched or gently taped closed to protect the cornea, and artificial tears (see page 174) may be used to keep the surface of the eye moist.

EAR

Earache

An earache may be caused by infection, injury, or a foreign body in the ear. For a discussion of ear squeeze (barotitis) that occurs with scuba diving, see page 363.

Ear Infection

Ear infection can be either internal (otitis media) or external (otitis externa) to the eardrum (tympanic membrane) (Figure 131).

Otitis media. Infection may occur that reddens and inflames the eardrum and causes blood, serum, or pus to collect behind the drum (see Figure 131, *B*). With otitis media (middle ear infection), there is no drainage from the external ear canal (unless the eardrum ruptures, which is unusual in an adult, although more common in a child) and the victim has a fever, often with a sore throat. In many cases, the victim has a history of prior infections. Most often, otitis media occurs in children; when it occurs in an adult, it may be associated with a sinus infection or functional obstruction of the eustachian tube (the pressure-release mechanism from the middle ear into the throat). A young child can rapidly become severely ill from otitis media; an infant may develop meningitis (see page 162) following an ear infection. In a few medical studies, children who chewed

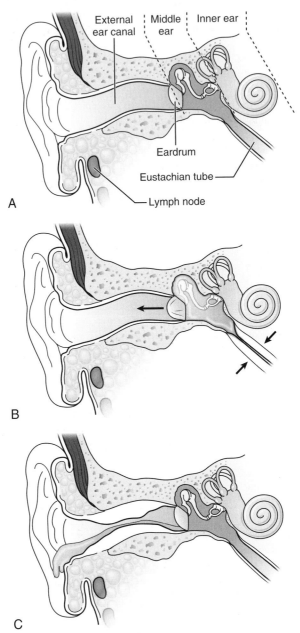

Figure 131. Ear infections. **A,** Normal ear anatomy. **B,** Otitis media (inner ear infection). The eardrum bulges outward as the middle ear fills with fluid. The eustachian tube narrows or closes. **C,** Otitis externa (external ear canal infection). The canal becomes swollen and drains pus.

sugarless gum containing xylitol (or who ingested syrup or granules containing xylitol—a sugar alcohol), which is derived from birch trees, may have had fewer ear infections. This is supposedly because xylitol inhibits the growth of certain bacteria that cause the infections. Neither this approach nor giving xylitol oral solution as a medication has been definitively proved effective at lowering ear infections. However, it's reasonable to advise children prone to ear infections to avoid table sugar–containing gum or candies.

Although many cases of otitis media in children are caused by viruses, such as respiratory syncytial virus, and resolve without antibiotic treatment, if you're distant from physician care and suspect otitis media, treat the child victim with an antibiotic. Adults and children should be treated with amoxicillin (80 to 100 mg/kg [2.2 lb] of body weight per day in three divided doses), amoxicillin–clavulanate (same dose of the amoxicillin component as for amoxicillin), cefdinir (14 mg/kg once daily or in two divided doses), cefpodoxime (10 mg/kg once daily or in two divided doses), cefuroxime (15 mg/kg in two divided doses), or clarithromycin for 10 days, or with azithromycin for 5 days. An additional antibiotic choice for adults is moxifloxacin 400 mg once a day for 10 days. An additional antibiotic choice for children is erythromycin–sulfisoxazole for 10 days. Other antibiotics that have been approved for treatment are cephalexin, cefprozil, loracarbef, and ceftibuten. Aspirin, ibuprofen, or acetaminophen should be used to control fever. *To avoid Reye syndrome (postviral encephalopathy and liver failure), don't use aspirin to control fever in a child under age 17.*

Otitis externa (swimmer's ear). Infection, commonly from the bacterium *Pseudomonas aeruginosa,* that develops in the external ear canal (often noted in swimmers and divers who don't keep the canal completely dry) rarely involves the eardrum (see Figure 131, C). When the external canal is kept moist, it's easier for bacteria to invade the skin and cause infection. The earliest symptom may be itching and a sensation of fullness. Subsequent symptoms include a white to yellow-green liquid or cheesy discharge from the ear, pain inside the ear, and decreased hearing. Not infrequently, the victim complains of exquisite tenderness when the external portions of the ear are tugged or with jaw motion and has tender, swollen lymph glands in the neck on the affected side. In a severe case, the victim may have a fever and appear toxic, and there may be cellulitis (see page 222) of the external ear and adjacent skin.

If the victim has only a discharge without fever, swollen lymph glands, or cellulitis, he may be treated with ear drops, such as acetic acid 2% solution (acetic acid otic); ascetic acid 2% with hydrocortisone 1% (Acetasol HC); or 2% nonaqueous acetic acid (VōSoL or Domeboro Otic). Household vinegar (approximately 5% acetic acid) diluted 1:1 with fresh water or with rubbing (isopropyl) alcohol (approximately 70%) can be used as a substitute. These ear drops should be administered four to five times a day for 7 days and may be retained with a cotton or gauze wick gently placed into the external ear canal, or by using an expanding foam ear sponge (such as a Speedi-Wick, Shippert Medical Technologies). To avoid injuring the eardrum, don't attempt to clean out the ear with a cotton swab or similar object. The solution should be retained in the ear for a minimum of 5 minutes with each application. If there is any suggestion that the eardrum may be punctured (e.g., the presence of bleeding), don't use this solution. After beginning to use the ear drops, most persons begin to feel significantly better within 48 to 72 hours, and have few or no symptoms within 7 days. If symptoms persist beyond a week, then continue therapy for up to 7 more days and see a doctor.

If the victim has a discharge with fever and/or swollen lymph glands, the ear drops should at a minimum contain hydrocortisone (VōSoL HC); he should also be given oral ciprofloxacin, levofloxacin, erythromycin, or penicillin. Antibiotic-containing ear drops that may be useful are ciprofloxacin 0.2% with hydrocortisone 1% (Cipro HC otic suspension);

ciprofloxacin 0.3% with dexamethasone 0.1% (Ciprodex); neomycin-polymyxin B-hydrocortisone (Cortisporin Otic); ofloxacin 0.3% otic solution (Floxin otic) 0.3%; and finafloxacin otic suspension (Xtoro). Ear drops are used three to four times a day for 7 days. If the discharge from the ear is gray or black, a fungal infection may also exist, in which case tolnaftate 1% solution may be added to the treatment regimen. Aspirin, ibuprofen, or acetaminophen should be used to control fever. *To avoid Reye syndrome (postviral encephalopathy and liver failure), don't use aspirin to control fever in a child under age 17.*

To prevent swimmer's ear, the external ear canal should be irrigated with VōSoL, Domeboro Otic solution (2% acetic acid, aluminum acetate, sodium acetate, and boric acid), diluted vinegar/alcohol (described earlier) or a 50:50 mixture, or an over-the-counter drying aid like Swim-EAR after each scuba dive or immersion episode in the water. Keep the solution in the canal for a full minute before allowing it to drain. Another product is ClearEars, which are earplugs that absorb moisture and are discarded after no more than a few uses.

The Mack's DryEar warm air ear dryer is a small, portable device to prevent and treat ear disorders by drying the ear canal. The airflow from this device runs for 80 seconds at a comfortable temperature and dries the outer ear canal. The device has a customized computer chip that directs a heater and fan to regulate the flow of warm air into the ear canal. The DryEar is equipped with a rechargeable lithium ion battery and can run 50 times before requiring a recharge. The device is not waterproof, so one must take care when carrying it near the water, and store it in a safe, dry location.

Referred Pain

"Referred" pain is pain that appears in one body region but actually originates in another. This occurs because different body regions are supplied with nerves that share common central pathways. In the case of ear pain, the cause may be a sore throat, tooth infection, or arthritic jaw. The ear pain will not disappear until the underlying cause is corrected.

Injury to the Eardrum

If something is poked into the ear, a hard blow is struck to the external ear, a diver descends rapidly without equalizing the pressure in his middle ear (see page 363), or a person is subjected to a loud explosive noise, the eardrum may be ruptured. This causes immediate intense pain and possibly loss of hearing, along with occasional nausea, vomiting, and dizziness. If the eardrum is ruptured, cover the external ear to prevent the ingress of dirt, and seek the aid of a physician. If debris has entered the ear, start the victim on penicillin or erythromycin by mouth. Don't put liquid medicine into the ear if you suspect that the eardrum is ruptured. If the dizziness is disabling, administer medicine for motion sickness (see page 411). Use appropriate pain medication.

Foreign Body in the Ear

A foreign body in the ear can be incredibly painful, particularly if it is dancing on the eardrum or resting against the sensitive lining of the ear canal. An inanimate foreign body (a piece of corn, peanut, foxtail, stone, or the like) can be left in the ear until an ear specialist with special forceps or irrigation equipment can remove it. If a live creature (cockroach, bee) enters the external ear canal and causes pain that's intolerable, the ear should be filled with 2% to 4% liquid lidocaine (topical anesthetic), which will (slowly) numb the ear and drown the bug at the same time. If lidocaine is not available, mineral oil can be used, with the caution that it will frequently cause the insect to struggle, which may encourage a sting or bite and incredible temporary pain. Rubbing alcohol will work, but may also cause pain. Once the animal is dead (a few minutes), a gentle attempt should be made with small tweezers to remove it. Don't attempt this unless you can see part of the bug, however. Don't push the bug in farther, or you might rupture the eardrum. If a dry bean or seed has become tightly trapped in the ear, don't use water to try to remove it, because the object will swell and become more impacted.

Wax in the Ear

If hearing is diminished in an ear because of a wax (cerumen) plug, the wax must first be softened with a solution such as Cerumenex or Debrox. Another useful wax softener is docusate sodium (Colace) solution. Put a few drops in the ear (retained by a wick or cotton) four to five times a day for 1 to 3 days. This will turn hard ear wax into mush. If none of these is available, household hydrogen peroxide might work. Then use a forceful stream of lukewarm water to flush out the wax. You can fashion a flushing device by attaching a plastic 18-gauge intravenous catheter (without the needle) to an 8 to 30 mL syringe. Don't try to clean out the ear with a cotton-tipped swab or other rigid object, because you may force the wax down deeper, perforate the eardrum, or scrape and cut the exquisitely sensitive skin that lines the external ear canal, setting up an infection. After the wax is removed, gently instill a few drops of vinegar or isopropyl (rubbing) alcohol in order to remove residual water and prevent external otitis (swimmer's ear) (see page 165).

EYE

The anatomy of the eye is shown in Figure 132. A proper eye examination is composed of an inspection for obvious injury to the eye or soft tissues surrounding the eye; assessment of the ability to see (visual acuity); muscular motion of the eyes; pupils for size, shape, equality, and whether they constrict when a bright light is shined into them; and the presence of blood or pus underneath the cornea. To check visual acuity, have the victim read something, one eye at a time, at a distance of about 16 inches. If the person uses glasses, have him wear them. If the victim cannot read, have him let you know the extent of his vision (e.g., can count fingers, detect hand motion, differentiate light from dark, or is blind).

When examining the pupils, note the following:

1. If the pupils are unequal, this might indicate an injury to the eye (see Figure 46). If the victim is unconscious and one or more pupils are widely dilated, it may indicate a brain

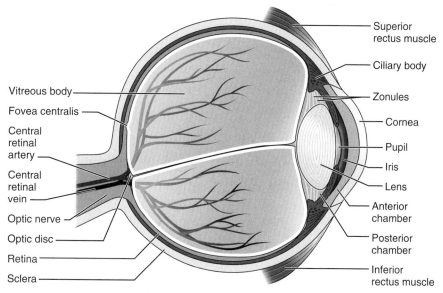

Figure 132. Anatomy of the eye.

injury. If one pupil is widely dilated and the victim is awake and seems otherwise normal, it might be the effect of having touched the eye with a medication.

2. If a bright light is shined in one eye, both pupils should constrict equally. Make note if this is not the case.

3. If the pupil is irregular (e.g., not round) in shape, there may be a penetrating injury to the eye.

Remember to protect your eyes in situations where they will be exposed to excessive ultraviolet (UV) light, wind, sand, dirt, flying objects (e.g., bungee cords or ice chips), toxic chemicals or plants, and so forth. This can be done by wearing sturdy goggles, sunglasses, or safety (shatter-proof) glasses.

Chemical Injury to the Eye

A chemical burn of the eye is a true emergency. If any acid, alkali, spitting cobra venom, skunk musk, or other chemical irritant is splashed into the eye, immediately flush the eye with cool water. Assist the victim in holding the eyelids open. Continue the irrigation for at least 30 minutes for exposure to acid and 60 minutes for alkali. Try to use at least 2 liters of liquid to irrigate the eye. It may take many more liters to remove acid or alkali, but these first 2 liters are a good start. Don't patch the eye closed, and seek immediate medical attention. If you are far from care, inspect the eye carefully for retained particles and remove them with a moistened cotton-tipped swab. Administer ofloxacin (Ocuflox) ophthalmic solution 0.3%, moxifloxacin 0.5% (Vigamox), or gatifloxacin 0.3% (Zymar) (1 to 2 drops four times a day) until the eye is healed.

If "superglue" comes in contact with the eyelids and they become glued shut, gently try to pull them apart. If this is not possible, apply Neosporin or bacitracin ointment to the eyelid margins and cover the eye with a patch. In 24 to 48 hours, the glue should dissolve and soften to allow the eyelids to separate. Don't use "superglue remover," which may contain acetone and is harmful to the cornea (clear surface of the eye). If antiseptic ointment is not available, patch the eye closed overnight with the eye pads presoaked with water. This may loosen the bond and allow the eyelids to be separated.

Foreign Body Under the Eyelid and Scratched Cornea; Corneal Ulcer

If a foreign body lodges on the cornea (the clear surface of the eye) without actual penetration of the eyeball, irrigate the eye copiously with an eyewash solution (use water if you don't have eyewash). If this is not successful, have the victim look downward, grasp his upper lid firmly by the eyelashes, and fold it up and inside out (evert it) over a cotton swab (Figure 133). You can lightly grease the swab with antiseptic ointment to keep it from sticking to the skin. If you can

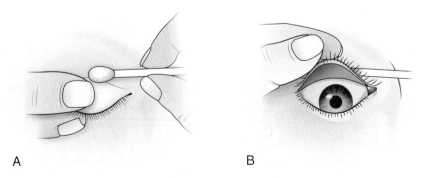

A   B

Figure 133. Eversion of the eyelid to locate a foreign body. **A,** The lid is grasped and pulled over a cotton swab or small blunt stick. **B,** The underside of the eyelid is inspected for a foreign body while the victim looks downward.

see the foreign body on the undersurface of the upper eyelid, gently wipe it away with a cotton swab or piece of moistened cloth. If you don't see the object, check between the lower eyelid and the eyeball. After the inspection, pull down on the eyelashes to unfold the lid.

Once you have removed the object, if the victim still feels as if something is in his eye, he may have suffered a scratch on the cornea (corneal abrasion). If the victim can tolerate the discomfort, don't patch the eye closed. Have the victim try wearing sunglasses to diminish the discomfort. If the discomfort does not allow the victim to remain safe (e.g., needs to walk along a trail with the potential for a serious fall), then it may help control the discomfort to patch the eye closed for 24 hours. However, be aware that this will not hasten healing, and because of the loss of binocular vision, may impair depth perception. Furthermore, *never patch an eye closed if there is any sign of an active infection* (pus or discharge). When the patch is removed, if there is residual pain, a gritty sensation, gooey discharge, or blurred vision, see a doctor as soon as possible. Tiny objects, such as the spine of a horse nettle (sand brier), can become embedded in the cornea and not be visible without the magnification available to an ophthalmologist.

To patch an eye, a ½-inch (1.3 cm) thick pad of soft cloth or bandage should be shaped to fit neatly over the eye socket, and affixed snugly to the face with tape or bandages extending across the patch onto the cheek below and the forehead opposite the affected eye (Figure 134). Prepackaged sterile elliptical eye pads are available. If only tape is available, the eyelids may be taped closed with a single small piece of tape.

Another way to hold an eye shield, patch, or padding around the eye is with a cravat (see page 170). First, place a strip of cloth approximately 2 inches (5 cm) wide and 15 inches (38 cm) long over the top of the head front-to-back, so that the face-side end hangs over the uninjured eye, near the nose. Place the patch, pad, or shield over the eye and hold it in place with a cravat, which should be wrapped horizontally around the head and then tied in position on top of the hanging cloth strip. Make the first tie (single loop or half square knot) in the cravat behind the head and at the base of the skull and keep wrapping it around to complete the final tie (square knot) where the ends meet. If the final tie will be over an eye, shift the cravat. Pull up the ends of the hanging cloth strip and tie them at the top of the head; this should lift the cravat up off the uninjured eye (Figure 135).

For a scratched cornea, administer an antibiotic in the unpatched affected eye until it is healed, which usually occurs in 3 to 5 days. Use ofloxacin (Ocuflox) ophthalmic solution 0.3%, moxifloxacin 0.5% (Vigamox), or gatifloxacin 0.3% (Zymar) one or two drops to the affected eye every 3 to 4 hours, or a ribbon of erythromycin ophthalmic ointment every 6 hours. If the scratched cornea is caused by contact lens overuse, instruct the victim to not wear contacts until

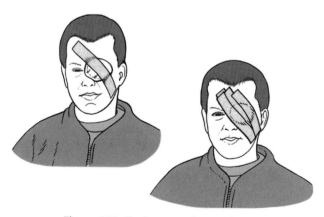

Figure 134. Taping a patch over the eye.

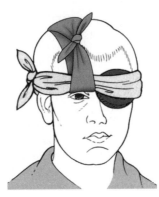

Figure 135. Holding an eye patch in place with a cravat. Hang a cloth strip over the uninjured eye. Hold the patch in place with a cravat. Tie the cloth strip to lift the cravat off the uninjured eye.

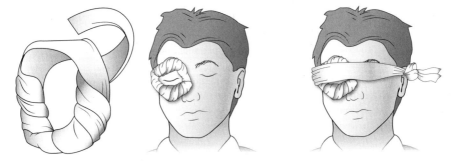

Figure 136. Bandage for the injured eye. A cravat or cloth is rolled and wrapped to make a doughnut-shaped shield, which is fixed in place over the eye.

the eye is completely healed. A topical anesthetic, such as tetracaine 1%, may be used safely for up to 24 hours as directed.

A corneal ulcer is an erosion, usually caused by a bacterial infection, that causes a "red eye," pain, and sometimes decreased visual acuity. It may follow a scratched cornea. The white of the eye is very reddened, and if you look closely, you may notice a small, round white or yellowish spot on the surface of the cornea. This is an emergency, because the ulcer may spread rapidly and cause permanent damage. If a corneal ulcer is suspected, immediately use ofloxacin (Ocuflox) ophthalmic solution 0.3%, gatifloxacin 0.3% (Zymar), or moxifloxacin 0.5% (Vigamox) two drops to the affected eye every 30 minutes for the first 6 hours, then every 4 hours and seek immediate medical attention. *Don't patch the eye if a corneal ulcer is seen or suspected.*

Injured Eyeball

If the eyeball is perforated, there will be a combination of loss of vision (ranging from hazy vision to blindness), pain, excessive tearing, a dilated pupil, and visible blood in the eye. There may be gelatinous material extruding from the eye, and the pupil will be irregular or jagged in appearance. Don't attempt to rinse out the wound vigorously; remove obvious dirt and debris without placing any pressure on the eye. Close the eyelid gently and cover the eye with a protective shield (not a patch under any sort of pressure). This can be fashioned by cutting gauze pads or soft cloth to the proper size, or by fashioning a doughnut-shaped shield with a cloth, cravat bandage, or shirt (Figure 136). Another good way to keep pressure off the eye is to cut an

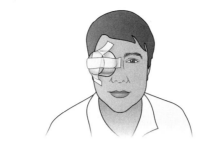

Figure 137. Using a cup to fashion an eye shield.

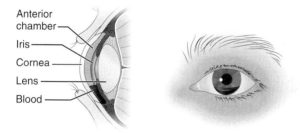

Anterior chamber
Iris
Cornea
Lens
Blood

Figure 138. Hyphema. Bleeding into the eye causes an accumulation of blood in the anterior chamber, where it settles into a layer behind the cornea. In severe cases, the pupil is obscured by red blood.

eye-sized hole in a stack of gauze pads and place the stack over the eye, taping or wrapping it in place. An eye shield can also be improvised by cutting off the bottom 2 inches (5 cm) of a paper cup and taping it over the eye. If tape is not available, a plastic or paper cup may be held in place by putting two small holes 1 inch from the lip on opposite sides of the cup and running a cord or strip of cloth through the holes across the cup such that the loose ends can be then wrapped around the head and tied off (Figure 137). Metal or plastic preshaped eye shields can be carried.

Don't exert pressure on the eyeball, because this can increase the damage. Instruct the victim to keep both eyes closed, and start him on ciprofloxacin, penicillin, doxycycline, cephalexin, or erythromycin. Seek immediate medical attention.

Bleeding into the Eye

If the eyeball has been struck (not torn or ruptured), there may be bleeding from small blood vessels within the eye into the clear liquid that fills the space directly behind the cornea and in front of the lens. Such bleeding is called a hyphema. It first appears as diffuse bloody (red) clouding of the fluid behind the cornea, which settles over the course of 6 to 8 hours into a clearly visible layer of blood (Figure 138). If such a condition is noted, the victim should have his eye patched closed (see the previous section) or wear sunglasses; he should be transported to an eye doctor. If possible, keep his head elevated and in an upright position and apply a rigid eye shield to protect the eye from being struck. The victim should avoid straining.

Finding a Displaced Soft Contact Lens

If a soft contact lens is displaced such that vision is blurred and the victim feels that it is still somewhere underneath an eyelid, you can attempt the following in sequence to try to find it:

1. Place a bit of downward pressure to the lower lid to retract it slightly from the eye. See if you can locate the contact lens.

2. Gently use a finger to lightly massage the upper lid with the motion directed toward the nose. See if that moves the lens to the nose-side of the eye such that you can see it. The massage may take a few minutes.
3. Evert the upper eyelid (see page 168) to get a better view of the top half of the eye.

All of these maneuvers may be facilitated by applying a few drops of artificial tears.

Removing Contact Lenses

If a victim is severely injured and wearing contact lenses, they should be removed. A contact lens remover may be used, or a slightly sticky surface of mini-marshmallow can be placed carefully against the lens to grasp it. Either soft or hard lenses can be removed by the following technique (Figure 139):

1. Slide the lens off the clear surface of the eye (cornea) over to the white area away from the nose.
2. Place one finger at the outside edge of the lower eyelid and pull the eyelid taut, while keeping the eye slightly open. This should lift the edge of the lens, so that you can pick it up. If you cannot remove the lens, position it so that as much as possible is over the white (and not on the cornea).
3. Place the lens in a container with contact lens solution, eyewash, or water (if possible, add 1 teaspoon [5 mL] of table salt per pint [473 mL] of water).
4. A soft contact lens can often be removed by simply pinching it gently between your thumb and index finger.

If you cannot remove a contact lens, it's best to close the eye gently, place a soft cloth or gauze pad patch over it, and tape it closed. Be certain that someone knows why this has been done (i.e., the lens is still in the person's eye).

Subconjunctival Hemorrhage

Bleeding into the white of the eye (subconjunctival hemorrhage) may occur spontaneously or after coughing, straining (vigorous exertion), vomiting, or strangulation (Figure 140). The bleeding is painless, does not interfere with vision (the cornea is not involved), and does not require any therapy. The blood will absorb over a period of a few weeks, as from any other bruise. If it does not, seek the care of an eye doctor.

Red Eye

A red or pink, itchy eye is usually caused by a viral infection. Other causes include bacterial infection, insect bite or sting, allergy (see page 192), overuse of contact lenses, corneal abrasion or ulcer (see page 168), foreign body (see page 168), irritation from chemicals or smoke, snow

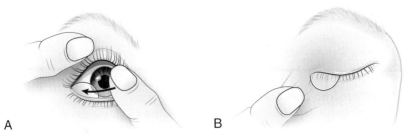

A   B

Figure 139. Contact lens removal. **A,** Push the lens gently to the lateral (away from the nose) white portion of the eye. **B,** A downward and outward pull on the skin at the lateral corner of the eye pops the lens free.

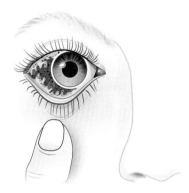

Figure 140. Subconjunctival hemorrhage. The red discoloration does not involve the cornea, which remains clear.

blindness (see page 174), glaucoma (see page 177), or injury (see page 170). If the infection is caused by a virus or bacteria, symptoms include itching, tearing, a gritty sensation, watery (viral) or thick (bacterial) discharge (runny yellow or greenish pus), crusted eyelashes and lids, and swollen eyelids, which are often stuck together on awakening in the morning. You may notice a swollen lymph gland in front of the ear. If fluid collects underneath the loosely attached (to the eyeball) conjunctiva (membrane-like external lining of the eyeball), it may cause it to swell up and balloon away from the eyeball.

If the cause is a known allergy or irritation from smoke, use eye drops with 0.025% oxymetazoline (OcuClear, Visine L.R.), antazoline phosphate 0.5% and naphazoline 0.05% (Vasocon-A), naphazoline 0.1% (Naphcon), or tetrahydrozoline (Visine) every 3 to 4 hours, so long as the victim does not have glaucoma.

If there is much yellowish discharge, suspect a bacterial infection and administer antibiotic eye drops (moxifloxacin 0.5%, gatifloxacin 0.3%, ciprofloxacin 0.3%, tobramycin or gentamicin 0.3%, ofloxacin 0.3%, trimethoprim plus polymyxin B, or sodium sulamyd 10%); the dose is two drops every 2 hours for 4 to 5 days while the victim is awake. Never use steroid-containing eye drops unless directed to do so by a physician. Antibacterial ointments are messy and may blur vision.

"Pink Eye" and Contact Lenses
"Pink eye" usually refers to a viral infection that causes redness, often accompanied by itching and a thick, yellow or green discharge. Often the lids are stuck together in the morning after sleeping. It's not uncommon to have "pink eye" develop in one eye and then rapidly be spread to the other eye, presumably because of touching the infected eye and then transferring the infection. Treatment consists of cool compresses applied three to four times a day, and sometimes antihistamine eye drops. Viral conjunctivitis is very contagious, so the victim should be advised to avoid close contact with others, including sharing implements of facial washing and hand towels or swimming in shared pools, for 2 weeks after the onset of the infection. Handwashing should be frequent and flawless.

Serious eye infections can be caused by fungus, such as that of the genus *Fusarium,* which has been discovered to grow in contact lens solution. Some experts believe that multipurpose solutions in general are more prone to transmitting infection, for reasons that have yet to be clearly determined.

Regardless of whether or not multipurpose solutions are riskier than single-purpose solutions, outdoor enthusiasts should note that contact lenses may be more difficult to manage in a wilderness environment for the following reasons:

1. Should a contact lens become displaced (e.g., fall out of the eye), it may be more easily lost than eyeglasses.
2. Contact lens solution can degrade or become contaminated by exposure to extreme temperatures, dehydration, or passing over dust and dirt that can accumulate on the threads of bottle caps.
3. Handling contact lenses with dirty hands can introduce bacteria and fungi to lenses or tissues of the eyes.
4. It may not be easy to change out contact lenses quickly if needed for a different refraction or environmental (e.g., sun or wind exposure) condition.
5. Once an eye becomes infected, contact lenses must be removed. They should not be reused if removed because of infection.

For these reasons, it's important to carry at least one, and preferably two, pairs of eyeglasses. At least one pair should be single-focus if you intend to be hiking or walking where you may trip or fall. If you need reading glasses, carry these as well. Also, be sure that you have sunglasses that block out as much ultraviolet light as possible. Include side shields if you are going to be at high altitude, on snowfields, on the water's surface, or traversing other highly reflective terrain, such as bright sand.

Dry Eyes

Dry eyes are common in dry environments, after prolonged exposure to wind, at high altitude, and associated with certain medical conditions in which tear production is diminished. Symptoms include a sensation of dryness, sensitivity to light, foreign body sensation, and blurred vision. Artificial tears, such as carboxymethylcellulose sodium 0.5% (Refresh Tears), or lubricating ointment (e.g., Lacri-Lube, containing mineral oil, white petrolatum, and lanolin alcohols) or gel (e.g., Refresh Liquigel, containing carboxymethylcellulose) may be soothing. Note that solutions to reduce redness, such as Visine, may worsen dry eyes. In the event that dry eyes persist despite administration of artificial tears, an ophthalmologist may prescribe cyclosporine (Restasis), an antiinflammatory medication that has been shown to increase production of the recipient's own tears and to relieve symptoms within 3 to 4 weeks. Avoid wearing contact lenses for prolonged periods of time. Consider using warm compresses or eye massage to unclog the meibomian glands, which are located on the edge of the eyelids and produce an oily substance that helps keep the tear film from evaporating. A device based upon this concept is Lipiflow (TearScience). Some persons report relief of dry, irritated, noninfected eyes from application of a cool or lukewarm moist teabag gently placed upon the closed eye. The tea that seeps into the eye contains tannins, which may be soothing.

Wearing wrap-around goggles or glacier glasses to diminish ultraviolet and wind exposure may help prevent dry eyes.

Blepharitis

Blepharitis is chronic flaking and irritation of the skin at the base of the eyelashes, affecting both eyes. It may become infected and be accompanied by fluctuating vision, itchy and burning eyes, and mucous discharge on awakening. Treatment is the application of bacitracin or erythromycin ophthalmic ointment thinly to the lid margins at bedtime for 4 weeks. Warm, moist compresses should be used a few times a day for 5 to 10 minutes at a time to loosen the debris, which is then gently wiped away. Artificial tears are useful to lessen the sensation of dry eyes.

Snow Blindness

Exposure to ultraviolet radiation (UVR) from the sun can lead to "sunburn" of the cornea (clear surface of the eye). This occurs when proper precautions are not used at high altitudes, where a greater amount of unfiltered (by the atmosphere) UVR is present; the exposure may be compounded by reflection from the snow. The intensity of ultraviolet energy increases by a factor of 4% to 6% for every 1000 ft (305 m) increase in altitude above sea level. Snow reflects 85% of ultraviolet B (UVB, the culprit wavelengths that cause snow blindness); dry sand reflects 17%, and grass or sandy turf reflects 2.5%. Water may reflect 10% to 30% of UVB, depending on the time of day and location.

The cornea absorbs UVR below 300 nanometers (nm), which includes a fair portion of UVB. Radiation of wavelengths longer than 300 nm is transmitted to the lens and, over time, can cause cataracts.

Exposure to UVB can cause a corneal burn within 1 hour, although symptoms may not become apparent for 6 to 12 hours. Symptoms include excessive tearing, pain, redness, swollen eyelids, pain when looking at light, headache, a gritty sensation in the eyes, and decreased (hazy) vision. Similar symptoms occur when the surface of the eye is physically scratched (corneal abrasion). Treatment consists of removing contact lenses and wearing sunglasses, or (less preferred) patching the eye closed (see page 169) after instilling a few drops of ophthalmic antibiotic solution (such as moxifloxacin 0.5%, gatifloxacin 0.3%, sodium sulamyd 10%, or gentamicin). The surface of the cornea will regenerate spontaneously in 24 to 48 hours. It's important to check the eye first for a foreign body (see page 168). After patching, the eye should be rechecked in 24 hours. If the eye appears to be infected with pus, it should be left unpatched; administer a topical antibiotic solution (see page 169) three to four times a day, and have the victim wear sunglasses. Pain medicine should be used as appropriate. If both eyes are involved and it's necessary to patch an eye in order to control the pain, only the more severely affected eye should be patched, so that the victim can continue to make his way.

Some experts recommend a topical nonsteroidal antiinflammatory or steroid solution to hasten the resolution of snow blindness. In a situation in which the diagnosis is certain and such medication is available, instillation may indeed improve things. However, if a topical steroid is applied to a misdiagnosed bacterial or viral infection—particularly herpes virus—the effect can be to worsen the situation. Since snow blindness is self-limited, the application of a topical steroid is not imperative and is best left to an ophthalmologist. Useful nonsteroidal topical solutions are ketorolac ophthalmic solution 0.5% (Acular) and diclofenac 0.1% (Voltaren), one or the other instilled 1 drop four times a day. External (e.g., applied to the closed eye) cool compresses may provide some pain relief.

Eye Allergies

Seasonal allergies commonly involve the eyes, often causing conjunctivitis. Allergic conjunctivitis causes symptoms of eyelid swelling, runny and itchy eyes, and redness, with or without a bumpy surface ("cobblestones") noted on the inside of the eyelids. This is treated with a variety of types of eye drops to counteract various components of the allergic reaction. Commonly prescribed are antazoline, ketotifen, azelastine, alamast, ketorolac, olopatadine and/or loteprednol or prednisolone. See page 193.

Protective Eyeglasses (Sunglasses)

The wavelengths of sunlight that appear to be most damaging to the eye are blue (400 to 500 nm), UVA (320 to 400 nm), and UVB (290 to 320 nm). Ultraviolet C (200 to 290 nm) is filtered out by the ozone layer of the atmosphere. Standards for ultraviolet protection in nonprescription sunglasses are set by the American National Standards Institute (ANSI). These state that such lenses should maintain UV absorption up to 400 nm and block 99.8% of UVB light and 95% of UVA. Lenses advertised for mountaineering or specifically for ultraviolet protection should meet these standards.

Sunglasses should be equipped with side protectors and, if necessary, optional nose guards. Frames should be prepared with wraparound temples and retaining straps or lanyards.

Polycarbonate lenses, which are lightweight, scratch resistant, and shatterproof, can be manufactured to absorb 99% of ultraviolet light. Most recreation supply companies manufacture or carry sunglasses and wraparound goggles that meet ANSI standards. At least one pair should be single-focus if you intend to be hiking or walking where you may trip or fall.

In general, amber, yellow, orange, brown, and rose lenses filter out blue light and increase the perception of contrast. Green and gray lenses soften glare and transmit a spectrum that does not increase contrast. Glass ambermatic or photochromic lenses (darker in bright sunlight), which contain millions of silver halide crystals, darken when exposed to ultraviolet light close to the visible spectrum. Polarized lenses improve vision by decreasing glare, but this does not decrease exposure to UV light.

Improvised sunglasses can be made by cutting small slits or puncturing pinholes in cardboard or two layers of a strip of duct tape after the adhesive sides have been stuck together. Fashion a shape that will fit across the eyes like a pair of sunglasses; tie in the back with a string attachment. The opening should be just large enough to allow adequate vision. This serves two purposes: limitation of ultraviolet transmission and creation of crude refraction to improve focus in a person who is nearsighted.

For safe driving, sunglasses should transmit at least 8% of visible light during daytime and 80% of visible light during darkness.

Vitreous Detachment

Floaters are small spots, lines, clouds, cobwebs, or veils that move around in the field of vision, especially when the eyes move. They can be in one or both eyes, but usually show up in one eye at a time. They are easiest to see when one looks at the sky or against a plain white background. Floaters are caused by tiny opacities inside the vitreous, which is the gel that fills the inside of the eye. In childhood and adolescence, the vitreous gel is clear, so that floaters are not seen. In adulthood, floaters can develop when the vitreous gel forms small clumps as part of the aging process. As light passes from the outside of the eye, through the cornea and lens, and then through the vitreous gel before it strikes the retina to record an image, the floaters can cast shadows on the retina. Floaters are annoying, but not dangerous, particularly if they have been present for a long time.

The sudden appearance of floaters can signify separation of the vitreous gel from the retina, which is the layer of tissue in the back of the eye on which visual images are recorded on specialized receptor cells. This occurs because the vitreous gel shrinks as it ages. If it shrinks enough, it begins to peel away from the retina, in what is called a vitreous separation or detachment. It's more common in nearsighted people and in persons who have had cataract surgery or injuries to their eyes or head. When a vitreous separation occurs, the floaters appear suddenly. As the gel peels away from the retina, it tugs on it, which can cause a person to experience the perception of flashes of light, usually on the outer (ear) side of the eye. These usually last no more than a second, and are caused by the nerves within the retina (which connect to the large optic nerve) being stimulated mechanically by the tug of the vitreous gel. Flashes are difficult to appreciate in daylight, but can be easily seen in the darkness. Moving the head or eyes can cause the flashes. Since flashes mean that the vitreous is pulling on the retina, this is a warning sign, because the traction can cause a retinal tear. If this happens, an ophthalmologist needs to perform laser surgery as soon as possible to prevent a full-blown retinal detachment.

The normal course for a vitreous separation is a 2- to 4-week process in which the separation is completed. This may be punctuated by intermittent addition of new floaters, but usually the burst of opacities is at the beginning of the process. Over time, most of the floaters diminish or disappear, but there may be some residual floaters. During the course of the separation, when a person first notices the floaters, and if a person suddenly develops new floaters, more frequent flashing lights, or a defect in a field of vision (often described as a "dark curtain"), an ophthalmologist should perform an examination to be certain that there is not a retinal tear or detachment. It's important to avoid sudden eye or head movements for several weeks after the onset of a vitreous separation, to decrease the likelihood of developing a retinal tear or detachment.

If a vitreous detachment is suspected, it's wise to begin to head toward civilization to undergo a proper eye examination. However, if it's likely that a retinal detachment has occurred (e.g., there is a "field cut," or a darkened area of vision as if a curtain was being pulled across the field of vision from any direction), it's prudent to evacuate immediately, including a more expensive mode of transportation if necessary, because treatment for retinal detachment is usually an operation by an ophthalmologist and time is of the essence. A progressive retinal detachment can lead to permanent loss of vision in the affected eye.

In terms of exercise, it's wise to avoid sudden head or eye movements, so no jogging or swimming with rapid head movements, wrestling, significant straining, and so on. Until the vitreous separation process is complete, a person should try to turn the head to look in a direction, rather than hold the head in a fixed position and move the eyes. All of this may be difficult in a precarious situation, such as rock climbing or kayaking, but one should just do the best he can given the particular circumstances.

Injury to the Retina

The retina is the thin inner posterior-surface tissue layer of the eye, the "screen" on which images are transmitted by light. From the retina, nerves from the eye carry signals to the brain. The retina can be injured by the transmission of unrestricted infrared rays (wavelengths of light beyond the red end of the visible spectrum). Usually, this occurs when someone views the sun directly during an eclipse or when a person stares at the sun while under the influence of hallucinogenic drugs. Symptoms include pain and blindness. If such an injury is suspected, sunglasses should be worn or the eye should be patched. The victim should be transported to an eye doctor.

Occasionally, a structural abnormality, the aging process, or a blow to the eye will cause the retina to become separated from the back of the eye (retinal detachment). Early symptoms include flashes of light and persistent floating spots in the field of vision ("floaters": see description in earlier section on vitreous detachment). As the retina peels off farther, a person loses vision painlessly, as if a curtain ("of darkness") was descending. Retinal detachment is a serious condition and requires emergency repair.

Optic Neuritis

Optic neuritis is inflammation of the optic nerve, which carries signals from the eye to the brain in the process of vision. It causes blurred vision of gradual onset, pain with eye movement, and an aching sensation in the affected eye. Commonly associated with multiple sclerosis, it can also be caused by infections (e.g., Lyme disease), cancer, and autoimmune syndromes. The treatment is high-dose steroids and other agents administered under the care of an ophthalmologist. In any circumstance when vision becomes impaired without an obvious cause such that it cannot be effectively treated in the wilderness, get the victim to an eye doctor as soon as possible.

Glaucoma

Glaucoma is a condition in which the pressure of the fluid within the eye is elevated. If this happens suddenly, the pressure can injure the nerves within the eye that record vision; blindness can result. Symptoms of an acute attack of glaucoma include severe pain, blurred vision or "halos" around lights, clouding of the cornea, intense reddening of the white of the eye, a dilated pupil that doesn't react to light, nausea, vomiting, and headache. If an attack occurs, the victim should be kept in a sitting or standing position and rushed to an ophthalmologist. If the victim is carrying medication(s), instill a drop of pilocarpine or carbachol *and* (depending on which medications are carried by the victim) a drop of timolol (or betaxolol, carteolol, levobunolol, or metipranolol), latanoprost (or travoprost, unoprostone, or bimatoprost), brimonidine (or apraclonidine), and/or dorzolamide (or brinzolamide) in the affected eye. If you are distant from care, and acetazolamide (Diamox) is available and there are no contraindications to its use (see page 307), it may be administered in a dose of 250 mg by mouth four times a day, or 500 mg sustained release by mouth twice a day. If prednisolone eye drops are available, instill one or two drops in the affected eye(s). Use ondansetron 4 to 8 mg oral dissolving tablet for nausea and vomiting.

Injured Eyelid
If the eyelid is injured, wash the eye carefully, apply bacitracin or mupirocin ointment, and then patch the eye closed (see page 169). If the eye cannot be covered with eyelid, apply a thick layer of antiseptic ointment to the eyelid and exposed eyeball and patch the eye. Seek immediate medical attention.

Stye and Chalazion
A stye (external hordeolum) is an infection of a small sebaceous gland that appears as a small abscess (see page 224) externally at the base of an eyelash. If the stye appears on the inside or within the eyelid, then it's likely an infection of the oil (meibomian) gland. The infection causes the eyelid to swell, redden, and become painful. The victim may notice increased tear production and the sensation of a foreign body in the eye. Usually, the stye comes to a head on the outside of the lid, but occasionally it will come to a head inside. If a stye begins to develop, the victim should hold warm, moist compresses to his eyelid for 30 minutes four times a day to soften the abscess. Erythromycin or other ophthalmic antibiotic drops or ointment can be applied to the stye twice a day for 7 days. The stye will either disappear or enlarge and come to a head. *Never squeeze an abscess on the face.* If the stye enlarges, comes to a head, and is extremely painful or interferes with vision, but will not open spontaneously, it can be carefully lanced with a sharp blade or needle to drain the pus. A physician should perform this procedure, unless the victim is more than 48 hours from medical attention and the infection has worsened to the extent that there is progressive swelling of the eyelid that impedes vision, or of the cheek or forehead. In this event, also administer dicloxacillin, erythromycin, or cephalexin. After the stye is incised, the pus can be expressed gently by pressing on opposite lateral sides with two cotton-tipped applicators.

A chalazion is an infected gland within the eyelid, rather than at the edge of the lid. It may also turn into an abscess. Treatment is the same as for a stye.

Eyelid Infection and Periorbital Cellulitis
If there is discharge and pain, with or without redness, from an eyelid on the side nearest the nose, this may be an infection in the tear duct. Apply warm compresses and administer amoxicillin–clavulanate, moxifloxacin, levofloxacin, ciprofloxacin, or cephalexin.

Redness and swelling of the eyelid and "soft" tissues around the eye (eyebrow, upper cheek) caused by infection is known as periorbital (around the orbit, or eye) cellulitis. This is extremely serious and must be treated aggressively, because the infection can spread to create an abscess in the brain. Treatment consists of administration of an antibiotic (moxifloxacin, levofloxacin, ciprofloxacin, cephalexin, clindamycin, amoxicillin–clavulanate, dicloxacillin, or erythromycin) and immediate evacuation to a hospital. To differentiate periorbital cellulitis from the swollen eyelids associated with an allergic reaction, note that with cellulitis, the onset will have been more gradual (typically associated with a less severe eye infection, such as conjunctivitis, or a local infection such as a stye or pimple), the affliction is only on one side, there are fever and chills, the soft tissues are painful, there is headache, and there is often a purulent (with pus) discharge from the eye. With an allergy, the eye is more "puffy," the onset is sudden, the eye is itchy and watering, there is no purulent discharge, and there are associated signs and symptoms of allergy (skin rash, generalized itching, swollen lips, etc.) (see page 64).

Orbital cellulitis involves a deep infection around the eye and presents as a swollen, red eye with significant pain on eye motion, decreased vision, and bulging of the eyeball in its socket. In contrast, victims of periorbital cellulitis have normal vision and painless motion of the eye. Orbital cellulitis is an emergency, so the victim should be started on the antibiotics listed previously and immediately evacuated to hospital medical care.

Pterygium

A pterygium is a noncancerous degeneration of the conjunctiva that occurs in persons who spend large amounts of time outdoors, particularly with exposure to ultraviolet light. It appears as a yellow, raised, "fleshy" knob of tissue that appears to begin in the nasal corner of the eye, and extends from there over the white part. It occasionally encroaches on the nasal margin of the cornea. It rarely grows further or requires treatment, because vision is usually not affected.

NOSE
Nosebleed

Nosebleed is classified as anterior or posterior, depending on where it originates within the nose. Generally, anterior nosebleed is less serious, because the victim will usually drain blood outward through the nostrils. Posterior nosebleed is more difficult to control, and the victim often drains blood back into the throat, with coughing and potential choking. Anterior nosebleed is more common and can usually be managed outside of the hospital. *If you suspect a posterior nosebleed* (bleeding from the nose accompanied by brisk bleeding into the throat, so that a lot of blood is continually swallowed, particularly after the anterior bleeding has been controlled), *immediately evacuate the victim to a hospital.*

The most frequent cause of a nosebleed is a small bleeding blood vessel or cut on the inner mucosal surface of a nostril. This is more common at high altitudes and in cold weather, because the drying effect causes the skin to become irritated and crack. One way to prevent nosebleeds is to keep the inside of the nose lubricated with an ointment such as mupirocin or bacitracin, or to spray regularly with saline solution (such as Ocean saline mist or drops with 0.65% sodium chloride). It's possible that nosebleeds are more common in persons whose blood pressure has risen out of control. People on prescription anticoagulant drugs are prone to nosebleeds.

To control an anterior nosebleed, attempt simple maneuvers first. Have the victim blow his nose to remove all clots. Keep him upright (sitting leaning forward) and calm, and firmly press both nostrils closed against the nasal septum (middle cartilage). Hold this position for 15 minutes without release; letting go before this time will only restart the bleeding, because it takes the small blood vessels and scratched surface a while to stop oozing. There are simple mechanical devices, such as the Nose Aid Emergency Nose Bleed Treatment, that accomplish this compression and free up the hands. After 15 minutes, let go or release the device and see if the bleeding has stopped. If not, gently but firmly pack both nostrils with a gauze or cotton roll moistened with phenylephrine 0.25% (Neo-Synephrine 1/4%) or oxymetazoline 0.05% (Afrin) and repeat the pinching maneuver for 20 minutes. Generally, this does the trick; if it doesn't, repeat the packing without the nasal spray. After the bleeding has stopped, leave the packing in place for 2 hours and then gently remove it. Cold compresses applied to the bridge of the nose or a roll of gauze or cotton placed beneath the upper lip are of limited help when dealing with a brisk nosebleed. Packing with hemostatic QuikClot NoseBleed gauze (Z-Medica Corporation) may be helpful. A useful device for packing the nose to stop a nosebleed is the Rhino Rocket (Shippert Medical Technologies), which is a compressed medical-grade foam sponge with applicator. The foam is guided into place, where it swells on contact with moisture (blood) to 8 to 10 times its compressed size. A string is attached to the sponge so that it can be easily removed. Weimert Epistaxis (nosebleed) Packing uses a similar approach. The Rapid Rhino 450 Epistaxis Device (ArthroCare Corporation) uses a hemostatic (stops bleeding) carboxymethylcellulose fabric over an inflatable balloon to apply compression within the nose. Merocel is a polyvinyl alcohol nasal tampon that is inserted into the nose, whereupon exposure to a topical vasoconstrictor (e.g., phenylephrine 0.25%) and saline causes it to expand and create pressure over the bleeding point. NasalCEASE (Catalina Healthcare) is a bundle of fine fibers made from brown seaweed (active ingredient calcium alginate) extract that can be inserted into the nose to aid clotting.

If the nose is packed, administer an antistaphylococcal antiseptic (such as dicloxacillin or trimethoprim–sulfamethoxazole) for the duration of the packing. The nasal packing should be kept moist with sterile saline or oxymetazoline (Afrin) spray.

After a nosebleed has thoroughly ceased and you're comfortable that you will not disrupt a blood clot and restart the bleeding, gently apply mupirocin or another antibacterial ointment to the affected nostril(s) two to three times per day to keep the interior of the nose moist.

If a person has a significant facial injury or brisk nosebleed, particularly if there is vomiting, allow him to sit in order to lean forward and drain these fluids without choking. If he needs to be recumbent, don't place him on his back. Rather, put him in the recovery position (see page 25).

Broken Nose

A fractured nose may or may not be deformed. If the nose is obviously depressed or pushed to one side, and the victim is having difficulty breathing through his mouth, the nose can be relocated, but this is usually quite painful. Grasp the bridge of the nose firmly and crunch it upward and back over to the midline. In the wilderness, it can be difficult to improvise an external splint. A malleable soft-aluminum nasal splint with adhesive ventilating foam is available as The Denver Splint Series 2000 (Shippert Medical Technologies). Treat any nosebleed as previously discussed. *The only reason to relocate the injury is to improve breathing if mouth breathing is inadequate.* The nasal bones won't begin to set solidly for 5 to 7 days; cosmetic manipulation can easily be performed after such a delay. If the skin is cut deeply over a broken nose, start the victim on an antibiotic (penicillin, cephalexin, or erythromycin).

Another risk from a broken nose is formation of a blood clot under the skin that lies over the nasal septum (cartilage) between the nostrils. If such a clot is not promptly drained, its resolution can cause collapse of the cartilage, infection, or erosion through the septum, leaving a hole through the septum. Anyone who has suffered a broken nose needs to be examined by a physician within 3 to 5 days of the injury, to avoid erosion of the nasal septum by a blood clot.

Foreign Body in the Nose

A small child will occasionally stuff a foreign object, such as a pebble or bead, into a nostril, where it will become stuck. Signs and symptoms include pain, a foul-smelling drainage, and sometimes fever. This can be a tough problem away from the hospital, because once the sensitive skin inside the nostril becomes irritated, it swells and traps the foreign object within a matrix of mucus, and sometimes blood or pus. If the object can't be easily seen and extracted without forcing it farther into the nostril or torturing the child, seek a physician's assistance. If you're carrying a flashlight and a small nasal speculum (a device for gently widening the nostril to facilitate access to the inside of the nose—Disposable Nasal Speculum, Bionix), you can attempt to look up the nose, but most small children will be extremely uncooperative, because this is pretty uncomfortable for them. One way to remove a nasal foreign body is to put a small dab of cyanoacrylate glue on the tip of a small stick (such as the rod portion of a cotton-tipped swab), and then hold the stick against the object until it is stuck, so that the stick can be used to pull out the object. If the object is metallic, try using a magnet. If fever is present, start the child on dicloxacillin or erythromycin.

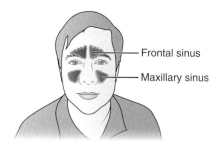

Figure 141. Location of the sinuses in the front of the skull and the face.

Sinusitis

The sinuses are spaces filled with air and lined with mucus-producing tissues found in the front of the skull and in the bones of the face (Figure 141). Sinusitis is a blockage and infection/inflammation of the lining of the sinuses, usually caused by bacteria and characterized by nasal congestion, headache, fever, decreased ability to smell, and tenderness in and over the involved sinus, with or without foul yellow or green discharge from the nose. Occasionally, the pain radiates to the eyes, bridge of the nose, and upper teeth. It's often made worse by bending forward. A person with sinusitis can become quite ill and suffer from excruciating headache, nausea, vomiting, and chills. Treatment involves administration of an antibiotic (first choice is amoxicillin–clavulanate (particularly in children), amoxicillin, azithromycin, or telithromycin; other choices include moxifloxacin, levofloxacin, clarithromycin, doxycycline, ciprofloxacin, trovafloxacin, levofloxacin, moxifloxacin, cefuroxime axetil, cefpodoxime, cefprozil, cefdinir, loracarbef, or erythromycin) and decongestants (oral pseudoephedrine and a nasal spray: phenylephrine 0.25% [Neo-Synephrine ¼%] or oxymetazoline 0.05% [Afrin]), as well as warm packs over the affected area(s). Don't use a topical decongestant for more than 3 or 4 consecutive days, to avoid "rebound" swelling of the inside of the nasal passages from chemical irritation and sensitization to the drug. Antihistamine drugs should not be routinely used, because they may dry out nasal and sinus secretions. Antihistamines and decongestants should both be avoided in children.

A person suffering from sinusitis should avoid rapid changes in ambient external pressure (such as scuba diving or air travel in unpressurized aircraft). If you use a neti pot or other vessel to perform nasal irrigation (which has never been proved to shorten the duration of sinusitis), be aware that there is a risk for bacterial contamination, such as from *Staphylococcus aureus,* particularly if the vessel has been used previously by you or another person. Tap water that's safe for drinking is not safe for using with a neti pot. Use only distilled or sterile (previously heated to at least 166.6° F (47° C) or previously boiled water. Rinse the neti pot after each use and allow it to air dry.

THROAT
Sore Throat and Tonsillitis

Sore throat (pharyngitis) is a common complication of viral infections (the common cold, infectious mononucleosis associated with Epstein-Barr virus), breathing dry air ("altitude throat"), or primary bacterial throat infection ("strep throat"). Symptoms of an infection include pain with swallowing, fever, swollen lymph nodes ("swollen glands") in the anterior neck, red throat, swollen tonsils, pus over the tonsils and throat (Figure 142), headache, fatigue, chills, fever, abdominal pain, and nausea and vomiting. Sometimes a person with streptococcal pharyngitis will have a fine, red skin rash, which usually spares the face and is known as scarlet fever.

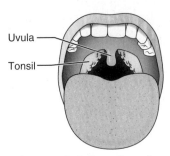

Uvula

Tonsil

Figure 142. Inflamed tonsils.

Because the symptoms of a viral throat and tonsil infection and a bacterial strep (group A beta-hemolytic streptococcus [GABHS]) throat are frequently identical, it is hard to make the differentiation without a throat-swab "rapid strep test" or bacterial culture. Below 3 years of age, a child rarely has a strep throat; in young adults, the presence of strep throat in the presence of classic symptoms (fever, pus, and swollen tonsils and lymph glands in the neck) is roughly 50%. However, because the risk for potential complications (heart disease [rheumatic fever], ear infection, peritonsillar abscess [see below]) from an untreated strep throat outweigh the complications of antibiotic use, it's advisable to treat persons older than 3 years of age (and particularly ages 3 to 15 years) with penicillin V or amoxicillin–clavulanate for a full 10-day course. Persons who are allergic to penicillin may take cefadroxil, cephalexin, or clindamycin for a full 10-day course, or azithromycin or clarithromycin for 5 days. Erythromycin for 10 days is fine, but may cause more gastrointestinal side effects than does azithromycin or clarithromycin. Even if the victim improves after 2 to 3 days, the antibiotic should be taken for the full course. Treating with antibiotics does not appear to reduce the risk for developing kidney disease (glomerulonephritis) after suffering streptococcal pharyngitis. Note that if the cause of the sore throat is mononucleosis (see page 183), treating with amoxicillin will very likely cause a bumpy spotted red skin rash, which is not an allergic reaction.

Adjuncts to care include saltwater gargles (½ teaspoon [2.5 mL] of table salt in 1 cup [237 mL] of warm water), throat lozenges, warm fluids (to moisten and soothe the throat), and aspirin or acetaminophen to control fever. *To avoid Reye syndrome (postviral encephalopathy and liver failure), don't use aspirin to control fever in a child under age 17.*

If a person develops an acute sore throat that rapidly becomes extremely uncomfortable (severe pain, difficulty swallowing), a single oral dose (8 mg for an adult; 0.6 mg/kg of body weight to a maximum of 8 mg for a child) of dexamethasone or its equivalent (see page 311) may be given along with an antibiotic, assuming the victim can swallow the medications. This may help decrease inflammation and somewhat hasten resolution of symptoms, but should not be given routinely for a "nontoxic," or run-of-the-mill, sore throat. *If someone with a sore throat has a high fever associated with difficult or noisy breathing, altered (e.g. hoarse) or muffled voice ("like talking with a potato in his mouth"), drooling, increasing difficulty opening the mouth or swallowing, stiff neck, or any visible swelling (bulging) in the back of the throat, he should be made as comfortable as possible and transported immediately to a hospital.* Such a condition may indicate an abscess in the back of the throat or next to a tonsil (peritonsillar abscess), infection and inflammation of the epiglottis (epiglottitis), or massively swollen tonsils. Any of these may rapidly obstruct the airway.

If a person develops tender swelling under the tongue and/or under the chin, particularly associated with swollen lymph glands in the neck, fever, difficulty swallowing, and foul breath, this may indicate an infection in the floor of the mouth. Treat the victim with an antibiotic as for a strep throat and seek immediate physician consultation.

A sore throat can be caused by overgrowth of the fungus *Candida albicans,* which leads to a condition known as "thrush." This occurs most commonly in persons who are immuno-suppressed, have recently taken broad-spectrum antibiotics, use inhaled or oral steroids, wear dentures or orthodontic appliances, have diabetes, or are elders. Symptoms include burning in the mouth and throat, white patches on the palate and in the mouth and throat, painful swallowing, heartburn, drooling, and loss of appetite. If thrush is suspected, it can be treated with nystatin (Mycostatin) oral suspension, swished and swallowed four times a day for 2 weeks, or with nystatin oral lozenges four to five times daily for 2 weeks. Another therapy is oral fluconazole 100 mg by mouth twice a day for 14 days, or itraconazole 100 to 200 mg daily for 7 days.

Infectious Mononucleosis

Mononucleosis ("mono") is a viral (Epstein-Barr virus) disease that most often afflicts persons in the second decade of life, and is commonly transmitted through infectious saliva ("kissing disease"). The normal incubation period is 30 to 50 days. Mononucleosis is characterized by low-grade (less than 101°F, or 38.3°C) fever, sore throat, swollen lymph glands (mostly in the neck, but occasionally in the armpits or in the groin), headache, fatigue, and, occasionally, skin rash, dark urine, muscle aching, and an enlarged spleen. Treatment consists of increased rest (it sometimes requires weeks for a normal energy level to return) and elimination of any physical activity that requires heavy exertion or risks abdominal injury (and thus rupture of the spleen) for at least 3 weeks after the onset of symptoms or 3 weeks after the date that fever disappears. The diagnosis is confirmed by a blood test; until that can be performed to confirm the presence of mononucleosis, it's reasonable to treat the victim for a possible strep throat (see page 181). Infected people should avoid sharing eating utensils and towels. Note that if the cause of a sore throat is mononucleosis, treating with amoxicillin will very likely cause a bumpy spotted red skin rash, which is not an allergic reaction.

Food Stuck in the Throat or Esophagus

If food becomes stuck in the throat or esophagus, it can be quite disconcerting. So long as the victim can breathe and speak easily, there is not an airway problem (see page 22). Ask the victim to swallow sips of liquid. Sometimes the food will soften over a few hours and pass to the stomach. If the food object feels sharp and stuck in the back of the mouth or throat, use a wooden tongue blade or handle of an eating implement (e.g., spoon) to push down the tongue and try to see it. If that's possible, it can perhaps be grasped with a long tweezers or loosened from its position by rubbing with a cotton-tipped swab. Often, what feels like a bone stuck in the throat is a scratch. So long as the victim can swallow liquids successfully and remain hydrated, it's fine to wait overnight to see if the foreign body sensation disappears.

Common Cold

See page 189.

MOUTH AND TEETH

Fever Blisters (Cold Sores)

Crops of blisters on the face, mouth, and lips that break out in times of stress (viral illness, emotional crisis, intense sun exposure) are often caused by reactivated herpes simplex virus (usually HSV-1). The blisters often weep and may become infected. If no topical medications are available, keep the blisters clean and dry. If the skin cracks and becomes painful, the blisters may be lubricated with bacitracin or mupirocin ointment. Cool compresses may help. Anesthetic ointment (e.g., lidocaine) or solution (see page 471) can be used. An effective topical treatment is an equal mixture of kaolin-pectin (Kaopectate) and diphenhydramine (Benadryl) elixir, with or without added 2% viscous lidocaine, to coat the area. Further sun exposure should be prevented with an adequate lip sunscreen (see page 213) of sun protection factor (SPF) 20 or greater.

Untreated, the lesions will disappear spontaneously in 10 to 15 days. Penciclovir 1% (Denavir) cream applied to the skin or lips every 2 hours while awake for 4 days may be prescribed to hasten resolution of the blisters. Alternatively, apply acyclovir (Zovirax) ointment thinly five times a day for a week. Another treatment is acyclovir 200 mg by mouth five times a day, or 400 mg three times a day, for 7 days. If the oral medication method is selected, consider valacyclovir (Valtrex) 2 g twice a day for 1 day, or famciclovir (Famvir) 500 mg by mouth twice a day for 7 days.

All herpes viruses are contagious. During times of visible blisters, eating and drinking utensils should not be shared. No kissing! To maximize prevention, use a high-SPF sunscreen and consider taking acyclovir (Zovirax) (400 mg twice daily by mouth) the day before and during intense ultraviolet light exposure. Docosanol (Abreva) cream applied to the skin at the onset of the prodrome of itching or burning (recognized by the sufferer) at the affected skin site may very slightly decrease the time to healing.

Canker (Mouth) Sores (Aphthous Ulcers or Stomatitis)

These painful gray-white round or oval patches with reddened (inflamed) edges form inside the mouth and may be associated with viral infections or an immune response to an infection or disease. They may be initiated by minor trauma, such as occurs with dentures or orthodontic braces, or by certain food allergies. Usually they are a chronic problem. Untreated, they last for 10 to 14 days. There are many different recommended therapies:

- Apply anesthetic lidocaine ointment 2.5% for a minute or two before eating to temporarily eliminate the pain.
- Swish and spit the antacid Maalox.
- Apply the anesthetic 20% benzocaine (HurriCaine, Beutlich Pharmaceuticals), which can be conveniently applied from a prepackaged dry handle swab.
- Apply lidocaine viscous gel 5% to ulcers four times daily for 2 weeks or until ulcers heal.
- Apply antiinflammatory amlexanox 5% oral paste (Aphthasol) four times a day to the affected area after brushing teeth for 2 weeks or until the ulcers heal.
- Apply a pinch of powdered alum (as in a styptic pencil) to initiate healing.
- Apply the topical bioadhesive carmellose (Orabase) four times daily for 2 weeks or until ulcers heal.
- A physician may advise one of these remedies: apply topical tetracycline or sucralfate; apply a mixture of fluocinonide 0.05% cream (Metosyn) and Orabase to the ulcer four times per day; or apply triamcinolone dental paste 1% (Adcortyl, or Kenalog in Orabase) to the ulcer four times per day.

The inside of the mouth should be rinsed thoroughly after eating to prevent food from becoming trapped in the sores. Antimicrobial mouthwashes, such as those containing chlorhexidine gluconate (0.12% or 0.2%), used three times daily may help prevent the onset of new sores. Triclosan is an antibacterial, antiinflammatory chemical contained in toothpaste (Colgate Total) that in certain circumstances might reduce the incidence of aphthous ulcers. Tell the sufferer to avoid spicy, acidic, or abrasive food. Any new sore in the mouth of an elderly person or frequent user of tobacco should be seen by a physician, who must consider a precancerous lesion or oral cancer.

Salivary Gland Infection/Inflammation

The parotid gland is located in front of the ear, the submandibular gland is located under the jawbone, and the sublingual glands are between the tongue and the bottom of the mouth. These salivary glands, which manufacture saliva, may become infected, inflamed, and/or obstructed.

This causes pain and swelling (with or without bad-tasting drainage into the mouth), fever, and chills. The pain and swelling may be worse after eating, which is a sign of obstruction. If inflammation/infection is suspected, have the person stay well hydrated, suck on hard candies (particularly lemon drops or flavors that promote salivation) or lozenges, and take amoxicillin-clavulanate or clindamycin for 7 to 10 days.

Black Tongue

Black "hairy" discoloration of the tongue may be caused by excessive growth of the papillae of the tongue. It may be associated with topical or systemic antibiotics, poor mouth and dental hygiene, smoking, drinking alcohol, or even certain mouthwashes. Usually, the only symptom is the discoloration, but some patients suffer nausea, bad breath, or altered taste of food. Treatment consists of brushing the tongue with a soft toothbrush. Black hairy tongue may be due to the presence of yeast (e.g., *Candida albicans*) infection and/or use of certain medications, such as bismuth (found in Pepto-Bismol) or doxycycline. If the discoloration does not resolve spontaneously, it may be treated with clotrimazole (10 mg troche dissolved in the mouth five times a day for 14 days) or with a 3-day treatment of fluconazole (150 mg by mouth once a day).

Sore Lips

Sore lips can have a variety of causes, usually related to being dry and sun-exposed. This condition can be prevented by a sunscreen-containing lip balm, such as ChapStick. If the skin at the angles of the mouth appears to be red and sore, particularly if there are small cracks in the skin, a person can apply a topical antifungal cream, such as ciclopirox olamine 0.77% (Loprox), followed in 3 hours by a topical steroid cream or ointment. Follow this routine once a day for a few days until the situation improves, then switch to ChapStick or something similar.

Toothaches and Tooth Inflammation/Infections

Toothaches occur most often in teeth that are decayed or have lost fillings. In this manner, the central pulp, which carries nerves and blood vessels, becomes inflamed (pulpitis). Symptoms of tooth inflammation or infection include pain in the tooth and jaw that occasionally travels into the neck and ear, pain on contact with cold or hot food or beverage, and headache. Sometimes it's difficult to localize the problem to a specific tooth, since it may not be sensitive when it is tapped. To identify the culprit tooth, apply an ice cube sequentially to each tooth until you elicit a painful reaction. Pain medication appropriate for the degree of suffering should be administered. Have the victim keep his head elevated. If a dental caries (eventually a "cavity" caused by decay) is early, it may be a brown or discolored area that is sensitive to cold for a minute or so after exposure. This can be treated with a high-fluoride or antisensitivity toothpaste and good oral hygiene.

If it hurts to bite down on a tooth, but nothing is obvious on inspection of it, there may be inflammation of the supporting structures. In this case, the victim can point to the affected tooth, or feel pain when you tap on a particular tooth. Treatment is a soft diet, pain medication, and something like a strip of leather positioned on the nonpainful (opposite) side to bite down upon, to create a space and prevent pressure on the affected tooth.

If an abscess (infection) (see page 224) develops in the root of the tooth or in the gum, there may be associated fever; swelling of the gum, jaw, or palate; and swollen lymph glands under the jaw and in the neck. If the abscess extends, the cheek and side of the face may swell. The victim should be started on penicillin, metronidazole, cephalexin, clindamycin, or erythromycin and given appropriate pain medication. If there is a soft, pointing abscess in the gum adjacent to a tooth and the victim is suffering, the abscess can be punctured with a scalpel or knife and drained (Figure 143). Hold snow or ice against the gum to provide some anesthesia before the incision. A gauze or cotton wick should be placed into the abscess cavity for a day or two (see

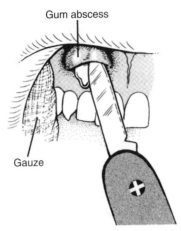

Gum abscess

Gauze

Figure 143. Incision and drainage of a gum abscess.

page 225). After this procedure, the area should be rinsed with salt water after each meal, at least four times a day.

To temporarily treat a cavity (decay) or site of a lost filling, dry the affected tooth carefully with cotton. Next, apply a cotton pad moistened with oil of cloves (eugenol) to the tooth cavity. In a pinch, you can use vanilla extract. Take care to keep eugenol off the gums, lips, and inside surfaces of the cheeks. Alternatively, topical benzocaine (Anbesol) can be applied to the gums. The patient needs to be taken to a dentist to have the tooth repaired or removed.

Another remedy for a cavity caused by decay or a lost filling is to fill the cavity with temporary filling material from a dental kit. Such materials include Cavit, which requires no mixing. It's applied directly to the tooth, using a wetted toothpick or cotton-tipped applicator as a packing and shaping instrument. Cavit is easiest to use if it is rolled a bit between the fingers in order to become warm and remain soft. Be sure to apply the material in between the teeth if there is a defect present in that location. Excess material can be removed by flossing. Intermediate restorative material (IRM) is prepared by adding a few drops of eugenol to powdered zinc oxide to make as dry a "dough" as possible. Zinc oxide–eugenol combination cements are advantageous in that they have an anesthetic effect and can be mixed to different consistencies, depending on whether they are to be used as filling material or adhesives. However, the eugenol can leak from its container, and the cement is sticky and more difficult to work with than Cavit. Temporary fillings such as these set after exposure to saliva and usually have to be replaced every few days. Another improvised filling is softened candle wax mixed with a few strands of cotton fiber, applied over a drop or two of eugenol.

If the gum line is inflamed or appears to be infected adjacent to a tooth, you can try to "break up" the infection by flossing vigorously or running a toothpick (probe) down into the space between the tooth and gum line. Administer an antibiotic, such as penicillin, metronidazole, or clindamycin.

Pericoronitis is an infection of the gum flap that overlies a tooth that has only partially advanced ("erupted") into the mouth. This is most common with a lower third molar and usually indicates an infection with *Streptococcus* bacteria. Symptoms include pain and a bad taste in the mouth. The treatment is to scrape and clean underneath and around the flap, initiate warm saltwater ($\frac{1}{2}$ teaspoon salt in a cup of water) rinses every 2 hours, and if the area is reddened such that it appears infected, begin the victim on dicloxacillin, clindamycin, cefuroxime, or erythromycin. Another good mouthwash would contain chlorhexidine 0.2%.

Good oral hygiene is the key to avoiding many tooth and gum problems. Teeth should be brushed twice a day using a soft-bristled toothbrush with a fluoride-containing toothpaste. Spit out excess toothpaste. Many experts recommend side-to-side brushing in the front of the teeth, and up-and-down brushing on the back surfaces. Flossing should be done at least once per day. Carry an antisensitivity toothpaste, such as Sensodyne.

Broken, Displaced, or Lost Tooth

If a tooth is cracked (with the root still present and in place), there is little for the victim to do other than keep his mouth clean and avoid contact with extremes of temperature. If air, saliva, the tongue, or temperature change coming into contact with an exposed nerve causes intolerable pain, a temporary cap (shield) can be created by mixing melted paraffin (candle wax) with a few strands of cotton. When the mixture begins to harden but can still be easily molded, press a wad onto the tooth, using the teeth on either side as anchors. A cap can also be fashioned from Cavit or IRM (see earlier instructions).

If a tooth is broken or a crown falls off, apply a little eugenol to the tooth for immediate pain control. For a displaced crown, determine its proper orientation and then press it back onto the tooth and see if the crown will hold without cement. If not, it will need to be replaced with an adhesive. First, carefully clean the inside of the crown, to remove any particles of old dried adhesive. This can be done by scraping with a safety pin or other similar object. Then, determine its proper orientation on the tooth. Dry the inside of the crown using a bit of cotton or tissue. Then, mix up a small amount of TempBond NE (a self-curing composite dental material) on top of a slightly waxy or other nonadherent surface and then apply it to the inside of the crown. Dry the top of the tooth. Reposition the crown and push it firmly onto the tooth. Have the victim bite down gently but firmly on a piece of cloth or gauze to be certain that the crown is pushed all the way back onto the tooth and is not elevated. If the bite is not proper, then this will cause problems such as a broken crown or underlying tooth. The TempBond NE will harden within the mouth in a minute or two. If TempBond NE is not available, apply a dab of Cavit and use it as a fastener, scraping away the excess. If that is not available, a dab of toothpaste will do. If all else fails, cover the tooth with paraffin or dental wax.

If a tooth is shifted out of its normal position, but is still embedded in the gum, it may need to be repositioned. If the tooth appears to be longer or off to one side, use a gloved hand, firmly grasp the tooth, and move it into proper alignment. If the tooth has been pushed into the gum and appears to be too short, don't move the tooth.

If an adult tooth is knocked cleanly out of the socket, it can sometimes be replaced successfully if the victim can reach a dentist within 2 hours. After that time, there is little hope for salvage of that particular tooth. Don't attempt to replace baby teeth. The best treatment for a tooth that has been out of the socket for 15 minutes or less is to *gently* rinse it clean (don't scrub the root of the tooth; handle it by the crown to avoid injuring the delicate periodontal ligament) and reinsert it with firm pressure into the socket to the level of the adjacent tooth. One way to improve alignment is to have the victim bite down gently on a piece of gauze or cloth after the tooth has been inserted.

Once the tooth is in proper position, it can be held in place by using a string or piece of dental floss to tie the affected tooth first to the tooth on one side of it, and then with a separate tie, to the tooth on the other side (Figure 144). Another method is to splint the tooth in place by fashioning a paraffin bridge or cap to the adjacent tooth. The bridge material should be applied to the front and back of the tooth, but not to where it contacts the occluding (e.g., lower versus upper) tooth. A better material for this purpose is Express Putty, which hardens within 4 minutes after equal amounts of the putty base and catalyst are mixed. Coe-Pak is also used for this purpose. A splint can be fashioned from a small piece of wire or thin, smooth-edged metal and attached using 2-octyl cyanoacrylate (e.g., DERMABOND ADVANCED Topical Skin

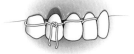

Figure 144. Tying a repositioned avulsed tooth in place with string or dental floss.

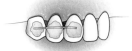

Figure 145. Holding a tooth next to an adjacent tooth using a splint and glue.

Adhesive) or Super Glue to the front of the replaced tooth and at least one adjacent tooth on each side (Figure 145). TempBond NE becomes brittle when it hardens, so is not optimal to use for this purpose. Dry the surfaces of the teeth before applying the glue. The splint should be left in place for 2 weeks. Daily hygiene should include gentle brushing with a soft toothbrush after each meal, and chlorhexidine 0.1% or other mouthwash rinse twice a day for 1 week.

The best storage solution for a tooth that has been knocked out and will be carried to a dentist is pH (acid-base) balanced (i.e., Hank's balanced salt solution). This is accompanied by a cushion to prevent injury to the microscopic ligament cells that hold the tooth in place and must reattach for the tooth to "take." The Save-A-Tooth or EMT Toothsaver storage device is recommended.

Alternatively, the tooth can be placed in a container and covered with a small amount of cool, pasteurized whole milk (not yogurt, low-fat milk, or powdered milk) for transport. Don't carry the tooth on a dry cloth or paper. Don't soak the tooth in tap water. A tooth can also be rinsed and carried by the victim in the space between his lower lip and lower gum (taking care not to swallow the tooth), although saliva is not particularly good for the periodontal ligament. *Don't place a tooth back into the socket unless an antibiotic (penicillin 500 mg four times a day or clindamycin 150 mg three times a day for 1 week) can be administered to avoid an infection, and tetanus toxoid given if necessary.*

If the socket of a broken, extracted, or lost tooth continues to bleed, apply direct pressure by having the victim bite on a gauze pack for at least 30 minutes. If there is a large blood clot, remove it manually or by rinsing, and then apply pressure. Keep the head elevated. If the bleeding does not stop after holding pressure for 30 to 45 minutes, biting on a dry tea bag (tannic acid) may help. Avoid sucking liquids through a straw or vigorous spitting, either of which might dislodge a blood clot that has formed in the socket. Once the bleeding is stopped, avoid rinsing, spitting, tooth brushing, and tobacco use for 24 hours. Gentle rinses with warm saltwater can be started after that time period.

"Dry socket" may occur 2 to 4 days after a tooth is extracted intentionally or accidentally lost. This is characterized by pain, foul odor, and a bad taste. Inspection of the tooth socket may show exposed bone. Treatment is gentle saltwater rinses followed by packing with a strip of eugenol-soaked gauze. The pack should be changed every 1 to 2 days until the symptoms are relieved, which may take up to 10 days. Another way to fill the socket and achieve pain relief is to use a paste of zinc oxide (Alvogyl) mixed with a crushed aspirin and a few drops of eugenol. This should be left in place by covering with a gauze or small piece of cloth for a couple of hours. Yet another anesthetic is topical diphenhydramine (Benadryl), which can be obtained by opening a capsule of the drug intended for oral administration. The powder should be carefully sprinkled into the socket and held in place with gauze. Note that if the powder distributes inside the mouth, areas of contact may become numb. During the recovery period, don't ingest alcohol or carbonated beverages. Taking 4 g of vitamin C by mouth each day has been cited to hasten recovery.

Wearing a properly fitted mouthguard is recommended if there is a high risk for injury to the teeth and the mouthguard will not inhibit success at the activity. Athletes wear them during contact sports, and they may also be used by mountain cyclists and stunt skiers.

Temporomandibular Joint Syndrome

The temporomandibular joint (TMJ)—where the jaw hinges into the face—can become tender if the jaw is struck, from forceful chewing or yawning, or from grinding the teeth at night. If this joint becomes irritated, the pain can be extremely distracting. Therapy consists of an NSAID, warm packs, and avoiding foods (such as beef jerky) that are difficult to chew. Don't chew gum or open the mouth excessively wide.

Mouth Ulcer (Canker Sore)

See page 184.

Trench Mouth

Trench mouth is an extreme case of gingivitis, in which a person's gums are severely inflamed. They are red in appearance and bleed easily. This is most commonly caused by poor oral hygiene, with or without concomitant poor nutrition. There may be a gray membrane between the teeth, and the teeth are often loose. Treatment is administration of oral tetracycline, doxycycline, penicillin, or erythromycin for 10 days, plus using antiseptic (e.g., chlorhexidine) mouthwash (swish and spit four times a day) combined with exquisite oral hygiene.

Broken or Snagged Braces

If a piece of skin or tongue becomes snagged in a sharp orthodontia wire, you need to use your ingenuity to unhook the skin. Sometimes this can be done by manipulating the lip(s) externally to slide them off the wire. You might need to use a forceps or tiny-tipped pliers to do the job. If you are successful, try to prevent the situation from happening again by carefully (don't break teeth) bending over any exposed sharp-edged wire so that it is facing inward toward the teeth, and then cover any rough or sharp exposed metal with wax, cotton, or even chewing gum. If a wire is loose and cannot be fixed into a non-irritating position, you may decide to remove it by cutting or breaking, taking extreme care to have a firm grip on it during the process so that it cannot be inhaled or swallowed.

UPPER RESPIRATORY DISORDERS

COMMON COLD

Most "colds" are upper respiratory tract infections caused by one of a host (at least 200) of viruses. It's not true that exposure to a cold climate ("catching a chill") causes a cold. Symptoms include runny nose, cough, sore throat, headache, muscle aches, fever, fatigue, weakness, and occasional nausea with vomiting and/or diarrhea. Unfortunately, there is no cure for the common cold. The best medicine is rest (although mild exercise may make you feel better), increased fluid intake to prevent dehydration and loosen secretions, and acetaminophen or aspirin for fever. *To avoid Reye syndrome (postviral encephalopathy and liver failure), don't use aspirin to control fever in a child under age 17. Use acetaminophen in preference to ibuprofen.*

Keep the victim warm (particularly the feet) and dry. For persons ages 6 years and older, treat nasal congestion with an oral decongestant and nasal spray (use the latter for 3 days maximum). Be aware that an oral decongestant can make a child hyperactive. For an infant, use saline nose drops ($\frac{1}{4}$ teaspoon [1.3 mL] of table salt in 1 cup [237 mL] of water) in a dose of two to three drops in each nostril a few times a day; the child will sneeze, or the drops can drain via gravity or be sucked out with a "baby bulb" syringe. When blowing your nose, be gentle, in order to avoid pushing mucus from the nose up into the sinuses.

A person who breathes steam (which has not been proved to improve a common cold) must be careful to avoid burns. There is no scientific evidence to support the use of chest rubs or megavitamins (specifically, vitamin C) in the prevention or diminution of viral illnesses. Probably the most important factor in rehabilitation is adequate rest.

Don't attempt to "sweat out" a cold with vigorous exercise. Such behavior causes worsened fever, dehydration, and debilitation. A person with a cold should see a doctor if he is ill for more than 3 weeks, his temperature elevation becomes extreme (see page 155), he develops a cough productive of yellow-green or darkened phlegm (see pages 45 and 192), or he develops chest pain associated with breathing, shaking chills, a severe earache, or a headache with a stiff neck (see page 162). Since colds are spread by contact, take particular care to wash and gel your hands after contact with an infected person.

The most common complication of a cold in a child is a middle ear infection. If a young child with a runny nose and cough begins to pull at his ear(s) or if a fever returns near the end of the course of a cold, consider treating the child for otitis media (see page 163). Pneumonia can also be a complication (see page 45). It should be suspected in any young child who appears short of breath (respiratory rate above 30 per minute in a child, or 40 per minute in an infant).

A cold can be differentiated from seasonal allergies on the basis of the following: cold—fever, chills, yellowish or green nasal discharge, sore throat, diarrhea, muscle aches; allergies—clear nasal discharge, repetitive sneezing, watery and itchy eyes.

Someone who has a chronic (lasts longer than 3 weeks) cough not clearly associated with a cold or other viral infection of the respiratory tract, who is coughing up blood, or who has another known problem such as pneumonia or lung cancer should seek the attention of a physician. The most common causes of a chronic cough are cigarette smoking, postnasal drip (often stimulated by seasonal allergies), unsuspected asthma, chronic sinus infection, or acid reflux from the stomach into the esophagus. In addition, persons who take angiotensin-converting enzyme (ACE) inhibitors to treat high blood pressure may develop a cough; this usually disappears a few days after the medicine is discontinued.

A U.S. FOOD AND DRUG ADMINISTRATION ADVISORY PANEL IN 2007 RECOMMENDED THAT THERE IS NO EVIDENCE THAT OVER-THE-COUNTER COLD AND COUGH MEDICINES WORK IN CHILDREN AND THAT THE PRODUCTS SHOULD NOT BE GIVEN TO CHILDREN YOUNGER THAN 6 YEARS OF AGE.

INFLUENZA

The influenza viruses (A, B, and C, with A being the most common and likely to cause pandemics) are responsible for seasonal epidemics of the flu, a predominantly respiratory disease. Variants of influenza A are known according to the host species (e.g., humans, swine, birds, horses) in which the viruses are most commonly found. In temperate climates, influenza is a cold weather disease. The illness is recognized by sudden high fever, sore throat, cough, nasal congestion, headache, muscle aches, weakness, and occasional (more common in children) nausea with vomiting and/or diarrhea. "Stomach flu" is a misnomer, because it is not caused by influenza virus, but rather, by other viruses and bacteria. Influenza is distinguished from a common cold by its intensity, particularly of the headache and muscle aches. The virus is transmitted from person to person via virus-laden large droplets (greater than 5 microns in diameter) generated when infected persons cough or sneeze or touch surfaces upon which the virus has come to rest. The incubation period is 1 to 3 days before a person becomes contagious, after which he sheds virus for up to another week.

Elderly or infirm individuals are at greatest risk for becoming severely debilitated or developing complications, such as pneumonia caused by bacteria. General therapy is the same as that for a cold: rest, adequate nutrition, increased fluid intake, and medicine for fever. Vaccines are prepared each year that are somewhat effective in the prevention of types A and B influenza (see page 426). Oseltamivir phosphate (Tamiflu) is a drug that's used for treatment of influenza types A and B for 5 days. In adults who have been ill for no more than 2 days, it is given in an adult oral dose of 75 mg twice daily. The pediatric dose is based on age and weight. For a child age 2 weeks to 12 years: weight less than 15 kg, 30 mg twice daily; 15 to 23 kg, 45 mg twice daily; 23 to 40 kg, 60 mg twice daily; weight greater than 40 kg or age greater than 12 years, 75 mg twice daily. For prevention of influenza, use the same dose once a day for 10 days. An alternative is zanamivir (Relenza) 10 mg inhaled twice a day for (1) treatment of persons older than 7 years of age for 5 days and (2) inhaled once a day for prevention for persons older than 5 years of age for 10 days. Persons at high risk (for severe influenza or complications) who should be treated with oseltamivir or zanamivir are children younger than 5 years of age (particularly younger than 2 years of age), adults older than 65 years of age, persons with chronic diseases (lung, heart, kidney, liver), diabetics, immunosuppressed, pregnant or within 2 weeks of having given birth, on chronic aspirin therapy, American Indians, Alaskan natives, morbidly obese, or residents of nursing homes or long-term care facilities. It should be noted that some experts have called into question the true benefit of treating influenza with oseltamivir or zanamivir, doubting whether the minimal reduction in duration of illness justifies the side effects and expense. So, recommendations for use of these drugs may change.

During an epidemic, victims have in the past benefited from administration of the oral drug rimantadine 200 mg by mouth daily for 5 to 7 days in adults, and 5 mg/kg of body weight per day (up to 150 mg) for 5 to 7 days in children. An alternative was amantadine in a dose of 100 mg twice daily for 5 days in adults, or 2.2 mg/kg of body weight (up to 75 mg) twice daily for 5 days in children. Note that these two medications are available by prescription for the prevention and treatment of type A influenza because they are ineffective against type B. They are also associated with several toxic effects and influenza viruses in the United States have become highly resistant to them, so they are not used routinely. They are mentioned here in the event that you find yourself in a situation outside of the United States where these are the only drugs available during an epidemic.

Avian influenza A (specifically H5N1, which exists in at least eight subgroups, or "clades") may be resistant to the adamantane drugs (rimantadine and amantadine), so would be treated with zanamivir or oseltamivir, the former in a dose of 75 mg and the latter in a dose of 150 mg by mouth twice a day for 10 days. This form of influenza is carried and spread by birds, notably poultry and perhaps wild birds. It has been found in other species, such as cats, tigers, leopards, pigs, ferrets, rabbits, rats, and emus, from which it might more rapidly mutate to a form more infectious to humans. Avian flu has a very aggressive profile, with a high (up to 60%) overall mortality rate in human victims. Infected humans show "typical" flu symptoms, followed rapidly by respiratory and multi-organ failure. There is little evidence for mild or asymptomatic human infections.

Undoubtedly, new strains of influenza A, such as H7N9, will continue to emerge, linked to animal origins and reservoirs for the viruses.

Influenza B less frequently causes severe disease, but it's certainly possible, usually in the form of heart disease. The two lineages of influenza B that circulate in the general population are Victoria-like and Yamagata-like.

With regard to protective masks, a properly fitted N95 face mask is supposed to have at least a 95% filtration capability at filtering a 0.3 micron droplet, which carries the virus, but not the virus particles individually.

BRONCHITIS

Bronchitis is inflammation of the air passages (bronchi), characterized by cough that persists for more than 5 days, production of sputum (clear [white], yellow or green phlegm, or "secretions"), fever, hoarseness, muscle aches, fatigue, and sometimes wheezing. Pneumonia is much more intense than bronchitis and involves severe, progressive pulmonary deterioration; bronchitis is a less debilitating condition. Cigarette smokers are prone to recurrent bouts of bronchitis, because they repetitively paralyze the defense mechanisms of the nose, throat, and lungs with cigarette smoke, and may have scarred lungs. Viruses and bacteria may cause bronchitis.

Treatment is controversial, since in the absence of a documented bacterial infection, no particular therapy has been shown to shorten the duration of bronchitis. If bronchitis persists for more than 2 to 3 weeks (particularly in persons who smoke cigarettes), or if the sputum changes in color from clear (white) to colored, then therapy may include administration of an oral antibiotic (first choice azithromycin, levofloxacin, or amoxicillin–clavulanate; others include moxifloxacin, amoxicillin, trimethoprim–sulfamethoxazole, doxycycline, cefixime, cefpodoxime, cefprozil, or erythromycin). With or without antibiotics, normal fluid intake, inhalation of humidified warm air (taking care to avoid steam burns) in order to loosen secretions and ease coughing, a drug to loosen secretions (e.g., guaifenesin [Mucinex] 600 mg by mouth every 12 hours), and acetaminophen or aspirin (the latter not for children under age 17 years) for fever may diminish symptoms. It's best to allow the victim to cough up secretions; however, if coughing fits become intolerable, a cough medicine (see page 470) may be used. Dextromethorphan is therefore often more effective than guaifenesin, which does not control coughing. A 7-day course of inhaled or oral corticosteroids may help. If wheezing and shortness of breath are problematic, an inhaled bronchodilator, such as albuterol, may be used. If pneumonia is suspected (see page 45), treat appropriately and seek immediate medical attention.

PLEURITIS

The lining of the lung, or pleura, is two layers of tissue separated by a thin film of lubricating fluid, which allows the lung to expand with a gliding motion when the chest wall moves outward during inhalation. When the pleura is irritated by an infection, most often caused by a virus, the inflammation may allow fluid to accumulate in this space and cause pain with breathing, localized to the area of irritation. The pain is sharp and worsened by a cough or deep breath. The treatment for viral pleuritis is rest and aspirin. Encourage the victim to breathe deeply. If he is weak or has a high fever, suspect deterioration into pneumonia (see page 45).

HAY FEVER

Hay fever ("rose fever," "catarrh") is an allergic reaction, often seasonal (hence the term "seasonal allergies") to dust, animal dander, plant (usually ragweed, sage, trees, and grasses) pollens, or other compounds found in the air. The victim suffers from red, itchy, and watery (from excessive tearing) eyes; swollen eyelids; white, ropey mucus discharge from the eyes; a runny nose with large amounts of clear mucus (allergic rhinitis); irritated nose with or without nasal congestion; sneezing; and general misery. In a severe case, a victim may suffer asthma, sinusitis, loss of smell, and fatigue. Fever is not a component. In most cases, the symptoms can be relieved by taking an antihistamine medication—although some of these have side effects, the most troublesome of which is drowsiness. Antihistamines that cause drowsiness include triprolidine (Actifed), diphenhydramine (Benadryl), and chlorpheniramine (Chlor-Trimeton). Nonsedating antihistamines, such as fexofenadine (Allegra), loratadine (Claritin), and cetirizine (Zyrtec), cause much less or no drowsiness. A nasal decongestant (such as oxymetazoline [Afrin]) will clear out the nose, but does not halt the allergic reaction. Furthermore, a nasal decongestant should not be used for more than 5 consecutive days, to avoid "rebound" nasal congestion from drug-induced inflammation. An allergy doctor can use skin tests to evaluate a victim for desensitization injections or patches. If allergies are debilitating and a change in environment is impossible, the victim will almost certainly benefit from a tapering dose of prednisone (see page 461). Nasal steroid sprays (such as fluticasone propionate 0.05% [Flonase], budesonide 32 mcg nasal spray [Rhinocort Aqua], or beclomethasone dipropionate [Beconase]) are a method for treating nasal irritation (blockage, runny nose, itching, and sneezing) from allergies, but usually require approximately 3 consecutive days use before a beneficial effect is noted. Cromolyn sodium nasal spray (NasalCrom), as recommended by some allergists, is another useful adjunct. This requires administration of up to four to six doses per day, and it may be 1 to 4 weeks before any benefit is noted.

Nonsteroidal eye drops for ocular allergy manifestations (seasonal allergic conjunctivitis) include 4% cromolyn sodium, ketorolac tromethamine 0.5% (Acular), lodoxamide 0.1% (stabilizes the cells that release histamine), and levocabastine hydrochloride 0.05% (histamine antagonist). While each of these is effective, it remains to be proved if any is more effective than cold soaks, artificial tears, or over-the-counter topical antihistamine (antazoline or pheniramine, combined with the blood vessel–constricting drug naphazoline hydrochloride) eye drops. Eye symptoms usually respond to oral medications used to treat systemic allergies.

DISORDERS OF THE GASTROINTESTINAL TRACT

DIARRHEA

Although diarrhea is included here in the "minor problems" section, severe diarrhea can be devastating. Diarrhea can be due to a number of causes, including bacterial infection, viral infection, protozoal infection (such as the protozoan *Cyclospora cayetanensis*, which can contaminate fresh berries, or *Cryptosporidium* species, which are waterborne), food poisoning from toxin(s), unusual parasites, inflammatory bowel disease, allergies, and anxiety. It's not always easy to determine the cause of loose bowel movements, but there is a general approach to therapy that ordinarily suffices until a precise diagnosis can be made. Diarrhea, with or without other manifestations of chronic illness, is a common complaint in travelers returned from foreign countries.

In all cases of diarrhea, a common discomfort is the irritated anus (particularly one that has been wiped with leaves or newspaper). Every traveler should carry a roll of toilet paper, baby wipes, and 1% hydrocortisone lotion or steroid ointment for an irritated bottom. Desitin diaper cream and A&D ointment also work well.

General Therapy for Diarrhea

Diet. If nausea and vomiting don't prevent eating, adjust the diet:

1. When diarrhea is severe, stick to clear fluids such as mineral water, soda, Kool-Aid, or broth. Electrolyte-containing sports beverages are fine. Apple and grape juices are good, but orange, tomato, pineapple, and grapefruit juices may irritate the stomach. Avoid milk products, tea, coffee, raw fruits and vegetables, and fatty foods. Don't take aspirin.
2. As soon as there is improvement (less frequent bowel movements, decreased cramping, increased appetite), begin solid foods, starting with broth, crackers, toast, gelatin, and hard-boiled eggs.

3. As the diarrhea subsides, add applesauce, mashed bananas, rice, boiled or baked potatoes, and plain pasta.
4. When stools begin to firm up, add cooked lean meat, cooked vegetables, yogurt, and cottage cheese. Avoid alcohol, spicy foods, and stewed fruit.

Dehydration can be estimated as follows:

1. Mild dehydration: Thirst, dry mucous membranes (mouth, eyes), dry armpits, dark urine, decreased sweating, normal pulse rate.
2. Moderate dehydration: The above plus sunken eyes, doughy skin, weakness, scant darkened urine, rapid and weak pulse rate.
3. Severe dehydration: The above plus altered mental status, elevated body temperature, no urine, no tears, no sweating, collapse, shock (see page 58).
4. In a baby, dehydration is manifest as dry diaper (decreased urine output), sunken eyes, sunken "soft spot" (fontanel) on the top of the head, dry tongue and mouth, rapid pulse, poor skin color (blue or pale), lethargy ("floppy baby"), and fast breathing (greater than 30 breaths per minute in a small child, or 40 per minute in an infant). For purposes of estimation, a normal pulse rate (per minute) in a newborn averages 120; at 2 years, 110; at 4 to 6 years, 100; and at 8 to 10 years, 90.

Fluid replacement. If fluid losses are significant (more than five bowel movements per day), begin to replace liquids as soon as you can. When in doubt as to the severity of dehydration, begin to replace liquids. If only fruit juice (without supplementation) is available, remember to cut it to half strength with water. Otherwise, the sugar content will be too high and may contribute to continued diarrhea. Estimation techniques to measure powdered ingredients (such as a "pinch" of table salt) are notoriously inaccurate, and can even be dangerous if you add excessive amounts. Use a proper measuring implement whenever possible. If nausea and vomiting are present to a degree sufficient to inhibit or prevent oral rehydration, consider administration of an antiemetic drug, such as ondansetron (Zofran: adult dose 4 mg oral dissolving tablet; pediatric dose 0.15 mg/kg body weight of the oral dissolving tablet every 8 hours).

1. *Mild diarrhea/dehydration:* Drink soda water, clear juices, broth, and electrolyte-containing sports beverages. Try to replace each diarrheal stool with 10 mL of oral rehydration salts (ORS) per 1 kg (2.2 lb) of body weight. If the child is vomiting, try to replace each episode of vomiting with 2 mL of ORS per 1 kg (2.2 lb) of body weight. Give ORS or any other replacement fluid slowly at first so that it is tolerated without vomiting. For small children, this may be a teaspoonful at a time; for adults it will be sips from a cup. If the patient vomits, then wait for 10 minutes and try once again to give ORS, but more slowly.
2. *Moderate diarrhea/dehydration:* Drink diluted (by half, with water) electrolyte-containing sports beverages, mineral water (bottled), or a homemade solution consisting of 1 quart or liter of disinfected water (or orange juice) plus ½ to 1 teaspoon (1.3 to 2.5 mL) of sodium chloride (table salt), ½ teaspoon of sodium bicarbonate (baking soda), ¼ teaspoon (0.6 mL) of potassium chloride (salt substitute), and glucose (6 to 8 teaspoons [30 to 40 mL] of table sugar, or 1 to 2 tablespoons [15 to 30 mL] of honey). Take care not to oversweeten (i.e., do not exceed 2% to 2.5% glucose) the solution with sugar, because this may worsen the diarrhea; too high a sugar concentration inhibits water absorption through the gastrointestinal tract. Each quart of this "home brew" should be alternated with ½ to 1 quart of plain disinfected water. Try to replace fluid losses at least every 2 hours.

   ORS that meet World Health Organization standards are available in a dry mix; use one packet per quart (liter) of water. One packet contains sodium chloride 3.5 g, potassium chloride 1.5 g, glucose 20 g, and trisodium citrate 2.9 g (or sodium bicarbonate 2.5 g). CeraLyte 70 ORS are based on a rice solution. One packet is mixed with a quart (liter) of water. After the solution is prepared, it should be consumed or discarded within 12 hours if kept at room temperature or 24 hours if kept refrigerated. *Rice-based electrolyte-containing drinks, such as CeraSport, are likely more effective than water in replacing fluid losses.* Other ORS products available over-the-counter include Pedialyte, Enfalyte, Naturalyte, and Rehydralyte. Elete is an electrolyte additive (to water) that contains sodium, chloride, potassium, zinc, and magnesium, but no glucose or carbohydrate.

In greater detail, try to get the victim to ingest a quart per hour until the frequency of urination begins to increase and the urine color becomes light-colored or clear. To begin, start with small (e.g., 5 mL or 1 teaspoon) amounts every 1 to 2 minutes, to avoid collection of a large amount of fluid in the stomach that might cause vomiting. A child should be given 1½ oz (44 mL) of ORS per pound (0.45 kg) of body weight over the first 4 hours, then 1 oz (30 mL) of ORS per pound of body weight per 8-hour period until the diarrhea resolves. Another estimate of fluid replacement for children is 100 mL (approximately 3 oz) of fluid per significant loose bowel movement. For an infant with diarrhea, decrease the amount of milk in the diet and add more water, diluted juices, half-strength sports beverages, and ORS. Sweetened carbonated beverages (soda pop) aren't good replacement fluids, because they contain too much sugar and little or no sodium and potassium. If the child is breast-fed, keep nursing (offer the breast more often). If the child is formula-fed, use ORS for 12 to 24 hours, and then try switching back to formula. If the diarrhea persists, switch back to ORS for another cycle. It's important to continue to provide nourishment with food (and calories) to children with diarrhea, not fluid alone. Avoid foods high in simple sugars (including tea, juices, and soft drinks). Try complex carbohydrates (rice, wheat, potatoes, bread, cereals), yogurt, lean meat, fruits, and vegetables.

If premeasured salts aren't available with which to supplement water, you can alternate glasses of the following two fluids, as recommended by the U.S. Public Health Service:
- Glass one—8 oz fruit juice with ¼ teaspoon (a "pinch") table salt and ½ teaspoon honey or corn syrup (237 mL juice, 1.3 mL table salt, 2.5 mL honey or corn syrup)
- Glass two—8 oz disinfected water with ¼ teaspoon baking soda (sodium bicarbonate) (237 mL water, 1.3 mL baking soda)

3. Another homemade fluid mixture is 1 teaspoon (5 mL) table salt and 1 cup (275 mL) rice cereal in a quart (liter) of water; this must be used within 12 hours or discarded. A small amount of artificial sweetener may make this mixture taste better.
4. *Severe diarrhea/dehydration:* Same as moderate. After a certain point, as with cholera, intravenous hydration may be lifesaving. See a physician as soon as possible.

Rehydration enema. When it is impossible to administer oral fluids, a rehydration enema can be lifesaving. Lubricate the anus, and then administer 1 pint of an enema solution of 1 liter of room temperature water mixed with 5 tablespoons of sugar and 1 tablespoon of salt. If the sugar and salt aren't available, use plain water. Have the person try to relax and retain the fluid for as long as possible before evacuating the residual. Try to administer 1 pint every 1 to 2 hours until the person is producing light-colored urine or is able to tolerate oral liquids.

Antimotility (decreased bowel activity) drugs. If fever, severe cramping, and bloody diarrhea are absent, it's safe to use antimotility drugs. They should be immediately discontinued if diarrhea lasts for more than 48 hours. If diarrhea lasts longer than 3 days, if the victim has a fever greater than 101°F (38.3°C), if he cannot keep liquids down because of vomiting, if there is blood in or on the stool, if the abdomen becomes swollen, or if there is no significant pain relief after 24 hours, seek a physician immediately.

The antimotility drug of choice is loperamide (Imodium A-D). The initial adult dose is 4 mg (two 2 mg capsules, or 4 teaspoons [20 mL] of the liquid), followed by 2 mg after each loose bowel movement, not to exceed 16 mg (eight capsules) per day or 2 consecutive days of administration. With uncomplicated (no fever or blood in stools), watery diarrhea, this drug can be given to children age 2 years and older. Give children a dose of 0.2 mg/kg (2.2 lb) of body weight every 6 hours. The liquid preparation contains 1 mg/teaspoon (5 mL).

For adults, diphenoxylate (Lomotil) is an alternative, but has side effects of dry mouth and urinary retention. Pepto-Bismol is another, less effective choice (see page 198).

Kaopectate (kaolin plus pectin) is of limited value. It does not shorten the course of diarrheal illness, and acts only to add a little consistency to stools. Lactobacillus preparations (acidophilus beverages or yogurt) don't shorten the course of acute diarrheal illness, but may be useful to repopulate the gastrointestinal tract with normal bacteria after a severe bout of diarrhea or administration of antibiotics used to treat diarrhea.

In non-U.S. countries, drugs that have been recommended to treat diarrhea in the absence of a specific diagnosis include chloramphenicol (Chloromycetin), Entero-Vioform, MexaForm, Intestopan, clioquinol, and iodoquinol. This may be dangerous, because these drugs can have adverse direct effects or side effects. Therefore, this approach should not be taken without a specific diagnosis for which these drugs are felt to be indicated.

Antibiotics. These should be used if diarrhea is moderate to severe (more than eight bowel movements per day), particularly if it is bloody and associated with severe cramping, vomiting, and fever.

Administer ciprofloxacin (Cipro) 500 mg twice a day, or trimethoprim–sulfamethoxazole (Bactrim or Septra) one double-strength pill twice a day for 3 days. These will treat *Escherichia coli* and *Shigella,* may be of use for *Salmonella,* and will not adversely affect the course of viral, *Staphylococcus,* or *Campylobacter* infections. If the person still suffers from diarrhea without improvement after 24 hours of this first antibiotic, add azithromycin (1 g single dose). The duration of cholera caused by *Vibrio cholerae* may be shortened by treating with azithromycin (1 g single dose), ciprofloxacin (1 g single dose; increasing resistance is being noted to this drug), or doxycycline (300 mg single dose) for adults, or trimethoprim–sulfamethoxazole (5 mg/kg, or 2.2 lb, of body weight, based on the trimethoprim component, for 3 days) for children, Other beneficial effects of antibiotic administration for cholera include diminished rate of "purging" diarrhea (often in the form of profound "rice water" stools), shortened period of being infectious, and less requirement for rehydration. The antibiotic is most effectively given after rehydration therapy has begun to take effect and vomiting diminished to the point that the antibiotic can be retained. Resistant strains are very common; for instance, in Bangladesh, cholera is resistant to tetracycline, erythromycin, and trimethoprim–sulfamethoxazole. Enteric fever caused by *Salmonella typhi* (typhoid fever) is best treated in adults with ciprofloxacin.

Alternative drugs include norfloxacin (Noroxin) 400 mg twice a day for 3 days, ofloxacin (Floxin) 200 or 300 mg twice a day for 3 days, or fleroxacin 400 mg once a day for 3 days. Another alternative drug is doxycycline (Vibramycin) 100 mg twice a day. Children younger than 12 years of age should not be given doxycycline, because it may cause discoloration of the permanent teeth. Because ciprofloxacin may affect bone growth in children, it should be given only to adults.

If the clinical picture clearly points to *Giardia lamblia* (see page 202), administer metronidazole (Flagyl) 250 mg three times a day for 7 days. A woman who is possibly pregnant should not use this drug except under the advice of her physician.

Sometimes diarrhea appears as a complication of antibiotic administration. This is called *Clostridium difficile*–associated disease, antibiotic-associated diarrhea, or antibiotic-associated colitis. It is caused by infection with the organism *C. difficile*, which thrives in the bowel after the normal germs are killed by the initial antibiotic therapy. Another causative factor may be administration of a proton pump inhibitor drug, which lowers gastric acid. This helps *C. difficile* to survive and therefore be able to elaborate its toxin. Therapy against *C. difficile* is metronidazole (Flagyl) 500 mg by mouth three times a day or 250 mg by mouth four times a day, or vancomycin 125 mg by mouth four times a day for 10 days. It's important to note that *C. difficile* spores aren't destroyed by disinfectant hand gels; thus handwashing remains extremely important to prevent the spread of this infectious organism. *C. difficile* infection is also observed in travelers without any history of prior antibiotic use.

Probiotics are harmless microorganisms (mostly bacteria and yeast) that are thought to provide health benefits. Examples include *Lactobacillus rhamnosus* and *casei*, which are found in certain yogurt products, and CULTURELLE, which is an all-natural dietary supplement containing the probiotic *L. rhamnosus* GG (LGG). Probiotics, therefore, are a class of "friendly" bacteria that live in the digestive tract, where they help to restore and maintain a healthy balance of "good" versus "bad" bacteria. They may be useful in helping the bowel recover its normal function if ingested during and after a bout of diarrhea, particularly if antibiotics are used to treat the victim. They may also slightly shorten the duration and symptoms of acute infectious diarrhea and lessen the propensity for a person to develop *C. difficile* infection after being treated with an antibiotic for gastroenteric infection.

Recovery from Diarrhea

After suffering from diarrhea, the recovering person will have a return of appetite and may wish to make up for lost time. That temptation to overeat should be resisted by using a "recovery diet" that progresses from easily digested foods such as crackers, gelatin, and "simple" carbohydrates; to eggs, potatoes, rice, bananas, and cooked vegetables; to dairy, meat, fatty foods, and raw fruits and vegetables. How quickly one progresses back to a normal diet depends on the reaction to the diet. If there is diminished gastroenteric upset accompanied by the presence of formed stools, then the diet can be advanced. One common problem that persons who have suffered from diarrhea may cause themselves is avoiding fiber and perceived irritating foods for too long to the extent that they now become constipated. After infectious diarrhea is resolved, one should optimally be able to get back to a normal diet and bowel pattern within a few days.

Traveler's Diarrhea

Traveler's diarrhea ("turista," "Kathmandu quickstep," "Montezuma's revenge," "Delhi belly," "Aztec two-step," "Hong Kong dog," and many other synonyms) is frequent, loose bowel movements (three or more loose stools in a 24-hour period) associated with one or more of nausea, vomiting, abdominal cramps, fever, urge to defecate, cramping and straining with defecation, or bloody or mucus-laden stools. It is caused by waterborne or food-borne pathogens, most commonly produced by forms of the bacterium *E. coli*, which is introduced into the diet as a fecal contaminant in water or on food. Someone has described it as "stool that fits the shape of the container." When caused by *E. coli*, symptoms usually occur 12 to 36 hours after ingesting the bacteria, and include the gradual or sudden onset of frequent (four to five per day) loose or watery bowel movements, rarely explosive, and far less violent than diarrhea associated with classic food poisoning (see later). Fever, bloating, fatigue, and abdominal pain are of minor to moderate severity. Nausea and vomiting are less frequently found than with viral gastroenteritis. Most traveler's diarrhea is caused by bacteria, but a small percentage may be caused by viruses or parasites.

The affliction will resolve spontaneously in 2 to 5 days if untreated, but may be hastened to a conclusion if an antibiotic is administered. The current recommendation is to treat adults with ciprofloxacin (Cipro) 500 mg twice a day for 1 to 3 days or a single dose of 1 g, norfloxacin 800 mg in a single dose, or azithromycin 1 g single dose (10 mg/kg [2.2 lb] of body weight in children once a day for 3 days). Trimethoprim–sulfamethoxazole (e.g., Bactrim or Septra) is no longer recommended for traveler's diarrhea, because of bacterial resistance. In Nepal, ciprofloxacin is very poorly effective for traveler's diarrhea, and azithromycin appears to be losing its effectiveness, all attributed to bacterial resistance. Fortunately, another effective drug (so far) is rifaximin in a dose of 200 mg by mouth three times per day for 3 days. For known traveler's diarrhea, the addition of loperamide (Imodium A-D) to the antibiotic regimen can be of significant benefit, with the precaution that it should be used only in the absence of high fever or bloody diarrhea. Alternatively, the diarrhea can be treated with bismuth subsalicylate (Pepto-Bismol); give two 262 mg tablets (or the liquid equivalent) every 30 minutes for eight doses, which may be repeated the second day. Kaolin and pectin given orally in combination may make the stools less runny, but don't shorten the duration of the diarrhea. Yogurt and lactobacillus preparations aren't effective treatments.

During the recovery period, it's fine to advance the diet fairly rapidly over a few days from clear liquids to bland foods to a normal diet.

To prevent traveler's diarrhea, a person traveling to high-risk regions with questionable hygiene and municipal water disinfection standards (developing countries of Latin America, Africa, the Middle East, and Asia) can take rifaximin 200 mg once a day or ciprofloxacin 500 mg (or norfloxacin 400 mg or ofloxacin 200 mg) once a day, during the journey. Southern Europe (Spain, Greece, Italy, Turkey) and parts of the Caribbean pose a lesser risk. Another drug that can be used is doxycycline (Vibramycin) 100 mg twice a day. This should be done under the guidance of a physician, who will explain the risks (allergic reactions, tendinitis, blood disorders, antibiotic-associated colitis, vaginal yeast infection, skin rashes, photosensitivity) versus the benefits (particularly for those prone to infectious diarrhea or who would suffer unduly from an episode of severe diarrhea). Ingesting lactobacilli may improve certain aspects of digestion, but does not prevent traveler's diarrhea.

Alternatively, it has been recommended that you can drink 4 tablespoons (60 mL) of Pepto-Bismol (bismuth subsalicylate) four times a day; this necessitates carrying one 8 oz bottle for each day. The tablets (two 262 mg tablets four times a day) are less palatable. However, this prophylaxis is not intended to substitute for dietary discretion. In addition, large doses of bismuth subsalicylate can be toxic, particularly to people who regularly use aspirin. Anyone with an aspirin allergy should not use bismuth subsalicylate. Side effects include blackened stools and a black tongue, nausea, constipation, and ringing in the ears.

People who would be advised to consider taking a drug to prevent infectious diarrhea include those with a significant underlying medical problem (such as acquired immunodeficiency syndrome [AIDS], inability to produce stomach acid, or inflammatory bowel disease) and those with an itinerary schedule rigid enough that it would be catastrophic to the mission to be laid up with diarrhea.

Prevention of Infectious Diarrhea

Some experts and the medical literature argue that conventional advice to avoid specific foods and liquids doesn't really help prevent traveler's diarrhea. However, on the chance that certain behaviors might be helpful, here are some commonly accepted notions of food safety.

General

- Wash your hands and use disinfectant gel before handling food during preparation or before eating.
- Stick to food that is served steaming hot.
- Dry foods, such as bread, are generally safe.

- Avoid casseroles, quiches, lasagna, and other foods that are prepared in advance and then allowed to sit for a prolonged period before consumption. During that time period, they can be contaminated by bacteria from fingers, insect legs, and contaminated serving utensils.
- As the World Health Organization simplifies its advice, "Peel it, cook it, or leave it."
- Spices (particularly originating from Mexico or India), including pepper, coriander, oregano, cumin, and curry, may be contaminated with bacteria such as *Salmonella*. Be certain to cook all foods seasoned with spices to a sufficiently high temperature.
- Cold foods should be maintained below 40°F (4.4°C). Hot foods should be maintained above 145°F (62.8°C).
- Foods with high sugar content, although not necessarily nutritious, are often safe to eat.
- Don't eat food taken from a leaking or swollen can (see Botulism, page 204). Inspect all food before eating for signs of obvious spoilage or contamination.
- Properly wash camp dishes and implements for eating (see page 200).

Food handling and storage
- Keep raw and cooked foods separate and discard all unused cooked food if there is no refrigeration.
- Refrigeration is considered to be 40°F (4.4°C) or below by any reasonable method.
- If you are thawing food, try to do so under cold conditions and not allow the food to become warm.
- Food should be prepared immediately before it is to be eaten. If the food is not refrigerated or maintained hot, it should be discarded after 1 hour.
- Foods of high hazard for spoilage or contamination are milk and milk products, meat and poultry, and fish and shellfish. When these foods are handled, take care to avoid cross-contamination via utensils, cutting boards, and so forth.

Fruits and vegetables
- Salads (particularly lettuce), raw vegetables, and unpeeled fruits and vegetables are risky business.
- Fresh produce should, when possible, be purchased not bruised or damaged. Produce should not be packed with raw meat, poultry, or seafood products.
- If you purchase already (presumably, fresh) cut produce, select items that are refrigerated or surrounded by ice. Perishable fruits and vegetables that are high risk if not refrigerated include strawberries, lettuce, herbs, and mushrooms.
- Remove any damaged or bruised areas on fruits and vegetables before eating. Discard rotten produce.
- Even if you plan to peel produce, wash or disinfect the surface first. Using a clean produce brush is recommended on the surface of firm produce, such as melons and cucumbers.
- Fruits and leafy vegetables should be washed in iodinated or chlorinated water, washed with dilute soap and previously boiled water, or immersed in boiling water for 30 seconds. Leafy vegetables can be immersed in a solution of chlorine in water at a concentration of 100 parts per million (add 1 tablespoon of liquid household bleach to a gallon of water). Remember to separate leaves and stalks before disinfection to allow better contact.
- Drying produce with a clean cloth or paper towel may further reduce bacterial count.
- In some underdeveloped countries, melons are injected with contaminated water to increase their weight before sale.
- Keep melons (with low acidity) cold. Consider all rinds to be dirty.

Meat and seafood
- Raw or undercooked meat (particularly hamburgers) and raw or undercooked snails or seafood are risky business.
- Refrigerated meat should be consumed within 2 days of purchase.

- Cooking temperature above 165° F (74° C) (particularly for poultry) is advised to kill germs that cause human illness.
- With regard to seafood, raw or undercooked products, particularly shellfish, are especially hazardous. *Vibrio* organisms—which cause, among other problems, cholera—frequently reside in crabs and oysters. Cook all shellfish for a minimum of 10 minutes of boiling, or 30 minutes of exposure to full steam.

Dairy and sauces
- Packaged butter and packaged processed cheese are usually safe to eat.
- Raw and unpasteurized dairy products should be avoided.
- Cold sauces, ice cream, fresh cheese, and spicy sauces in open containers are risky business.

Water and beverages
- Tap water and ice are risky business. Stick to boiled or properly disinfected water.
- Carbonated beverages in sealed bottles or cans should be safe. Alcohol in mixed drinks does not disinfect water.
- At high altitudes and in pristine wilderness environments, it may be safe to brush your teeth with mountain water, so long as you spit and don't swallow. However, it's safer to use properly disinfected water.

Dining out
- Be cautious with buffets, food from street vendors, and the salads served on flights that originate from developing countries.
- Food prepared in restaurants in developing countries probably poses greater risk than does self-prepared food. Patronize reputable establishments.

The Importance of Hand Hygiene

If possible, wash your hands with soap and water before, during, and after preparing food; before eating food; after using a toilet or latrine; after handling a diaper, cleaning a person who has defecated, or disposing of feces (particularly those of children); after blowing your nose, coughing, or sneezing; after touching an animal, animal feed, or animal waste; after handling garbage; before and after caring for someone who is sick; and before and after treating a cut or wound. If a disinfectant gel (at least 60% alcohol-based) or lotion is available, use it, even after handwashing. This will significantly reduce the risk for transmission of bacteria and viruses that cause infections. Disinfectant gels don't provide protection, however, against spore-forming bacteria, such as *C. difficile*, so handwashing retains its importance when this bacterium is a possible environmental contaminant.

In addition to proper handwashing (or wiping with disinfectant gel or cream) and disinfection of drinking water, there are a number of important actions, such as "food rules" (proper washing, cooking, and serving; what foods to avoid—see earlier), bathroom hygiene, not sharing items such as towels and toothbrushes, and so on.

Washing Dishes and Cooking/Eating Utensils

One important topic is how best to wash dishes and cooking/eating utensils to remove diarrhea-causing bacteria and viruses. One effective washing-up system is removal of most food residue with detergent (5 mL or 1 teaspoon) in the water in Bowl One (containing 5 liters of water), followed by a finishing wash (scrub until clean) with bleach (10 mL or 2 teaspoons of 4% chlorine bleach) in the water in Bowl Two (5 liters), followed by a final rinse in drinkable water in Bowl Three (5 liters). The final rinse is felt to remove the taste of the detergent and bleach (the latter considered to be a disinfectant). A few final recommendations are to use hot water in Bowl One, use a scouring pad or brush in Bowl Two with the bleach to avoid contamination of the scourer, allow all utensils to air dry after washing, and clean the washing-up bowls and allow them to dry between uses. Use up to 100 mL or 20 teaspoons (3 teaspoons = 1 tablespoon) of bleach in Bowl Two if there is a current outbreak of diarrhea and vomiting. This increases the disinfection power of the second bowl.

Sometimes it will be necessary to create a chlorine solution for disinfection of hands and skin, floors, clothes, bedding and equipment, or bodily fluids, particularly if someone has suffered diarrhea. For instructions, see page 481.

Water disinfection is discussed on page 406.

Viral Diarrhea

Traveler's diarrhea can also be caused by viruses. Viral gastroenteritis (commonly caused by rotaviruses [perhaps the most common cause of severe gastroenteritis in children less than 5 years of age] or Norwalk-like viruses) includes diarrhea as a symptom. Norovirus (for which there is not yet a licensed vaccine) is a problem with outbreaks of diarrhea on cruise ships, in long-term care facilities, and in schools. Viral gastroenteritis is often associated with nausea and vomiting, fever, stomach cramps, copious rectal gas, and a flu-like syndrome. The diarrhea is typically watery, frequent (up to 20 movements per day), often foul-smelling, discolored (green to greenish brown), and without significant mucus or blood. Generally, the victim will have cyclic waves of lower abdominal cramps, relieved by bowel movements.

It's critical to keep the victim from becoming dehydrated. What comes out below should be replaced from above. Therapy requires continual oral hydration with clear liquids such as apple juice or broth. If they are available, drink electrolyte-containing beverages.

The cramps can be controlled with propantheline bromide (Pro-Banthine), loperamide (Imodium A-D), or diphenoxylate (Lomotil), which will also help limit the diarrhea. It should be noted, however, that these drugs will slow down the activity of the bowel and allow any toxins that are in the gut to remain in contact with the bowel wall. With certain bacterial and viral infections, these drugs may prolong the carrier state and actually increase the severity and duration of the disease. Therefore, it's prudent to avoid the use of loperamide or diphenoxylate unless the intake of fluids cannot keep pace with the diarrhea and dehydration is becoming a real concern. *Never give an antimotility agent to an infant.* Loperamide can be used in children age 2 years and older if the diarrhea is watery and nonbloody, there is no associated fever, and diarrhea is leading to debilitating dehydration. Give a child a 0.2 mg/kg (2.2 lb) of body weight dose every 6 hours. The liquid preparation contains 1 mg/teaspoon (5 mL).

Cryptosporidiosis

Cryptosporidiosis is caused by *Cryptosporidium parvum* or *hominis*, which are commonly found in surface water in the United States. It is also commonly associated with non-U.S. travel. Infection is caused by ingestion of the oocysts and manifested by watery diarrhea, abdominal cramps, nausea and vomiting, fatigue, and low-grade fever. The cysts are 2 microns in diameter. Symptoms begin 2 to 10 days after ingestion, and may last for up to 2 weeks, with a carrier state of up to 2 months. Treatment is nitazoxanide 500 mg by mouth twice a day for 3 days in adults, and 100 mg twice a day in children up to age 12. Another effective treatment is azithromycin 500 mg by mouth once a day for 5 days in adults or paromomycin 500 mg three times a day for 7 days.

Food Poisoning

Food poisoning is caused by toxins that are produced by a number of bacteria, with the most common being *Staphylococcus*. Improper preservation (generally, lack of refrigeration) of food allows bacterial proliferation, which is not corrected by cooking. Typically, the symptoms occur 2 to 6 hours after eating and consist of severe abdominal cramps with nausea and vomiting. Diarrhea may be delayed by an hour or two, or may occur simultaneously with the nausea and vomiting. The diarrhea is often explosive. As with viral gastroenteritis, the bowel movements may be foul-smelling and blood-tinged. The disease is self-limited, and generally subsides after 6 to 12 hours. Treatment consists of rehydration with clear liquids. Antimotility drugs, such as loperamide (Imodium A-D) or diphenoxylate (Lomotil), may prolong the disorder, and should not be used unless the victim cannot replenish fluid losses.

Escherichia Coli O157:H7

E. coli O157:H7 is a bacterium that has been transmitted by as few as 10 bacteria in raw or undercooked hamburger meat, fruit juices, and other food with fecal contamination. It can be spread person to person, and has also been transmitted by petting animals, contacting animal manure, and swimming in recreational pool water. As has been noted previously, in the presence of someone with any cause of diarrhea, excellent handwashing technique should be observed. If a person is ill with a diarrheal illness, he or she should not prepare food for others or share common bodies of swimming or bathing water. Try to not swallow lake or swimming pool water.

After ingesting the bacteria, an infection may occur after an incubation period of 1 to 10 days, with 3 days being the average delay between exposure and illness. It causes a syndrome of fever or no fever, abdominal pain, vomiting, and nonbloody diarrhea, followed in a few days by bloody diarrhea, dehydration, weakness, anemia, and kidney failure. There is not yet an effective treatment with antibiotics. In fact, therapy with some antibiotics may contribute to more severe illness (see later). Prevention means strict handwashing before eating and cooking ground beef until it is no longer pink (160°F [71°C]). Don't mix raw and cooked foods, particularly meat. After you cook meat, don't serve it on the unwashed dish that carried the raw food. Since raw meat, especially beef, can be a problem, be certain to wash hands, cooking utensils, cutting boards, dishes, and counters after they have been in contact with raw meat. Milk and fruit juices prepared from crushing processes require pasteurization. Understand that in the absence of pasteurization, which is a heating process, no product can be guaranteed to not be contaminated with the bacteria normally killed in the pasteurization process. Many of us like to drink fresh fruit juice. When we do so, we take a risk, usually quite minor, that it may be contaminated.

For treatment of known or highly suspected *E. coli* O157:H7 infection, antibiotics are not recommended. This is because in some cases, antibiotics may worsen the affliction. The precise reason this happens is not known, but one suggestion is that by causing rapid death of large numbers of bacteria, large amounts of the Shiga toxin (also known as verocytotoxin) are released, which causes the medical problems. Antidiarrheal agents, such as loperamide (Imodium), are also not recommended, because they are thought to possibly keep the bacteria in contact with the bowel for longer periods of time. Most patients recover without antibiotics in approximately a week. Severely dehydrated individuals may require intravenous fluids. Children infected with *E. coli* O157:H7 are at higher risk than are adults for developing hemolytic-uremic syndrome, in which they may suffer kidney failure.

The difficulty with the recommendation to withhold antibiotics is that it's very difficult to make a precise field diagnosis of any particular cause of diarrhea. So, antibiotics are often given until confirmation of the infectious agent is reported by a laboratory.

Giardia Lamblia

G. lamblia is a flagellate protozoan (one-celled organism) that has become a worldwide problem, particularly in wilderness settings in the western United States, Nepal, and the Soviet Union. It is transmitted as cysts in the feces of many animals, which include humans, elk, beavers, deer, cows, dogs, and sheep. Dormant *Giardia* cysts enter water, from where they are ingested by humans. Cysts can live for up to 3 months in cold water.

If more than 10 to 25 cysts are swallowed, the organisms establish residence in the duodenum and jejunum (first parts of the small bowel), and after an incubation period of 7 to 20 days emerge in another form (trophozoite) to cause stomach cramps, flatulence, a swollen lower abdomen, often explosive and foul-smelling watery ("floating") diarrhea, "rotten" (sulfurous) belching, and nausea. Fever and vomiting are unusual except in the first few days of illness. Foul flatus and abdominal cramping are common. Because of the delay in onset after ingestion of the cysts, many a backpacker develops "backpacker's diarrhea" or "beaver fever" after he returns to civilization, and does not recognize the causal link to the recent journey. If the diarrhea becomes chronic, the victim can lose appetite and weight and become weak. Diagnosis is made by a physician who recognizes trophozoites or microscopic cysts in the stool of the victim, takes a sample of mucus from the duodenum, or is confident with a clinical diagnosis.

Untreated, the illness usually resolves after about 6 weeks. However, the diarrhea may go on for months. Therapy for *Giardia* infestation is administration of metronidazole (Flagyl) 250 to 500 mg three times a day for 7 to 10 days; the pediatric dose is 5 mg/kg (2.2 lb) of body weight to a maximum of 250 mg per dose administered three times per day. Another excellent drug is tinidazole (Tindamax, Tiniba, Fasigyn), which is taken in a 2 g dose for 1 or 2 days; the pediatric dose is 50 mg/kg (2.2 lb) of body weight in a single dose. Another prescription therapy is quinacrine hydrochloride (Atabrine) 100 mg twice a day for 7 days; the pediatric dose is 7 mg/kg (2.2 lb) of body weight per day in three divided doses for 7 days. Unfortunately, quinacrine has side effects (which occur in 1 to 4 out of every 1000 people) that include making the person psychotic (lose touch with reality) for up to a few weeks. A good therapy for children is furazolidone (Furoxone) 6 mg/kg of body weight in four divided doses for 7 days. There have been mixed reports of success with albendazole given in a dose of 400 mg per day for 3 to 5 days. Particularly when an expedition will not reach civilization for 3 to 4 weeks, there is no reason to withhold treatment awaiting a definitive diagnosis. If the field diagnosis is correct, in most cases drug therapy will cause dramatic relief from symptoms within 3 days. There is no prophylactic drug that is recommended to prevent infestation.

Other Infectious Diarrheas

Diarrhea can be caused by a number of parasites and other infectious agents, which include *Campylobacter, Shigella, Salmonella, Yersinia, Vibrio, Cryptosporidium,* and *Entamoeba histolytica* (and other protozoa that cause amebiasis). *Campylobacter jejuni* are the bacteria that most commonly cause diarrhea in the United States, often noted after eating contaminated poultry. Although up to a quarter of persons who are infected are without symptoms, those who become ill frequently exhibit nausea, severe diarrhea, and abdominal pain. *Campylobacter upsaliensis* causes bloody diarrhea in dogs. *Campylobacter* infection is treated with azithromycin 500 mg by mouth once a day for 3 days. The pediatric dose is 10 mg/kg (2.2 lb) of body weight up to 500 mg by mouth once a day for 3 days. *Campylobacter* infection may also be treated with erythromycin 500 mg four times a day for 5 days.

Amebic dysentery is caused by *E. histolytica*, the symptoms of which are the (usually) gradual onset of diarrhea (watery or bloody, frequent, copious, and sometimes with fever) that does not respond to antibiotics, characterized by severe lower abdominal pain and a swollen abdomen. In an endemic area, presumptive field treatment is with metronidazole 750 mg by mouth three times a day for 10 days or tinidazole 600 mg by mouth for 5 days. This is accompanied by eradication of the cyst forms remaining in the bowel wall with a drug such as paromomycin (25 to 35 mg/kg body weight in 3 divided doses for 10 days) or diloxanide furoate (500 mg by mouth three times a day for 7 days). *Cryptosporidium* infection is treated with nitazoxanide (Alinia) in a dose of 500 mg by mouth twice a day for 3 days. Algal diarrhea (a cause of diarrhea more commonly noted in Nepal and Peru) is caused by *Cyclospora cayetanensis,* and is treated with trimethoprim–sulfamethoxazole one double-strength tablet twice a day for 7 days. *Cystoisospora belli* infection is treated with trimethoprim–sulfamethoxazole one double-strength tablet four times a day for 10 days.

Diarrhea-causing pathogens cause a constellation of fever, chills, nausea, vomiting, diarrhea (with or without mucus and blood), weakness, and abdominal pain. Because the clinical picture can be similar with infection from any of these organisms, the differentiation between them frequently relies on examination of the stool under the microscope and/or culture of the stool to identify the specific pathogen. For the sake of the brief expedition, the treatment is the same: rehydration with copious amounts of balanced electrolyte solutions, and antimotility agents only when essential to prevent severe dehydration. If the victim suffers from high fever with shaking chills, has persistent bloody or mucus-laden bowel movements, or is debilitated by dehydration, he should seek the care of a physician. Meanwhile, administration of ciprofloxacin (Cipro) 500 mg two times a day (or 750 mg once a day) or azithromycin 1 g once a day for 3 days will treat *E. coli* and *Shigella*. Infection with *Salmonella* can be treated with levofloxacin 500 mg (or another fluoroquinolone antibiotic) once a day for 7 to 10 days. The pediatric dose for either ciprofloxacin or azithromycin for this purpose is 10 mg/kg (2.2 lb) of body weight up to the adult dose, given twice a day by mouth. As soon as the victim of persistent diarrhea returns to civilization, he should visit a physician for a thorough evaluation. If the ova or parasitic forms of amoebae are seen during microscopic examination of stool, other drugs, such as tinidazole, metronidazole, diloxanide furoate, paromomycin, or diiodohydroxyquin, may be prescribed. If the ova or parasitic forms of worms are seen, drugs such as ivermectin, mebendazole or pyrantel pamoate may be prescribed. Treating the "chronic carrier" condition in which a person harbors typhoidal salmonella involves 4 to 6 weeks of antibiotic treatment.

Botulism

Botulism is a neurotoxic affliction caused by the bacterium *Clostridium botulinum* or certain other *Clostridium* species. Botulism can afflict a person who ingests or inhales the toxin or spores. Wound botulism occurs when a wound is infected with *C. botulinum*. Home-canned foods (particularly vegetables, meat, and seafood) are often the cause if there is a low acid content. Fermented foods, such as fish, herb-infused oils, potatoes baked in aluminum foil and then stored at room temperature before consumption, and sauces (particularly cheese) are also common causes. Infants may ingest botulinum spore–contaminated honey. After an incubation period of 12 hours to 3 days, adults afflicted with foodborne botulism show initial gastroenteric symptoms of constipation, vomiting, and abdominal pain; diarrhea is less common. Neurologic symptoms include blurred or double vision, drooping eyelids, slurred speech, difficulty swallowing, and muscle weakness. This can lead to an inability to breathe. Infants may show symptoms of weakness, sleepiness, tiredness, poor feeding, weak cry, constipation, and diminished head control. If botulism is suspected, the treatment is trivalent antitoxin. This counteracts botulinum toxins A, B, and E, which cause most cases in the United States. There is also a bivalent antitoxin to counteract botulinum toxins A and B. Botulism Antitoxin Heptavalent treats botulism A, B, C, D, E, F, and G.

Irritable Bowel Syndrome

Irritable bowel syndrome (IBS, sometimes called spastic colitis, nervous colon, or irritable colon) is characterized by abdominal distention, the passage of flatus, cramping (pain) relieved by defecation, onset associated with change in frequency and/or form of the stool, and mucus-laden diarrhea. This can be debilitating. The sufferer may also complain intermittently of constipation. The onset of IBS is often associated with a change of the form of the stool (commonly loose or watery, or sometimes pellets). It is more common in women than men, and can be triggered by psychological stress. Many sufferers carry their own antidiarrheal or antispasmodic medication, such as loperamide or clidinium bromide with chlordiazepoxide (Librax). Constipation may be treated with laxatives such as lactulose or polyethylene glycol solution (see Constipation, later). Drugs that diminish hyperactivity of the bowel include dicyclomine hydrochloride and hyoscyamine sulfate. Diarrhea is treated with loperamide. Alosetron is used only for severe diarrhea-predominant IBS that does not respond after 6 months to conventional therapies.

Irritable bowel is a diagnosis of exclusion that should be made by a physician. If a person is known to suffer from IBS with a constipation component, he should be encouraged to eat adequate fiber (indigestible plant carbohydrate: bran, steamed vegetables, or 20 to 30 g fiber supplement) and avoid coffee (caffeine), alcohol, fatty foods, and gas-producing vegetables. A useful prophylactic measure may be regular ingestion of a probiotic (e.g., *Lactobacillus* or *Bifidobacterium infantis* 35624) preparation. Regular exercise also appears to be helpful for some individuals. There are numerous therapies under investigation for persons with IBS that's refractory to all of these measures. These include antidepressants, serotonin-3 and serotonin-4 receptor antagonists, antibiotics, herbal therapy (including peppermint oil), and other agents to reduce the sensitivity and motility of the bowel. For instance, rifaximin, a minimally absorbed antibiotic that is sometimes used to treat infectious diarrhea (see page 475), has been reported in a medical study to have been used successfully to treat IBS without constipation to relieve symptoms of bloating, abdominal pain, and loose or watery stools. Linaclotide is a drug used to treat constipation-predominant IBS. A "low FODMAP" diet, which eliminates certain carbohydrates that are felt to perhaps be fermented in the bowel and contribute to IBS, may be helpful to reduce symptoms.

CONSTIPATION

If a person becomes constipated (straining, difficult bowel movements with hard stools), the retention of stool and discomfort can be severe. Significant contributing factors to constipation are diet, dehydration, and lack of exercise. During outdoor activities, take care to drink fluids at regular intervals. In addition, sufficient fiber (20 to 30 g per day in any form: bran, whole-grain cereals, vegetables, fruits, fiber supplements) must be maintained in the diet. The "city backpacker" diet of chocolate bars, peanuts, and cheese sandwiches will turn the most irascible bowels into mortar. Regular, preemptive doses of a stool softener such as docusate sodium (Colace), or a bulking agent such as psyllium seed hydrophilic mucilloid (Metamucil), must be ingested with at least two glasses of water to be effective. Consider eating foods like chia seeds with copious amounts of water. Eat plenty of fruits and vegetables.

To relieve the victim of mild constipation, try the following measures:

1. Force fluids.
2. Adjust the diet (more for prevention than treatment).
3. Consider the use of a stool softener (mineral oil; docusate sodium: Colace, Regulax SS, Surfak); bulking agent (psyllium: Metamucil, Perdiem, Fiberall; methylcellulose: Citrucel; polycarbophil: Fibercon, Equalactin, Konsyl); osmotic laxative (magnesium hydroxide: Phillips' Milk of Magnesia; magnesium citrate: Evac-Q-Mag; sodium phosphate: Fleet Enema, Fleet Phospho-Soda, Visicol), natural laxative (prune juice), poorly absorbed sugar (lactulose: Cephulac, Chronulac, Duphalac); polyethylene glycol and electrolytes: Colyte, GoLYTELY, NuLYTELY; polyethylene glycol: MiraLAX, and/or stimulant laxative (cascara sagrada: Colamin, Sagrada-lax; senna: Senokot, Ex-Lax; castor oil: Purge, Neoloid, Emulsoil). Peri-Colace is a combination of the stool softener docusate sodium and casanthranol, a laxative. Other drugs are listed on page 468.
4. In general, it's best to avoid the use of repetitive enemas or potent laxatives, because they can cause large fluid losses. A useful enema is a Colace 5 mL (200 mg) "microenema." A child may benefit from a plain glycerin suppository. In general, enemas can cause cramping and bloating. If they contain electrolytes, such as magnesium or phosphate, they can cause elevated levels of these in the bloodstream. Typical enemas include 6 to 12 ounces of milk and an equal portion of molasses; 2 tablespoons of Epsom salts per quart of lukewarm water; 45 mL of Phospho-Soda with 2 quarts of water; 9 mL packet of Castile soap in 2 quarts of tap water; 30 mL of mineral oil in 1 to 2 quarts of water; and 1 to 2 quarts of warm (body temperature) tap water.

5. If a victim becomes impacted (has not had a bowel movement for 5 to 10 days due to constipation), using stool softeners will probably be ineffective, and piling on an ingested load of bulky fiber is just dumping more backfill behind the dam. Unfortunately, to break the roadblock, you may have to perform the physical removal of stool from the rectum, using a softening enema first and then a gloved finger for the extraction. This should be done gently, to prevent injury to the anus and walls of the rectum. Two fingers are used to dilate the anus, then the stool is broken up with a scissoring motion. After as much stool as possible is removed manually, an enema should be used.

On a prolonged expedition, you should carry the stimulant laxative drug bisacodyl (Dulco-lax). This is administered in oral (5 mg) or glycerin suppository (10 mg) form, with onset of effect in a few hours. Bisacodyl causes the bowel to contract, which can be extremely uncomfortable in someone with a large fecal impaction.

A very useful drug to treat constipation is polyethylene glycol solution (MiraLAX) given as 17 g powder (1 heaping tablespoon) dissolved in 8 oz (240 mL) of water taken daily for up to 4 days to initiate a bowel movement. Another method is lactulose syrup 10 mg per tablespoon (15 mL) of syrup. Administer 1 or 2 tablespoons per day.

An elderly person with any significant change in bowel habits should see a physician on return to civilization.

HEMORRHOIDS, ANAL FISSURE, AND RECTAL PROLAPSE

Hemorrhoids are enlarged veins that are found outside (external hemorrhoids) or inside (internal hemorrhoids) the anal opening (Figure 146). They cause problems that range from minor itching and skin irritation to excruciating pain, inflammation, and bleeding. The bleeding is noticed as bright red blood either on the outside of the stool (not mixed in with the excrement), in the toilet water, or on the toilet paper. Bleeding is usually sporadic, associated with difficult bowel movements (constipation) with straining, and passage of hard stools. To avoid problems, keep stools soft (see page 205). Anal itching can be controlled with good hygiene, witch hazel compresses, a steroid preparation, and ice packs. If hemorrhoids flare, the treatment is sitz (sitting) baths in warm water for 30 minutes three times a day, and application of medication in the form of cream, ointment, or suppositories (Preparation H [essentially a petrolatum lubricant]; Anusol or Tronolane [with pramoxine 1% for pain and itching] or Anusol HC-1 [without pramoxine, but with hydrocortisone 1% for inflammation]; Nupercainal [1% dibucaine]; pramoxine hydrochloride 1% with hydrocortisone acetate 1% [ProctoCream-HC];

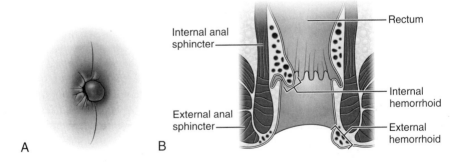

Figure 146. Hemorrhoids. **A,** External view of the anus with an enlarged external hemorrhoid. **B,** A cross-sectional view of the anus and rectum shows dilated veins that protrude into the rectum (internal hemorrhoids) and externally from the anus.

ELA-Max 5 [lidocaine 5%] anorectal cream; Analpram-HC cream or ointment [hydrocortisone and pramoxine]). Unless bleeding is severe, it can be managed with sterile pads and gentle pressure. If the victim develops a fever associated with severe rectal pain or cannot pass a bowel movement, a physician should be sought.

A thrombosed hemorrhoid is one in which the blood has clotted within the dilated vein and formed a visible and palpable enlarged, hardened, and dark blue-purple knot. Pain is generally severe, and the victim may be unable to complete a bowel movement. The treatment usually involves incision through the wall of the vein and removal of the clot. Until the victim can be brought to a physician, warm soaks may ease the discomfort. Don't sit on a donut cushion because this might worsen the problem. Generally, all elderly people with rectal bleeding should be fully evaluated by a physician, to be sure that there is not another, more serious, cause. Sometimes a small grape-like cluster of dilated veins will protrude from the rectum. If this occurs, have the victim go onto his hands and knees or onto his side, and then apply gentle steady direct pressure to the protruding tissue until it slides back inside the rectum. If this is successful, have the victim lie still for about an hour.

An anal fissure is a crack of the skin that appears at the top (usually) or bottom of the anal opening. The most common cause is stretching of the skin beyond its ability. The fissure becomes an open sore and may become painful and raw, sometimes with bleeding. Apply the best possible hygiene after each bowel movement and attempt to keep the fissure covered with petrolatum, bacitracin ointment, or zinc oxide ointment. Try to keep the stools soft (e.g., avoid constipation—see page 205) and maintain a brisk fluid intake. If it's possible to soak in a warm sitz ("sitting") bath from time to time, then do so. If the fissure is making it difficult to have a bowel movement because of the pain, then try using a topical analgesic, such as lidocaine. A doctor may prescribe topical nitroglycerin ointment, which in some fashion promotes wound healing.

Anal itching is a common problem. It is usually caused by less-than-perfect hygiene, although there are other more serious causes, so if it is persistent, you should have a medical practitioner inspect the area. In the outdoors, if the skin area around the anus is moist or soiled, particularly if it is already irritated and itchy, then the first approach should be to try to keep the skin clean and dry. Wash daily with soap and water, and if possible, use antibacterial soap. Avoid alcohol-based wipes, tight underpants, or constrictive thermal undergarments. A small piece of absorbent cotton, non-perfumed talcum powder, or powdered cornstarch may be used to absorb moisture. For the itching, a zinc oxide–based ointment (such as would be used for diaper rash) may be helpful. Dietary avoidance of coffee, tea, cola beverages, chocolate, citrus, and dairy products has been recommended, but there is no proof that this helps. Using 1% hydrocortisone cream might help, but stronger steroid preparations or repeated use of any steroid can predispose to infections or cause the skin to become thinner. Because people tend to scratch during their sleep, keep fingernails trimmed.

Rectal prolapse is a condition in which a person's "insides" (in this case, the rectum portion of the bowel) have extruded through the anus. This usually occurs in elders, commonly during a bowel movement in which there has been straining. If it's not possible to bring the victim to medical care, then one method used to reduce swelling of the prolapsed rectum and allow it to be pushed back inside the victim is to cover the prolapsed rectum with a thick layer of granulated ("table") sugar and allow everything to rest for 15 to 30 minutes. Don't use a sugar substitute. After that time period, gentle pressure is used to allow the bowel to slide back within the victim. If the maneuver is successful, place the victim on a non-constipating diet.

FLATUS

The rectal passage of bowel gas offers relief and occasional embarrassment. If stomach cramps are due to excessive gas production, the drug of choice is simethicone (Mylicon or Mylicon-80), which causes dissolution of large gas collections and eases the passage of flatus. Charcoal Plus tablets and Flatulex tablets contain simethicone combined with activated charcoal, an absorbent. Beano food enzyme dietary supplement contains the enzyme alpha-galactosidase, which is advertised to be effective in preventing gas formation from vegetables, beans, and grains that contain indigestible sugars that ferment in the bowel to create gas. Because intestinal gas (methane) can be flammable, don't attempt to ignite rectal gas or direct the stream of gas into a campfire. Backflashes and minor burns are a real risk.

HEARTBURN

Heartburn is a manifestation of esophageal reflux (in medical parlance, sometimes called gastro-esophageal reflux disease [GERD]), in which stomach contents containing acid and food travel backward from the stomach into the esophagus. This causes irritation and pain, which is typically sharp or burning and located under the breastbone and/or in the upper abdomen. It may be associated with belching, a sour taste in the mouth, and/or near-vomiting. When severe, the pain may be confused with angina (see page 46). Omeprazole (Prilosec) is a drug that suppresses gastric acid secretion. It can be prescribed for a 1- to 2-week period by a physician for GERD or for up to a 4- to 8-week period for severe erosive inflammation of the esophagus (adult dose 20 to 40 mg by mouth in the morning and 20 mg in the evening). Other drugs in this category ("proton pump inhibitors") are pantoprazole (Protonix) and rabeprazole (AcipHex). Mild heartburn is often managed with antacids, particularly Gaviscon, which forms a "foam" that floats on the stomach contents and protects the esophagus from refluxed acid. Metoclopramide hydrochloride (Reglan) helps control muscle tone at the sphincter (junction) between the stomach and the esophagus, and thus helps prevent reflux. Nizatidine 75 mg (Axid AR ["acid reducer"]) is an H2-blocker drug (see page 469) that inhibits gastric acid secretion. It is swallowed 30 to 60 minutes before eating, and can be used up to twice in 24 hours. Cimetidine (Tagamet) 200 mg can be used in a similar manner. Famotidine (Pepcid AC) 10 or 20 mg twice a day (preferably ingested 15 to 60 minutes before eating) for up to 6 weeks is another therapy.

Keep meals small, and don't eat them immediately before reclining (no bedtime snacks). Known gastric irritants (e.g., alcohol, cigarettes, pepperoni sandwiches) should be avoided. If possible, sleep with the head of your bed or sleeping bag elevated. Occasionally, it's necessary to sleep in the sitting position, to counteract the forces of gravity and a loose esophageal sphincter. Wear loose-fitting clothing around the stomach. Weight loss is advised for overweight or obese persons.

NAUSEA AND VOMITING

Nausea and vomiting may arise from causes as simple as anxiety, or may represent a serious problem such as appendicitis, ingestion of a poisonous plant, or response to a head injury. When vomiting is secondary to a serious underlying disorder, the basic problem must be remedied. Any victim with nausea and vomiting who suffers from altered mental status, uncontrollable high fever, extreme abdominal pain, or chest pain that might represent heart disease—or who is either very young or very old—should be evacuated promptly. Anyone who vomits blood should be taken to a hospital immediately. Vomiting in children is particularly worrisome if it accompanies head trauma (see page 59) or abdominal trauma (see page 116). Severe vomiting (which might represent a bowel obstruction [see page 122] or appendicitis [see page 121]) is concerning. Lethargy or confusion that accompanies vomiting might indicate an infection or poisoning.

If nausea and vomiting due to gastroenteritis become excessive, they can be managed with an antiemetic. One effective drug is ondansetron (Zofran). The adult dose is one 4 mg dissolving tablet every 8 hours; the pediatric dose is 0.15 mg/kg of body weight of the oral dissolving tablet every 6 to 8 hours. The adult dose may be safely repeated after 5 minutes if the first dose is not effective. Alternative drugs are prochlorperazine (Compazine), which can be administered orally or as a suppository, promethazine (Phenergan), which comes in suppository form, metoclopramide (Reglan), or trimethobenzamide (Tigan), which can be taken orally or by suppository. If the victim is so ill that he cannot keep anything in his stomach, it makes no sense to administer an oral medication, so an injection or suppository must be used. After multiple episodes of vomiting, the victim may suffer from dehydration (see page 194), particularly if there is associated diarrhea as part of a gastroenteritis. Fluid replacement is essential. The diet should be advanced slowly as the victim's hunger returns.

Nausea and vomiting due to motion sickness are discussed on page 411. Cyclical vomiting is a disorder in which the victim experiences fatigue and nausea, and perhaps sweating and pale skin color for approximately 90 minutes before onset of explosive vomiting, which may last for up to 24 hours in children and 3 days in adults. The victims may vomit up to six times per hour. This disorder, which may sometimes be accompanied by abdominal pain, can be triggered by stress, upper respiratory tract infection, menses, sleep deprivation, certain foods, asthma attacks, motion sickness, or environmental allergies. Treatment is supportive and based on symptoms. If an attack is severe, the victim may require intravenous hydration.

VOMITING BLOOD

Bleeding from the gastrointestinal tract can cause the victim to vomit blood (either bright red, or dark brown "coffee grounds"). If the blood is not vomited, it passes through the bowels and emerges as dark black tarry stools (melena) or occasionally as maroon clots or bright red blood. Brisk bleeding in the stomach or bowels may be painless; any bleeding should be considered serious. Even if the bleeding episode is brief (except for bleeding from known hemorrhoids), the victim should be evacuated immediately to a hospital. If the victim is known to have ulcer disease and ceases vomiting, antacids should be given by mouth.

Persistent retching can cause the stomach wall to tear and begin to bleed. For this reason, persistent nausea and vomiting from any cause should be controlled with medications, if possible.

ULCER DISEASE

A gastric ulcer is an erosion into the stomach. A peptic ulcer is an erosion into the duodenum (first portion of the small bowel) that's worsened by the constant assault from gastric acid and digestive juices. Many ulcers are caused by infection of the inner lining of the stomach and bowel with the microorganism *Helicobacter pylori*, which can be eradicated with an intensive course of multiple antibiotics. Such therapy is undertaken not in the field, but under the supervision of a physician.

The major symptom of ulcer disease is burning, sharp, or aching pain in the upper abdomen that's usually relieved by the ingestion of food or antacids, although the latter alone may be therapeutic. Classically, the pain occurs when the stomach is empty, particularly during times of emotional stress. Because the greatest amounts of acid are secreted following meals and between the hours of midnight and 3:00 AM, these are times when pain is most frequent.

If the victim is strongly suspected or known to have an ulcer, and can control the pain readily with medications, the journey can continue. Make every attempt to keep on a regular meal schedule and to take medication properly during waking hours. As noted below, cigarette smoking and alcohol ingestion are strictly prohibited. If pain is not immediately controlled, or if there is any suggestion of bleeding or perforation, rapid transport to a hospital is indicated.

Therapy

1. *Antacids.* These are the traditional mainstay of therapy and should be taken in a dose of 2 to 3 tablespoons (30 to 45 mL) 1 and 3 hours after meals, at bedtime, and as necessary to control pain. Liquids are generally more effective than tablets. Solid food and milk are not recommended as antacids. While they may decrease pain briefly, they actually stimulate the secretion of acid.

2. *Drugs to inhibit the secretion of acid.* Medications used to decrease acid secretion (antagonists to histamine H2 receptors and proton [acid] pump inhibitors) decrease bowel activity and cramping. An example of the former is famotidine 20 mg by mouth daily; an example of the latter is omeprazole 20 to 40 mg by mouth daily.
3. *Drugs to protect the lining of the gastrointestinal tract.* Sucralfate (Carafate) is a drug that binds with the ulcer and protects the bowel lining from further erosion. Because it requires the presence of acid in the ulcer crater to be activated, it should not be given at the same time as antacids.
4. *Avoidance of alcohol, tea, coffee, tobacco, and known gastric irritants.*
5. *Don't use household baking soda to neutralize acid in the stomach.* Baking soda (bicarbonate) reacts with the acid to liberate heat and gas.

HEPATITIS

Hepatitis is inflammation of the liver that's caused by viral infection or parasitic infestation, drugs, toxic chemicals, alcohol abuse, or autoimmune disease. Type A infectious (short-incubation) hepatitis is the more commonly encountered viral form. The virus is excreted in urine and feces and contaminates drinking water and food products (such as raw shellfish). Type B infectious (long incubation) hepatitis is caused by a virus found in many bodily fluids (blood, saliva, semen) and is spread by direct person-to-person contact. Type C infectious hepatitis is most commonly associated with blood transfusions. Multiple other forms of viral hepatitis have been discovered by medical researchers. Hepatitis D is found only in persons who are currently or previously infected with hepatitis B. Hepatitis E is likely the most common cause of acute hepatitis and jaundice in the developing world, and is transmitted to humans mostly by eating meat and organs of pigs, boars, and deer. Hepatitis F and G are recently described and of as yet unknown significance.

Hepatitis causes the victim to have a constellation of signs and symptoms, which include yellow discoloration of the skin and eyes (jaundice—from the buildup of bilirubin pigment, which the diseased liver cannot process properly), nausea and vomiting, fatigue, weakness, fever, chills, darkened urine, diarrhea, pale-colored bowel movements (which may precede the onset of jaundice by 1 to 3 days), abdominal pain (particularly in the right upper quadrant over the swollen and tender liver), loss of appetite, joint pain, muscle aching, itching, and red skin rash. A young child may suffer from type A infection, yet show only a mild flu-like illness.

Anyone suspected of having hepatitis should be placed at maximum rest and transported to a physician. Avoid alcohol and medication ingestion, because the metabolism of many drugs is altered in the victim with a diseased liver. He should be encouraged to avoid dehydration and should maintain adequate food intake. If the cause of hepatitis is viral, the victim's disease may be contagious for his first 2 weeks of illness. Don't share eating utensils or washrags. Body secretions (saliva and waste products) frequently carry the virus; therefore, pay strict attention to handwashing. Sexual contact should be avoided during the infectious period. In no case should a needle used for injection of medicine into one person be reused for another individual.

Protection against hepatitis is best accomplished by prevention of virus transmission through good hygiene. Hepatitis A vaccine is available (see page 425). In countries of high hepatitis incidence (poor sanitation, infested water or food), pooled immune serum globulin (ISG, or gamma globulin) injections are advised (see page 425); these protect unimmunized people against hepatitis A, and diminish symptoms in infected people. In a study that compared hepatitis A vaccine against ISG for postexposure prophylaxis against hepatitis A in persons who had not been previously immunized, it appeared that they were roughly equivalent, with the ISG being slightly more effective at preventing hepatitis A. Hepatitis B vaccine (see page 425) is intended for health care workers or those who will visit or reside in regions of high endemicity. It is of little benefit against hepatitis A.

SKIN DISORDERS

SUNBURN

The solar radiation that strikes the earth includes 50% visible light (wavelength 400 to 760 nanometers [nm]), 40% infrared (760 to 1,700 nm), and 10% ultraviolet (10 to 400 nm) (Figure 147). Energetic rays (e.g., cosmic rays, gamma rays, and x-rays) with wavelengths shorter than 10 nm don't penetrate to the earth's surface to any significant degree. Sunburn is a cutaneous photosensitivity reaction caused by exposure of the skin to ultraviolet radiation (UVR) from the sun. There are four types of UVR: vacuum UVR is 10 to 200 nm (absorbed by air and unable to penetrate Earth's atmosphere), UVA is 320 to 400 nm, UVB is 290 to 320 nm, and UVC is 100 to 290 nm. UVC is filtered out by the ozone layer of the atmosphere. UVB is the culprit in the creation of sunburn and cancer. UVA is of less immediate danger but is a serious cause of skin aging, drug-related photosensitivity, and skin cancer. Furthermore, persons taking immunosuppressive agents for medical reasons (e.g., AIDS or cancer) may be more predisposed to skin cancer caused by UVA.

Ultraviolet exposure varies with the time of day (greatest between 9 AM and 3 PM because of increased solar proximity and decreased angle of light rays), season (greater in summer), altitude (8% to 10% increase per each 1000 ft, or 305 m, of elevation above sea level), location (greater near the Equator), and weather (greater in the wind). Snow or ice reflects 85% of UVR, dry sand 17%, and grass 2.5%. Water may reflect 10% to 100% of UVR, depending on the time of day, location, and surface. However, UVR at midday may penetrate up to 24 inches (60 cm) through water. Clouds absorb 10% to 80% of UVR, but rarely more than 40%. Most clothes reflect (light-colored) or absorb (dark-colored) UVR. A dry white cotton shirt has a maximum sun protection factor (SPF) of 8 (see Sunscreens, below). However, it's important to note that wet cotton of any color probably transmits considerable UVR.

Skin darkening occurs immediately on UVA exposure, as preformed melanin is released, and lasts for 15 to 30 minutes. Tanning occurs after 3 days of exposure, as additional melanin is produced. If the skin is not conditioned with gradual doses of UVR (tanning), a burn can

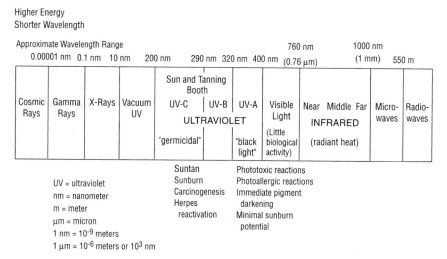

Figure 147. Solar radiation.

be created. A person's sensitivity to UVR depends on his skin type and thickness, the pigment (melanin) in his skin, and weather conditions. Well-hydrated skin is penetrated four times as effectively by UVR as is dry skin, because the moist skin does not scatter or reflect UVR as well.

Depending on the exposure, the injury can range from mild redness to blistering and disablement. Rapid pigment darkening from immediate melanin release is followed by the redness with which we are all familiar, caused by dilation of superficial blood vessels. This begins 2 to 8 hours after exposure and reaches its maximum (the "burn") in 24 to 36 hours, with associated itching and pain.

Wind appears to augment the injury, as do heat, atmospheric moisture, and immersion in water. "Windburn" is not possible without UVR or abrasive sand. Since windburn is due in part to the drying effect of low humidity at high altitudes, it can be helpful to protect the skin with a greasy sunscreen or barrier cream.

People may be more sensitive to UVR after they have ingested certain drugs (such as tetracycline, doxycycline, fluoroquinolones, vitamin A derivatives, nonsteroidal antiinflammatories, sulfa derivatives, minoxidil, diltiazem, nifedipine, thiazide diuretics, hypoglycemic agents, chloroquine, dapsone, quinidine, carbamazepine, chemotherapeutic drugs, and barbiturates) or have been exposed to certain plants (such as lime, citron, bitter orange, lemon, celery, parsnip, fennel, dill, wild carrot, fig, buttercup, mustard, milfoil, agrimony, rue, hogweed, Queen Anne's lace, and stinking mayweed). Your eyes may become more sensitive to light (e.g., you may need to wear sunglasses at a lower UV threshold) if you're taking certain medications, such as digoxin, quinidine, tolazamide, or tolbutamide.

For a mild sunburn in which no blistering is present, the victim may be treated with cool liquid compresses, cool showers, a nonsensitizing skin moisturizer (such as Vaseline Intensive Care), and aspirin or an NSAID, to decrease the pain and inflammation. Topical anesthetic sprays, many of which contain benzocaine and/or diphenhydramine, should in general be avoided, because they can cause sensitization and an allergic reaction. Menthol-containing lotions may be helpful. Topical steroids don't appreciably diminish a sunburn.

If the victim is deep red ("cooked lobster") without blisters, a stronger antiinflammatory drug, such as prednisone, may be given. A 5-day course of prednisone (80 mg on the first day, 60 mg the second, 40 mg the third, 20 mg the fourth, and 10 mg the fifth) may decrease the discomfort of "sun poisoning," which is the constellation of low-grade fever, chills, loss of appetite, nausea, and weakness that accompanies an extensive nonblistering total-body first degree sunburn. He should be forced to drink enough balanced electrolyte-supplemented liquids to avoid dehydration (see page 194). Corticosteroids should always be taken with the understanding that a rare side effect is serious deterioration of the head ("ball" of the ball-and-socket joint) of the femur, the long bone of the thigh. Corticosteroids are interchangeable to a certain degree. If you must substitute, here is a rough measure of equivalence: 20 mg prednisone equals 16 mg methylprednisolone equals 3 mg dexamethasone.

Topical steroid creams, such as pramoxine with hydrocortisone (Pramosone cream or lotion) may be used if blisters aren't present. Pramoxine alone (Prax) is a nonsensitizing topical anesthetic. Topical steroid preparations should not be applied to blistered skin, because wound healing may be delayed and infection made more likely. On the other hand, aloe vera lotion or gel may be soothing and promote healing. Vitamin E is an antioxidant that, when mixed with aloe vera, may soothe the skin. However, this hasn't been proved to promote healing any better than aloe vera alone. Other remedies that have been suggested include bathing in a tub of water augmented by baking soda or oatmeal, or applying 0.1% diclofenac gel.

With a severe sunburn in which blistering is present, the victim has by definition suffered second-degree burns (see page 108) and should be treated accordingly. Gently clean the burned areas and cover with sterile dressings. Administer appropriate pain medication.

SUNSCREENS

Sunscreens (available as lotions, creams, waxes, ointments, and oils) either absorb light of a particular wavelength, act as barriers, or reflect light. "Broad-spectrum sunscreens" protect against both UVA and UVB rays. There is no evidence that any ingredients in sunscreens cause skin damage or cancer. Choose sunscreens based on your estimated exposure and on your own propensity to tan or burn. There is no such thing as a "safe tan," even when sunscreens are used, because sun exposure is directly linked to skin cancer. In addition, long-term exposure to UVR from sunlight causes premature skin aging and loss of skin tone. The term *photoaging* refers to these effects—increased wrinkles, loose skin, brown spots, a leathery appearance, and uneven pigmentation.

Dermatologists classify sun-reactive skin types (based on the first 45 to 60 minutes of sun exposure after winter or after a prolonged period of no sun exposure) as follows:

Type I: Always burns easily, never tans. Fair-skinned people with a high number of moles are at the greatest risk for melanoma.

Type II: Always burns easily, tans minimally.

Type III: Burns moderately, tans gradually and uniformly (light brown).

Type IV: Burns minimally, always tans well (moderate brown).

Type V: Rarely burns, tans profusely (dark brown).

Type VI: Never burns, is deeply pigmented (black skin).

In all cases it's wise to overestimate the protection necessary and to carry a strong sunscreen. To protect hair from sun damage, wear a hat.

Para-aminobenzoic acid (PABA) derivatives, which are water soluble, are sunscreens that absorb UVB (not UVA) and that accumulate in the skin with repeated application. The most commonly used PABA derivative is padimate O (octyl dimethyl PABA). The most effective method of application is to moisturize the skin (shower or bathe) and then apply the sunscreen. For maximum effect, chemical sunscreens should be applied liberally (most people only apply $\frac{1}{4}$ to $\frac{1}{2}$ of what they need) at least 15 to 30 minutes before exposure, and the skin should be kept dry for at least 2 hours after sunscreen application. Sun blockers, such as titanium, are effective essentially immediately.

When PABA itself is used, a recommended preparation is 5% to 10% PABA in 50% to 70% alcohol. However, PABA is now used infrequently because its absorption peak of UVB at 296 nm is too far from 307 nm, where UVB exerts its greatest effect. Furthermore, it causes skin irritation—a stinging sensation—and can stain cotton and synthetic fabrics. PABA derivatives are less problematic.

Benzophenones (e.g., avobenzone) are sunscreens that are more effective against UVA. These should be used in 6% to 10% concentration. Because they aren't well absorbed by the skin, they require frequent reapplication. Photoplex broad-spectrum sunscreen lotion contains a PABA-ester combined with a potent UVA absorber, Parsol 1789. This is an excellent sunscreen for sensitive people, particularly those at risk for drug-induced photosensitivity. Other effective UVA blockers include ecamsule and micronized titanium dioxide or zinc oxide.

Sunscreens come in different concentrations (such as PreSun "8" or "15"). A higher SPF number indicates a greater degree of protection against UVB. SPF ranges from 2 (absorbs 50% of UVB) to 50 (absorbs 98% of UVB). "Minimal erythema dose" (MED) is the amount of UVR exposure required to redden the skin. SPF is derived by dividing the MED of skin covered with sunscreen by the MED of unprotected skin. Thus, an SPF of 15 indicates that it requires 15 times the UVR exposure to achieve a sunburn as it would without protection. The SPF number assumes a liberal (approximately $1\frac{1}{4}$ oz, or 37 mL, per adult) application of the sunscreen. Because sunscreens are rarely perfectly applied, it's best to assume a markedly lower (approximately 50%) SPF than stated on the label. In general, a sunscreen with an SPF number of 8 or less will allow tanning, probably by UVA exposure. There is no standard for measuring UVA protection. Persons with sensitive or unconditioned skin should use a sunscreen with an SPF number of 10 or greater. Fair-skinned people who never tan or who tan poorly (types I, II, or III) or mountain climbers (there is more UV exposure at higher altitudes, and more is reflected off snow) should always use a sunscreen with an SPF number of 15 or greater. Most sun exposure occurs before 18 years of age, so it's very important to apply sunscreens to children and young adults.

Substantivity refers to the ability of a sunscreen to resist water wash-off. Layering sunscreens doesn't work well, because the last layer applied usually washes off. Current specialty sunscreens with high substantivity include Bullfrog Water Pro Body Gel, Aloe Gator Total Sun Block Lotion, and Dermatone Ultimate Fisherman's Sunscreen. Water resistance claims on sunscreen labels must indicate whether the sunscreen remains effective for 40 minutes or 80 minutes while swimming or sweating.

Sunscreens are first applied to cool, dry skin for optimal absorption; wait 15 to 30 minutes before water exposure. Reapply them liberally and often, particularly after swimming or heavy perspiration. In general, most sunscreens should be reapplied every 20 minutes to 2 hours. Be aware that the concomitant use of insect repellent containing DEET (see page 336) lowers the effectiveness of the sunscreen by a factor of one third. Although many sunscreens are designed to bond or adhere to the skin under adverse environmental conditions, there are certain situations in which *any* sunscreen should be reapplied at a maximum of 3- to 4-hour intervals:

- Continuous sun exposure, particularly between the hours of 10 AM and 3 PM
- Exposure at altitude of 7000 ft (2135 m) or higher
- Exposure within 20 degrees latitude of the Equator
- Exposure during May through July in the Northern Hemisphere, and December through February in the Southern Hemisphere
- Frequent water immersion, particularly with toweling off
- Preexisting sunburn or skin irritation
- Ingestion of drugs, such as certain antibiotics, that can cause photosensitization

Some authorities recommend using sunscreens of at least SPF 29, with the rationale that most people underapply or improperly apply them. Bald-headed men should protect their domes. All children should be adequately protected. However, avoid PABA-containing products in children less than 6 months old. Persons sensitive to PABA can use Piz-Buin, Ti-Screen, Sawyer Products Stay-Put Sun Block, Uval, and Solbar products. Eating PABA does not protect the skin.

For total protection against ultraviolet and visible light, a preparation can be composed from various mixtures of titanium dioxide, red petrolatum, talc, zinc oxide, kaolin, red ferric oxide (calamine), and ichthammol. These preparations or similar commercial products ("glacier cream") are used for lip and nose protection. Micronized titanium dioxide and zinc oxide can be prepared in an invisible preparation (such as Ti-Screen Natural 16 and Neutrogena Chemical Free 17) that does not cause skin irritation. In this regard, Blue Lizard Australian Sensitive Sunscreen SPF 30+ is an excellent product. Sunscreens that prevent infrared transmission may help prevent flares of fever blisters caused by herpes virus. An improvised sunscreen can be made by preparing a sludge of ashes from charcoal or wood, or from ground clay. In a pinch, axle grease will work to some degree.

If you're concerned about jellyfish stings, a useful product is Safe Sea Sunblock with Jellyfish Sting Protective Lotion (www.buysafesea.com), which is both a sunscreen and jellyfish sting inhibitor.

Substances that are ineffective as sunscreens and that may increase the propensity to burn include baby oil, cocoa butter, and mineral oil. Promising antioxidant substances under investigation as effective sunscreens are vitamins A, C, and E, and chemicals found in green tea.

Although "tanning tablets" or "bronzers" induce a pigmentary change in the skin that resembles a suntan, they provide minimal, if any, true protection from the effects of ultraviolet exposure. Like the sun, indoor tanning machines induce skin changes that lead to premature skin aging and cancer. The best tan derived from the natural sun's UVB carries an SPF of approximately 2; a tanning bed supplies UVA and therefore no protection. Furthermore, tanning beds don't stimulate enough natural production of vitamin D to be worth the risk of developing skin cancer.

Taking aspirin or an NSAID at 6-hour intervals three times before sun exposure may help protect the sun-sensitive person.

Many effective sunscreens, particularly those advertised to stay on in the water, are extremely irritating to the eyes, so take care when applying these to the forehead and nose. Near the eyes, avoid sunscreens with an alcohol or propylene glycol base. Instead, use a sunscreen cream.

There are also sunscreen/insect repellent combinations, such as Coppertone Bug & Sun. Avon Bug Guard contains Skin-So-Soft (mostly mineral oil) in combination with picaridin or IR3535, and in at least one version, it is enhanced by a sunscreen.

Sun protection from clothing is determined by the nature of the material, color (dark is better), moisture (dry is better), and tightness of weave. A line of medical clothing, Solumbra by Sun Precautions, is advertised to be "soft, lightweight and comfortable," and offers 100+ SPF protection. Solar Protective Factory also manufactures high-SPF protective clothing. Women's hosiery has an unacceptably low SPF. The ability of Lycra to block UVR varies depending on whether it is lax (very effective) to stretched (nearly ineffective). Dry, white cotton (T-shirt) has an SPF of 5 to 8. The ultraviolet protection factor (UPF) is a measure of UVR protection provided by a fabric. Thus, a UPF of 15 indicates that $\frac{1}{15}$ of the UVR that strikes the surface of the fabric penetrates through to the skin. A chemical UVR protectant, Tinosorb FD (Rit Sun Guard), may be used as a laundry additive, increasing the UPF of washed clothing up to 50.

UVR protection provided by hats depends on the style. Broad-brimmed hats and "bucket" hats provide the most protection for the face and head. Sunday Afternoons manufactures comfortable broad-brimmed hats with neck shields advertised to block 97% of UV. Legionnaires hats do a decent job of protection, but baseball caps leave many facial areas exposed. If you are wearing a helmet, add a visor.

To summarize the most important ways to have sunscreens be effective:

1. Apply sunscreens liberally and cover all exposed areas. Use at least 2 to 3 tablespoons to cover your body and 1 tablespoon to cover your face. Reapply every few hours in dry conditions.
2. Apply sunscreens at least 1 hour in advance of exposure.
3. Reapply sunscreens after swimming, bathing, sweating, or otherwise washing them off the skin.
4. Insect repellent applied at the same time as a sunscreen reduces effectiveness of the sunscreen.
5. Anticipate intense UVR exposure at high altitude, on the water, and even on cloudy days.

Photolyase is an enzyme harvested from plankton extract that is reported to lessen damage to the DNA of cells that is caused by UVR exposure. There is evolving science indicating that this may become an important ingredient in topical lotions or creams applied after UVR exposure has occurred. There are "DNA repair" products on the market (promoted for anti-aging) that might one day be recommended to minimize or prevent cell damage and the inflammatory response that are part of sunburn.

Sunglasses for eye protection against UVR are discussed on page 175.

MELANOMA

Melanoma is a type of skin cancer that can be caused by ultraviolet light exposure, with UVB more causative than UVA. Indeed, regular use of a sunscreen with an SPF of at least 15 during the first 18 years of life may reduce the lifetime risk of developing melanoma by more than 75%. People with white skin and a tendency to burn rather than tan are at increased risk for developing melanoma. Tanning bed use is thought to be associated with increased risk for melanoma, particularly in young women.

Although you wouldn't self-treat a melanoma, it's important for those who spend a great deal of time outdoors to recognize the features of skin cancer. Regularly inspect existing moles, birthmarks, and other skin lesions. Since melanoma is often found on a person's back or other area that cannot be easily inspected, it's important to have a knowledgeable person (such as a dermatologist) inspect all suspicious skin lesions from time to time.

Warning signs within a skin lesion (particularly a mole) include the following:

1. Irregular, ragged, jagged, notched, or blurred border.
2. Asymmetrical appearance (one portion different from the rest, with respect to color, darkness, or texture).
3. Change in appearance or features (size, color, texture, sensation); onset of pain in a lesion; rapid growth of a lesion. If a mole looks different than others on the body, it is suspicious.
4. Recent growth, bleeding, itching, scaling, or tenderness. Melanomas are usually greater in diameter than a pencil eraser, but can sometimes be smaller.
5. Variation in color within the lesion or discoloration (black, dark brown, tan, blue, red, white, mottled).

If you note any of these features, see a dermatologist for a proper evaluation. Basal cell carcinoma and squamous cell carcinoma are two other types of cancer associated with UVR exposure.

POISON IVY, SUMAC, AND OAK (GENUS *TOXICODENDRON*)

The rashes of poison ivy, poison sumac, and poison oak are caused by a resin (urushiol) found in the resin canals of leaves, stems, vines, berries, and roots (Figure 148). The resin is not found

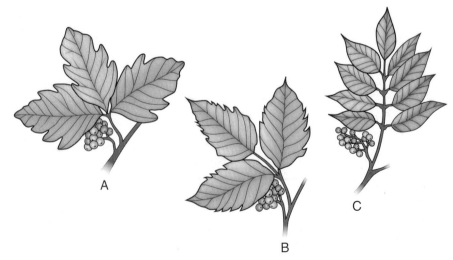

Figure 148. A, Poison oak. **B,** Poison ivy. **C,** Poison sumac.

on the surface of the leaves. The potency of the sap does not vary with the seasons. In its natural state, the oil is colorless; on exposure to air, oxidation causes it to turn black. Because the plant parts have to be injured to leak the resin, most cases are reported in spring, when the leaves are most fragile. Dried leaves are less toxic, because the oil has returned to the stem and roots through the resin canals. However, smoke from burning plants carries the residual available resin in small particles and can cause a severe reaction on the skin and in the nose, mouth, throat, and lungs.

The poison oak group does not grow in Alaska or Hawaii, and it rarely grows above 4000 ft (1219 m). Other plants or parts of plants that contain urushiol include the India ink tree, mango rind, cashew nut shell, and Japanese lacquer tree. A smaller number of reactions are caused by the poisonwood tree found in the southern tip of Florida. Because the resin is long lived, it can be spread by contact with tents, clothing, and pet fur.

Sensitivity to the resin varies with each individual, and can present for the first time at any age. The first exposure produces a rash in 6 to 25 days. Subsequent exposures can cause a rash in 8 hours to 10 days, with 2 to 3 days most common. Unless the resin is removed from the skin within 10 minutes of exposure, a reaction is inevitable in sensitive individuals. It is generally accepted that the resin binds to the skin within 30 minutes, is completely bound to the skin within 8 hours, and is likely impossible to remove effectively with soap and water after just 60 minutes. Some highly sensitive persons will suffer a reaction even if the resin is washed off within 1 minute of exposure.

The rash begins with itching followed by redness, followed by lines of reddened bumps and blisters. The skin may swell, blisters grow, and weeping/oozing lesions develop. Swelling of the tissues can be quite severe. After approximately a week, the rash begins to dry, and scabs begin to form, particularly if the victim has done much scratching and rubbing. This is followed by thickening and darkening of the skin, which may last for many weeks.

After exposure, it is usually most convenient to remove the resin with soap and cool water, but to be most effective, washing must occur within 30 minutes. Rubbing alcohol is a better solvent for the resin than is water. Zanfel Poison Ivy Wash (Zanfel Laboratories) is a soap mixture of ethoxylate and sodium lauroyl sarcosinate surfactants that binds to urushiol on the skin so that it can be washed off. The instructions for use (to treat an area the size of an adult hand or face) are to wet the affected area; squeeze a minimum $1\frac{1}{2}$ inch ribbon of Zanfel into one palm and then wet and rub both hands together for 10 seconds to work the product into a paste; rub both hands on the affected area for up to 3 minutes to work the Zanfel into the skin until there is no itching; and rinse the area thoroughly. If the itch returns, repeat the process. Tecnu Outdoor Skin Cleanser (alkane and alcohol) (Tec Labs) works quite well when applied soon after exposure, rubbed in for 2 minutes, and rinsed off, with a repeat of the entire sequence. Tecnu Extreme Medicated Poison Ivy Scrub is advertised to be effective after a 15-second application. Another wash designed to remove urushiol is Dr. West's Ivy Detox Cleanser, which contains magnesium sulfate. Herbal remedies that have been claimed (but never proven) to be effective are jewelweed (*Impatiens capensis*, which is an ingredient in Burt's Bees Poison Ivy Soap), witch hazel bark, and aloe plant.

For treatment of the skin reaction, shake lotions such as calamine are soothing and drying, and they control itching. A good nonsensitizing topical anesthetic is pramoxine hydrochloride 1% (Prax cream or lotion). Caladryl contains calamine and pramoxine. Avoid topical benzocaine, and tetracaine. Avoid topical diphenhydramine in children under the age of 2 years. Antihistamines (such as diphenhydramine [Benadryl]) control itching and act as sedatives. Nonsedating antihistamines, such as fexofenadine (Allegra) or loratadine (Claritin), may also diminish itching. A soothing bath in tepid (not hot) water with half a 1 lb box of baking soda, 2 cups (551 mL) of linnet starch, or 1 cup (275 mL) Aveeno oatmeal is excellent. If Aveeno is not available, a woman's nylon stuffed with regular (not instant) oatmeal can be thrown in the tub. Aluminum acetate in water (1:20) soaks may be soothing, as might aluminum subacetate (Burow's solution, Domeboro), which comes as a 5% solution that should be diluted to a 1:40 concentration. When these soaks are used, they should be applied as cotton-soaked wet dressings three to four times a day for 15 to 30 minutes per application to dry out the weeping rash. Topical steroid creams are generally of little value. Potent topical steroid ointments aren't effective unless they are applied before the appearance of blisters and continued for 2 to 3 weeks, so aren't recommended. Alcohol applications are painful and don't hasten resolution of the rash. There are topical agents, such as pimecrolimus (Elidel) 1% cream and tacrolimus (Protopic) 0.03% or 0.1% ointment, which modulate the immune system and are effective without causing skin atrophy, as would be caused by a superpotent topical steroid.

If the reaction is severe (facial or genital involvement or intolerable itching), the victim should be treated with a course of oral prednisone (80 to 100 mg each of the first 3 days, then decreased by 10 mg every 2 days until the final dose is 10 mg—80, 80, 70, 70, 60, 60, and so on). Corticosteroids should always be taken with the understanding that a rare side effect is serious deterioration of the head ("ball" of the ball-and-socket joint) of the femur, the long bone of the thigh. At the end of the course of corticosteroids, the victim may suffer a "flare-up" of the rash and symptoms, which may be treated with a repeated course of medication. Corticosteroids are interchangeable to a certain degree. If you must substitute, here is a rough measure of equivalence: 20 mg prednisone equals 16 mg methylprednisolone equals 3 mg dexamethasone.

Once the resin has been removed from the skin, the rash and blister fluid are not contagious. However, if the resin is still present, touching the involved skin will allow resin to be transferred to other areas. All clothes, sleeping bags, and pets should be washed with soap and water, because the resin can persist for years, particularly on woolen garments and blankets.

For prevention, there are few commercially available topical chemical preparations that act as effective barriers, although it appears that activated charcoal, aluminum oxide, and silica gel may work. Multi Shield (Interpro) is a protective agent for sensitive individuals. It should be applied over any sunscreen, and must be washed off carefully after use according to instructions. Stokogard Outdoor Cream is a linoleic acid dimer barrier cream preparation that is advertised to provide up to 8 hours of skin protection. Hollister Moisture Barrier and Hydropel may prove useful as barriers. IvyBlock (Enviroderm Pharmaceuticals) contains bentoquatam, which acts as a barrier. It is applied at least 15 minutes before going outdoors and then every 4 hours. Antiperspirants are used anecdotally as barriers, but have not been proven effective.

Other Irritating Plants

Poodle-dog bush *(Eriodictyon parryi)* is a purple-flowered plant that when touched can cause a reaction ranging from mild skin irritation with or without blistering to breathing difficulty. It is treated like a poison oak exposure.

Some plants produce thorns/spines/spicules, fluids, or crystals that act as primary irritants to the skin, in a nonallergic reaction, causing combinations of burning sensation, itching, and swelling. These plants include buttercup, croton bush, spurge, manchineel, beach apple, daisy, mustard, radish, pineapple, lemon, crown of thorns, milkbush, candelabra cactus, daffodil, hyacinth, stinging nettle, itchweed, dogwood, barley, millet, prickly pear, snow-on-the-mountain, primrose, geranium, meadow rue, narcissus, oleander, opuntia cactus, mesquite, tulip, mistletoe, wolfsbane, and horse nettle.

The skin should be thoroughly washed with soap and water. If barbs are embedded in the skin, removal may be easiest if you apply the sticky side of adhesive tape to the skin, and then peel the barbs off embedded to the tape.

Small cactus spines or the spicules of a stinging nettle can be removed by applying the sticky side of adhesive (duct) tape and peeling it off, or spreading a facial gel (mask or peel) or rubber cement, allowing it to dry, and peeling it off. Large spines can be removed with forceps. This may be necessary if the barbs on the cactus spine inhibit easy removal with the adhesive-tape method. A single cactus thorn can be as sharp as a needle and penetrate easily through the skin without leaving an external mark.

Medicated soaks recommended by dermatologists for plant-induced skin irritation include aluminum acetate solution (1:20) or Dalibour (Dalidane) solution (copper and zinc sulfate and camphor). Administration of corticosteroids (such as prednisone) is not useful for a primary (nonallergic) skin irritation.

RASHES INCURRED IN THE WATER
Seaweed Dermatitis

There are more than 3000 species of alga, which range in size from 1 micron to 100 meters in length. The blue-green algae *Microcoleus lyngbyaceus* is a fine, hairlike plant that gets inside the bathing suit of the unwary aquanaut in Hawaiian and Floridian waters, particularly during summer months. Usually, skin under the suit remains in moist contact with the algae (the other skin dries or is rinsed off) and becomes red and itchy, with occasional blistering and/or weeping. The reaction may start a few minutes to a few hours after the victim leaves the water. Treatment consists of a vigorous soap-and-water scrub, followed by a rinse with isopropyl (rubbing) alcohol. Apply hydrocortisone lotion 1% twice a day. If the reaction is severe, oral prednisone may be administered in a dose similar to that for a severe poison oak reaction (see page 218).

Swimmer's Itch

Swimmer's itch (clamdigger's itch) is caused by skin contact with cercariae, which are the immature free-swimming larval forms of parasitic schistosomes (flatworms) found throughout the world in both fresh and salt waters. Snails and birds are the intermediate hosts for the flatworms; the worms don't colonize humans. They release hundreds of fork-tailed microscopic cercariae into the water.

The affliction is contracted when a film of cercaria-infested water dries on exposed (uncovered by clothing) skin. As the water begins to dry, the cercariae penetrate the outer layer of the skin, but die immediately. An allergic response causes itching to be noted within minutes. Each schistosome that enters the skin causes a single red raised spot. Shortly afterward, the skin can become diffusely reddened and swollen, with an intense rash and, occasionally, hives. Blisters may develop over the next 24 to 48 hours. If the area is scratched, it may become infected and the victim develop impetigo (see page 222). Untreated, the affliction is limited to 1 to 2 weeks. Those who have suffered swimmer's itch previously may be more severely affected on repeated exposures, which suggests that an allergy might be present.

Swimmer's itch can be prevented by briskly rubbing the skin with a towel immediately after leaving the water, to prevent the cercariae from having time to penetrate the skin. Once the reaction has occurred, the skin should be lightly rinsed with isopropyl (rubbing) alcohol and then coated with calamine or Caladryl lotion. Additional remedies are baking soda or anti-itch oatmeal tub baths. If the reaction is severe, the victim should be treated with oral prednisone as if he suffered from poison oak (see page 218).

Because the cercariae are present in greatest concentration in shallow, warmer water and in weed beds (where the snails are), swimmers should seek to avoid these areas.

Sea Bather's Eruption

Sea bather's eruption, often misnamed sea lice (which are true crustacean parasites on fish), occurs in seawater and often involves bathing suit–covered areas of the skin in addition to exposed areas. The skin rash distribution may be similar to that from seaweed dermatitis, but no seaweed is found on the skin. The cause is stings from the nematocysts (stinging cells) of thimble jellyfish, such as *Linuche unguiculata*, and the larval forms of certain anemones. The victim may notice a tingling sensation on exposed skin or under the bathing suit (breasts, groin, cuffs of wet suits) while still in the water, which is made much worse if he takes a freshwater rinse (shower) while still wearing the suit. The rash usually consists of red bumps, which may become dense and confluent. Itching is severe and may become painful. Treatment is often not optimal, because application of vinegar or rubbing alcohol to stop the envenomation may not be very effective. An agent that may work better is a solution of papain (such as unseasoned meat tenderizer), which may be applied using a mildly abrasive pad. Another remedy that may be effective is lidocaine hydrochloride 4%. After the decontamination and a thorough freshwater rinse, apply hydrocortisone lotion 1% twice a day to treat the inflammatory component of the skin reaction. If the reaction is severe, the victim may suffer from headache, fever, chills, weakness, vomiting, itchy eyes, and burning on urination, and should be treated with oral prednisone as if he suffered from poison oak (see page 218). Topical calamine lotion with 1% menthol may be soothing.

The stinging cells may remain in the bathing suit even after it dries, so once a person has sustained a sea bather's eruption, his clothing should undergo a machine washing or be thoroughly rinsed in alcohol or vinegar, then be washed by hand with soap and water.

To prevent sea bather's eruption, an ocean bather or diver should wear, at a minimum, a synthetic nylon-rubber (Lycra [DuPont]) "dive skin." Safe Sea Sunblock with Jellyfish Sting Protective Lotion (www.buysafesea.com) is both a sunscreen and jellyfish sting inhibitor that may be used to diminish the incidence and severity of jellyfish stings.

Soapfish Dermatitis

The tropical soapfish *Rypticus saponaceous* is covered with a soapy mucus. When exposed to this slime, the victim's skin becomes red, itches, and undergoes mild swelling. Treatment involves a thorough wash with soap and water, followed by cool compresses, application of calamine lotion, and treatment for a mild allergic reaction similar to that for hives (see below).

Fish Handler's Disease

When cleaning marine fish or shellfish, the handler frequently creates small nicks and scrapes in his skin, usually on his hands. If these become infected with the bacteria *Erysipelothrix rhusiopathiae*, a skin rash may develop within 2 to 7 days. The rash appears as a red to violet-colored area of raised skin surrounding the small cut or scrape, with warmth, slight tenderness, and a well-defined border. The sufferer should be treated with penicillin, cephalexin, or ciprofloxacin for 1 week.

Seal Finger

Seal finger is a unique infection (suspected to be due to *Mycoplasma*), usually of a finger, caused by exposure to seals, walruses, and sea lions. The human victim contacts the skin or a mucous membrane of the animal to initiate the infection, which is characterized by swelling and pain that starts as a small nodule. Swelling and stiffness of the finger progresses to involve the joint, which can lead to bone and cartilage damage. Treatment is with oral tetracycline. The initial dose is 1.5 g, followed by 500 mg four times a day for 4 to 6 weeks. Ciprofloxacin may be used if tetracycline or doxycycline is not available.

HIVES

Hives are one skin manifestation of an allergic reaction, or may develop as part of a nonallergic reaction (such as to a medication). Hives appear as raised, red, and irregularly bordered welts or thickened patches of skin (Figure 149). Often, the victim will also complain of itching and/or fever. The treatment for hives presumed to be caused by allergy is to administer an antihistamine (such as diphenhydramine [Benadryl]) at 6-hour intervals until the rash has begun to

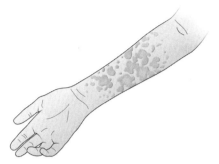

Figure 149. Hives.

subside and the itching is relieved, and to observe the victim closely for progression to a serious allergic reaction. Hives can appear in moments, yet take days to completely resolve. If the victim complains of shortness of breath or wheezing, or has a swollen tongue (muffled voice) or lips, anticipate a more serious allergic reaction (see page 64). Be prepared to administer epinephrine (see page 444).

Hives can also be induced by exposure to cold or during rewarming of cold skin (cold urticaria). Accompanying the skin lesions can be fatigue, headache, shortness of breath, rapid heart rate, and, rarely, full-blown anaphylaxis (see page 64). Avoidance of cold may not be totally preventive, since the rate of cooling seems to be as important a factor as the environmental temperature. Avoidance of sudden temperature changes and cold exposure are advised. Certain drugs, such as cyproheptadine (Periactin), may be prescribed by a physician as treatment.

Skin-colored swelling (sometimes severe and called angioedema, indicating fluid collection in the deep skin and subcutaneous tissues) of the lips, eyes, and mucous membranes occurs in 2 to 20 per 10,000 new users of angiotensin-converting enzyme (ACE) inhibitors (a type of drug used to treat hypertension). This is also seen with penicillin allergy and may portend difficulty breathing, so should be treated aggressively, as for a severe allergic reaction (see page 64).

HEAT RASH

Heat rash is a skin irritation composed of small raised spots that coalesce to form large areas of redness, particularly in the groin, under the arms, in the creases of the elbows, over the chest, under the neck, and under the breasts. It is rarely itchy; more often, it becomes irritated, particularly with rubbing. It should be treated with cool compresses; with light cotton clothing that will absorb sweat; and, if painful, with thin applications of 0.5% to 1% hydrocortisone lotion twice a day.

INTERTRIGO

Intertrigo is softening and maceration of skin caused by moisture and rubbing where two skin surfaces are in continual close contact, such as in the creases underneath a woman's breasts, in the groin, or in skinfolds of obese persons. Attempts to keep the area dry are usually unsuccessful in hot and humid environments. To soothe the rash, apply a thin layer of antiseptic ointment, such as bacitracin or mupirocin. If the rash begins to show a white curdish discharge, it may be a yeast infection (see page 126) and may respond to an antifungal preparation.

CHAFE

Chafe occurs between the thighs and in the groin creases, particularly in runners and cyclists. The skin is reddened and painful. The best way to treat it is to avoid the offending activity and to lubricate the affected skin with something greasy, such as petrolatum or a nonsensitizing antiseptic ointment, such as bacitracin. Treatment and prevention include wearing clean, absorbent pants and underwear.

IMPETIGO

Impetigo is a highly contagious, superficial skin infection caused by the bacteria *Staphylococcus*, with or without an antecedent *Streptococcus* infection. It is most often seen in warm and humid climates, and presents as discrete weeping sores, with honey-yellow crusted scabs (with or without yellow pus) of the sort often associated with infected insect bites, small scrapes, or areas frequently scratched. The rash may start as pinhead-sized blisters filled with white or yellow pus. Once a few sores have become infected and ruptured, they coalesce and crop up all over the body (particularly in children), and can cause fevers, fatigue, and swollen regional lymph glands. In the blister form of impetigo, the victim shows large, superficial, and fragile blisters that are commonly seen on the trunk, limbs, armpits, and other skinfold areas.

The skin should be washed twice a day with pHisoHex scrub (not for infants and children under 2 years of age), a half-strength solution of hydrogen peroxide, or soap and water, and the sores covered with a thin layer of mupirocin ointment or cream, bacitracin (less effective) ointment, or retapamulin 1% ointment. Before applying the ointment (three times a day until all lesions have cleared), remove the crusts with warm soaks. Methicillin-resistant *Staphylococcus aureus* (MRSA)–related infections (see later) may be treated with bacitracin (alone or in combination with polymyxin and neomycin), mupirocin, or retapamulin, although topical therapy may not be sufficient to treat the infection. Note that oral antibiotics, in the absence of MRSA, offer no particular benefit over proper topical therapy. If an oral antibiotic is used, treatment involves administration of oral dicloxacillin, cephalexin, azithromycin, erythromycin, or amoxicillin/clavulanate for 7 to 10 days. If there is resistance to these antibiotics or a high concern for MRSA, use trimethoprim–sulfamethoxazole (particularly for children under 8 years old), doxycycline, or minocycline (the latter two are contraindicated in children younger than 8 years).

If a person is prone to impetigo, he may be a chronic carrier of *Staphylococcus* bacteria inside his nose. This can be controlled for up to 3 months by an intranasal application, using a cotton-tipped swab, of mupirocin calcium ointment 2% (Bactroban Nasal) four times a day for 5 days.

CELLULITIS, INCLUDING METHICILLIN-RESISTANT *STAPHYLOCOCCUS AUREUS*

Cellulitis is inflammation of soft tissues of the body, commonly involving the skin and subcutaneous (under the skin) structures. Signs and symptoms include reddened skin, swelling, tenderness, blistering and "weeping" from the skin (in severe cases), tender and swollen lymph nodes, and fever and chills (severe cases). It is often caused by the bacteria *Streptococcus* or *Staphylococcus*. Many other germs can cause cellulitis, particularly if it follows a dog bite, injury in the aquatic environment, or scratch from a thorn or plant, or if the victim suffers from immunosuppression. Fever, swollen lymph glands, and red streaking that travels in a linear fashion from the infected site toward the trunk indicate the spread of infection into the lymphatic system (lymphangitis, or "blood poisoning") (Figure 150). Cellulitis associated with air that can be felt by an examiner in the soft tissues, often described as "Rice Krispies," is indicative of a rapidly advancing and potentially life-threatening infection, known as necrotizing fasciitis (caused by "flesh-eating bacteria").

An increasing cause of cellulitis and abscesses is MRSA, which can generate prolonged and debilitating infections. These bacteria are resistant to all currently available penicillins and cephalosporins. If MRSA infection is a possibility, the antibiotics of choice in the outdoors are trimethoprim–sulfamethoxazole, clindamycin, doxycycline, or minocycline. Other drugs that may be prescribed by a physician once that diagnosis is confirmed include daptomycin, linezolid, or rifampin, the latter as part of a combination therapy. The disadvantages of clindamycin are

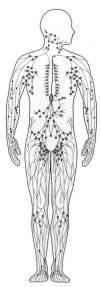

Figure 150. General location of lymph nodes within the lymphatic system. Tenderness and enlargement of the nodes mark inflammation in the lymph nodes; red streaking can sometimes be appreciated.

its association with subsequent diarrhea caused by *Clostridium difficile* and the emergence of bacterial resistance. If trimethoprim–sulfamethoxazole or doxycycline/minocycline is prescribed because of suspicion for a MRSA infection, it's prudent to add a beta-lactam antibiotic (such as cephalexin) to cover possible infection with group A *Streptococci*. Trimethoprim–sulfamethoxazole used alone for MRSA has met with mixed results. Rifampin is sometimes used in combination with trimethoprim–sulfamethoxazole or doxycycline to treat MRSA infection, but this is not based on scientific data. Fluoroquinolone antibiotics, such as ciprofloxacin (Cipro), should not be used to treat skin and soft tissue infections caused by community-acquired MRSA, because of bacterial resistance. High-risk persons for MRSA infection include contacts of a person with a MRSA infection, children, male homosexuals, soldiers, prisoners, athletes (especially in contact sports), Native Americans, Pacific Islanders, previously infected individuals, and intravenous drug users. If MRSA is not a consideration (unfortunately, this will probably soon never be the case), antibiotics for cellulitis may include cephalexin, dicloxacillin, or amoxicillin–clavulanate.

If cellulitis is associated with human or animal bite (see page 368), the initial antibiotic should be amoxicillin–clavulanate; if it's associated with exposure to fresh water or salt water (see page 347), ciprofloxacin or doxycycline should be administered along with an antibiotic to cover *Staphylococcus*; if it's associated with exposure to raw meat, fish or clam processing, or animal handling, infection with *E. rhusiopathiae* ("fish handler's disease") should be suspected and the initial antibiotic treatment should include amoxicillin or ciprofloxacin.

Important measures to prevent the spread of any skin infection, and in particular MRSA infection, include covering all draining wounds with clean bandages, washing hands after contact with a contaminated wound, laundering clothing after it has been contaminated, bathing regularly using soap, avoiding sharing items (such as towels, clothing, razors, etc.) that may be contaminated, and cleaning equipment with effective agents (such as detergent or disinfectant, such as a quaternary ammonium compound or dilute bleach). For MRSA in particular, prevention measures also include applying 2% mupirocin ointment to the inside of the nostrils with a cotton-tipped swab twice a day for 5 days, and washing intact (not open wounds, the face, or mucous membranes) skin with 4% chlorhexidine gluconate solution, followed by a thorough water rinse, once a day for 5 days.

ABSCESS

An abscess (boil) is a collection of pus. Although it can occur anywhere on or in the body, it's most frequently noticed on the skin, particularly in an area of high perspiration, friction, and bacteria (particularly *Staphylococcus*) accumulation, such as associated with hair follicles under the arm (Figure 151) or in the groin. The early abscess first appears as a firm, tender red lump, which progresses over the course of a few days into a reddish-purple, soft, tender, raised area, occasionally with a white or yellowish cap ("comes to a head") (Figure 152). The surrounding skin is reddened and thickened, and regional lymph glands may be swollen and tender. Fever, swollen lymph glands, and red streaking that travels in a linear fashion from the infected site toward the trunk indicate the spread of infection into the lymphatic system (lymphangitis, or "blood poisoning") (see Figure 150).

Treatment involves drainage of the pus and dead tissue from within the core of the soft abscess. This is performed by taking a sharp blade and cutting a line into the roof of the abscess at its softest point (Figure 153, *A*). The incision must be large enough (generally, at least half the size of the soft area) to allow all of the pus to drain. On rare occasions, the pus inside the abscess will squirt from the incision, so take care to protect your eyes and clothes. After the pus is allowed to drain, the cavity should be rinsed well and then packed snugly with a small piece of gauze

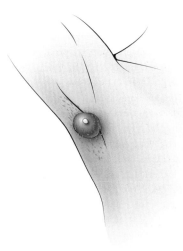

Figure 151. External appearance of an abscess in the armpit.

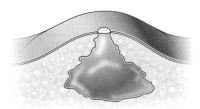

Figure 152. Cross section of a pus pocket, with a soft cap.

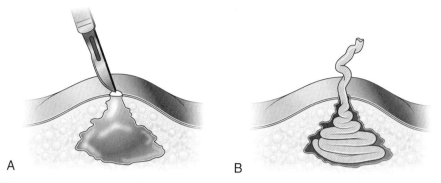

Figure 153. A, To drain an abscess, a stab wound is made in the center of the softest area. **B,** After the pus is removed and the cavity is rinsed, a gauze wick is layered into the cavity.

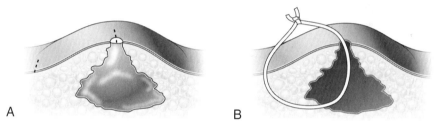

Figure 154. A, Two incisions are placed approximately 1 inch apart to allow the loop technique for abscess drainage. **B,** The rubber is tied off to create a loose loop.

(see Figure 153, *B*) to prevent the skin from sealing closed over the created empty space (and thus merely reaccumulating pus, rather than healing). Each day, the packing is removed (yank it out quickly to minimize pain) and the wound irrigated and then repacked until the cavity shrinks to a small size. If the abscess remains open while it's healing such that continuous drainage is ensured, packing is not necessary. If the abscess is adequately drained, there is no need to begin antibiotic administration.

Another method to manage an abscess is the "loop technique." In this method, the abscess is incised and drained as above, but with a smaller incision. After the abscess is rinsed, instead of packing the abscess, another incision about ¼ to ½ inch in length is made about 1 inch from the center of the abscess (Figure 154, *A*). A small flexible rubber drain, or the finger of a surgical glove, is inserted into the center incision and pulled out from the lateral incision, then tied off (knotted) so that a loose loop of rubber drain is created (see Figure 154, *B*). This loop should slide freely within the abscess cavity. It is left in place to promote drainage until the abscess ceases draining and appears to be healing well (usually 3 to 5 days), then it is untied or cut and removed, after which warm compresses may be applied a few times a day to complete the healing process.

Don't squeeze an abscess to cause rupture, particularly not on the face. This may force bacteria into the bloodstream and create a much more serious infection elsewhere (such as behind the eye or in the brain). After you make an incision into the top of an abscess and it is draining freely, it's all right to push the sides gently to express the pus.

If the abscess has not yet softened, but is still red, painful, and hard, begin the victim on warm soaks and administer dicloxacillin, erythromycin, or cephalexin. If MRSA is suspected, use an antibiotic recommended previously (see Cellulitis, earlier). Continue the soaks until the abscess softens and a white or yellow cap becomes apparent. If the abscess is soft, but there is evidence of lymphatic infection (see earlier), administer an antibiotic. If the abscess is near the anus, there is a risk that it can extend to become adjacent to the rectum. Suggested antibiotics for a perianal abscess are metronidazole in combination with amoxicillin–clavulanate.

Draining an abscess or dealing with a large wound infection may involve some nasty odors. If you cannot tolerate the smell, try rubbing a bit of toothpaste underneath your nose. If you have a face mask that covers the mouth and nose, such as an N95 face mask, wear it over the toothpaste, or if you have a dry teabag, place it inside the face mask instead of using the toothpaste.

INGROWN TOENAIL

An ingrown toenail occurs when the lateral edge of a nail penetrates into the skin alongside or outside the groove in which it normally advances during growth. This can be caused by an injury to the nail or toe, improperly fitting footwear, fungal infection, or improper trimming. Redness, pain, and swelling are common, and an infection may develop.

Treatment involves relieving the pressure created by the toenail on the soft tissues that surround it. Soak the affected toe for 30 minutes in a basin or bucket of warm water, preferably with a squirt of disinfectant such as povidone–iodine solution. Using a blunt, stiff tweezer, needle driver (see page 248), scissors, or nail clipper, rotate (extract) the ingrown portion of the nail out of the nail bed, and clip or cut it off (Figure 155). If this is impossible because of pain, which is common when there is an infection, you may need to first administer pain medication. To prevent the nail from growing back into the groove and once again becoming ingrown, pack the groove with cotton or layered strips of gauze or clean cloth. Change the packing every few days until the nail has grown back correctly or you can no longer keep the packing in place. Apply a thin layer of antiseptic ointment, such as bacitracin, underneath the packing or after nail extraction, even if a bandage is not available.

If you don't have any tools to trim the nail and wish to relieve the pressure, try taking a piece of tape and placing one edge on the soft tissue of the toe against, but not touching, the edge of the ingrown nail (Figure 156). Wrap the tape underneath the toe while pulling, to separate the soft tissue from the nail and relieve the pressure. This is a temporary measure at best.

If there are signs of an infection (see page 222), administer dicloxacillin, cephalexin, or erythromycin for 5 to 7 days and continue the warm- or hot-water soaks two or three times a day.

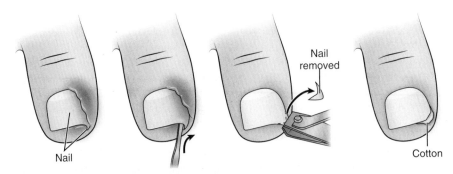

Figure 155. Removing an ingrown toenail.

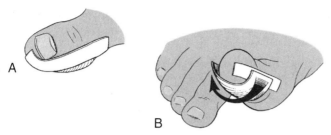

Figure 156. Relieving the pressure on an ingrown toenail. **A,** Place a strip of tape next to the painful ingrown toenail. **B,** Wrap the tape under the toe to separate the tissue from the nail.

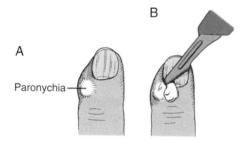

Figure 157. A, Paronychia. **B,** Draining a paronychia.

FINGERTIP CRACKS

Annoying fingertip skin cracks occur in cold, dry climates or after repeated exposure to saltwater and abrasion. They can be prevented by using skin moisturizers and limiting handwashing. Healing can be accelerated by applying a greasy (petrolatum-based) ointment and covering with a bandage. If the crack is resilient, it can be closed with a small amount of Super Glue (e.g., ethyl-2-cyanoacrylate). Medicinal tissue adhesives that should be used, if available, in preference to ethyl-2-cyanoacrylate are 2-octyl-cyanoacrylate (e.g., DERMABOND ADVANCED Topical Skin Adhesive) or n-2-butylcyanoacrylate (e.g., Histoacryl Blue or GluStitch). After you apply the glue and let it set, apply a fingertip bandage to keep the wound dry for 2 to 3 days. As the crack heals, the shed skin carries away the glue. If the glue is dislodged by accident before the crack heals, reapply it.

PARONYCHIA

A paronychia is a small abscess (see page 224) at the base of a nail (just beyond the cuticle) in the space between the soft tissue and the nail. It commonly appears as a red or yellowish, soft, and tender swelling in one corner at the base of the nail (Figure 157, A). If the nail feels mobile, there may be an underlying abscess.

If the area is firm, it may not yet be ready for incision and drainage, so begin warm water soaks. To treat a soft or draining paronychia, soak the affected finger in nonscalding hot water with a squirt of disinfectant (such as povidone–iodine) for 30 minutes. To drain the collection of pus, slide the tip of a no. 11 scalpel blade or an 18-gauge needle underneath the cuticle, holding the blade flat against the nail, to puncture the pocket and allow drainage (see Figure 157, B). If you don't have a scalpel, you can use a clean, small knife blade, or even the prong of a fork. Lift

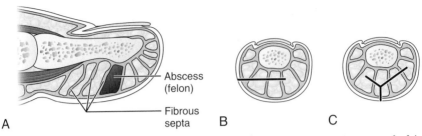

Figure 158. A, Felon. **B,** Linear incision through the pad of the finger for drainage of a felon. **C,** L-shaped incision to allow improved drainage of a felon.

the tissue gently off the nail. The abscess will be no more than ¼ inch (0.6 cm) below the margin of the cuticle; if you have penetrated that far without the obvious release of pus, cease your digging, start the victim on dicloxacillin, cephalexin, amoxicillin–clavulanate, or erythromycin, and continue with hot-water soaks three times a day. If pus is released, jam a 1 inch (2.5 cm) wick of gauze into the pocket, if the victim will tolerate it; with or without the wick, continue the soaks for a few days to keep the pocket draining.

FELON

A felon is a severe infection (abscess) of the pulpy tip of a finger (Figure 158, *A*), usually caused by infection with *Staphylococcus* or *Streptococcus* bacteria. It can arise from a nick in the skin, extension of a paronychia, infected hangnail, or puncture wound. The finger becomes swollen and extremely tender, with throbbing pain. Occasionally, there is extension of the infection via the lymphatic system (see page 223), with swollen lymph glands behind the elbow and in the armpit. It is possible to develop a fever because of a felon.

Merely soaking the felon in hot water will not help much. The definitive treatment is drainage, but this can be extremely painful. An incision needs to be made that allows extensive drainage from the fingertip. The most common incision is linear through the pad of the fingertip, sometimes with extension in an L shape to enter into and allow drainage from all the pockets of pus (see Figure 158, *B*). It may also be performed as a single longitudinal incision from the side of the finger into the depth of the abscess. This may sometimes be extended completely through the finger and out the other side with placement of a gauze or rubber "drain." Following the incision, warm water soaks are undertaken and antibiotics administered. The victim should be started on dicloxacillin, cephalexin, amoxicillin–clavulanate, or erythromycin.

BLISTERS

Blisters are the bane of hikers. These clear fluid–filled or blood-filled vesicles have probably ended more outings than all major illnesses combined. The cause of a friction blister is the repeated action of skin rubbing against another surface. As the external contact, such as a coarse, sweat- and dust-impregnated sock, moves across the skin, the opposing force is called the frictional force (Ff). The combination of the magnitude of the Ff and the frequency of the rubbing of the object across the skin determines the probability of blister development. Therefore, the greater the Ff, the lower the number of rubbing cycles needed for blister development. In terms of foot blister formation, shear forces extend horizontally between skin layers, between the skin and sock interface, between socks, and between socks and footwear. When the forces within a shoe or boot overcome resistance, sliding occurs. Repeated sliding at a friction point causes irritation that may be perceived as an initial sensation of heat—the so-called "hot spot." Further

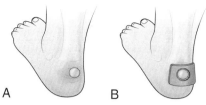

Figure 159. A, Blister on the heel. **B,** A cushion of moleskin protects the area from further irritation.

friction on a hot spot causes blister formation. The separated space in the area under the blister roof quickly fills with fluid. Thick skin like that found on the palms and soles is more likely to undergo blister formation.

Spontaneous blister healing is rapid if one can reduce further friction and worsening of the injury. In a mere 24 hours after blister formation, there is regenerative growth in the blister wound, and at 48 hours, evidence of healing. However, in the presence of continued friction and pressure, as is often the case in the backcountry, the body certainly benefits from medical attention that provides healing assistance.

The best protection for a blister is its own roof. Small intact blisters that aren't causing significant discomfort should be left intact (Figure 159). To assist in protecting this roof, a small adhesive bandage or pad can be applied. Be certain to place a first layer of paper tape under any cloth adhesive tape, so you don't inadvertently unroof the blister when removing the tape.

The pain from a blister is due to pressure on the incompressible fluid trapped between skin layers. As the abrasion and pressure builds, there is further weakening and separation of skin layers and increased potential for rupturing the blister. When a blister opens, raw skin is exposed. If a blister is punctured with a needle and drained, it will often refill within a few hours. If a large hole is made that allows continuous fluid drainage, there is risk for tearing off the roof and leaving a large damaged area.

Blisters deep to a callus should not be drained, as this is a painful and difficult process. These subcallus blisters quickly refill with fluid after drainage, and the process can introduce bacteria that cause infection. Likewise, blood-filled blisters should be left intact, because of a similar concern for infection.

Any blister with murky fluid, that is draining pus, or that is associated with warm, red skin or red streaking toward the heart may be infected. If the blister appears to be infected, it should be unroofed entirely, an appropriate dressing applied, and the victim treated with dicloxacillin, erythromycin, or cephalexin for 5 days or until the skin appears normal. If the dressing (such as Curad Hydro Heal) keeps the blister slightly moist, it may be less prone to drying out and cracking.

If a blister is caused by a thermal burn (see page 108), it should be immediately immersed in cold water (don't apply ice directly to the burn) for 10 to 15 minutes, to relieve pain and lessen the ultimate injury. Then dry the wound and apply a soft, sterile dressing. Unless there is a reason to suspect infection (cloudy fluid or pus, fever, redness and swelling beyond the blister edges, swollen lymph glands), burn blisters should be left intact. Opening an uninfected blister or sticking a needle into it risks introducing bacteria that can cause an infection. Topical antibacterial creams such as silver sulfadiazine or mupirocin, or ointments such as mupirocin or bacitracin, should be applied if the blister is broken or to prevent the dressing from sticking to the wound. Alternatively, apply a layer of Spenco 2nd Skin or Aquaphor gauze underneath a sterile gauze dressing.

There is no one correct way to manage a blister. For every technique and product mentioned, there are at least several different options. The following blister treatments assume that you must continue on your feet, because resting and staying off your feet is not an option.

Basic Blister Treatment (for Intact Blisters)

1. Cut moleskin (or a basic blister care product) into a donut of diameter $\frac{1}{4}$ inch to $\frac{1}{3}$ inch around the blister. The blister should fit inside the hole in the donut.
2. Place a patch of Spenco 2nd Skin in the donut hole directly over the blister.
3. Cover the moleskin donut with another layer of moleskin and patch with benzoin and tape.
4. Note that this "traditional" moleskin/donut treatment may cause further pressure points either directly under the moleskin or by transferring pressure and subsequent increased friction to the opposite side of the foot.

Basic Blister Draining

1. Cleanse both the blister skin and a safety pin with an alcohol pad. The diameter of a safety pin is large enough to allow continuous drainage, yet not so large as to risk unroofing the blister. If alcohol is not available, you can disinfect the needle by heating it to red hot and then allowing it to cool.
2. Puncture the blister with the pin at several points at the margin of the blister (generally on the outside of the foot), rather than via one large hole. This will allow natural foot pressure to continually squeeze out fluid, limiting the risk for unroofing the blister.
3. Gently push out fluid with your fingers.
4. Blot away the expressed fluid.
5. Cover the drained blister with paper tape (protects the blister roof from being torn away when any other overlying tape is removed).
6. Cover the paper tape with benzoin, and then with shaped adhesive tape. All tape should have trimmed and rounded edges to minimize "dog ears" and peeling.
7. Reaccumulated fluid can be drained through an intact bandage.

Treatment of Open and Torn Blisters

1. Using small scissors or another sharp object, carefully unroof the blister, completely trimming off the dead skin.
2. Place Spenco 2nd Skin on raw skin.
3. Cover the Spenco 2nd Skin with paper tape.
4. Apply a benzoin coating.
5. Cover with Elastikon or another tape product.

Toe Blister

1. Drain the blister with an alcohol-cleansed safety pin.
2. Use one piece of Micropore tape to encircle the toe (leaving the torn tape end at the top of the foot to avoid irritating neighboring toes).
3. Pinch the tape closed.
4. Trim sharp edges or wrinkles in the tape. Avoid cloth tape or Elastikon on the toes, as the abrasive nature of these tape varieties may cause blisters on adjacent toes.

To Prevent Blisters

1. Minimize friction generated by the normal biomechanical forces of walking and the contributors to friction. Reduce the carried load, whether that means losing personal

weight or shedding pounds from the backpack. Use a padded insole or arch support to help evenly distribute pressure over the bottom surface of the foot.

2. Increase or decrease the ease with which two surfaces rub against each other.

3. Shoes or boots should fit properly and comfortably. Shoes that are too tight increase contact points of pressure on the foot. Those that are too loose allow excess movement that allows generation of friction. Overly narrow shoes typically cause blisters on the large and small toes. Loose shoes can create blisters on the tips of toes from sliding and jamming the tips into the toe box. A toe box that's too shallow can cause blisters on the tops of the toes.

4. Fit (size) shoes in the evening, because feet tend to swell throughout the day. When trying on shoes or boots, make sure to wear the same socks and/or insoles or orthotics that you will be using on the trails. Size boots to compensate for thicker socks.

5. Allow for ample time to break in new footwear. This will stretch the material, sometimes loosen it, and increase flexibility. The breaking-in period also conditions the skin itself by causing the outermost layer to thicken.

6. Soft and supple feet are better able to withstand frictional stress than are cracked and horny feet. Many podiatrists recommend preparing feet with Bag Balm, a moisturizer, petrolatum, or other softening agent. Calluses should be filed down and toenails kept trimmed short and beveled downward.

7. Create a weak shear layer by using two pairs of socks. The goal is to have friction occur between the layers of socks, not between the skin and the socks. Wear a smooth, thin, snug-fitting synthetic sock as an inner layer with a thick, woven sock as an outer layer. The thinner synthetic liner sock will also assist in moisture control by wicking moisture and perspiration away from the skin surface.

8. Barriers are best used as preventive measures before blisters form, either at the beginning of the day or as soon as a hot spot develops. The barrier needs to be adhesive so it can remain fixed to skin, despite the action of friction, warmth, and/or moisture. Blist-O-Ban bandages (SAM Medical Products), Micropore paper tape, cloth tape, Elastikon elastic tape, moleskin, Spenco Blister Pads, Band-Aid Blister Block, and duct tape are methods to prevent blister development. Using an adhesive such as tincture of benzoin or Pedi-Pre Tape Spray will help keep the barrier adherent to the skin. Another way to eliminate friction from a potential hot spot is to use a sandwich bag. Cut off a corner of the bag, put a lubricant between the two surfaces, then tape the prepared bag to the skin in the desired location (Figure 160).

9. A cardinal rule of taping is to smooth out any wrinkles, and cut off "dog ears" that might lead to further pressure points. ENGO Blister Prevention Patches are slick fabric-film composite patches that are placed on the inside of the shoe or insole. Silicon gel toecaps and sheaths reduce friction between the toes.

10. Keep the skin clean and dry to minimize friction. Skin hydration leads to increasing contact area and friction, so moist skin results in more frequent blisters. However, very wet skin has a low incidence of blister formation, likely due to the lubricating effects of water on the skin surface. High-technology oversocks combine waterproof materials with traditional socks to help keep feet dry when repeatedly exposed to water. Combining GORE-TEX oversocks with wicking liner socks and foot antiperspirant is a method to reduce foot moisture. If your feet are often moist or sweaty, change socks frequently.

11. Consider the addition of gaiters to help eliminate dirt, gravel, sand, and rocks from entering the sock-shoe system.

12. Drying powders decrease moisture for short periods of time and are useful in the evening to dry out feet, but after about 1 hour may actually increase the friction between surfaces. Lubricants have been developed that are more advanced than traditional Vaseline, which

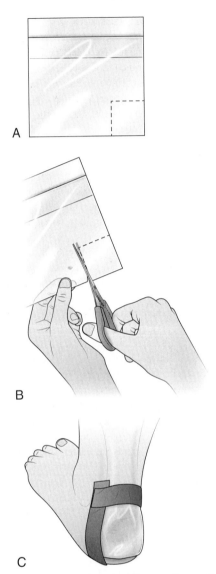

Figure 160. Using a sandwich bag to eliminate friction from a "hot spot" that might turn into a blister. **A,** Mark a corner of the bag to the size desired to cover the blister with a decent margin. **B,** Cut the bag, taking care to include both thicknesses (double layer, so that the plastic can slide on itself). **C,** Tape the plastic in place to cover the entire "hot spot" without applying any tape directly to the irritated skin.

is greasy and tends to trap grit particles, which are irritating and may increase friction and blister production. Advanced lubricants that combine silicone and petrolatum have a silky feel, prevent friction, and repel moisture from the skin. Lubricants can be applied preemptively, or over tape after hot spots develop. However, after about 3 hours, friction is increased as the lubricants are absorbed into the skin and socks. Lubricants should be tested before use on the trail to assess for allergic reaction, and reapplied frequently.

13. Antiperspirants irritate and block sweat ducts, reducing the amount of perspiration. People who suffer from a condition called hyperhidrosis experience excessive foot perspiration and subsequently have extremely moist feet. These people may benefit the most from antiperspirants. If possible, wash and dry your feet each day. To control foot sweating—which leads to blisters, fungal infections, and foot odor—spray your feet daily with an aluminum chlorhydrate antiperspirant, unless a fissure or crack appears in the skin, in which case spraying must be discontinued until the skin is healed. An alternative is to use a drying, deodorant foot powder.

14. Blisters or reddened skin may also be caused by an allergic ("contact") reaction to chemicals such as formaldehyde or rubber. If a rash is confined to the soles of the feet (shoe inserts) or top of the feet (shoe tongue dye), suspect this problem. In this case, the footgear must be changed.

PLANTAR WARTS

Plantar warts occur on the soles of the feet and are attributed to viruses. They may appear in weight-bearing areas and show themselves as thickened skin, sometimes raised from the surface and strewn with black dots, which are tiny clotted blood vessels. If they are in locations that cause pain with walking, they should be very carefully shaved with a sharp-edged blade or "sanded" down with a nail file so that they are flush to the surrounding skin, without exposing sensitive underlying tissue or causing a bleeding, infection-prone wound. They can ultimately be removed by using a salicylic acid plaster, freezing, topical imiquimod cream, or laser.

ATHLETE'S FOOT, RINGWORM, AND JOCK ITCH

Athlete's foot, ringworm, and jock itch are all caused by fungal infections. These more commonly develop in warm, moist areas, such as between the toes and in the groin. Athlete's foot (tinea pedis, or "foot") can be recognized as a red rash, moist or scaling, with small blisters and frequent weeping. Itching is the major symptom. Ringworm (tinea corporis, or "body") appears as one or more ring-shaped red areas on the torso. The rash spreads outward in an enlarging circle; the central area may clear slightly as the fungus in the center dies. There is scaling and itching, and occasionally tiny blisters at the expanding margin. Jock itch (tinea cruris, or "groin") is a red rash with a well-demarcated border that causes itching and irritation in the groin and occasionally over the genitals.

These rashes are more common in summer, particularly among those who do a lot of sweating and bathe infrequently. They are managed with antifungal cream (terbinafine 1% [Lamisil], butenafine [Lotrimin Ultra], ketoconazole 2% [Nizoral], econazole [Spectazole], naftifine 1% (Naftin cream or gel), or miconazole [Micatin or Lotrimin AF]) and antifungal powder, such as tolnaftate (Tinactin) or clotrimazole 1% (Lotrimin), applied two or three times a day. If the rash is refractory to topical therapy, a physician can prescribe an oral antifungal agent, such as fluconazole 150 mg by mouth once a week for up to 4 weeks. Because a fungal infection is contagious, socks and underwear should not be shared. If possible, wear cotton underclothing that absorbs sweat.

Sometimes a person can have horrible foot odor from wearing the same sweaty socks repeatedly combined with bad hygiene. This may be due to isovaleric acid formation. If the smell is horrible, one way to quickly eliminate it from the feet is to soak the feet in an antacid liquid (e.g., Mylanta or Maalox). Follow that with a brisk soap and water scrub.

TINEA VERSICOLOR

Tinea versicolor (sometimes called pityriasis versicolor) is a superficial infection caused by yeasts of the *Malassezia* species that creates skin discoloration with minimal itching or scaling. It appears as multiple discolored (white, gray, pink, or darkened [like a tan]) spots or patches on the shoulders, arms, chest, and back. It is treated with topical applications of selenium sulfide (Selsun) solution for 15 minutes a day for 10 days. Another way to apply Selsun is to moisten the affected area at bedtime, allow it to dry, and then wash it off in the morning. If that's ineffective, it may be treated with topical antifungal preparations (see earlier) or an oral dose of ketoconazole (Nizoral) 400 mg prescribed by a dermatologist. Alternatively, it can be treated with itraconazole (Sporanox) 800 to 1000 mg daily for 5 days.

ONYCHOMYCOSIS

Onychomycosis is a fungal infection under a nail, most commonly a toenail. This causes the nail to become discolored and deformed. The condition may be associated with chronic fungal infection in the skin, either as an itchy, scaling, or moist rash, or as recurrent blisters between the toes and on the sole of the foot.

A physician may prescribe the antifungal medication itraconazole (Sporanox) 200 mg once a day for 12 weeks or twice a day for 1 week per month for 3 consecutive months, or terbinafine (Lamisil) 250 mg per day for 3 months. Because these medications can induce side effects—such as headache, liver and gastrointestinal disturbances, and skin rash—and because they may interact adversely with certain drugs (such as terfenadine, cisapride, midazolam, triazolam, cimetidine, and rifampin), their administration should strictly be guided by a physician. Topical therapies, such as amorolfine, ciclopirox nail lacquer, and tioconazole, may be effective in cases where less than half of the nail is involved. Tavaborole topical solution 5% (Kerydin) has recently been approved for treatment of toenail onychomycosis. It is applied once daily for 48 weeks to the affected toenail(s). Another new therapy, topical efinaconazole 10% solution (JUBLIA), is available.

Prevention involves excellent foot hygiene and avoidance of fungal infection between the toes (athlete's foot) (see page 233). Each day, gently massage your feet and apply antifungal powder. Keep your nails trimmed. When hiking, use two pairs of socks—an inner thin liner sock of polypropylene or polyester and a thicker outer sock densely woven from a wool (or similar material) blend.

DIAPER RASH

If a baby develops a diaper rash, keep the diaper area clean and dry. For redness alone, apply Desitin diaper cream or A&D ointment. If a fungal infection is suspected, as evidenced by a more intensely red rash, raised bumps, and faint whitish discharge in the groin creases, add an antifungal cream, such as miconazole (Micatin). Don't apply steroid cream or ointment preparations, which can cause an infant's skin to atrophy. If the rash persists and circumstances permit, it may be helpful to have the child go without diapers, particularly during nap time.

ARMPIT ODOR

Armpit odor is common. Most of the time, adequate hygiene and deodorants are sufficient to eliminate this problem. However, sometimes the odor (particularly with sweating) becomes rancid and also causes staining of light-colored shirts. If the armpit is inspected and yellow, red, black, or cream-colored granular material is seen to be adherent to the armpit hairs, it may represent a superficial corynebacterial infection. Treatment is to shave the hair and to use for a few weeks a topical preparation of 15% aluminum chloride and/or topical 2% erythromycin solution. Prevention includes using an aluminum chloride–based antiperspirant and/or washing-gelling with benzoyl peroxide (e.g., Clearasil), or shaving the armpit hair.

LICE

In a situation of poor hygiene and shared living quarters, particularly overseas, you may acquire head and/or body lice, which make their homes predominantly in hair-covered areas of the body.

The overwhelming symptom is itching. To search for head lice, inspect the scalp carefully. On close inspection, you may discover nits (white, ovoid 0.5 to 1 mm empty egg cases) attached to the hair shaft, or tiny 3 to 4 mm crawling adult forms in the scalp, or rarely on the eyelashes. The nits remain attached to the hair and move out with hair growth at a rate of approximately 0.4 inch (1 cm) per month. A common finding is swollen lymph glands behind the ears or running down the back of the neck. Body lice and their nits live in the seams of clothing. The bites are most abundant on the shoulders, trunk, and buttocks. The pubic louse, or "crab" louse, prefers to reside in pubic hair, but may also appear on the eyebrows, on the eyelashes, or under the arms. Bites are hard to find, but if the infestation has been present for a few weeks, steel gray–colored spots may be seen on the trunk and thighs.

Fortunately, lice cannot leap or fly. It's often difficult to identify lice and mites by simple visual inspection of the scalp. A fine "nit comb" run through the scalp is better for detection. Wetting the hair may help. The treatment is to lather the body and scalp vigorously with crotamiton 10% (Eurax) lotion, leave the lather in place for 10 minutes, and then rinse. For pubic lice, it may be necessary to rub crotamiton lotion into the affected area daily for several weeks to destroy hatching ova.

For head lice, children may be treated with 5% permethrin (Elimite) cream in a single application; this is safe for infants over 2 months of age. Rub the cream into the skin and scalp, and wash it off after 8 to 12 hours. Thoroughly comb the hair in a direction toward the scalp to remove all nits. To be most effective, the process should be repeated in 1 week.

One percent permethrin cream rinse (Nix) or 0.5% malathion lotion (Ovide; approved for age 2 years and older) is also effective for removing lice from the hair. Apply it after the hair has been washed and towel-dried, leave it on for 10 to 20 minutes, and then rinse it off. Use a fine-toothed comb to remove the nits after rinsing. Comb again in 1 to 2 days. Repeat the treatment in 10 days to eliminate emerging lice. Another head lice treatment for persons ages 4 years and older is spinosad (Natroba) topical suspension 0.9% applied for 10 minutes, and repeated a week later if live lice are still seen. A treatment for resistant head and body lice is 0.3% pyrethium and 3% piperonyl butoxide (R and C shampoo, or RID) applied to all affected areas and washed off after 10 minutes. Other pyrethrins are A-200, Licide, and Pronto. Pubic lice may be treated with the same medications used for head lice. Topical ivermectin 0.5% lotion (Skilice) applied for 10 minutes to dry louse-infested hair has been effective when other methods failed. Benzyl alcohol lotion (Ulesfia) suffocates head lice. If it is used, it should be repeated in 10 days.

All hats, scarves, clothing, and bedding (including sleeping bags) should be washed thoroughly with laundry soap in hot water or dry-cleaned. All people in close contact should be evaluated for lice and treated if necessary.

Lindane 1% (Kwell) shampoo and other lindane-containing products have been banned in the state of California.

SCABIES

Scabies is caused by the human scabies mite *Sarcoptes scabiei* var. *hominis,* which completes its entire life cycle on the skin of a human. It's usually acquired during sexual contact, but can also be acquired from clothing and bedding. The usual manifestations are severe nocturnal itching, which is provoked by body warming, such as occurs from the heat of a fire. A serpentine burrow is seen on the surface of the skin, which is created as an impregnated adult female burrows into the skin and deposits eggs along a path that usually does not exceed $\frac{1}{5}$ to $\frac{1}{3}$ inch (5 to 10 mm) in length. Common sites for infestation are the web spaces between fingers, sides of fingers, wrists, elbows, buttocks, feet, ankles, and belt line. Infants may be infested on the scalp and soles of the feet.

Untreated, the disorder can persist indefinitely. Permethrin cream 5% (Elimite) rinsed off after 8 to 14 hours is an effective therapy approved for use in infants over 2 months of age. A cure can be effected with a single 8-hour application of 1% gamma benzene hexachloride (Kwell) lotion or cream, but this product should not be used in children or pregnant women. Other treatments available in Europe are benzyl benzoate 10% or 25% lotion rinsed off after 24 hours, and allethrin 0.6% aerosol rinsed off after 12 hours. Symptoms may persist (up to a month) after the mites have been killed, until the uppermost layer of skin is shed. The chemical should also be applied beneath the fingernails, where mites may be deposited during scratching. Other therapies are crotamiton ointment or cream 10% for 2 consecutive nights (not very effective), or sulfur in petrolatum (5% to 10%) for 3 consecutive nights.

CREEPING ERUPTION

Creeping eruption is the common term for cutaneous larva migrans, which is caused by the larvae of hookworms *(Ancylostoma species)* that infest cats and dogs. Humans pick up the larvae on exposure to dirt, particularly moist, sandy soils or beach sand following a rainfall. The larvae invade the skin, most commonly on the feet, lower legs, hands, and buttocks (from sitting). The larvae tunnel through the top layer of skin, leaving a serpentine, threadlike trail of inflamed (red) tissue, which itches and may be slightly painful. The trail may extend up to a few centimeters per day. Usually, the affliction heals without treatment. However, if one wishes to treat, the remedy is albendazole 200 mg by mouth twice a day, or ivermectin 200 mcg/kg (2.2. lb) of body weight in a single daily oral dose for 2 days (noting that ivermectin is not yet approved by the U.S. Food and Drug Administration for this indication). Another therapy is topical thiabendazole four times a day for 2 weeks. If the topical medication is not available, thiabendazole can be administered in an oral form in a dose of 22 mg/kg (2.2 lb) of body weight, not to exceed 1.5 g per dose, twice a day for 2 days. Oral therapy appears to be much more effective than topical therapy. If the rash doesn't completely resolve within 72 hours after therapy, repeat the treatment.

SHINGLES

Shingles is the common name for herpes zoster, a skin eruption with activation often related to stress. Individuals carry the varicella-zoster virus (the same agent that causes chickenpox [varicella] in children) dormant in nerve roots. On stimulation, usually in an elderly individual or someone with impaired immunity, it causes outcropping of a series of blisters in patterns that correspond with skin areas served by particular nerve roots originating from the spinal cord (Figure 161). Classically, the victim will have a day or two of unexplained itching or burning pain in the area that is going to break out and then will notice the onset of the rash, which appears as crops of clear blisters over 3 to 5 days. Symptoms that occur before the appearance of the rash often include headache, aversion to light, and fatigue. The discomfort can be tremendous and may necessitate liberal use of pain medication. The rash itself should be kept clean and dry and covered with a light, dry dressing to prevent further irritation from rubbing or the sun.

The disorder is self-limited and resolves spontaneously over the course of approximately 10 days to 4 weeks, as the blisters become cloudy, crust over, and then disappear. If the victim becomes moderately ill (fever, chills, severe headache) or if the rash involves the eyes, mouth, or genitals, see a physician, who may prescribe acyclovir (Zovirax) 800 mg five times a day, valacyclovir (Valtrex) 1 g three times a day, or famciclovir (Famvir) 500 mg three times a day for 5 to 7 days. There is some early evidence that promptly treating with an antiviral agent might decrease the risk for suffering a stroke within 6 months following the episode of herpes zoster. Unfortunately, after the rash resolves, the pain ("postherpetic neuralgia") may persist for 1 to 3 months, or even for years. Topical lidocaine 5% patches, capsaicin 0.075% cream, and oral gabapentin (Neurontin) or pregabalin (Lyrica) are treatments that may be prescribed by a physician to treat postherpetic neuralgia.

Zostavax is a vaccine to reduce the risk for herpes zoster in adults ages 60 years and older. Because it contains live attenuated virus, it should not be given to anyone who is

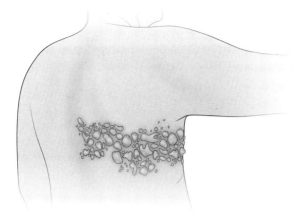

Figure 161. Shingles (herpes zoster) eruption.

immunosuppressed for any reason. It is given as a single dose subcutaneously. It appears to be quite effective in preventing shingles in persons who have never before suffered from this condition.

HERPES SIMPLEX VIRUS GENITAL INFECTION

Herpes simplex virus 1 infection is associated with lesions (e.g., fever blisters) on the face and mouth, whereas herpes simplex virus 2 infection typically causes infection in the genital region, as well as occasionally on the face. After an incubation period of 2 to 10 days from the time of sexual contact, the victim suffers 1 or 2 days of tingling and burning pain precisely where the sores will develop. These skin irritations are painful or itchy and may be reddened patches of blisters or ulcers. The victim may also suffer headache, fever, muscle and joint aches, and nausea and vomiting. The recommended treatment for a first episode is acyclovir 400 mg by mouth three times a day or 200 mg by mouth five times a day, famciclovir 250 mg by mouth three times a day, or valacyclovir 1 g by mouth twice a day for 7 to 10 days. A recurrent episode is treated for 5 days.

FEVER BLISTERS

See page 183.

MINOR BRUISES AND WOUNDS

BRUISES

A bruise is a collection of blood that develops in soft tissue (muscle, skin, or fat), caused by a direct blow to the body part, a tearing motion (such as a twisted ankle), or spontaneous bleeding (ruptured or leaking blood vessel). With trauma, tiny blood vessels are torn or crushed and leak blood into the tissue, so that it rapidly becomes discolored. Pain and swelling are proportional to the amount of injury. People on anticoagulants (such as warfarin) and hemophiliacs tend to develop larger bruises; elders and those taking steroid medications tend to bruise easily, often spontaneously.

The immediate (within the first 48 hours) treatment of a bruise is to apply cold compresses or to immerse the injured part in cold water (such as a mountain stream). This decreases the leakage of blood, minimizes swelling, and helps reduce pain. Cold applications should be made for intermittent 10-minute periods until a minimum total application time of 1 hour is attained. To avoid frostbite, don't apply ice directly to the skin. Wrap the ice in a cloth before application.

If the swelling progresses rapidly (such as with bleeding into the thigh), an elastic bandage can be wrapped snugly to try to limit the swelling. Continue cold applications over the wrap. It's important to keep the wrap loose enough to allow free circulation. Fingertips and toes should remain pink and warm; wrist and foot pulses should remain brisk. Elastic wraps can be helpful if pain and swelling will not allow the victim to extricate himself to seek medical attention.

Elevation of the bruised and swollen part above the level of the heart is essential, to allow gravity to further keep swelling to a minimum.

Never attempt to puncture or cut into a bruise to drain it. This is fraught with the risk of uncontrolled bleeding and the introduction of bacteria that cause infection. The exception to this rule is a tense and painful collection of blood under the fingernail (see below).

After 48 to 72 hours, application of moist or dry heat will promote local circulation and resolution of swelling and discoloration. Heat ointments, balms, and liniments don't transfer real heat. They are chemical or botanical substances that make the skin feel warm by stimulating nerve endings in the outermost layers of the skin and sometimes causing small blood vessels to dilate. This does not hasten healing, but may help a bit with soreness and stiffness. These substances should only be used on intact skin and never on mucous membranes.

People who have prolonged blood-clotting times and/or who have large bruises should avoid products that contain aspirin, which might cause increased bleeding. A hemophiliac who sustains an expanding bruise will likely need to be transfused with a blood-clotting "factor" to promote coagulation; transport to a medical facility should be prompt.

A severe bruise, usually caused by a direct blunt force, can on rare occasion develop into a compartment syndrome (see page 69).

BLACK EYE

A black eye is a darkened blue or purple discoloration in the region around the eye. It can be caused by a direct blow (bruise) or by blood that has settled into the area from a broken nose, skull fracture, or laceration of the eyebrow or forehead. "Raccoon eyes" are black eyes caused by a skull fracture. If a black eye is due to a direct injury (with swelling and pain), first examine the eyeball for injury (see page 170). The skin discoloration may be treated with intermittent cold compresses for 24 hours.

BLOOD UNDER THE FINGERNAIL

When a fingertip is smashed between two objects, there is frequently a rapid blue discoloration of the fingernail, which is caused by a collection of blood underneath the nail. Pain from the pressure may be quite severe. To relieve the pain, it's necessary to create a small hole in the nail directly over the collection of blood, to allow the blood to drain and thus relieve the pressure. This can be done during the first 24 to 48 hours following the injury by drilling a small hole in the nail by twirling a scalpel blade, sharp knife, or needle. As soon as the nail is penetrated, blood will spurt out, and the pain will be considerably lessened. Another technique is to heat a paper clip or similar-diameter metal wire to red-hot temperature in a flame (taking care not to burn your fingers while holding the other end of the wire; use needle-nose pliers, if available). Quickly and steadily press the glowing-hot wire through the nail until it is penetrated (Figure 162). Before and after the procedure, the finger should be washed carefully. If the procedure was

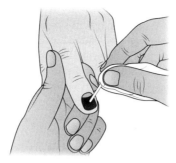

Figure 162. Hot paper clip technique to drain blood from under the fingernail.

not performed under sterile conditions, administer dicloxacillin, erythromycin, or cephalexin for 3 days.

TORN FINGERNAIL

If a fingernail is torn in such a manner that it is partially removed from the nail bed, carefully clean the wound and decide whether you can leave the nail in place as is or whether you need to trim it in order to make it easier to apply a clean dressing. If you decide to trim the nail, take care to not cut away any of the nail root (lowest portion of the nail that tucks under the skin). If the nail has been torn off, then cover the nail bed with something nonadherent, such as a piece of Vaseline gauze, or bacitracin underneath a nonstick piece of Telfa. If you use a dressing that sticks to the nail bed, it will become encrusted and be difficult to remove without soaking, and become painful to remove.

PUNCTURE WOUNDS

Puncture wounds are most frequently caused by nails, tree branches, thorns, fishhooks, and the like. Because they don't drain freely, these wounds carry a high risk for retained bacteria and subsequent infections. A puncture wound should be irrigated copiously with the cleanest solution that's available and left open to heal. Bleeding washes bacteria from the wound, so a small amount of bleeding should be encouraged. Never suture or tape a puncture wound closed, unless necessary to halt profuse bleeding; doing so promotes the development of infection. Similarly, don't occlude the opening of a puncture wound with a "grease seal" or plug of medicinal ointment; apply any antiseptic sparingly. If the wound is more than $\frac{1}{4}$ inch (0.6 cm) at its opening, you can leave a piece of sterile gauze in the wound as a wick for a day or two, to allow drainage and prevent formation of an abscess cavity (see page 224). If the wound becomes infected (see page 222), apply warm soaks four or more times a day. Treat the victim with dicloxacillin, erythromycin, or cephalexin for 4 days.

IMPALED OBJECT

See page 57.

SCRAPES

Scrapes (abrasions) are injuries that occur to the top layers of skin when it is abraded by a rough surface. They are generally very painful, because large surface areas with numerous nerve endings are involved. Bleeding is of an oozing, rather than free-flowing, nature.

An abrasion should be scrubbed until every last speck of dirt is removed. Although it hurts just to think about this, scrubbing is necessary for two reasons. The first is the infection potential when such a large area of injured skin is exposed to dirt and debris. The second is that if small stones or pieces of dirt are left in the wound, these in essence become like ink in a tattoo, leaving the victim with permanent markings that sometimes require surgical excision. Soap-and-water scrubbing with a good final rinse should be followed with an antiseptic ointment such as bacitracin or mupirocin, or cream such as mupirocin, and a sterile nonadherent dressing or Spenco 2nd Skin. You can also place Hydrogel occlusive dressing over an abrasion; it will absorb up to $2\frac{1}{2}$ times its weight in fluid weeping from the wound. It should be covered with a dry, light dressing. This technique is useful for burns as well. If the surface area is not particularly large or is on a difficult-to-bandage area, such as the nose or ears, the bandage (not the ointment) may be omitted.

The pain of cleansing can be relieved by applying pads soaked with lidocaine 2.5% ointment to the abrasion for 10 to 15 minutes before scrubbing. To avoid lidocaine toxicity, don't do this if the surface area of the abrasion exceeds 5% of the total body surface area (an area approximately five times the size of the victim's fingers and palm). In some cases, particularly when there is deeply embedded grime that will be extremely painful to remove, it's useful to inject the wound with a local anesthetic (see page 242).

CUTS (LACERATIONS)

Remove all clothing covering a wound to determine the origin and magnitude of any bleeding. Try to wash your hands with soap and water and then don protective gloves before contacting blood or other potentially infectious bodily fluids. After you have cared for a cut or wound, you should wash your hands again.

1. *Control bleeding.* This can be done in almost every instance by direct pressure (see page 50). Apply firm pressure to the wound using a wadded sterile compress, cloth, or direct hand contact (wearing surgical gloves, if possible; if you're allergic to latex, use nonlatex synthetic, such as nitrile). Hold pressure for a full 10 to 15 minutes without release. If this does not stop the bleeding, apply a sterile compress and wrap with an elastic bandage, taking care to not wrap so tightly as to occlude the circulation (check for warm and pink fingers and toes). If bleeding is not controlled with pressure alone, you may need to apply a hemostatic (stops bleeding) dressing or compress. These are described on page 50. During all of these maneuvers, keep the victim calm and elevate the injured part as much as possible.

   To control bleeding from a cut finger in order to allow its inspection and cleaning, sometimes pressure is not sufficient. In this case, one may improvise a tourniquet effect by wrapping the base of the finger tightly with a piece of tape, using the donned single finger cut from a rubber glove and then rolled back from the tip upon itself (Figure 163), or applying a commercial donut-style finger tourniquet (e.g., Tourni-Cot, Mar-Med Co.).

2. *Clean the wound.* In many cases, "the solution to pollution is dilution." After you have controlled the bleeding, the minor wound(s) should be properly cleansed. If you have needed to use hemostatic gauze or other blood-stopping agent to control the bleeding, you should wait for at least 60 minutes before attempting to clean the wound. Otherwise, brisk bleeding may reoccur. Wear sterile, nonpermeable, nonlatex (such as nitrile) gloves if these are available; if you're not allergic to latex, then latex gloves are acceptable. If sterile gloves aren't available, wear nonsterile gloves. Examine the wound and remove all obvious foreign debris.

   The best way to clean a wound is to irrigate away the dirt and bacteria. Along with removing foreign bodies from within a wound and dirty or destroyed tissue from the wound edges, irrigation is the most important factor in preventing wound infections. The irrigating stream should be forceful enough (approximately 8 to 10 pounds per square inch) to dislodge the foreign material without injuring the tissues beneath the stream or forcing harmful material deeper into the wound. Use the cleanest disinfected water

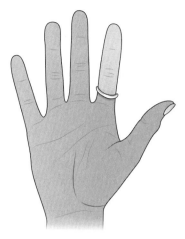

Figure 163. To control bleeding, cut a single finger from a rubber glove, then place it on the bleeding finger. Cut a small hole in the tip, then roll it back down over the finger so that it becomes tight at the base of the finger.

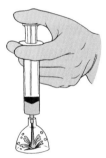

Figure 164. Using a Zerowet Splashield attached to a syringe to irrigate the open wound.

available. The best irrigants are "normal" saline (0.9% NaCl) solution (add 1½ level teaspoon [9 g] of table salt per quart or liter of disinfected saline or water) or plain disinfected water. Tap water without the addition of povidone–iodine is fine for irrigation purposes. Addition of no more than 1 fluid oz (30 mL) of povidone–iodine (Betadine) solution (not soapy "scrub") into a liter of irrigating fluid has been recommended in the past, but has fallen out of favor. Certainly, don't use a povidone–iodine solution to irrigate eyes, and don't drink this stuff. Hydrogen peroxide and other antiseptics are tissue toxic. Try to use at least 500 mL (roughly 1 pint) of irrigation fluid per wound. There is no benefit from soaking a wound in water, disinfected or not. Soaking may actually increase the bacterial count. If there is grease in the wound, it is best to avoid commercial degreasing agents; use soap and water, followed by water irrigation.

Use a syringe (30 to 60 mL is best, but any size can be used) with a 16- to 20-gauge (18-gauge is best) plastic catheter or steel needle attached to draw up the irrigating fluid and act as a "squirt gun." This creates a stream of the appropriate force (range of 5 to 12 pounds per square inch). Wound irrigation syringes with blunt tips are available commercially. Another way to obtain the appropriate stream diameter and force is to attach a Zerowet Splashield or Supershield (www.zerowet.com) to a plastic syringe (Figure 164). A complete wound irrigation system (Klenzalac) with a 10 mL syringe, fill stem, and Splashield is also available. This technique protects the operator from splash

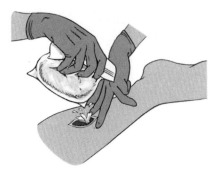

Figure 165. Using a small plastic bag filled with water to irrigate a wound.

exposure to blood and tissue fluid. Another pump for irrigating a wound might be a water disinfection filter, if a properly sized tip to direct the stream can be connected. If you don't have these supplies, you can fill a small (as sturdy as possible) plastic bag with the irrigating solution, punch a tiny hole in the bag, and squeeze out the liquid (Figure 165). Irrigate the wound until it appears clean, usually with at least a pint to a quart (½ to 1 liter) of liquid. Take care to avoid splashing yourself.

Sometimes irrigation isn't enough to remove all of the dirt from the wound, or you won't be carrying irrigation equipment. In that case, the wound needs to be scrubbed out with a gauze or cloth, using a disinfectant solution or hand soap and the cleanest disinfected water available. This can be painful, so get everything ready in advance and then try to accomplish the task as quickly as possible. Rinse the wound thoroughly when you are finished.

Don't forcefully irrigate a puncture wound, because you may push fluid deeper into the tissues and force germs and other contaminants further into the wound.

Scrubbing and irrigation will often cause a wound to begin bleeding again as blood clots are dislodged from tiny blood vessels. After cleaning the wound, stop this bleeding by holding absorbent gauze with pressure against the wound.

Don't pour tincture of iodine, rubbing alcohol, merthiolate, mercurochrome, or any other over-the-counter antiseptic into the wound (except for potentially rabid animal bites—see page 368). These preparations inhibit wound healing and are extremely painful. Although recommended by healers in ancient civilizations, herbal doctors, and professional woodsmen, the use of butter, pine sap, ground charcoal, hard liquor, or wine as an antiseptic is not recommended.

3. *Anesthetize (numb) the wound.* Most laypeople will never be called on to sew (suture) or staple a wound closed. However, for the benefit of rescuers who might need to employ advanced skills, here are the basics:

Local anesthesia of a wound can be achieved by injecting sterile 1% lidocaine or 0.25% bupivacaine solution into the edges of the wound using a 25-, 27-, or 30-gauge needle attached to a 10 mL syringe. There will be less stinging sensation with injection if you add 1 mL of 8.4% sodium bicarbonate solution to each 10 mL of the lidocaine solution before using it, and also if you allow the product to come to room temperature if it was previously refrigerated. Bicarbonate should not be added to bupivacaine, because it causes precipitation if the solution is not used immediately. Once bicarbonate has been injected, the shelf life of the multidose vial of anesthetic decreases considerably, so this maneuver may not be practical in the field. Whenever possible, use a new ampule or vial of anesthetic for each episode (event, or victim). This minimizes the risk of injecting a contaminated (with bacteria) product and causing a wound infection. *Never* share needles between victims.

To draw up medication into a syringe, follow the instructions given for intramuscular injection on page 444. The onset of anesthesia from injection of lidocaine or bupivacaine is 2 to 5 minutes, with duration of action 1 hour for lidocaine and 4 hours for bupivacaine. The maximum safe adult dose (volume) of 1% lidocaine is 30 mL; for 0.25% bupivacaine, it is 70 mL. For a child, the maximum safe dose for 1% lidocaine is 0.4 mL/kg (2.2 lb) of body weight, up to 30 mL; the maximum safe dose for 0.25% bupivacaine is 1 mL/kg, up to 70 mL. Of course, it's best to stay as far as possible below the maximum safe dose.

The wound should be cleansed of all major debris and dirt before injecting an anesthetic, so as not to plunge the needle through grime. Inject through the open (cut or torn) portion of the wound, rather than through the surface of the skin, unless this is necessary to avoid gross contamination. One useful technique is to insert the short needle up to its hub, and then inject while you slowly withdraw the needle back out from the skin, rather than injecting during entry. As with any other medical intervention, it's important to have practiced ahead of time before attempting to numb a wound by injecting it with an anesthetic.

Numbing a wound can be done before it is definitively cleansed and irrigated, particularly if the cleansing process will be extremely painful (as when an abrasion needs to be scrubbed). In order to not have to reinject the wound because the anesthetic has worn off, have all of your supplies gathered and your helpers ready to assist before you inject.

Reapproximate the anatomy (close the wound) as best as possible. Most cuts don't involve tissue loss, so that edges fit together like a jigsaw puzzle. Because of the infection risk away from the hospital or doctor's office (a relatively germ-free environment), don't close a wound tightly with stitches of thread (sutures) unless absolutely necessary. Instead, bring the wound edges together with paper tape with adhesive specifically made for wound closure (such as elastic or nonelastic Steri-Strips) or with butterfly bandages (see page 246, Taping a Wound Closed). The latter can be fashioned from regular surgical adhesive tape (Figure 166). A small scar is preferable to a wound infection caused by tight closure that requires hospitalization for surgical management of the infection. If nothing else is

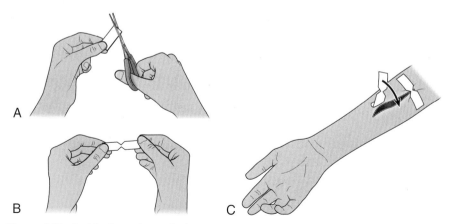

Figure 166. Fashioning a butterfly bandage. **A,** Fold a piece of tape so that the smooth (nonadhesive) sides are touching (e.g., don't let the tape stick together) and cut off both corners at the crease. **B,** The straightened tape reveals the "butterfly." **C,** The bandage is used to hold the wound edges close together.

available to hold together the edges of a widely gaping wound that prevents the victim from seeking help, use one or more safety pins.

No matter what method you use to close a wound, the best way to make the opposite sides match up properly, and to take tension off the wound while the remainder of the closure is completed, is to place the first piece of tape, staple, or suture (thread) at the midpoint of the wound ("halve the wound") (Figure 167). The second fastener should then "halve the halves" (Figure 168), so that the wound is now quartered, and so forth until the closure is complete. A final long locking strip can be placed over the ends of the crossing strips to complete the closure (Figure 169).

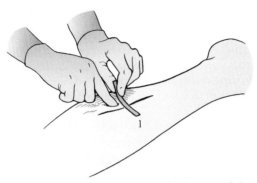

Figure 167. "Halving" a wound for the first act of closure.

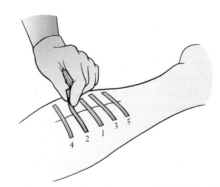

Figure 168. Halving a half, or "quartering the wound." This helps keep the wound in alignment and prevent mismatched sides (of different lengths).

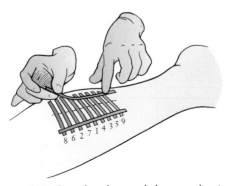

Figure 169. Completed wound closure using tape.

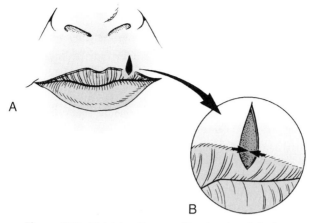

Figure 170. Matching the vermilion border of the lip.

When aligning the two sides of a cut lip, be sure to match the vermilion border (the line where the skin of the lip meets the skin of the face) perfectly (Figure 170). The same concern holds for aligning a laceration of the eyebrow. Never shave an eyebrow, because it might not grow back! In fact, there is no absolute need to shave hair from the skin around any wound. Shaving hair may increase the risk for infection, because you create micro-nicks in the skin with your razor or knife edge.

Regardless of which technique you choose to close the wound, it's useful to splint the repair (see page 70) for at least a few days, to allow healing to begin without the wear and tear of motion, particularly across a joint.

One way to close a laceration of the scalp is to twirl hair (if it is at least 1.2 inches [3 cm] in length) on direct opposite sides of the wound to form strands, pull these strands toward each other to pull the skin together, and then twirl them around each other. Then put a drop of rapid-cure cyanoacrylate glue (such as Super Glue) at the lowest junction of the strands while you are holding them together, and allow the glue to set up, which will occur very quickly. If a cyanoacrylate glue is not available, another way to do this is to first lay a long piece of string or dental floss along and beyond the length of the wound. Then, twirl the hair to form the strands, and twirl the strands together as described above. Next, use the string to tie the hair strands together (see Figure 47). Repeat the gluing or tying process as necessary to account for the entire open length of the wound. If the wound is large and you don't have a cyanoacrylate glue or any string, you may be able to hold the edges together by directly tying the twirled hair taken from opposite sides of the wound, but this is usually quite difficult.

SKIN FLAPS AND AVULSIONS

If a cut occurs at an oblique angle to the skin, so that a very thin layer of skin is "shaved" away, the wound should be cleaned carefully and the flap repositioned and held in place with tape (see later). If the flap is extremely thin or if its base of attachment is small, the blood supply may not be sufficient to allow survival of the tissue. In this circumstance, it will turn dusky blue and then blacken, harden, shrivel, and fall away. Unless there is an underlying infection—in which case the obviously dead or dying tissue should be removed—the flap may provide a biologic covering, much like a skin graft, to allow the underlying tissue to proliferate and heal. Since it's difficult to tell which dusky flaps will survive and turn pink and which will deteriorate and "mummify," it's best to give the flap at least a few days before trimming to see which way things are headed.

If a large chunk of skin is cut away entirely, or avulsed, the wound must either be closed, allowed to fill in as it heals with new tissue, or covered with a skin graft. The first two options are available to you in the field. If fat or muscle is showing and the wound edges will not easily pull together for field closure, the wound should be cleaned carefully, a sterile bandage (see later) applied, and the victim transported to definitive medical care.

TAPING A WOUND CLOSED

To apply tape to a wound, prepare the skin surrounding the cut by drying it thoroughly. Next, apply a thin layer of tincture of benzoin using a cotton-tipped swab, taking care not to get any into the open wound (it will sting like crazy). Another product that makes skin sticky and allows tape to adhere is Mastisol Liquid Adhesive. Push the two sides of the wound together so that they are perfectly opposed, and then lay the first adhesive strip across the wound at the midpoint of its length. Continue to apply strips perpendicular to the long axis of the wound until it is closed. Use diagonal or crisscross strips for extra strength.

If you don't have an assistant and it's difficult to hold the wound edges together and lay down an adhesive strip at the same time, you can attach a strip to one side of the wound, attach a second strip immediately next to the first one on the opposite side, and then use the two loose ends to pull the wound together (Figure 171). If the strips keep popping off the skin because it's slippery or too much tension is required to keep the edges together, you can run a strip of adhesive tape or duct tape longitudinally along the wound edges on either side of the gash about ¼ inch (0.6 cm) away from the opening, and use these as anchors for the crossing strips (Figure 172).

Another method of wound closure using tape, which may be more appropriate for a longer wound, is to cut two strips of adhesive tape 1 inch (2.5 cm) longer than the wound. Fold one quarter of each strip of tape over lengthwise (sticky to sticky) to create a long nonsticky edge on

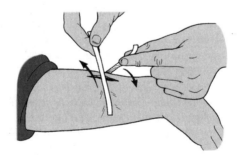

Figure 171. Using opposite-facing tape strips to pull a wound closed.

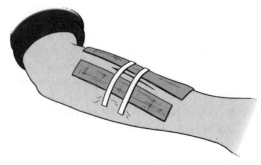

Figure 172. Longitudinal tape strips used as anchors for the cross (closing) pieces.

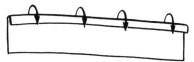

Figure 173. Folding a longitudinal piece of tape to prepare for a suture anchor strip.

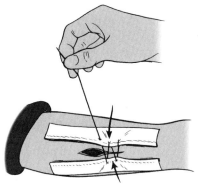

Figure 174. Sewing the tape suture strips together to close the wound.

each piece (Figure 173). Attach one strip of the tape on each side of the wound, ¼ to ½ inch (0.6 to 1.3 cm) from the wound, with the folded (nonsticky) edge toward the wound. Using a needle and thread, sew the folded edges together, cinching them tightly enough to bring the wound edges together properly (Figure 174). The tape will stick much better if you first apply a thin layer of benzoin or Mastisol Liquid Adhesive to the skin. Don't apply antiseptic ointment to a wound before trying to tape it closed, because after you apply the ointment, the tape (or "butterfly" bandages) will not stick.

If you don't have adhesive tape, you can fashion strips from cloth or sturdy nylon-like material. Use superglue to attach the first end and allow it to dry. Pull the strip across the wound to achieve closure and then glue the other end in place. Take care to keep the glue out of the open wound.

If you intend to apply antiseptic ointment to a wound, don't apply it before attempting to tape it closed, because the tape will not stick. It should be applied sparingly only after the tape closure has been completed.

SEWING (SUTURING) A WOUND CLOSED

In general, it's best to avoid sewing (suturing) a wound closed outside of the sterile environment of the hospital. However, sometimes this is necessary, particularly if the wound is large and cannot be closed with taping methods.

Sutures come in a variety of sizes attached to many different types of needles, depending on their purpose. For an expedition kit intended for use by a layperson, I recommend carrying nonabsorbable 3/O monofilament nylon suture (such as Ethilon, Dermalon, or Prolene) attached ("swaged on") to a large curved "cutting" needle, and 4/O monofilament nylon suture attached to a large curved cutting needle. The 3/O suture is larger in diameter, and should be used to close large wounds on the scalp, trunk, and limbs. The smaller-diameter 4/O suture is used to close smaller wounds on the trunk, limbs, hands, and feet. Although there are other suture types (such as nonabsorbable silk and absorbable gut and synthetics), sizes (thick to so fine [ophthalmic] that it requires a magnifying glass to see them), and needles (such as small curved and straight), these two suture setups will suffice for most situations in which a layperson might wish to stitch a wound. Ideally, you would use 5/O and 6/O (smaller diameter) suture material on the face, but this is more difficult to manipulate and tie if you're inexperienced.

Absorbable sutures can also be used to close skin surface wounds and have the added benefit that they will eventually dissolve and fall out. Fast-absorbing gut suture material absorbs in 5 to 7 days and can be used on the face; plain gut absorbs in 8 to 9 days and can be used on the torso and limbs.

The instrument used to push the needle through the skin is a needle holder (Webster-style "needle driver"). It has finger handles like scissors, and clamps open and shut with finger pressure to hold the needle firmly in its finely grooved jaws. It is held in a certain way to allow the wrist rotation that forces the curved needle through the skin.

The goal of stitching a wound is to bring the skin edges neatly together without excessive tightness, which would be manifested by a wound that's puckered up and stitches that become buried. Most wounds swell a bit; thus, it's not necessary to cinch them closed with too much tension. After a wound is stitched, it should lie flat.

Wear sterile, nonlatex (such as nitrile), nonpermeable surgical gloves if they are available. If you aren't allergic to latex, then latex gloves may be worn. If sterile gloves aren't available, nonsterile gloves are acceptable. The needle should be placed into the jaws of the needle driver so that it can be clamped just behind (toward the suture) the midpoint of the curve (Figure 175). The needle should be oriented perpendicular to the skin and pushed through using a gentle rotating motion at the wrist; this pushes it out into the base of the wound (Figure 176). Then release the needle, reach down into the wound and regrip the needle that has exited into the wound, and pull the needle and suture through the wound until a 2 inch (5 cm) tag is left outside

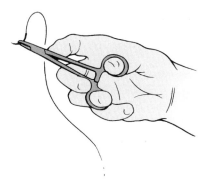

Figure 175. Gripping a suture needle with a needle driver.

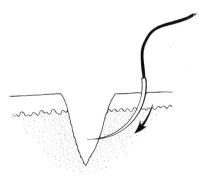

Figure 176. Pushing the needle through the skin and out into the base of the wound.

the skin (Figure 177). The needle is once again grasped with the needle driver as before, pushed into the opposite side of the base of the wound at exactly the same depth as it entered into the wound on the other side (Figure 178), and rotated out through the external skin surface on the same side (Figure 179). Now, once again release the needle from the needle driver. The ideal suture placement is square or bottle-shaped (U shaped) (Figure 180). As shown in this figure,

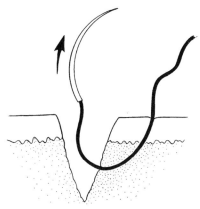

Figure 177. Pulling the suture through the first side of the wound.

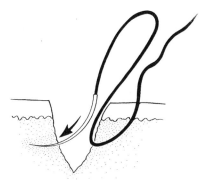

Figure 178. Pushing the needle into the base of the opposite side of the wound.

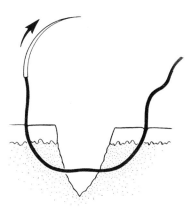

Figure 179. Rotating the needle out through the second (final) side of the wound.

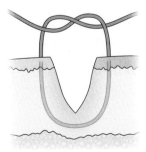

Figure 180. The U shape of proper suture placement.

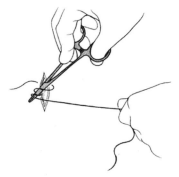

Figure 181. To tie a suture, first loop it around the needle driver twice.

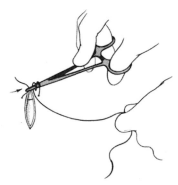

Figure 182. Grab the short end of the suture with the needle driver.

the suture ideally crosses the wound close to its deepest point; slightly above (see Figures 177 to 180) or below (see Figure 180) is acceptable.

To tie a modified square knot, the long end (with the needle) of the suture is looped around the needle holder twice (Figure 181); then the short end of the suture—which was left as a 2 inch (5 cm) tag—is grasped and lock-clamped tightly in the jaws of the needle driver (Figure 182). Holding the needle in one hand and the needle driver in the other, lay the double loop down flat against the skin to pull the wound together (Figure 183). To complete the knot, a single loop is thrown around the needle driver in the direction opposite the first (clockwise versus counterclockwise, or "over" versus "under") (Figure 184), the short end of the suture once again

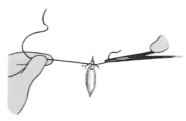

Figure 183. Laying down the first loop of a knot.

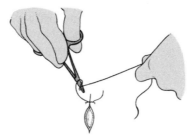

Figure 184. Creating the second loop of a square knot over the needle driver.

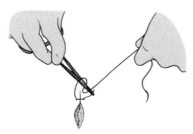

Figure 185. Once again, grab the short end of the suture with the needle driver.

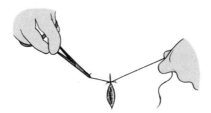

Figure 186. Completing the first square knot.

grasped with the needle driver (Figure 185), and the knot pulled tight; cross your hands properly to lay the second loop-tie down flat ("square") against the first (Figure 186). The knot completion process should be repeated three more times for a total of five "throws" to ensure that the knot won't unravel. Cut the long ends ¼ inch (0.6 cm) from the knot.

Place the stitches close enough together (approximately ¼ inch [0.6 cm]) so that the wound is closed and there is no fat showing from underneath the skin. A nice way to close a wound is to place enough stitches to bring the wound edges into reasonable approximation and support the tension, and then close the remainder with cloth or paper adhesive strips. Put the first stitch at the midpoint of the wound, then at the midpoints of the remaining segments, and so forth. If you begin stitching at one end and work your way to the other, you run a much greater chance of misaligning the wound edges and ending up with a tear-shaped "dog-ear" that can't be easily closed; this might force you to remove all of the stitches and begin all over again.

Sometimes the skin wound that you wish to close is in the midst of very thin skin, such as the delicate skin found on the arms or legs of older people. It's usually impossible to pull these skin edges together with a needle and stitches without tearing through the skin. One method to make this possible is to put adhesive wound closure strips (such as Steri-Strips) over the skin in a parallel orientation on opposite sides of the wound close to the wound edges in an attempt to bolster the skin. Then sew through the skin-strip combination.

After you stitch a wound, it may ooze blood from the needle holes or the center of the wound. Apply firm, direct pressure with a gauze bandage or cloth for 10 to 15 minutes. To dress the wound, apply a thin layer of bacitracin or mupirocin ointment and an absorbent sterile bandage. Inspect the wound daily for signs of infection (see page 222). If an infection develops, remove a few stitches over the worst area to see if any pus is released. Allowing the wound to drain in one area may allow you to keep the other stitches in place for the normal duration of healing. When in doubt, however, take all of the stitches out and let the wound heal open or under loose approximation with adhesive strips.

Try to keep the wound dry for at least 4 days. Stitches are left in place for 14 days across the joints of the finger and hand, 10 days on the arms and legs, 7 days on the trunk and scalp, and 4 days on the face. After you remove a stitch, you can reinforce a wound with adhesive strips for a week to allow a margin of safety for healing.

If you're going to carry sutures with the intention of sewing a wound, you should have a skilled medical practitioner teach you how to suture before you need to do it yourself. You can practice the technique on a pig's foot, a chicken leg, or even a thick-skinned orange.

To remove a stitch from a healed wound, wash the wound carefully and then cut the stitch on one side only of the visible knot. If you cut on both sides of the knot, you may not be able to retrieve the buried portion of the stitch. Grasp the knot with tweezers and pull the stitch out of the skin. If a crust has formed over the stitch, soften it up by applying moist compresses for 30 minutes before removing it.

STAPLING A WOUND CLOSED

An excellent technique for closing relatively straight lacerations on the arm, leg, trunk, and scalp is stapling. A disposable surgical stapler, such as the Precise 5-, 15-, or 25-staple Disposable Skin Stapler (3M Medical-Surgical Division), allows precise placement of stainless-steel staples. The proper technique takes practice. Hold the skin edges together and press the business end of the stapler against the wound closure line, and then squeeze the stapler to discharge a staple into the skin (Figure 187). The recipient feels a quick pinprick. The closure is rapid and sturdy. The staples are left in place for 7 days on the scalp and trunk, and 10 days on the arm or leg. A disposable scissors-handle staple remover or smaller pinch-handle-style staple remover (Precise SR-1, 3M) is used to painlessly remove the staples (Figure 188).

If you're going to carry surgical staples with the intention of stapling a wound, you should receive proper instruction before the journey.

GLUING A WOUND CLOSED

Topical tissue adhesives ("glue"), which can be applied in a thin layer on top of a wound (*not* within the wound) to bond the edges together, have been recommended for superficial cuts. The two classes of these adhesives marketed in the United States are the octyl-cyanoacrylates (e.g., DERMABOND, DERMABOND ADVANCED, and SurgiSeal) and butyl-cyanoacrylates

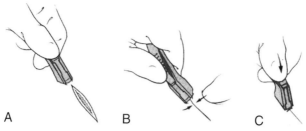

Figure 187. A, Preparing to staple a wound. **B,** Pressing the surgical tissue stapler against the skin while pushing the wound edges together. **C,** Squeezing the stapler in order to discharge the staple into the skin.

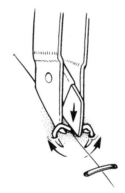

Figure 188. Removing a surgical staple.

(e.g., Histoacryl Blue, Indermil, GluStitch, and LiquiBand). In a recent evaluation, DERM-ABOND ADVANCED was the strongest and most flexible, and set in the shortest time, but this may not make a difference in terms of the totality of wound healing. DERMABOND ADVANCED is available in a ProPen applicator that makes this product quite easy to apply (see later). Other brands of over-the-counter tissue glue products are likely not as strong as prescription items, but may be quite adequate for outdoor use. Industrial (nonmedical) super-glues are nonsterile and may cause a bit of skin irritation, but are likely relatively effective and safe.

Tissue adhesive wound closure creates a closure that, while not initially absolutely as strong across a highly stressed area, like the skin overlying a finger joint, ultimately results in a similar cosmetic outcome to sewing the skin together. It cannot be used on the eye, inner moist surfaces of the mouth and lips, or areas with dense body hair.

To glue a wound shut, first clean it carefully, then blot it dry. Push the wound edges together so that they are perfectly aligned. The goal is to apply the glue so that it touches external skin only and does not enter the wound. Have an assistant apply a thin layer of glue over the surface while the edges are held evenly together and the wound is flat. Allow that layer to dry, then repeat two or three more times. When using the DERMABOND ADVANCED topical skin adhesive applicator, follow these instructions:

1. Hold the applicator away from the patient with the tip pointed downward.
2. Squeeze the bulb to crush the ampule inside, then release the pressure.
3. Gently squeeze the bulb again to moisten the internal filter with adhesive.
4. Hold the wound edges together with a gloved (if possible) hand or tweezers.

5. Apply DERMABOND ADVANCED in a single continuous layer while maintaining steady bulb pressure. Don't push the applicator into an open wound.

6. Hold the skin edges together for 60 seconds. The adhesive sets fully in about 90 seconds.

   Routine tape-strip reinforcement is recommended, and topical ointments should be avoided, as they will weaken the bond between the glue and the skin. After the wound is closed with tissue adhesive, the victim may wash off or shower, but should not soak the wound, swim, or bathe in a tub, because prolonged moisture loosens the bond. Blot, rather than wipe, the area dry. Superglue should not be used to close deep wounds, because if it leaks into the wound, it can cause an intense inflammatory reaction.

7. *Dress the wound.* This is generally done in layers. The first layer is antiseptic cream or ointment, which should be sparingly applied to the surface of the wound, provided that there is good drainage and there are no large, open (deep) pockets in the wound. A thick antiseptic grease seal that prevents drainage may actually promote the development of a deep-space infection. Antiseptic ointment may soften and weaken a tissue glue closure. If an antiseptic is not available, honey applied topically on a wound may reduce infection and promote wound healing. It's also useful for infected wounds. Medical-grade honey is "manuka" honey, a honey derived from *Leptospermum* trees. Honey intended for human consumption is fine for wound care purposes.

   A nonadherent next (inner) layer of a bandage keeps the overlying dressing from sticking. This should be nonstick (preferably sterile) Telfa or an impregnated (with petrolatum, for instance) gauze. If an antiseptic ointment or cream will prevent adhesion of the bandage, a prepackaged square of fine-mesh gauze can be used, but be advised that the ooze from a wound usually negates the lubricating features of most creams and allows bandages to stick. A nonadherent dressing can be improvised by applying antiseptic ointment, petrolatum, or honey to a gauze pad.

   Special wound coverings include Spenco 2nd Skin, an inert hydrogel composed of water and polyethylene oxide. It absorbs fluids (so long as it doesn't dry out), which wicks serum and secretions away from the wound and promotes wound healing. Other occlusive hydrogel-type dressings are NU-GEL (preserved polyvinyl pyrrolidone in water) and Hydrogel, which can absorb up to $2\frac{1}{2}$ times its weight in fluids exuded from the wound.

   The next layer is composed of absorbent sterile dressings, such as dry gauze pads (see Bandaging Techniques, page 255). If these aren't available, use clean white cloth (the more absorbent, the better). Apply the entire bandage assembly snugly enough to control bleeding, but not to impede circulation (as judged by warm and pink fingers and toes). Keep dressings in place with conforming rolled gauze, which can also allow some air circulation. If a prepackaged rolled gauze is not available, one can be created by taking a tee shirt and cutting a continuous strip in a spiral from the bottom of the shirt. All dressings should be changed as frequently as they become soaked; if there is no significant drainage, they should be changed daily. If the skin is becoming macerated (wrinkled and pale colored; kept perpetually moist), lighten up on the ointment or cream and apply a less occlusive dressing, while still keeping the wound protected.

   Another technique for relatively "dry" wounds (nonseeping and nonbleeding) is to apply a layer of Tegaderm—a thin, semi-transparent dressing material through which a wound can "breathe." This is also available as a small patch packaged with a short ($2\frac{3}{8}$ inch) Steri-Strip in a Wound Closure System (3M).

   If you use tape to secure a dressing, you can apply tincture of benzoin or Mastisol Liquid Adhesive to increase the stickiness of the skin. Don't let any benzoin run into the wound—it really stings. When dressings are applied, keep the body part in the position of function (normal resting position) (see Figure 49). Check all dressings daily for soaking, a snug fit, and underlying infection. If you wish to remove a dressing that's stuck to a wound, soak it off by moistening it with warm water or a brief application of hydrogen peroxide. Bandaging techniques are addressed in the next section.

8. *Splint the wound* (see page 70). For instance, if the injury involves the hand, also place the arm in a sling to minimize motion of the injured part. Movement delays healing and promotes the spread of infection.

9. *There is always the risk of infection.* If the wound is lengthy (more than 2 inches [5 cm]) or very deep, is an animal bite (particularly of the hand or foot), is on the hand or foot, is a puncture wound, has inadequate drainage, is within the mouth, is deep or complex (e.g., with visible bone or tendon; entering into a joint), is sustained by someone who is immunosuppressed (e.g., human immunodeficiency virus [HIV] infection, diabetes, chronic corticosteroid use), has resulted from a crush injury, or is very dirty (particularly if contaminated with soil)—or if you are more than 24 hours from medical care—the situation carries a high risk for infection and the victim should be treated with an oral antibiotic (dicloxacillin, erythromycin, or cephalexin) until the wound is healed or help is reached. For a cat (feline) bite, use ciprofloxacin in addition; a physician may substitute cefuroxime or cefoxitin.

10. *Seek appropriate medical attention.* Field cleansing and dressing are no substitutes for proper irrigation, trimming, and wound management undertaken in a medical facility. Small nicks don't require fancy intervention, but if you are in doubt as to the seriousness of the injury, get good advice. The nuances of optimal wound healing are many, but general basics to remember are that it may require many months to a year for scars to contract into their final appearance; topical silicone gel (available over-the-counter) combined with gentle massage may keep a scar soft and minimize its size; vitamin E is unproven as a beneficial topical substance to promote wound healing or minimize scar formation; and sunscreen should be applied to all "red" scars to protect them from ultraviolet light exposure for at least a year after the wound appears to be healed.

BANDAGING TECHNIQUES

Bandage application is an art form. The only way to become proficient is to practice. There is no inviolable rule other than to avoid excessive tightness, which might compromise circulation. Use square knots to tie bandage ends securely. Signs that a bandage is too tight are blue discoloration of the fingernails/fingertips/toenails/toes, cool and pale skin color, tingling or loss of feeling beyond the bandage, difficulty moving the fingers or toes, and pain underneath or beyond the bandage.

A triangular bandage is a three-cornered bandage, usually approximately 42 inches (1 m) across the base. A cravat is a triangular bandage folded two or three times into a long strap (Figure 189).

Finger bandage. Fold a 1 inch (2.5 cm) rolled gauze back and forth over the tip of the finger to cover and cushion the wound (Figure 190). Then wrap the gauze around the finger until the bandage is snug and not overly bulky. On the last turn around the finger, pull the gauze over the top of the hand, so that it extends beyond the wrist. Split this tail lengthwise. Tie a knot at the wrist, and wrap the two ends around the wrist; tie again to secure the bandage. Another technique involves not splitting the tail, wrapping it around the wrist twice, and then bringing it up over the top of the hand around the base of the finger from the side opposite where it originated, looping it over the hand back to the wrist, and tying it off (Figure 191).

Hand bandage. The hand should be bandaged as if for a fracture, in the position of function (see Figure 49). Take care to place gauze or cotton padding between the fingers to separate and cushion them. Use a simple figure-of-eight wrap across the palm.

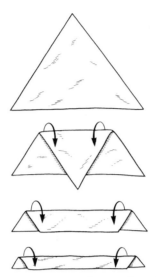

Figure 189. Making a cravat from a triangular bandage.

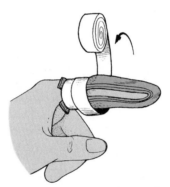

Figure 190. To begin a finger bandage, place layers of gauze over the fingertip.

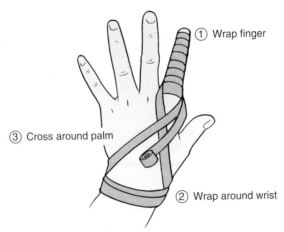

① Wrap finger

③ Cross around palm

② Wrap around wrist

Figure 191. To complete a finger bandage, wrap the gauze around the finger, then bring it across the palm and around the wrist to tie off.

Wrist bandage. Begin by wrapping the wrist two to three times (Figure 192). Continue over the top of the hand, and then through the space between the thumb and fingers, across the palm. Repeat the process in a figure-of-eight pattern until the desired thickness and rigidity is obtained.

Arm or leg bandage. Cover the wound(s) with a gauze pad(s). Overwrap the wound using simple spiral turns of rolled gauze or a figure-of-eight pattern (Figure 193). Secure the bandage with adhesive tape in a spiral pattern to avoid a tourniquet effect. Whenever possible, don't apply tape directly to the skin.

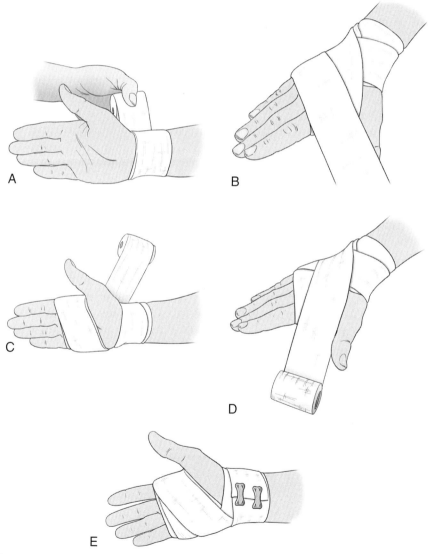

Figure 192. Creation of a wrist bandage. **A,** First, wrap around the wrist a few times. **B,** Continue across the top of the hand and then in the "web space" between the thumb and index finger. **C,** Continue back across the top of the wrist, and then **(D)** continue back over the hand in **(E)** a figure-of-eight pattern.

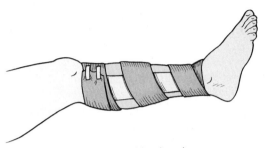

Figure 193. Spiral leg bandage.

Thigh and groin bandage. Wrap a 6-inch elastic bandage around the mid-thigh in an inner to outer direction and continue up toward the pelvis (Figure 194). At the groin crease, continue up and around the waist one time. This anchors the bandage. Then proceed back down the thigh to complete the figure-of-eight pattern. If the injury is to the quadriceps ("quads") or hamstrings ("hammies") muscles, put additional wraps on the thigh. If the injury is to the groin, alternate wrapping around the hip with wrapping the thigh. Since this is a large bandage, a double-length wrap serves best.

Foot bandage. The foot should be bandaged as if wrapped for an ankle sprain, using gauze instead of elastic wraps (see page 266).

Shoulder bandage. To make a shoulder bandage (Figure 195) from a triangular bandage, lay the base over the shoulder at a downward diagonal across the chest (front and back) with the apex pointed down the arm. Roll or fold the apex back down a few turns to create the beginning of a cravat; tie this just in front of the opposite armpit. Roll or fold the apex up the arm in the same manner until the bandage achieves the desired coverage, and then tie off this smaller cravat segment with the knot visible on the outside of the arm.

Chest bandage. To wrap the chest with gauze, circle the chest and upper abdomen for a few turns. To keep the bandage from slipping toward the hips, bring it up over the shoulder every third or fourth turn. Secure with adhesive tape.

Head bandage. Place the base edge of a triangular bandage just over the eyes (Figure 196). Fold the base edge 1 inch (2.5 cm) under to create a hem. Allow the bandage to fall back over the top of the head, with the apex point (tail) dropping over the back of the head. Then cross the other two free corners (at the ends of the hem) over the tail and tie them in a single turn (half of a knot). Continue to bring them around to the forehead and tie a complete square knot. Tuck the hanging tail over and into the half knot behind the head. If more pressure is necessary, tie a cravat directly over a gauze or cloth bandage.

Another way to secure a bandage to the side of the head, ear, or chin is to lay a cravat over the wound at the cravat's midpoint, and then wrap it vertically over the head and under the chin (Figure 197). Cross the cravat on the side of the head at ear level, and wrap the ends in opposite directions horizontally so that one side loops across the forehead. Tie the knot behind the ear.

Eye bandage. See page 170.

Bandages are changed for wound inspection and to avoid infection. If it's difficult to remove tape adhered to the skin, this may be accomplished by lifting up one edge and then swiping at the stuck adhesive margin with an alcohol wipe or cloth soaked in rubbing alcohol. Take care to keep the alcohol out of any open wound. An excellent way to avoid this situation is to tape bandage-to-bandage, if possible, by using rolled gauze to secure the bandage.

WOUND INFECTION

Despite your best efforts, a wound may become infected. The most common bacteria that cause wound infections are *Staphylococcus aureus* and *Streptococcus pyogenes*. Common signs of an

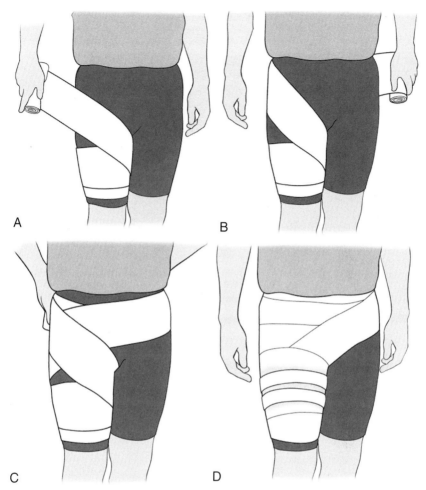

Figure 194. Creation of a thigh and groin bandage. **A,** Wrap a long 6-inch elastic bandage around the mid-thigh in an inner-to-outer direction working upward. **B,** At the groin crease, continue to wrap around the waist one time, then **(C)** wrap back down the thigh. **D,** Finish by wrapping around the thigh.

infection include redness and swelling surrounding the wound, pus or cloudy discharge (pink, green, or cream colored), foul odor (this is variable), fever, increased wound tenderness, red streaking that travels to the trunk from the wound, and swollen lymph nodes in the vicinity of the infection (see Figure 150).

If a wound is infected, its edges should be spread apart to allow the drainage of any pus. To do this, you need to remove some or all fastening bandages (such as butterfly bandages). The wound should then be irrigated copiously and dressed with a dry, absorbent, sterile bandage without bringing the wound edges tightly together. Begin to apply warm, moist compresses, using disinfected water, to the wound at least four times a day; also begin the victim on an antibiotic (dicloxacillin, cephalexin, or erythromycin). For a cat bite, use amoxicillin–clavulanate, cefuroxime axetil, azithromycin, clindamycin plus ciprofloxacin, or penicillin plus dicloxacillin. For a wound incurred in ocean, river, or lake water, administer ciprofloxacin or trimethoprim–sulfamethoxazole as an additional antibiotic.

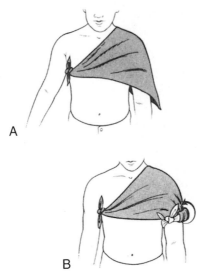

Figure 195. Shoulder bandage. **A,** Drape a triangular bandage over the shoulder. Begin to form a cravat and tie off in front of the opposite armpit. **B,** Complete the bandage.

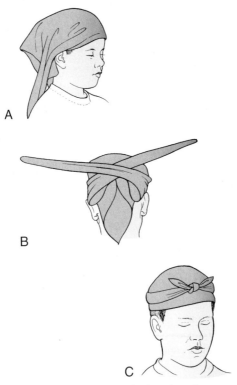

Figure 196. Head bandage. **A,** Drape a triangular bandage just over the eyes. **B,** Create a hem and cross behind the head, tying with a half knot in order to **(C)** fashion a square knot in the front. Tuck the tail that remains behind the head into the half knot.

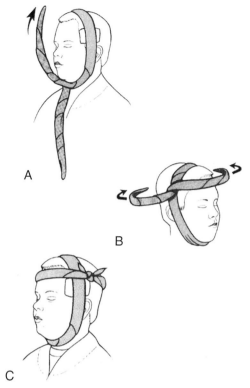

Figure 197. Securing a bandage to the side of the head. **A,** Lay a cravat over the wound. **B,** Cross the cravat and **(C)** tie it off behind the ear.

If a wound infection is advancing, the victim should be brought rapidly to a physician. If you see gas bubbles in a wound, if it's draining foul reddish-gray fluid, and/or if there is a feeling of "Rice Krispies" (crepitus) in the skin surrounding a wound, it may be the onset of necrotizing ("flesh-eating," leading to cell death) tissue infection, resulting in gangrene. This is a life-threatening infection and requires immediate surgical attention.

ABSCESS (BOIL)
See page 224.

SCALP LACERATION (CUT ON THE HEAD)
See page 63.

FISHHOOK REMOVAL
See page 446.

SPLINTER REMOVAL
See page 447.

BLISTERS
See page 228.

MUSCULOSKELETAL INJURIES

OVERUSE SYNDROMES

Whenever a muscle is overused—that is, exercised past its state of conditioning—there is actual destruction of the muscle tissue and generation of lactic acid. Given a reasonable rest period, the products of metabolism are carried away in the circulation and the muscle tissue regenerates to a healthy, sometimes even stronger, condition. However, if the exercise has been vigorous and unrelenting, the participant may suffer from a variety of aches and pains that are generally categorized as overuse syndromes.

Carpal Tunnel Syndrome

Carpal tunnel syndrome is caused by elevated pressure in the carpal tunnel, which is a space at the base of the wrist through which pass nine tendons that flex (bend toward the palm) the fingers, along with the median nerve. It can be caused for a number of reasons, which include forceful, repetitive use of the wrist. People with short, wide hands and square-shaped wrists may be at greater risk to develop this syndrome. The pressure causes the median nerve to have diminished function, which leads to the signs and symptoms. These include pain, numbness, tingling, and/or burning sensation on the palm side of the thumb, index finger, middle finger, and thumb side of the fourth finger. The "pinkie" side of the fourth finger and entire fifth finger are spared, as they are serviced by the ulnar nerve, which lies outside the carpal tunnel. Treatment is to avoid the offending activity and to splint the wrist in a "neutral" position of function (see page 69), both night and day if possible. An NSAID may be helpful. If the case is severe, a physician may prescribe oral steroids or inject steroids into the carpal tunnel. Medical evidence does not support the use of vitamin B_6. If carpal tunnel syndrome persists and the victim shows loss of nerve function or muscle wasting at the base of the thumb, surgery may be advised to decrease the pressure.

Cyclist's Palsy

If a cyclist leans on the handlebars for an extended period of time, he may compress the ulnar nerve as it passes through the wrist. Symptoms include numbness and tingling of the fifth finger and the outside half of the fourth finger. Treat with a wrist splint and administration of an NSAID. On rare occasion, steroid injection or surgical decompression of the nerve is necessary.

Saturday Night Palsy

This occurs if a person sleeps with his arm draped over the back of a chair or against a hard object, such as a log. The radial nerve is compressed as it wraps around the upper long bone (humerus) of the arm. Symptoms include diminished or no sensation on the top of the hand over the first and second fingers, as well as over the thumb. When the hand is held straight out, palm down, the hand drops down at the wrist into a limp position (Figure 198). Even though it may have only taken one night to affect the nerve, it may take a few weeks for recovery, so the wrist should be splinted in a position of function (see page 69). Add a sling if necessary to support the forearm and hand.

Rotator Cuff Tendinitis

The rotator cuff comprises four muscles: supraspinatus, infraspinatus, teres minor, and subscapularis. Each of these muscles is connected to the scapula, traverses over the shoulder, and

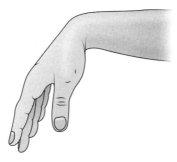

Figure 198. Position of the hand when suffering from "Saturday night palsy."

attaches to the upper arm bone. These muscles stabilize the shoulder and lift and rotate the arm. When they are stretched or strained, motion at the shoulder can be quite painful. Rest, avoiding painful motion, intermittent cool compresses or ice packs, and taking an NSAID are recommended for relief and recovery. If the pain persists, then there may be a rotator cuff tear that requires surgical repair.

Turf Toe

Turf toe refers to a condition in which the ligaments around the metatarsophalangeal joint (large joint) of the great toe are sprained by overuse. This is usually seen in athletes, but sometimes in long distance walkers, hikers, and climbers. Pain, swelling, and decreased joint movement at the base of the great toe are the most common symptoms, with occasional bruising and altered gait, leading to difficulty with ambulatory activities. Treatment includes diminishing or eliminating the offending activity and using rest, application of cold, and administration of nonsteroidal antiinflammatory medication. With proper therapy, it may take a few weeks to return to normal.

Muscle Fatigue

Simple fatigue, with depletion of energy stores within the muscle, is manifested as weakness, pain on exertion, soreness to the touch, and cramping. In many cases, this is compounded by dehydration, deficiencies of electrolytes (usually sodium and/or potassium), lack of sufficient caloric intake, or a specific injury. The sufferer has been informed by his body that it's time to rest. Sufficient time should be allowed to remove waste products, restore energy sources, correct dehydration, and regenerate muscle tissue. The victim should avoid vigorous physical activity for 12 to 24 hours and should eat and drink amply. For overuse syndromes, pharmaceutical muscle relaxants are of little value and pain medication is generally not necessary. Massage of the involved muscle groups is relaxing, although it probably does not hasten recovery.

Shin Splints

Shin splints is the term used to describe a painful disorder (medial tibial stress syndrome) generated by excessive walking, running, or hiking. The sufferer has irritated the thin membrane that connects the two lower leg bones along the longitudinal axes where the membrane attaches to the bones. With every footstep, there is further irritation of the membrane, so that it can become impossible to walk rapidly. Rest is the most important treatment. The victim should attempt to curtail running or vigorous walking activity, and may benefit from administration of aspirin or an NSAID. A shoe that is well cushioned (particularly its ball and heel) is very important for prevention and recovery. More complex orthotics may be required.

Taping may help. Find the area of maximal tenderness by pressing on the skin. Place a foam or thick cloth pad over that spot, and hold the pad in place by first using pre-wrap (preferably)

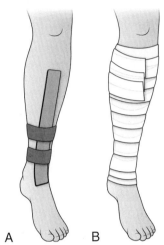

Figure 199. Taping for shin splints. **A,** Place a foam pad on the affected area. **B,** Cover the foam with pre-wrap and tape.

(Figure 199, *A*), then covering the pre-wrap with tape from the tops of the malleoli to the lower calf (see Figure 199, *B*).

Plantar Fasciitis

Plantar fasciitis is inflammation of the fascia (tough connective sheath tissue) that encloses the muscles and tendons that traverse the bottom of the foot. It is a syndrome of overuse, caused by excessive walking or running, particularly associated with repetitive impact on the bottom of a foot that's improperly cushioned or without appropriate arch support. There is pain in the bottom of the foot (ball, arch, and/or heel) that is worsened by repetitive weight bearing. The pain is often worse with the first steps in the morning or after a period of inactivity. It occurs commonly in athletes and long-distance hikers, particularly if they wear poorly fitting shoes or boots. When examining the foot, pain may be elicited by applying pressure to the forward-inside area of the heel. If heel pain was sudden in onset and included a tearing sensation, then the plantar fascia may have been torn. This is more serious and mandates rest.

Treatment consists of rest, elevation of the foot with cold (ice packs) applied to the tender areas at the end of the hiking day, wearing orthotics, gentle stretching (e.g., pulling back the toes and front part of the foot), and administration of an NSAID. Worn at night, a splint that holds the foot in neutral position—thus keeping the plantar fascia slightly stretched—may help, as may avoiding walking barefoot or in flat-soled shoes.

If the victim must continue to walk on the painful foot, it can be taped to provide arch support. This is accomplished as follows: Apply a thin layer of benzoin or spray tape adhesive onto the bottom of the foot. Fix an anchor strip of ¾ inch (1.9 cm) adhesive tape in a U shape around the heel from just under the malleoli (prominences of the ankle) up to just behind the level of the "knuckles" of the toes (Figure 200, *A*). Next, lay fairly tight cross-strips of ½ inch (1.3 cm) tape across the bottom of the foot, with the ends torn to lay on the anchor strip (see Figure 200, *B*). This creates a "sling" of tape under the foot for support. Finally, apply another U-shaped piece of tape around the heel that crosses under the center of the arch and locks down the crosspieces (see Figure 200, *C*).

Prevention of plantar fasciitis includes wearing properly fitted shoes and boots, performing Achilles tendon stretch exercises, avoiding harsh impacts to the bottoms of the feet, and maintaining proper body weight. It's too soon to tell if wearing minimalist footwear designed with

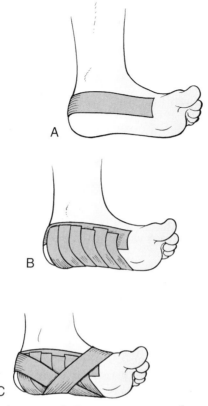

Figure 200. Taping for arch support. **A,** Fix an anchor strip under the heel. **B,** Attach strips across the bottom of the foot. **C,** Lock the crosspieces.

less, or even no cushioning will increase the incidence of plantar fasciitis or other foot conditions affected by different types of support. It has been observed that barefoot-style running encourages a forefoot, rather than a heel-strike, landing, which consumes additional energy. The extrapolation of this observation to the trekking condition remains to be determined.

Torn Muscle

A torn muscle ("pulled" muscle) is recognized as sudden pain in a muscle group associated with a particular vigorous exertion, such as sprinting or lifting a heavy object. Depending on the severity of the injury, there may be associated bruising, swelling, loss of mobility, and/or weakness. For instance, a small tear in the deltoid muscle of the shoulder may cause minor discomfort on lifting the arm over the head, while complete separation of the quadriceps group in the anterior thigh will cause inability to straighten the leg at the knee, extreme local pain, blue discoloration of the knee, and a defect in the shape of the muscles above the knee that's easily felt and seen.

In general, a minor muscle injury can be distinguished from a bone injury by evaluating active and passive range of motion. Active range of motion is the range of normal activity the victim can manage without rescuer assistance; this will be painful with both muscle and bone injuries. Passive motion is movement of a body part performed only with the aid of the rescuer; no effort is provided by the victim, who should attempt to relax the muscle completely. If there is no pain on passive (assisted) motion, but pain is present on active motion, the injury is most likely muscular, because an injured bone will hurt no matter how it is moved. If there is pain on passive motion, with or without pain on active motion, suspect a bone injury.

Minor muscle injuries should be treated in the first 24 hours with immobilization, application of cold (insulated ice packs or chemical cold packs; don't apply ice directly to the skin) for 30 to 45 minutes every 2 to 3 hours, and elevation. After 48 to 72 hours, application of heat (warm water or a heating pad, *not* ointments) and gentle movement should be started. If a significant injury is suspected (e.g., complete tear of the biceps muscle or quadriceps muscle group), the injury should be immobilized as for a fracture (see page 70) and the victim transported to a physician.

The best way to prevent a pulled muscle is to be flexible at baseline and to stretch and warm up adequately. This allows local blood flow to increase and minimizes the risk for small tears that can cause spasm, which in turn leads to decreased flexibility.

Sprains and Strains
Sprains and strains are injuries to ligaments (which attach one bone to another) and tendons (which attach muscle to bone) that are incurred by twisting, direct blunt trauma, or overexertion. Symptoms include pain, swelling and/or deformity, decreased range of motion secondary to pain, and bruising. The treatment is the same as for a suspected fracture. The injured part should be elevated, immobilized (see page 70), and treated with cold applications for the first 24 to 48 hours ("RICE": rest/rehabilitation, ice, compression, and elevation). After 72 hours, heat may be applied. It's important to prevent reinjury (ankles are notorious) by proper wrapping or application of a splint. Because the injured joint is immediately weakened, it should not be relied on for great exertion.

The most common sprain is of an ankle. It can be challenging to tell the difference between an ankle sprain and a broken ankle. The Ottawa Ankle Rules help physicians determine whether or not to obtain ankle x-rays and can also be useful to help decide to what degree a person is injured. It's more likely than not that a person may have suffered a broken ankle if there is:
1. Bony pain over the medial or lateral malleoli
2. Bone pain along the distal (toward the ankle) 6 cm of the posterior edge of the tibia ("shinbone"), which is the larger and stronger of the two bones in the leg below the knee (the other being the fibula) and connects the knee with the ankle bones
3. Pain at the tip of the medial malleolus
4. Bone tenderness along the distal 6 cm of the posterior edge of the fibula
5. Pain at the tip of the lateral malleolus
6. Inability to bear weight both immediately and for four walking steps

While taping or otherwise immobilizing an ankle sprain may not affect the long-term ankle function, it may allow a person to bear weight and walk sooner and with less assistance. If the injury is minor (no chance of a fracture) and/or if the victim needs to put weight on the ankle to seek help, the ankle may be wrapped snugly with an elastic wrap in a figure-of-eight method (Figure 201) or taped in a crisscross weave (Figure 202). Elastoplast bandaging is a good alternative to an elastic wrap.

Another method to tape an ankle is that favored by athletic trainers (Figure 203). The taping is focused on keeping the ankle from turning inward (inverting). This method uses anchor strips of tape on the lower leg and foot; then stirrups running from the inside of the ankle, underneath the foot, and then to the outside of the ankle; and a figure-of-eight technique.
1. Position the ankle at 90 degrees, and apply a ring of tape high above the ankle.
2. Apply three strips of tape as stirrups, with a slight fanning to achieve width.
3. Apply horizontal strips to cover the malleoli and the Achilles tendon.
4. Apply the first figure-of-eight strip of tape. Run the tape across the front of the ankle in the left-to-right direction.

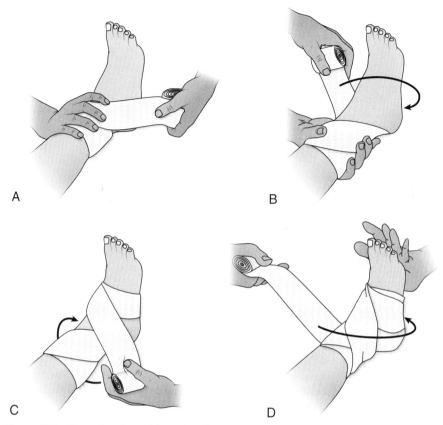

Figure 201. Wrapping the ankle with a figure-of-eight bandage. **A,** Start above the ankle and **(B)** wrap down under the foot. **C,** Cross back and forth over the top of the foot and **(D)** continue in a figure-of-eight pattern to secure the ankle.

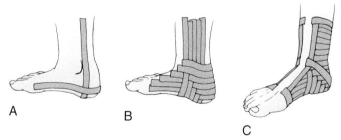

Figure 202. Taping a sprained ankle. **A,** Strips of adhesive tape are placed perpendicular to each other to **(B)** lock the ankle with a tight weave. **C,** The tape edges are covered to prevent peeling.

5. Continue to wrap the tape under the foot to the opposite side, and then cross back over the top of the foot.
6. Finish off the strip by wrapping around the leg and tear or cut the tape in front of the ankle.
7. Repeat the figure-of-eight process with a new strip, applying it this time in the right-to-left direction. Alternate directions once or twice more with new strips, then use

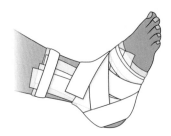

Figure 203. Ankle taping method favored by athletic trainers.

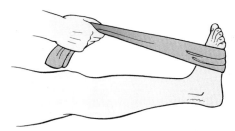

Figure 204. Pulling up on the toes to attain proper ankle position for wrapping.

circumferential tape wraps to fill in the gaps and finish off the entire process to the desired thickness and support.

During the wrapping or taping, have the victim point his toes and ankle upward by passing a slender rope or strap around the ball of the foot and pulling toward the body (Figure 204). This allows the ankle to be strapped with the foot perpendicular to the leg and the ankle ligaments in the shortened position in which they should heal. A splint can be fashioned from a SAM Splint (see Figures 303 to 305) to provide additional support. If the sprain is severe, splint the ankle as for a fracture. An Aircast Air-Stirrup or AirSport ankle brace is excellent for in-shoe support.

The Achilles tendon, which runs from the heel into the lower calf, may become irritated or inflamed due to recurrent impact or repetitive stretching, particularly if the heel is not well padded. An inflamed Achilles tendon that's painful should be protected against further irritation by limiting vigorous exercise and using a heel cup or extra padding underneath the heel to reduce stretch forces on the tendon. Achilles tendon rupture is usually caused by a sudden forceful impact on the foot that is "flexed," with toes pointed down, commonly during a jumping activity. There is pain and a sensation that something has torn or "popped." The victim has difficulty walking and pushing down with the forefoot. A simple test that can detect a complete Achilles tendon rupture is to have the victim lie face down with the leg bent at the knee. Squeeze his calf and see if the foot moves in such a way that the toes point downward. If there is no motion (in comparison to the uninjured side), the tendon may be ruptured. For treatment, splint the foot and ankle with the toes pointed slightly downward, and try to eliminate weight bearing. If they are available, insert heel lifts in both shoes.

Knee sprain is discussed on page 105.

ARTHRITIS

Arthritis is irritation and inflammation of a joint that can be caused by overuse, infection, or various diseases (such as gout, caused by deposition of uric acid crystals). Symptoms include pain in the joint with motion, swelling (fluid collection), redness, and warmth. If there is an infection within the joint, the condition can rapidly become serious. Generally, people with such infections have high fever, shaking chills, weakness, a recent infection elsewhere in the body, or recent direct injury (often penetrating through the skin) to the joint. Differentiating between an arthritic and an infected joint is often impossible until a physician inserts a needle to see if bacteria-laden fluid or pus is present within the joint, and to obtain fluid for a culture. If infection is a possibility, the victim immediately should be started on dicloxacillin, erythromycin, or cephalexin.

If there is little chance of infection and you know the joint problem is due to overuse, have the victim take aspirin or an NSAID. Rest the affected joint, keep it elevated if it is swollen, and adjust goals for the trip accordingly. If the victim is known to have gout and experiences an acute flare, he may be treated with an NSAID, with colchicine 1.2 mg followed by 0.6 mg in 1 hour, or with prednisone 30 to 60 mg by mouth per day for 2 days, with a tapering dose over a 10-day period. Corticosteroids are interchangeable to a certain degree. If you must substitute, here is a rough measure of equivalence: 20 mg prednisone equals 16 mg methylprednisolone equals 3 mg dexamethasone.

Glucosamine and chondroitin are dietary supplements taken by some persons who suffer arthritis, particularly osteoarthritis, or overuse syndromes. These are natural substances reputed to repair and maintain cartilage by suppressing inflammation and stimulating cartilage growth, strength, and resilience. The evidence for benefits is more on the "not effective" than "effective" side, so that most testimonials are anecdotal. These supplements are generally considered to be safe, but can carry side effects of headache, drowsiness, abdominal pain, constipation, diarrhea, heartburn, nausea, skin rash, insulin resistance, and (rarely) allergic reaction.

BURSITIS

Bursitis is irritation and inflammation of the lubricating sac (bursa) that allows muscles to move freely around a joint. Common areas of irritation include the shoulder (irritated by arm swinging), the sac in front of the kneecap (irritated by prolonged kneeling), on the outside of the hip (irritated by walking, hiking, or falling), and behind the elbow (irritated by a fall) (Figure 205). Evaluation and treatment are the same as for arthritis.

VENOUS THROMBOSIS AND THROMBOPHLEBITIS

Thrombophlebitis is inflammation in a vein associated with the development of a blood clot (known as venous thrombosis: "DVT" means deep venous thrombosis). This occurs in conditions of injury to the veins (cuts, bruises) or after periods of prolonged rest in a single position (sitting on a plane, cramped in a cave). Other factors include genetic predisposition, pregnancy, tobacco use, cancer, and varicose veins. A blood clot irritates the lining of the vein and causes local redness or purplish discoloration, swelling, warmth, and pain. If the clot enlarges, an entire limb length can become affected. These clots are most common in the lower leg, so the calf muscle may be tender to compression or there may be pain in the calf when the foot is flexed upward (toes toward the head). If the clot is in a deep vein, it may break off and travel to the lungs, where it causes a serious condition known as pulmonary embolism (see page 44).

It's easy to confuse the presentation of thrombophlebitis with that of an infection. If you suspect the former, have the victim elevate the limb and apply hot packs or soaks for 60 minutes every 3 hours. Seek immediate medical attention. If you're more than 24 hours from help and not absolutely certain whether you are treating infection or inflammation, administer an antibiotic (dicloxacillin, erythromycin, or cephalexin).

To avoid venous thrombosis, avoid prolonged periods of inactivity; get up and walk around once an hour when traveling on a plane, bus, or train; remain fit, active, and well hydrated; consider support hose if you have varicose veins or a history of blood clot formation in your legs or pelvis; and don't use tobacco products.

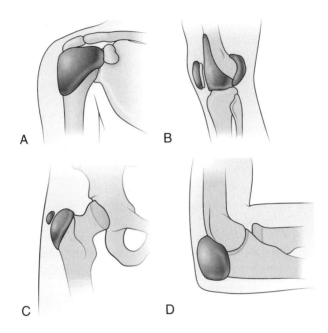

Figure 205. Bursitis affects the lubricating sacs (bursae) near the **(A)** shoulder, **(B)** knee, **(C)** hip, and **(D)** elbow.

BACK PAIN

Back pain is a common medical complaint. It may be caused by an anatomic abnormality (e.g., scoliosis), or acute or chronic injury of muscle, bone, intervertebral disk, or other anatomic structure. It may be indicative of a kidney infection (see page 273) or aortic dilation/rupture (see page 124).

The most common back injury is muscle strain. Symptoms include muscle pain and spasm adjacent to the vertebrae. If these occur in the lumbar (lower back) region, treatment consists of maximum rest while lying supine on a firm supporting surface. The knees may be drawn up to straddle a pillow or rolled blanket. All possible lifting and forward bending should be discontinued. The victim should take aspirin or an NSAID to control pain and inflammation, and additional pain medicine as necessary. Gentle massage and alternating applications of ice packs and heat are sometimes soothing. Corsets and lower back braces aren't particularly helpful. For severe muscle spasm, a physician may prescribe a skeletal muscle relaxant, such as metaxalone (Skelaxin) 800 mg by mouth three to four times per day.

After the pain is gone, which may take a few days to a week or more, consider beginning stretching exercises, particularly for the hamstrings, and strengthening the abdominal muscles. These activities may help reduce back problems in the future. Other useful exercises include lying flat while doing ankle pump repetitions, single-leg (alternating) knee-to-chest raises (while relaxing the back and neck), and partial sit-ups. Under the guidance of a physical therapist, you may be instructed to do toe raises and back-against-the-wall partial squats, as well as back arches ("cat humps") or prone press-ups to a forearm rest position.

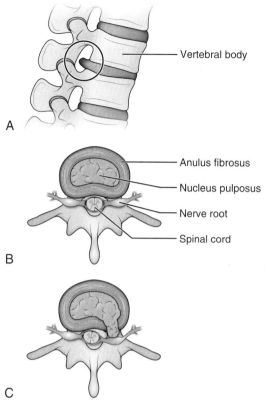

A

Vertebral body

Anulus fibrosus

Nucleus pulposus

Nerve root

Spinal cord

B

C

Figure 206. Herniated (slipped) disk. **A,** Posterior protrusion of the disk into the spinal (cord) canal. **B,** Cross section of the normal disk. **C,** Protruding disk impinges on the nerve root.

For any treatment regimen intended to improve back pain, if it worsens the back pain, then stop. While you're on the mend, avoid forward-bending toe-touches, straight-leg or full sit-ups, leg lifts ("squats"), or any exercise that involves heavy lifting and straining.

If one of the cushioning intervertebral (between the vertebrae) disks has been injured (Figure 206), additional symptoms may be noted. These include numbness and/or tingling of parts of the leg (indicating impingement of the disk on a nerve root arising from the spinal cord), shooting pains through the buttocks and posterior leg (indicating irritation of the sciatic nerve [sciatica]), leg weakness, foot drop, constipation, or difficulty with urination. The acute treatment is the same as for muscular back strain. If there is weakness or altered sensation in the leg or foot, bowel or bladder dysfunction, or numbness in the perineum and/or buttocks, seek immediate medical attention.

Lumbar spinal stenosis is a condition in which there is narrowing of the spinal canal in such a fashion that the spinal cord or nerve roots originating from the spinal cord and exiting the spinal canal are compressed. The most common symptom is discomfort that radiates from the back into the buttocks, thigh(s), and lower leg(s), made worse by walking, prolonged standing, and arching (extending) the back, and lessened by rest and bending (flexing) forward. Sitting usually provides relief, whereas walking and hiking worsen the pain. Exercises in which the person leans forward, such as cycling, may be better tolerated. Treatment is with an NSAID. More severe cases require injection of anesthetic into the space immediately outside the spinal cord, or surgery to widen the bony space(s) through which pass the affected nerve root(s).

If a person with back pain develops a fever, then infection should be suspected. This may involve a bone, soft tissue (such as an abscess adjacent to the spinal cord), or kidney. Fever with severe or unrelenting back pain is a reason to seek medical attention.

Backpacks are the quintessential symbol of trekking and mountaineering. A well-fitted, sturdy and durable backpack gives the user the freedom of the hills. Along with hiking boots, a backpack is essential for any sort of expedition in which someone is responsible for carrying his or her supplies. What is less well known is that a poorly fitted backpack can contribute to significant back pain, inefficient travel, or even the ruin of a trip. A backpack that weighs on its carrier can cause muscle spasm, sore neck and shoulders, numbness and tingling in the hands and fingers, sore hips, and irritated skin.

Features in a backpack that will allow it to fit properly, distribute weight evenly and across the correct body parts, and withstand extremes of environment are, in no particular order:
1. Proper size. It fits the torso closely, in particular the upper part of the body. When the padded waist strap is tightened, the weight of the pack should be distributed evenly across the hips.
2. The shoulder straps should be wide and well padded, to avoid compressing the front of the shoulders and armpits. They should be easily loosened and tightened. There should be a connecting strap that can be opened, closed, and adjusted traversing the front of the chest attached to and between the shoulder straps.
3. Adjustable straps to fine-tune the tightness of the waist strap and the proximity of the pack to the back of the wearer are desirable.
4. Multiple compartments allow rational storage, ease of finding carried items, and more even weight distribution than possible with a single-compartment pack. Side pockets, top pockets, tie-down loops, an adjustable top cover, and other features to partition objects into discrete locations while protecting them from the elements are all good to have.
5. The pack should be designed so that it can be donned from a sitting or standing position, using the legs for stabilization. If it can be put on only by hoisting it and slinging it across the back, muscle strain is inevitable.
6. For a child-carrier pack, be certain that it is designed so that an active child can't easily self-extricate from the pack and wind up dangling or on the ground.

Outdoor enthusiasts have a unique set of activities that may cause back pain. Advice for them to avoid this condition includes:
1. Learn how to lift heavy objects using the deep knee bend, positioning the weight properly on the torso, minimizing rotation or twisting when lifting, and lifting with a controlled, measured pace.
2. Be particularly careful with overhead lifts, which require more strength and balance.
3. If multiple persons are involved in a lift, perfect communications are important to coordinate movements.
4. If a heavy object is falling, don't attempt to catch it or slow its fall.
5. Use mechanical hoist systems when feasible.
6. If minor back pain is present, avoid any heavy lifting.

DISORDERS OF THE KIDNEYS, BLADDER, AND PROSTATE

BLADDER INFECTION

Bladder infection (cystitis, sometimes called urinary tract infection [UTI]) occurs frequently in females, because the shorter female urethra does not protect the bladder from bacteria as efficiently as does the male organ. A person with a bladder infection complains of discomfort (sharp pain, cramping, or burning) on urination, urge to urinate ("urgency"), frequent urination, difficulty initiating urination, lower abdominal cramping, and sometimes bloody urine, which may be as severe as small clots. Similar symptoms may be suffered by males who harbor infections in the prostate gland.

Treatment involves administration of an antibiotic and increased oral fluid intake. Because many antibiotics are well concentrated in the urine, there are a number of acceptable treatment regimens. For the sake of simplicity, the female victim may be treated (in order of preference) with nitrofurantoin monohydrate/macrocrystals (Macrobid) 100 mg capsule twice a day for 5 days (safe in pregnancy) with meals; trimethoprim–sulfamethoxazole (Bactrim or Septra) in one double-strength tablet twice a day for 3 days, or two double-strength tablets in one dose; fosfomycin trometamol (Monurol) 3 g sachet single dose; ciprofloxacin 250 mg twice a day for 3 days, or 500 mg in one dose; levofloxacin 250 or 500 mg once a day for 3 days; ofloxacin 200 mg twice a day for 3 days, or 400 mg in one dose; norfloxacin 400 mg twice a day for 3 days; lomefloxacin 400 mg; trovafloxacin 100 mg; cefpodoxime 100 mg twice a day for 7 days; or amoxicillin–clavulanate 500 mg/125 mg twice a day for 7 days. If the victim is diabetic or older than 65 years of age, or if the symptoms don't completely resolve or they recur within a few days of therapy, use the same or a different drug for 7 to 10 days. If the victim is pregnant, use nitrofurantoin, amoxicillin, ampicillin, cephalexin, cefadroxil, or trimethoprim–sulfamethoxazole. However, don't use trimethoprim in the first trimester.

Chlamydia are bacterium-like "germs" that are increasingly the cause of reproductive tract infections in women and genitourinary tract infections in men. Because the penicillins (such as ampicillin) aren't effective against *Chlamydia,* any male with a bladder infection should be treated with tetracycline (500 mg four times a day), doxycycline (100 mg twice a day), or trimethoprim–sulfamethoxazole (one double-strength tablet twice a day) for 10 days, or with azithromycin 1 g in a single dose. Any male who develops a bladder or prostate infection (see page 275) should be seen by a physician when he returns from his journey.

Some persons believe that the incidence of bladder infections in women may be decreased by a daily 8 oz (237 mL) glass of cranberry juice, or by ingesting cranberry juice capsules or tablets. This has never been scientifically proved.

It may not be convenient for a woman to squat in order to urinate outdoors. There are devices available to facilitate a woman's urinating while standing or squatting. The Whiz Freedom is advertised as a hydrophobic (repels water), antibacterial, and ecofriendly urine director. This device fits over the pudendal region so that urination can be accomplished when standing or sitting outdoors (or indoors) in such a manner that the urine stream is captured and directed away from the body. Another product intended for the same purpose is the "Lady J."

KIDNEY INFECTION

Kidney infection (pyelonephritis) is considerably more serious than bladder infection. Symptoms may include all of those for bladder infection, as well as flank or lower back pain, severe abdominal pain, fever, chills, nausea and vomiting, weakness, and cloudy urine with or without a foul odor. The pain is characterized as aching and may become pronounced if you punch the victim gently just under the ribs adjacent to the spine on the affected side.

The field treatment is to administer an antibiotic. Begin the victim on ciprofloxacin (500 mg twice a day or 1 g [extended release] once a day for 7 days), levofloxacin (750 mg once a day for 5 days), trimethoprim–sulfamethoxazole (one double-strength tablet twice a day for 14 days), or any of the following for 10 days: norfloxacin (400 mg twice a day), ofloxacin (200 to 300 mg twice a day), lomefloxacin (400 mg once a day), moxifloxacin (400 mg once a day), amoxicillin–clavulanate (875/125 mg twice a day), or cefadroxil (500 mg twice a day). The victim may require hospitalization for an intravenous antibiotic(s). Therefore, anyone who is suspected to have a kidney infection should be evacuated immediately.

KIDNEY STONE

See page 128.

BLOOD IN THE URINE

Blood in the urine is caused by bladder or kidney infection, overuse of NSAIDs, the passage of a stone(s), blunt or penetrating injury to the flank (kidney region), bleeding disorder, or tumor of the genitourinary tract. After heavy exertion or high fever, a person may break down muscle tissue and release myoglobin (an oxygen-carrying protein found in muscle) into the bloodstream. In cases of burns, severe injury, or certain infections, red blood cells can be destroyed and will release their oxygen-containing protein (hemoglobin) into the bloodstream. Hemoglobin and myoglobin are filtered through the kidneys and may be concentrated in the urine, giving it a pink to reddish-brown hue. If the urine is not made dilute (by drinking large amounts of fluid to increase its volume), the concentration of these pigments in the kidney can clog the filtration system and cause sudden kidney failure. Although after vigorous exercise some individuals may normally pass a small amount of reddish urine, anyone who develops darkened urine after fever or exertion should be placed at maximum rest, cooled to a normal body temperature (see page 296), encouraged to drink as much fluid as possible, and rapidly transported to a medical facility. If you are more than 24 hours away from a doctor, the urine rapidly clears with rest and increased fluids, and the victim appears in good health, the journey may continue.

Urine can also be discolored by ingestion of certain chemical agents, such as urinary tract anesthetics (blue-green or orange), beets (pink-red), or bile pigments (brown, seen with hepatitis).

ACUTE URINARY RETENTION

There are occasions when a person cannot urinate and the bladder becomes distended with urine. This is seen more often in males than females, because a common cause is obstruction of the urethra where it passes through the male prostate gland. If the gland is enlarged (benign prostatic hypertrophy [BPH]), which occurs in elderly males almost exclusively, the passageway for urine can be narrowed to the point where it becomes obstructed. Early symptoms, which develop as the passage narrows, are difficulty initiating a stream, a weak stream, dribbling (leakage of urine), and urinating small amounts. On occasion, it may become painful to urinate. If the obstruction becomes complete, it causes urine to collect in the bladder, which becomes painfully distended and can be felt as a hard mass in the lower abdomen. Unless the obstruction can be relieved, this is an emergency. The usual treatment is to pass a small tube (catheter) through the penis directly into the bladder. This can be difficult and should be attempted only by someone trained in the technique. It's a good idea for someone properly trained to carry a urinary catheter(s) and lubricant on any expedition that will include elderly males as participants.

If a male has an enlarged prostate, drugs that are anticholinergic (such as certain antispasmodics) or that contain atropine and its derivatives can precipitate acute urinary retention. For instance, an elderly male with BPH on a diving expedition who takes anti–motion-sickness medication may suffer urinary retention as a side effect of the medication. A medication that relieves the symptoms of BPH in some men is tamsulosin (Flomax 0.4 mg capsule once daily), which relaxes the prostate muscles around the urethra, allowing urine to flow more freely out of the bladder. This medication can create its own side effects of dizziness and low blood pressure on arising, similar to what is seen with dehydration. Therefore, it's important for people using this medication to stay well hydrated and avoid situations in which a dizzy spell or fainting might create a serious injury.

PROSTATE INFECTION

Bacterial infection of the prostate gland (prostatitis) is usually abrupt in onset, with fever, urgency and frequency of urination, pain on urination that may radiate to the lower back, chills, weakness, and sometimes difficulty urinating leading to urinary retention. While there may be a sensation of burning on urination, there is usually scant or no discharge from the urethra. "Bicycle seat prostatitis," from prolonged pounding on the prostate caused by lengthy cycling, is not uncommon. Until the diagnosis is confirmed, the victim should begin to take an oral anti-biotic such as ciprofloxacin, levofloxacin, trimethoprim–sulfamethoxazole, or amoxicillin-clavulanate. On a prolonged journey, if an antibiotic appears to be effective within a few days, it should be continued for a minimum of 3 weeks. If prostatitis is suspected and an antibiotic started, add ibuprofen to the treatment plan for the first few days. In a young, sexually active male, suspect gonorrhea or chlamydial infection (see page 273).

MALE GENITAL PROBLEMS

PAINFUL TESTICLE

If a male complains of a painful testicle, examine both testicles. Look for discoloration or swell-ing. If a testicle has been injured by a blow, provide support with an improvised jockstrap and apply ice packs. If a testicle suddenly becomes painful, particularly in an adolescent, and appears swollen and/or discolored, usually without a penile discharge, it may be twisted, or "torsed." If a painful testicle appears to be resting in a higher position than the other testicle, particularly if it appears swollen and/or has a horizontal orientation, suspect testicular torsion. Since this usually happens if the testicle rotates inward (toward the midline) (Figure 207), gently see if you can rotate it outward (looking from above, like opening a book) within the scrotum. If this causes a dramatic relief of pain, you may have saved the testicle. If the testicle rotates easily but the severe pain is not reduced, be prepared to continue the outward rotation, because the testicle may have torsed itself by rotating completely, up to twice around. If the maneuver increases the pain and appears to shorten the "hang" of the testicle, you may be worsening the torsion and might attempt rotating the testicle in the opposite direction.

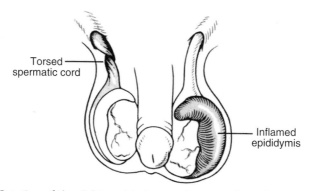

Figure 207. Rotation of the right testicle in a torsion; an inflamed epididymis of the left testicle.

If you believe an unresolved torsion is present, this is an emergency and the victim should be rushed to a physician. If a torsion is not resolved within the first 4 to 6 hours, the testicle may be lost. The pain is usually followed by swelling in the scrotum and groin region. Sometimes the affected testicle is seen to be slightly higher than the uninvolved testicle. The pain may be of a severity to cause the victim to become nauseated or vomit, and to feel faint.

If a testicle is swollen and the victim complains of pain or burning on urination, he may suffer from infection or inflammation of the epididymis, which is part of the sperm-collection pathway (see Figure 207). Other symptoms include lower abdominal, flank, or groin pain. If the case is severe, the victim may suffer fever, chills, nausea, and muscle aches. This should be treated with doxycycline (100 mg twice a day), tetracycline (500 mg four times a day), ciprofloxacin (500 mg twice a day), levofloxacin (250 mg daily), norfloxacin (400 mg twice a day), or trimethoprim–sulfamethoxazole (one double-strength tablet twice a day) for 10 days. Another diagnosis to consider, particularly in an adolescent male, is a sexually transmitted disease (see Penile Discharge, below). If epididymitis is diagnosed, the victim will require decreased activity or bed rest for a few days, and scrotal support using an athletic garment.

One way to help distinguish epididymitis from testicular torsion is to gently elevate the scrotum—in general, with epididymitis the pain is diminished, whereas with torsion it is commonly increased, although this is not absolute.

PENILE DISCHARGE

If a male complains of a discharge from his penis, particularly if it follows sexual intercourse by a few days and is yellow or greenish in color, you must suspect gonorrhea. It's generally safest to treat the victim for both gonorrhea and a chlamydial infection, because people frequently carry both infections simultaneously. In a doctor's hands, a sufferer of gonorrhea will be treated with an intramuscular injection of ceftriaxone 250 mg *plus* either a single oral dose of either azithromycin 1 g or oral doxycycline 100 mg twice a day for 7 days (to treat *Chlamydia*). Away from professional medical care, if more than 24 hours will pass before a doctor can be reached, to treat the gonorrhea, administer cefixime 400 mg orally as a single dose. Alternative single-dose therapies for gonorrhea are cefpodoxime 200 mg, cefuroxime 1 g, ciprofloxacin 500 mg, ofloxacin 400 mg, azithromycin 2 g, or norfloxacin 800 mg. To attempt to treat gonorrhea and chlamydial infection with one medication at the same time, you can use the single-dose 2 g azithromycin therapy. Syphilis may also have been transmitted, so the victim should be tested on return to civilization, even if the victim was treated with a 2 g dose of azithromycin, since there is occasionally resistance of the causative spirochete *(Treponema pallidum)* to this drug.

If there has been no sexual intercourse and a penile discharge develops, particularly if it's white or clear, treat with doxycycline or azithromycin.

In this day and age, no person should engage in casual unprotected sexual intercourse. A man should wear a latex (not lambskin) condom that has been stored in a cool, dry place. If he or his partner is allergic to latex, then a nonlatex synthetic condom should be used. The package should show no evidence of leakage. The spermicide nonoxynol-9 (condom lubricant or vaginal foam) offers additional protection against viruses.

INFECTION OF THE FORESKIN (BALANITIS)

An uncircumcised male may develop an infection of the foreskin, which usually appears as redness of the head (glans) of the penis and of the underside of the foreskin, sometimes with excessive moisture, small bumps, and whitish discharge (likely yeast). To treat this condition, wash the penis twice each day and apply a topical antifungal cream, such as clotrimazole after each washing. If the situation does not resolve within a week, then administer metronidazole 500 mg by mouth twice a day for 7 days.

PSYCHIATRIC EMERGENCIES

The wilderness experience can be quite stressful, or a member of the party may behave in an unusual fashion. This may be directly related to the events at hand or reflect an underlying psychiatric disorder. It's imperative that someone recognize warning signs early and evacuate anyone who cannot retain mental stability, to avoid placing the impaired individual and his traveling companions at risk for injury. Don't be afraid to inquire about a past history of psychiatric illness.

ANXIETY

Anxiety is the most common psychiatric symptom and may range from appropriate and adaptive minor doubts about success to a full-blown panic reaction. Minor anxiety is expressed as general apprehension about a situation that is perceived in some way to be dangerous. The excessive worrier may become timid and withdrawn, and may lose his enthusiasm for participation. His anxiety may be clothed in criticism of plans or refusal to cooperate. Some people suffer from general, free-floating anxiety. It's important that every member of the expedition voice fears and objections at the outset, so as not to be caught in a panic when crossing treacherous terrain or performing rescues.

The treatment is reassurance and support. Frequently, practice sessions that build up to a completed effort will relieve anxiety and improve the performance of the group. In no case should anyone be made to feel ashamed of his fears. Rather, the leader should seek to help the victim conquer them.

Approach what problems you can directly. Most people do much better if fear is identified and managed than if it is never confronted.

In certain circumstances, in which anxiety must be conquered to allow extrication, rescue, or even survival, judicious use of an antianxiety drug, such as lorazepam (Ativan) 0.2 to 2 mg, alprazolam (Xanax) 0.5 mg, or diazepam (Valium) 2 to 5 mg, may be useful.

PANIC

Panic is anxiety in the extreme. Signs and symptoms may include heart palpitations, sensation of pounding heart, rapid heart rate, sweating, trembling or shaking, shortness of breath or a sensation of "smothering," choking sensation, chest discomfort, nausea, dizziness, fainting, a sensation of loss of reality, and fear of dying. The victim loses all judgment and becomes consumed with efforts at escape and self-preservation. Panic renders the victim unable to make reasonable decisions and immediately places him and all around him at risk for injury. The rescuer must assume a strong authoritative posture with the panic victim, assuring him in no uncertain terms that the situation is under control and the panic behavior is detrimental. Depending on the situation, this can be done with verbal explanations, convincing arguments, or demonstrations of safety. As for anxiety, antianxiety drugs such as diazepam, lorazepam, or alprazolam may be helpful. If the victim places other individuals at immediate risk for injury, he should be subdued, with force if necessary.

Persons who use cocaine, marijuana, phencyclidine (PCP, angel dust), methamphetamine (speed), or hallucinogens are prone to panic reactions under conditions of stress. The management of these reactions is little different from that previously outlined; the exception is the risk of violent behavior from anyone under the influence of cocaine, methamphetamine, or PCP. If a person appears to be under the influence of psychotropic drugs, do your best to keep him from hurting anyone, but be careful not to become injured yourself in the process.

HYPERVENTILATION

One manifestation of anxiety that verges on panic is the hyperventilation syndrome, in which the victim, overcome by his fears, begins to breathe at a rate of 40 to 100 times per minute. This causes the level of carbon dioxide in his blood to fall precipitously and to render the blood alkaline (from its normal neutral state). The symptoms are dizziness; fainting spells; numbness and tingling in the hands, feet, and around the mouth; muscle spasm in the hands and wrists; and, occasionally, seizures. If you're certain that the victim is hyperventilating because of anxiety (that is, there is no reason to suspect a collapsed lung [see page 39], pneumonia [see page 45], asthma [see page 42], diabetic ketoacidosis [see page 135], or other medical problem), encourage slow regular breathing. The old-fashioned therapy used to be to place a paper bag or similar device over the mouth and nose for about 5 minutes and have the victim breathe in and out of this bag to rebreathe his own expired carbon dioxide, theoretically allowing more rapid normalization of the level in the bloodstream and correction of symptoms. However, since insufficient oxygen is available to the victim while rebreathing from the bag, this technique may be dangerous for persons with heart or lung disease. If there is a clean length of wide tubing (e.g., garden hose) of approximately 12 to 18 inches, the victim can breathe through the tubing to increase the amount of retained carbon dioxide while still having access to adequate oxygen, until symptoms abate. However, since this tubing is not likely to be present, the most important intervention will probably be to attempt to calm the victim in order to lessen the breathing rate. After the episode, make an attempt to identify the cause of the anxiety.

DEPRESSION

Depression occurs in the outdoor setting in response to situations that are perceived as hopeless. Some victims who are injured, lose their way, or are weakened by starvation and exposure may lose the will to continue. They become listless, fatigued out of proportion to their physical condition, uninterested, inattentive, without appetite, sleepy, and tearful. Clearly, the rescuer must encourage all party members to maintain their survival instincts, continue to help others, and help themselves. In a cold environment, remember that hypothermia (see page 281) is a significant cause of apathy and should be corrected if possible. An individual with chronic depression may go on a vacation trip with the enthusiastic expectation that his psychiatric disease will be alleviated or that his most recent depression has lifted. The sudden realization that such expectations are not fulfilled may put that person at risk for severe mood depression. Don't be afraid to inquire about a past history of psychiatric illness. It's encouraging to note that in certain circumstances, self-esteem may be improved by successfully participating in outdoor activities, such as mountaineering.

PSYCHOSIS

Psychosis (which includes schizophrenia) is a change in behavior in which the victim loses touch with reality and may suffer from any combination of auditory or visual hallucinations; paranoid (extremely fearful) behavior; extreme agitation (including combative behavior) or, conversely, profound lack of activity (catatonia); disorganized thoughts and speech; and inability to care for self (inattention to the activities of daily living, such as eating, bathing, sleeping, etc.). This can be due to a medical problem, drug effect, or psychiatric disorder. A person with psychosis should be evacuated promptly, while protecting the person from harming himself or others. Always consider low blood sugar (see page 133), meningitis (see page 162), hyperthermia (see page 296), and hypothermia (see page 281) in any person with altered mental status. It's possible that a person with psychosis may benefit a bit from a dose of diazepam (Valium), but this may not be effective.

REACTION TO AN INJURY OR ILLNESS

People's reactions to stress differ. They may become irrational, angry, apathetic, confused, or withdrawn following an accident or harsh environmental exposure. The most common reaction, given the presence of a strong leader, is to become dependent. It's crucial for the rescuer to bolster the victim's self-confidence and self-esteem at every opportunity, for it may take extraordinary physical and mental effort to survive a catastrophe in the wilderness.

Try to individualize your approach to each person. To best understand the changing needs of victims and families, try to maintain regular dialog intended solely for the purpose of psychological support. Stay with the victim as much as possible. Use frequent touch and reassurances to relay your sense of concern and offer comfort. As best as possible, involve the victim in his treatment and rescue, so that his thoughts are attuned to survival rather than to fear or grief.

When you're under stress, do your best to be supportive to others with less emotional control. Anger is rarely successful and commonly worsens an already difficult situation.

Equally important, the rescuer must constantly be alert for true medical problems that masquerade as psychological disorders. The uninterested victim may be hypothermic, the belligerent climber hyperthermic, the intoxicated hiker hypoglycemic, or the irritable child stricken with acute mountain sickness.

POSTTRAUMATIC STRESS DISORDER

Posttraumatic stress disorder (PTSD) is a condition of anxiety in which the victim who has been exposed to an extreme stress or event, to which he may have reacted with fear and helplessness, reacts in a manner that includes reliving the event, avoiding reminders of the event, and/or showing a condition of hyperarousal. Reliving the event can include nightmares or flashbacks. Symptoms of avoidance include eliminating any locations, persons, or situations that serve as reminders or showing loss of memory for the event. Hyperarousal means difficulty sleeping, being irritable or short-tempered, having difficulty concentrating, or being exceptionally fearful. Furthermore, a person suffering from PTSD may be having difficulty with activities of daily living, be apathetic, and become fatalistic.

This condition is different from the less complicated responses of fear, grief, anxiety, panic, and even depression. In a wilderness setting, it's more likely to follow a natural disaster with many casualties than one in which there were a small number of victims. Personal pain and violence contribute to the propensity for PTSD, as perhaps do extreme environmental exposures. Certain parts of the brain, including the hypothalamus, hippocampus and amygdala, are felt to be involved with PTSD.

Treatment includes habituation that allows confrontation with and understanding of fears, creating an environment of education and support, and stress reduction, including the techniques of prolonged exposure and cognitive therapy. In some situations, antidepressant and antianxiety medications have been recommended, but whether or not they are useful is controversial.

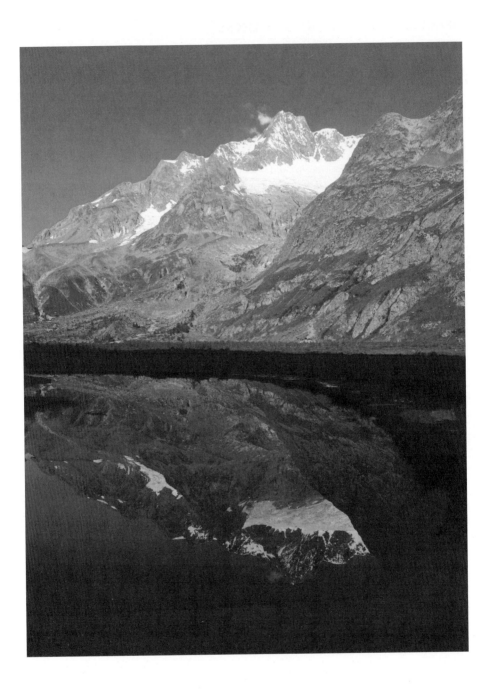

PART FOUR

Disorders Related to Specific Environments

INJURIES AND ILLNESSES DUE TO COLD

HYPOTHERMIA (LOWERED BODY TEMPERATURE)

The body generates heat through metabolic processes that can be maximized with involuntary shivering to roughly 5 times the basal level (up to 10 times with maximum exercise). However, shivering is abolished after a few hours of exposure, because of exhaustion and depletion of muscle energy supplies. When a victim loses the ability to shiver, the cooling process becomes quite rapid. Skin, surface fat, and superficial muscle layers then act as an insulating "shell" for the core of vital organs (heart, lungs, liver, kidneys, and so on). People are tropical beings—that is, when they are naked and at rest, the environmental temperature at which body heat is neither gained nor lost is 82°F (28°C). Normal oral temperature is 98.6°F (37°C). Normal skin temperature in cool weather is 90°F to 93°F (32.2°C to 33.9°C); this can drop to 70°F to 73°F (21.1°C to 22.8°C) before core cooling begins. Accidental hypothermia occurs when there is an unintentional decrease of 3.6°F (2°C) from the normal core (measured rectally) body temperature of 98.6°F to 99.9°F (37°C to 37.7°C). Mild hypothermia is considered to occur when the core temperature is between normal and 91.4°F (33°C); moderate hypothermia is core body temperature below 91.4°F (33°C) down to 85.2°F (29°C); severe hypothermia is core body temperature below 85.2°F (29°C) down to 71.6°F (22°C); and profound hypothermia is below 71.6°F (22°C).

Heat is lost from the body to the environment by direct contact (conduction), air movement (convection), infrared energy emission (radiation), conversion of liquid (sweat) to a gas (evaporation), and exhalation of heated air from the lungs (respiration). It's important to note that the rate of heat loss via conduction is increased 5-fold in wet clothes and at least 25-fold in cold-water immersion. Windchill (Figure 208) refers to the increase in the rate of heat loss (convection) that would occur when a victim is exposed to moving air. This chill can be compounded further if the victim is wet (conduction, convection, and evaporation).

At a core body temperature of 96.8°F (36°C), metabolic rate, blood pressure, and preshivering muscle tone increase. At 95°F (35°C), the body reaches its maximum effectiveness at generating heat by shivering.

Immersion hypothermia refers to the particular case in which a victim has become hypothermic because of sudden immersion into cold water. Again, water has a thermal conductivity approximately 25 times greater than that of air, and a person immersed in cold water rapidly transfers heat from his skin into the water. The actual rate of core temperature drop in a human is determined in part by these phenomena and in part by how quickly heat is transferred from the core to the skin, skin thickness, the presence or absence of clothing, the initial core temperature, gender, fitness, water temperature, drug effects, nutritional status, and behavior in the water.

A sudden plunge into cold water causes the victim to hyperventilate (see page 278), which may lead to confusion, muscle spasm, and loss of consciousness. Cold water rapidly cools

WIND SPEED   TEMPERATURE (°F)

Calm	40	35	30	25	20	15	10	5	0	−5	−10	−15	−20	−25	−30	−35	−40	−45
5 mph	36	31	25	19	13	7	1	−5	−11	−16	−22	−28	−34	−40	−46	−52	−57	−63
10 mph	34	27	21	15	9	3	−4	−10	−16	−22	−28	−35	−41	−47	−53	−59	−66	−72
15 mph	32	25	19	13	6	0	−7	−13	−19	−26	−32	−39	−45	−51	−58	−64	−71	−77
20 mph	30	24	17	11	4	−2	−9	−15	−22	−29	−35	−42	−48	−55	−61	−68	−74	−81
25 mph	29	23	16	9	3	−4	−11	−17	−24	−31	−37	−44	−51	−58	−64	−71	−78	−84
30 mph	28	22	15	8	1	−5	−12	−19	−26	−33	−39	−46	−53	−60	−67	−73	−80	−87
35 mph	28	21	14	7	0	−7	−14	−21	−27	−34	−41	−48	−55	−62	−69	−76	−82	−89
40 mph	27	20	13	6	−1	−8	−15	−22	−29	−36	−43	−50	−57	−64	−71	−78	−84	−91
45 mph	26	19	12	5	−2	−9	−16	−23	−30	−37	−44	−51	−58	−65	−72	−79	−86	−93
50 mph	26	19	12	4	−3	−10	−17	−24	−31	−38	−45	−52	−60	−67	−74	−81	−88	−95
55 mph	25	18	11	4	−3	−11	−18	−25	−32	−39	−46	−54	−61	−68	−75	−82	−89	−97
60 mph	25	17	10	3	−4	−11	−19	−26	−33	−40	−48	−55	−62	−69	−76	−84	−91	−98

Figure 208. Windchill determination. To determine windchill, find the ambient air temperature on the top line, then read down the column to the line that corresponds with the current wind speed. Example: When the air temperature is 10° F and the wind speed is 20 mph, the rate of heat loss is equivalent to −9° F under calm conditions. To convert to metric or Celsius, use the following: 1 mile = 1.61 kilometers; C = 5/9 (F − 32).

muscles, and the victim loses his ability to swim or tread water. Muscles and nerves may become ineffective within 10 minutes. Over the ensuing hour, shivering occurs and then ceases. Anyone pulled from cold water should be presumed to be hypothermic.

The progression of hypothermia leads to predictable physiologic responses, which roughly correspond to different body temperatures. Although not invariable, the signs and symptoms are as follows:

91.4-98.6° F (33-37° C). Mild hypothermia. Sensation of cold; shivering; increased heart rate; urge to urinate; slight incoordination in hand movements; increased respiratory rate; increased reflexes (leg jerk when the knee is tapped); red face; muscular incoordination, stumbling gait, maladaptive behavior, rapid heart rate converting to slow heart rate, apathy.

85.2-91.4° F (29-33° C). Moderate hypothermia. Stupor; decreased or absent shivering; weakness; apathy, drowsiness, and/or confusion; poor judgment; slurred speech; inability to walk or follow commands; paradoxical undressing (inappropriate behavior); complaints of loss of vision; amnesia; rapid heart rate converting to slow heart rate; rapid breathing rate converting to shallow breathing; loss of shivering; possible nonreactive or dilated pupils, abnormal heart rhythms, diminished breathing.

71.6-85.2° F (22-29° C). Severe hypothermia. Minimal breathing; coma; decreased respiratory rate; decreased neurologic reflexes progressing to no reflexes; no voluntary motion or response to pain; very slow heart rate, low blood pressure; maximum risk for ventricular fibrillation. The victim no longer can control his body temperature and rapidly cools to the surrounding environmental temperature.

Below 71.6° F (22° C). Profound hypothermia. Rigid muscles; barely detectable or absent blood pressure, heart rate, and respirations; dilated pupils; risk for ventricular fibrillation; appearance of death.

The first principle of therapy is to suspect hypothermia. Any person who is found in a cold environment should be suspected of suffering from hypothermia. The definition of "cold environment" is variable. Someone who is wet, improperly dressed, and intoxicated with alcohol can become hypothermic in 70° F (21° C) weather. Don't use yourself as an indicator of warmth—you may be perfectly comfortable while your companion is lapsing into hypothermia.

Unless the victim is found frozen in a block of ice or has been recently pulled from frigid waters, the most likely clue to a hypothermic state is altered mental status. The winter hiker who gradually loses interest and lags behind the group ("Just leave me behind. I'll catch up."), who dresses inappropriately for the weather or begins to undress, or who begins to stumble and make inappropriate remarks should be immediately evaluated for low body temperature. A hypothermic individual may become anxious, repeat himself, or even become delusional. *Never leave a victim of even mild hypothermia to fend for himself.*

The second principle of therapy is to measure the victim's temperature. This should be done, if possible, with a thermometer calibrated to read below 94° F (34.4° C), which is the cutoff for most standard oral thermometers. Hypothermia thermometers with a range of 75° F to 105° F (23.9° C to 40.5° C) are available. Temperature ideally should be measured rectally, although this is often impractical. Oral and axillary (armpit) temperatures are unreliable in this situation and should be used only to screen for low body temperature. That is, if they are normal, the victim will have at least a normal body temperature, but could be hotter. However, if they are low, they may grossly understate how cold the victim really is and should be followed with a rectal measurement. Digital electronic eardrum scanners used to measure temperature may also yield a false (compared to the core) reading.

Unless the victim has suffered a full cardiopulmonary arrest, the hypothermia itself may not be harmful. Unless tissue is actually frozen, cold is in many ways protective to the brain and heart. However, if a hypothermic victim is improperly transported or rewarmed, the process may precipitate ventricular fibrillation, in which the heart does not contract, but quivers in such a fashion as to be unable to pump blood. *The burden of rescue is to transport and rewarm the victim in a way that does not precipitate ventricular fibrillation.*

The following general rules of therapy apply to all cases:

1. Handle all victims gently. Rough handling can cause the heart to fibrillate (cause a cardiac arrest). Secure the scene and avoid creating additional victims via unstable snow, ice, or rock fall.

2. If necessary, protect the airway (see page 22) and cervical spine (see page 35). Stabilize all other major injuries, such as broken bones. Cover open wounds.

3. Prevent the victim from becoming any colder. Provide shelter. Remove all his wet clothing and replace it with dry clothing. Don't give away all of your clothing, however, or *you* may become hypothermic. Replace wet clothing with sleeping bags, insulated pads, bubble wrap, blankets, or even newspaper. Products from Blizzard (www.blizzardsurvival.com) or GrabberWorld (www.grabberworld.com) can be used to provide protection from the elements. These include familiar items such as the SPACE Brand Emergency Blanket. If a hypothermia prevention and management kit (containing a ready-heat blanket and heat-reflective shell, is available, use it. An excellent (but much more expensive) product is a Hypothermic Stabilizer Bag. An improvised insulation wrap can be prepared (Figure 209).

Cover the victim's head and neck. This is very important. Insulate the victim from above *and below* with blankets. Don't change blankets unless necessary to keep the victim dry. If possible, put him in a sleeping bag sandwiched between two warm rescuers. Another technique is to use skin-to-skin contact by having a warm human rescuer lie inside a sleeping bag with the victim. But remember that in this situation, no heat is really contributed by the bag itself. Don't count on a sleeping bag to be adequately prewarmed by a normothermic rescuer's body heat. Another method is to blow warm air from an electric hair dryer into the bag with the victim. Hot water in bottles, *well insulated with clothing to*

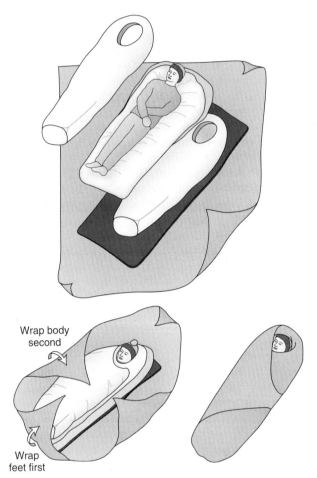

Figure 209. Improved insulation wrap.

prevent skin burns, may be placed next to the victim in areas of high heat transfer, such as the neck, chest wall, and groin. A great deal of warmth may be conserved by using a thin liner bag inside a normal sleeping bag. Don't apply commercial heat packs, hot-water-filled canteens, or hot rocks directly to the skin; they must be wrapped in blankets or towels to avoid serious burns.

4. Don't attempt to warm the victim by vigorous exercise, rubbing the arms and legs, or immersing in warm water. This is "rough handling" and can cause the heart to fibrillate if the victim is severely hypothermic. If warm water (no hotter than 104° F [40° C]) is available and can be kept warm, the victim's hands and feet can be immersed.

5. Seek assistance as soon as possible.

Mild Hypothermia

The victim of mild hypothermia is awake, can answer questions intelligently, and complains of feeling cold. He may or may not be shivering.

Prevent the victim from becoming any colder. Get him out of the wind and into a shelter. If necessary, build a fire or ignite a stove for added warmth. Gently remove wet items of clothing and replace them with dry garments. This is very important, even if the victim will be very briefly exposed out in the open. If no dry replacements are available, the clothed victim should be covered with a waterproof tarp or poncho to prevent evaporative heat loss. Cover the head, neck, hands, and feet. Insulate the victim above and below with blankets. If the victim is coherent and can swallow without difficulty, encourage ingestion of warm sweetened fluids. Good choices include warm gelatin (Jell-O), juice, or cocoa, because carbohydrates fuel shivering. If only cool or cold liquids are available for drinking, this is fine. Avoid heavily caffeinated beverages. If a dry sleeping bag is available, one or more rescuers should climb in with the victim and share body heat. However, this technique may not be very effective, and great care must be taken not to cause the victim to become wet (e.g., from the rescuer's sweat). Try to keep the victim in a horizontal position until he is well hydrated. Don't vigorously massage the arms and legs, because skin rubbing suppresses shivering, dilates the skin, and does not contribute to rewarming.

Moderate Hypothermia

The victim of moderate hypothermia has become apathetic and mildly confused, wishes to be left behind, and is uncooperative. Speech is often slurred, and logic is on the wane. The victim rapidly becomes uncoordinated and clumsy, often stumbling. He has ceased to shiver, and shows signs of muscle stiffness. Unless you have a thermometer to measure this victim's temperature, you must assume that he is severely hypothermic or will soon become so. Follow the directions for mild hypothermia, with the added caution that it's best not to allow this victim to walk about until he is fully alert; in addition, don't give him fluids to drink until he becomes wide awake and understands what is going on. When the victim can drink fluids, these should be sweetened with sugar to avoid the complication of low blood sugar (hypoglycemia).

Severe and Profound Hypothermia

Depending on the body temperature, a victim who appears to be asleep may be in a complete coma. Below 86°F (30°C), humans become poikilothermic, like a snake, and take on the temperature of the environment.

Examine the victim carefully and gently for signs of life. Listen closely near the nose and mouth and examine chest movement for spontaneous breathing. If the victim's breathing is very shallow, you may not see a vapor trail. Feel for at least 1 minute at the groin (femoral artery) and neck (carotid artery) for a weak and/or slow pulse (see page 30).

If the victim shows any signs of life (movement, pulse, respirations), don't initiate the chest compressions of cardiopulmonary resuscitation (CPR). If the victim is breathing regularly, even at a subnormal rate, his heart is beating. Because hypothermia is protective, the victim does not require a "normal" heart rate, respiratory rate, and blood pressure. Pumping on the chest unnecessarily is "rough handling," and may induce ventricular fibrillation. Administer supplemental oxygen (see page 405) by face mask if it is available.

If the victim is breathing at a rate of less than 6 to 7 breaths per minute, you should begin mouth-to-mouth breathing (see page 28) to achieve an overall rate of 12 to 13 breaths per minute.

If help is on the way (within 2 hours) and there are no signs of life whatsoever, or if you're in doubt (about whether the victim is hypothermic, for instance), you should begin standard CPR (see page 30). If possible, continue CPR until the victim reaches the hospital. Rescue breathing should take priority over chest compressions, particularly in the victim of cold-water immersion. There have been documented cases of "miraculous" recoveries from complete cardiopulmonary arrest associated with environmental hypothermia after prolonged resuscitation, presumably because of the protective effect of the cold. Remember, "no one is dead until he is warm and dead." In the absence of an obvious fatal injury (such as decapitation), resuscitation and transport to a hospital should be undertaken. Fixed and dilated pupils, failure to identify a pulse or breathing, skin mottling of any sort, and stiff muscles all may be mistaken for the condition of death in the setting of hypothermia. Hypothermic victims with the appearance of death have been resurrected in the hospital, after they have been rewarmed.

A victim of severe hypothermia cannot be rewarmed in the field. If a hypothermic victim suffers what you determine to be a cardiac arrest in the wilderness, transport should be the first priority. If enough rescuers are present to allow CPR and simultaneous transport, do both. If you are the only person present, don't bother with CPR, because you will not be able to resuscitate the victim until he is rewarmed. Your only hope is that the victim is in a cold-protected state ("metabolic icebox") and that you can extricate him (as gently as possible) to sophisticated medical attention.

In any case of severe hypothermia, transport should be undertaken as soon as possible. Take care to cover the victim with dry blankets and to handle him as gently as possible.

Preparing a Hypothermic Victim for Transport

1. Keep the victim dry. Replace all wet clothing. If there is no replacement clothing available, wring out the wet clothing, including gloves and mittens, and then put it back on the victim. Lay the victim on a sleeping bag and then cover him with a layer of blankets. If necessary, use bubble wrap or some other insulating material. If the hands are extremely cold, pull them out of the sleeves of clothing in order to put the hands in the victim's armpits for warming. See the earlier discussion about emergency waterproof blankets and bags. Cover everything with a plastic sheet.
2. Keep the victim horizontal. Don't allow massage of the extremities. Don't allow the victim to exert himself. Rapid rewarming or restoration of circulation will release cold, acid-laden blood from the limbs back to the core organs, which may cause a profound deterioration of the victim.
3. Splint and bandage all injuries as appropriate. Cover all open wounds.
4. Limit rewarming to methods that prevent further heat loss. Place insulated (e.g., with clothing) hot-water bottles in the victim's armpits and groin. Take care to not burn the skin. Keep his head and neck covered.

A Special Note About the Victim of Cold-Water Drowning

If a victim is pulled from icy waters and appears to be clinically dead (fixed dilated pupils, no respirations, no detectable pulse), perform CPR until a qualified medical person is available to intervene or you become exhausted. Because of the physiology of cold-water immersion, the victim may be sufficiently protected to survive the event.

Prevention of Hypothermia

1. Carry adequate food and thermal wear, such as Thermax, Capilene, and/or polypropylene ("polypro") or wool undergarments. Anticipate the worst possible weather conditions. Dress in layers so that you can adjust clothing for overcooling, overheating, perspiration, and external moisture. Use a foundation layer to wick moisture from the body to outer layers. The first layer (such as CoolMax) should keep the skin cool and dry (to avoid perspiration). Add an insulation layer to provide incremental warmth. For shirts, use wool, fleece, Capilene, or polypropylene. Consider a turtleneck or neck gaiter. For pants, wear wool or pile, with a Velcro, zipper, or button fly. Carry windproof and waterproof outer garments, mittens or gloves (with glove liners), socks, and a hat. In very cold weather, up to 70% of generated heat may be lost by radiation from the uncovered head. Boots should be large enough to accommodate a pair of polypropylene socks ("liner socks") plus at least one pair of heavy wool socks without cramping the toes.
2. Stay dry. Avoid sweating.

3. Keep hands and feet dry. This is important to avoid frostbite as well. Hand Sense is a cream that can be applied to the hands to keep them dry by reducing perspiration. It was designed as a topical protectant, and is not a moisturizer. For the feet, aluminum chlorohydrate–containing antiperspirant sprayed onto the skin can help control sweating. Do this three times a week for the first week of winter, then once a week after that. Avoid leather boots that become soaked with moisture and don't dry out easily.
4. Don't exhaust yourself in cold weather. Don't sit down in the snow or on the ice without insulation beneath you.
5. Seek shelter in times of extreme cold and high winds. Don't sit on cold rocks or metal. Insulate yourself from the ground with a pad, backpack, log, or tree limb. Carry a properly rated (for the cold) sleeping bag stuffed with PolarGuard, Quallofil, or down. Consider using a bag in which the down has been treated to achieve water repellency. Insulate hands and feet well, even when you are in your sleeping bag, which should be fluffed up before entry. Don't enter a sleeping bag if you're wet without drying off first if possible.
6. Don't become dehydrated. In the cold, dehydration is caused by evaporation from the respiratory tree, increased urination, and inadequate fluid intake. Drink at least 3 to 4 quarts (liters) of fluid daily. During extreme exercise, drink at least 5 to 6 quarts (liters) per day. Ingesting snow is an inefficient way to replace water, because it worsens hypothermia. Drink cold water from a stream in preference to eating snow. Don't skip meals. Don't consume alcoholic beverages. They cause an initial sensation of warmth because of dilation of superficial skin blood vessels, but this same effect contributes markedly to heat loss. At night, fill a canteen or Nalgene water container with at least 1 quart (liter) of water, and sleep with it to keep it from freezing.
7. Consume adequate calories.

WHAT TO DO IF YOU FALL THROUGH THE ICE

In terms of survival, the "1-10-1 Principle" states that when a person is plunged into very cold water (32°F or 0°C), he or she has 1 minute to control breathing (e.g., to stop hyperventilating from the "gasp reflex"), 10 minutes of purposeful movement before the muscles are numb and not responsive, 1 hour before hypothermia leads to unconsciousness, and 2 hours until profound hypothermia causes death.

1. When a person falls into extremely cold water, he begins to gasp and hyperventilate. Control your breathing. Calm down and slow your breathing rate, so that you are not hyperventilating. This generally takes 30 seconds to 2 minutes.
2. Keep clothing on in the water—it contributes to insulation and helps with flotation.
3. Keep your hands and arms on top of the ice and kick your feet vigorously, to bring your body to a horizontal position and propel you up onto the ice. Otherwise, keep swimming at a minimum. If you are able to slide your body out of the water onto the ice, don't stand up. Roll or slide your body away from the opening onto thicker ice, where you may then stand. Try to leave in the direction from which you first approached, as this ice has already proved that it can withstand your weight.
4. If you cannot exit the water, try to hold your arms on top of the ice, so that they freeze to the ice, which will prevent you from submerging under the surface of the water. This may give you an extra hour of survival time.

HOW TO ASSIST SOMEONE WHO HAS FALLEN THROUGH THE ICE

If someone has fallen through the ice, it is an urgent and dangerous situation. Although it's important to rescue the victim, it is equally important to not create additional victims.

1. Recognize that ice conditions are unsafe. No one else should approach the area.

2. Resist the urge to rush up to help the victim, so that you don't also fall through the ice. Encourage the victim to remain calm and not panic. Direct the victim to an area of strong ice and to attempt a self-rescue, as described above.

3. If self-rescue is not accomplished, you can throw a buoyant object to the victim to help him remain floating. Before it is thrown, tie a rope or cord to the object, so that if the victim can hold onto it, you might be able to pull the victim. If only a rope is available, tie a large loop at the end, which the victim can grab. Instruct the victim to put the loop over his body and under his arms, put one arm through the loop and bend his elbow around the rope, or just hold on.

4. The victim might be reached with a long tree branch, ladder, or other object that can be pushed along the surface of the ice. It's important for the rescuer to not get too close to the hole in the ice.

5. If the victim cannot be removed from the water using the techniques above, he should be instructed to hold the arms up on the ice for the purpose of letting them freeze to the ice while help is summoned.

6. To avoid falling through ice in the first place, you should look for signage that might indicate its safety or unsafety; check with local authorities if they have any information; travel across ice under observation of someone else; bring safety equipment; wear a life jacket or other flotation device; avoid traveling on ice at night; select "blue ice" over white ice or gray ice; and avoid ice with cracks or slushy areas.

WINTER STORM PREPAREDNESS

Outdoor, and indeed urban, travelers should always plan for the unusual and unexpected. Tools include familiarity with weather forecasts, strategizing worst-case scenarios, carrying emergency items, avoiding solo travel, and leaving notice of the projected route and expected time of return. With good planning, deteriorating weather or a forced unexpected night outdoors might then become more of an inconvenience than a life-threatening ordeal. While we usually consider a life-or-death situation related to the elements to be associated with a remote expedition or natural disaster, it can happen during a routine drive along the highway on the way to a ski destination.

Winter storm preparedness is essential for anyone who drives a motor vehicle in snow country. One must always be aware of the possibility of spending an unplanned night out in a vehicle. Causes include bad weather, breakdown, having an accident, running out of fuel, becoming lost, and getting stuck. Winter driving is especially hazardous because of the dangers of driving on snow or ice, losing visibility and orientation, fewer people on the road from whom to receive assistance, and the threats of frostbite and hypothermia. Accepting the possibility of trouble, carrying a vehicle survival kit (see later), and giving some thought to survival strategies will help prevent a night out in your car from deteriorating into a life-threatening experience.

Most travelers dress to arrive at a destination and not to survive a night out; in other words, they dress "to arrive, not to survive." A vehicle survival kit (listed later) should include extra clothing, blankets or sleeping bags, food, water, signaling equipment, and communications equipment (cell phone, citizen's band radio, etc.). It's also always better to stay with the vehicle, which provides significant protection and is more visible to rescuers than a person on foot. Most laypersons are not experienced trail-blazing in wilderness environments, particularly when landmarks are obscured by rain or snow, and darkness and cold weather conspire to alter orientation and judgment.

In cold weather, and especially for long-distance travel, drivers should keep their vehicles in the best possible mechanical condition. Drivers should use winter-grade oil, the proper amount of radiator antifreeze, deicer fluid for the fuel tank, and antifreezing solution in the windshield-cleaning fluid. Windshield wiper blades that are becoming worn should be replaced, and special snow-and-ice–resistant blades used when available. A combination snow brush and ice scraper should be carried. A can of deicer is useful for frozen door locks and wiper blades. Snow tires, preferably studded (illegal in some states), are desirable, but even with special tires and/or four-wheel drive, chains should be carried. All-wheel drive or four-wheel drive is optimal, and front-wheel drive is superior to rear-wheel drive. The battery should be kept charged, the exhaust system free of leaks, and the gas tank full ("drive on the upper half of your tank").

Despite best efforts, you may become stranded or lost. If that happens, tie a brightly colored piece of cloth (such as a length of surveyor's tape) to the antenna. At night, leave the inside dome light illuminated so that it may be seen by snowplow drivers and rescuers. Headlights use too much current, so use the dome light. If necessary for heat, the standard recommendation has been that the motor and heater can be run for 2 minutes each hour (after checking to see if that exhaust pipe is free of snow). However, a more recent recommendation is that since it takes more gasoline to start a cold engine than a warm one, one should initially turn the heat up all the way and run the car engine until the inside is comfortable. Then, shut off the engine and wait until it becomes uncomfortably cold inside the car (which could be 10 to 30 minutes depending on outside temperature). The engine, however, will still be "warm." Start the engine again and run the heater until the occupants feel warm. Keep repeating this process.

Keep the tailpipe free from snow pack. Carbon monoxide poisoning can be a threat, so don't go to sleep inside the car with the engine running; if the engine is running, keep a downwind window cracked 1 to 2 inches in case there is a carbon monoxide leak into the interior of the vehicle. A reusable carbon monoxide detector is a wise addition to the survival kit. One or two large candles ("fat Christmas candle" size) should be carried to provide heat and light if the gasoline supply runs out, since two lit candles can raise the interior temperature well above freezing. However, resources should be used sparingly because you're never sure how long you will be stranded.

Foresight enough to include heavy clothing and blankets or sleeping bags in the cold-weather vehicle survival kit is better than relying excessively on external heat generation. Don't smoke tobacco products or drink alcohol. If you have to exit the vehicle in a snowstorm, put on additional windproof clothing and snow goggles, and tie a lifeline to yourself and the door handle before moving away from the vehicle.

You must decide whether to wait for rescue or attempt to walk out under your own power. If rescue is possible, it's almost always better to remain in a snug shelter and conserve your strength. If you decide to leave, you must effectively mark your trail, to aid rescuers and enable you to return to the site if necessary. Travel should never be attempted in severe or extremely cold weather, or in deep snow without snowshoes or skis. If no chance of rescue exists, prepare as best as possible, wait for good weather, and then travel in the most logical direction.

The best way for a lost or stranded person to aid potential rescuers is to do everything possible to draw attention to his or her location. Most modern rescues utilize ground parties, helicopters, and fixed-wing aircraft. Besides radios, cell phones, and other electronic equipment, signaling devices are either auditory or visual. Three of anything is a universal distress signal: three whistle blasts, three horn blasts, three fires. The most effective auditory device is a whistle. Blowing a whistle is less tiring than shouting, and the distinctive sound can be heard farther than a human voice. An effective visual ground-to-air signal device is a glass signal mirror with a sighting device, which can be seen up to 10 miles away but requires sunlight. Special rescue beacons are available and can be carried as emergency equipment. These include strobe lights, laser signal lights, special beacons with both signaling and GPS capability, and personal locator beacons (PLBs).

Smoke is easily seen by day and a fire or flashlight by night. On a cloudy day, black smoke is more visible than white; the reverse is true on a sunny day. White smoke stands out well against a green forest background but not against snow. Black smoke can be produced by burning parts of a vehicle, such as rubber or oil, and white smoke by adding green vegetation to a fire. The lost person who anticipates an air search should keep a fire going with large supplies of dry, burnable material (wood and brush) and have a large pile of cut green vegetation close by. When an aircraft is heard, the dry materials are placed on the fire and allowed to flare, and then armloads of the green vegetation are piled on top. This produces lots of smoke and a hot thermal updraft to carry it aloft.

A vehicle cold weather survival kit should include the following items:

1. Sleeping bag or two blankets for each occupant
2. Extra winter clothing, including gloves, boots, and snow goggles, for each occupant
3. Emergency food
4. Metal cup
5. Waterproof matches
6. Long-burning candles, at least two
7. First-aid kit
8. Spare doses of personal medications
9. Swiss army knife or Leatherman-type multitool
10. Three 3 lb empty coffee cans with lids, for melting snow or sanitary purposes
11. Toilet paper
12. Cell phone and/or citizen's band radio, with chargers
13. Portable radio receiver, with spare batteries
14. Flashlight with extra batteries and bulb
15. Battery booster cables and/or car battery recharging unit (plugs into cigarette lighter)
16. Extra quart of automobile oil (place some in hubcap and burn for emergency smoke signal)
17. Tire chains
18. Jack and spare tire
19. Road flares
20. Snow shovel
21. Windshield scraper and brush
22. Tow strap or chain
23. Small sack of sand or cat litter
24. Two plastic gallon drinking water jugs, full
25. Tool kit
26. Gas line deicer
27. Flagging, such as surveyor's tape (tie to top of radio antenna for signal)
28. Duct tape
29. Notebook and pencil/marker
30. Long rope (e.g., clothesline) to act as safety rope if you leave the car during a blizzard
31. Carbon monoxide detector
32. Axe
33. Saw
34. Full tank of gas

SAFE SLEDDING

In terms of injuries, sledding leads the list for winter sports activities. This includes a large number of head injuries. To avoid sledding mishaps:

1. Select a safe hill:
   a. Not too steep
   b. Long, flat run-out at the bottom to allow a safe stop

   c. Does not end near a roadway, parking lot, fence, stream, lake, or drop-off

   d. Free from obstacles, including trees, dips, bumps, rocks, and stumps

   e. Little or no ice

2. Sled in conditions of good visibility (daytime, no fog, excellent lighting at night).
3. Dress for the cold. Dress for protection. Don't wear any dangling clothing that can get caught up in the sled.
4. Wear a helmet (e.g., ski helmet).
5. Use a well-constructed sled for which you can control the direction and speed. Understand that your risk for an accident is greater when tubing, sitting on a sheet of cardboard, or flying down the hill on a plastic saucer or toboggan that cannot be steered.
6. Sit on the sled face-forward toward the bottom of the hill. Don't sled while standing or facing backward. Never sled head-first.
7. An adult should accompany a small child on the sled.
8. Don't pile more than one person on a sled, except for an adult with a small child.
9. Keep arms and legs inside the border of the sled.
10. Avoid sudden sharp turns.
11. Don't attempt to go over a jump.
12. If you lose control of the sled, roll off it and get out of the way.
13. Don't ride a sled pulled by a motor vehicle.
14. Don't sled under the influence of alcohol or mind-altering drugs.
15. Don't sled across a frozen body of water unless it is known to absolutely be safe.

FROSTBITE

Frostbite is an injury caused by the actual freezing of tissues. Factors that predispose a person to frostbite include poor circulation (caused by previous cold injuries, tobacco use, alcohol ingestion, diseases of the blood vessels, constricting garments, poorly fitting boots, old age), fatigue, and extremes of cold exposure. Windchill contributes markedly to frostbite risk. For instance, at an air temperature of 15°F (−9.4°C), a 55 mph (88 km/hr) wind causes the same rate of heat loss as a 5 mph (8 km/hr) breeze at an air temperature of 0°F (−17.8°C). Furthermore, since a human in motion creates his own wind (while riding a snowmobile, for example), the risk for frostbite for such a person increases. Humidity and wetness also increase the propensity for frostbite.

During exposure, once the temperature of a hand or foot drops to 59°F (15°C), the blood vessels maximally constrict and minimal blood flow occurs. As the limb temperature declines to 50°F (10°C), there may be brief periods of blood vessel dilation, alternated with constriction, as the body attempts to provide some protection from the cold. This is known as the "hunting response" and is seen more commonly in the Inuit (Eskimos) and persons of Nordic descent. Below 50°F (10°C), the skin becomes numb and injury may go unnoticed until it's too late. Tissue at the body surface freezes at or below a temperature of 24.8°F (−4°C) because of the effect of underlying warm tissue. Once circulation is abolished, the skin temperature may drop at a rate in excess of 1°F (0.56°C) per minute. Once tissue freezes, it cools rapidly to attain the temperature of the environment.

The major immediate symptom of a frostbite injury is numbness, occasionally preceded by itching and prickly pain. The frostbitten area will appear to be white, with a yellow or bluish (grayish) waxy (sometimes mottled) tint. If the injury is superficial, as commonly occurs on the face, the skin is firm and may indent with a touch, because the underlying tissue is still soft and pliable. If the injury is deep, the skin may feel hard and actually be frozen solid. A hand or foot may feel clumsy or absent. The areas most commonly affected are the fingertips and toes (particularly in cramped footwear), followed by the earlobes, nose tip, cheeks, and other exposed skin. These parts have little heat-generating capability and no significant insulation. Male joggers have had their genitals frostbitten.

In general, persons should not walk on frostbitten feet unless this is necessary to save one's life. Rapid rewarming is the standard therapy. However, *don't thaw out a frostbitten body part if it cannot be kept thawed.* In other words, if you come upon a lost hiker 10 miles (16 km) back in the woods who has frostbitten toes, don't use your stove to heat water to thaw out his feet if he will then have to put his wet boots back on and hike out—refreezing his toes in the process. Frostbitten tissue is severely damaged and is prone to reinjury; refreezing causes an injury that will far exceed the initial frostbite wound. It's much better to walk out on frostbitten toes until safety is reached than to thaw and allow refreezing. Thus, if a victim needs to be transported to another site for rewarming, don't allow "slow" or partial rewarming, particularly if there is a chance that the tissue will be allowed to refreeze. Pad the affected body part, apply a protective splint, and hustle the victim to the site where the definitive thaw will take place. Don't allow tobacco or alcohol use. Don't rub frozen tissue with snow or ice, or massage the tissue.

Once the victim has reached a location (shelter) where refreezing will not occur, remove all constrictive jewelry and wet clothing. Replace wet clothes with dry garments. Immerse the frostbitten part in water heated to 104°F to 108°F (40°C to 42.2°C). Some authorities advise using water heated to 98.6°F to 102°F (37°C to 39°C), which decreases pain associated with rewarming while just slightly reducing rewarming time. Don't induce a burn injury by using hotter water. You can estimate 108°F (42.2°C) water by considering it to be water in which normal skin can be submerged for a prolonged period with minimal discomfort. Heated tap water may be too hot. Never use a numb frostbitten finger or toe to test water temperature. It's best to use your own hand or the victim's uninjured hand to test the temperature. Circulate the water to allow thawing to proceed as rapidly as possible. When adding more hot water, take the body part out, add the water, test the temperature, and then reimmerse the part. It's best to use a container in which the body part can be immersed without touching the sides; for instance, a 20-quart (20-liter) pot will accommodate a foot. If the skin is frozen to mittens or metal, use heated water to remove them. *Never rewarm the tissues by vigorous rubbing or by using the heat of a campfire, hand warmers, meals ready-to-eat (MRE) heaters, camp stove, or car exhaust,* because you have a high likelihood of damaging the tissues.

If the victim is hypothermic, attend first to the hypothermia. Thawing should not be undertaken until the core body temperature has reached 95°F (35°C) (see page 281).

Thawing of the tissues usually requires 30 to 45 minutes. It is complete when the skin is soft and pliable, and color (usually quite red; rarely, bluish) and sensation have returned. Allowing the limb to move in the circulating water is fine, but massage may be harmful. Moderate to extreme burning pain may occur during the last 5 to 10 minutes of rewarming, particularly if the frostbitten tissue was numb before rewarming.

Thawed frostbite may be present in a number of stages, much like a burn injury. These are recognized as follows:

First degree: Numbness, redness, and swelling; no tissue loss.

Second degree: Superficial blistering, with clear (yellowish) or milky fluid in the blisters, surrounded by redness and swelling. There is little, if any, tissue loss.

Third degree: Deep blistering, with purple blood-containing fluid in the blisters. There is usually tissue loss.

Fourth degree: Extremely deep involvement (including bone); induces mummification. There is always tissue loss.

Sensation may remain until blisters appear at 6 to 24 hours after rapid rewarming. These often don't extend to the ends of fingers and toes (Figure 210). Leave these blisters intact. After thawing the skin, protect it with fluffy, sterile bandages (aloe vera lotion, gel, or cream should be applied, if available). Pad gently between the digits with sterile cotton or wool pads, held in

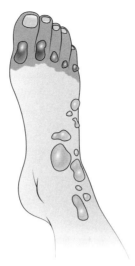

Figure 210. Blisters of frostbite may not extend to the ends of fingers and toes.

place by a loose, rolled bandage. Transport the victim to a medical facility. Administer ibuprofen 400 to 800 mg three times a day. If ibuprofen is not available, administer aspirin 325 mg once a day. If frostbite involves the feet, try to minimize walking. Don't allow tobacco use or the drinking of alcohol. Keep the victim well hydrated with warm beverages. Administer pain medications as needed.

After the thaw, if the victim is days away from hospital care, manage the wound as follows:

1. If you don't have sufficient sterile bandages to re-dress the wounds at least once a day until you reach a hospital, allow blisters to remain intact. Apply topical aloe vera gel or lotion twice a day. Cover with sterile gauze.
2. If white or clear blisters begin to leak, trim them away and apply antiseptic ointment (mupirocin or bacitracin) or cream (mupirocin). If tense or white or clear blisters prohibit evacuation by walking (e.g., they will rupture spontaneously), then drain and cover them with bandages. Don't drain bloody blisters. If antiseptic ointment is not available, continue with aloe vera gel or lotion. Cover with a sterile dressing (see page 254), taking particular care to pad with cotton or gauze between fingers and toes.
3. If at all possible, keep purple or bloody blisters intact, because they provide a covering that keeps the underlying damaged tissue from drying out. Apply topical aloe vera gel or lotion twice a day. Cover with sterile gauze.
4. Elevate the affected part.
5. Apply a protective splint (see page 70) if necessary to surround the bulky cushion dressing.
6. For the first 72 hours after the injury, administer dicloxacillin, cephalexin, or erythromycin, particularly for larger wounds.
7. If the skin blackens and begins to harden, apply topical mupirocin or bacitracin ointment, or mupirocin cream, daily to the margin where the dying skin meets the normal skin.

Throbbing pain may begin a few days after rewarming and continue for up to a few weeks. After the pain subsides, it's not unusual for the victim to notice a residual tingling sensation. If there is no tissue loss, the duration of abnormal sensation may be only a month; with extensive tissue loss, it can exceed 6 months. Intermittent burning pain or electric current–like sensations may be present.

Tissue that has been destroyed by frostbite will usually harden and turn black in the second week after rewarming, forming a "shell" over the viable tissue underneath. If the destruction is extensive, the affected area will wither and shrivel beneath the blackness and self-amputate over 3 to 6 months. If the victim cannot seek medical care in that interval, the wound should be kept clean and dry, and signs of infection (see page 222) treated appropriately with antibiotics.

The corneas can be frostbitten if people (such as snowmobilers) force their eyes open in situations of high windchill. Symptoms include blurred vision, aversion to light, swollen eyelids, and excessive tearing. The treatment is the same as for a corneal abrasion (see page 168).

Prevention of Frostbite

1. Dress to maintain body warmth. Wear adequate, properly fitting (not tight) clothing, particularly boots that can accommodate a pair of polypropylene socks and at least one pair of wool socks without cramping the toes or wrinkling the socks. Dress your feet for the temperature of subsurface colder snow, not the "warm" snow at the surface. Take care to cover the head, neck, hands, feet, and face (particularly the nose and ears). Wear mittens in preference to gloves, to decrease the surface area available for heat loss from the fingers. Mitten shells and gloves should be made of synthetics or soft, flexible, dry-tanned leather (e.g., moose, deer, elk, caribou) that won't dry stiffly after it becomes wet. Don't grease the leather. Mitten inserts and glove linings should be made of soft wool. Tie mittens and gloves to sleeves or string them around the neck, so they aren't dropped or lost.
2. Carry pocket, hand, and/or foot warmers and use them properly. Choices include fuel-burning warmers or chemical (such as Grabber hand warmer) packs, reusable sodium acetate thermal packs, or air-activated, single-use hand and pocket warmers. Don't rely upon a single warmer to reduce cold exposure. Carry several warmers to compensate for failures and short duration of warming. Don't expect the devices to work if they become wet. The heavier device, the longer the heat production.
3. Keep the head warm to help prevent reflex blood vessel constriction in the fingers and toes.
4. Keep clothing dry. Avoid perspiring during extremely cold weather. Keep skin dry and avoid moisturization.
5. Don't touch bare metal with bare skin. Certain liquids (such as gasoline) become colder than frozen water before they freeze, and can cause frostbite. Cover all metal handles with cloth, tape, or leather. Take care when handling cameras. For brief periods of exposure when dexterity is required, wear silk or rayon gloves.
6. Don't maintain one position in the cold for a prolonged period of time. Avoid cramped quarters.
7. Wear a sunscreen with a cream or grease base to prevent windburn.
8. Stay well hydrated. Eat enough food to maximize body-heat production. Avoid becoming fatigued.
9. Don't overwash exposed skin in freezing weather. The natural oils are a barrier to cold injury. Shave sparingly or not at all for cosmetic reasons. If skin becomes exceedingly dry, apply a thin layer of petrolatum-based ointment.
10. Don't drink alcohol or use tobacco products.
11. Keep fingernails and toenails properly trimmed.
12. Don't climb during extreme weather conditions.

FROSTNIP

Frostnip is reversible ice-crystal formation that occurs on the surface of the skin. It is distinct from frostbite in that actual freezing of the tissues does not occur. However, because the symptoms (numbness, frosted appearance) may resemble those of frostbite, it should be taken as a serious warning that the skin is not adequately protected.

IMMERSION FOOT (TRENCH FOOT)

Immersion, or "trench," foot (affecting lower limbs) is caused by prolonged (hours to days) exposure to cold water or to conditions of persistent cold (32° F to 59° F, or 0° C to 15° C) and high humidity, without actual freezing of tissues. Symptoms include itching, tingling, and eventually numbness. At first, the skin appears blanched, yellowish-white or mottled, but rarely blistered. It is not painful, but muscle cramps may be present.

If you suspect immersion foot, carefully cleanse and dry the limb, and rewarm it. After the limb has initially been fully rewarmed, it may become very reddened, warm to the touch, swollen, and painful. Then, maintain it in an environment in which the victim can be kept warm while the injured limb(s) can be kept cool (not cold). Don't rub the limb. Pain reaches its maximum intensity in 24 to 36 hours, and may be worsened at night. If the limbs are held in a dependent position, they may turn purplish in color; when raised, they may blanch. Treat the injury as a combination of frostbite and a burn wound, using daily dressing changes, topical antiseptic ointments, and antibiotics if necessary to treat any infection. If left unattended, immersion foot can lead to prolonged disability. In a severe case, the skin may become gangrenous.

Prevention of immersion foot involves keeping the feet dry and warm. Check the feet every day. Change socks as often as necessary to keep them dry, and attempt to promote circulation to the feet. Avoid constrictive or nonventilated (rubber) footwear. Wear properly fitted boots. Silicone ointment applied to the soles may be preventive. There are special boots (OTB by New Balance) designed with perforations through the sole to drain water. These should be considered in special circumstances.

CHILBLAIN (PERNIO)

Chilblain is less severe than immersion foot. It mostly afflicts women, who develop patches of redness or blue discoloration, nodules, and, rarely, blisters or ulcerations on the lower legs, feet, thighs, toes, hands, and ears. The skin changes appear approximately 12 hours after cold exposure and are accompanied by intense itching and burning or tingling sensations.

Treatment involves rewarming the affected skin, keeping it washed and dried, gentle massage, and covering the nodules with dry, soft, and sterile bandages. Affected limbs should be elevated to minimize swelling. Rewarming should not exceed 86° F (30° C), to minimize pain. In a severe case, nifedipine 20 mg by mouth three times a day for a few days has been shown to be effective. Ibuprofen 400 to 600 mg by mouth two or three times a day may be helpful. After rewarming, the tender blue skin nodules may persist for up to 3 weeks. Once healing has occurred, the skin may remain darkened.

Women with a past history of pernio or history of Raynaud's phenomenon (constriction of small blood vessels, leading to painful hands and feet that become pale or blue on exposure to cold—see below) seem to be more prone to an episode. A topical lanolin-based lotion or emollient (hydrating) cream may be helpful in prevention. Pernio might possibly be prevented or lessened by taking ibuprofen 400 to 600 mg by mouth two or three times a day.

RAYNAUD'S PHENOMENON

Raynaud's phenomenon is constriction of tiny blood vessels ("vasospasm") in the fingers and/or toes after exposure to cold or an emotionally stressful situation. The initial appearance is one of severely blanched (whitened) or bluish skin, often with a sharp "cutoff" margin in the midportion of the digit(s). This is caused by decreased circulation. The episode ends with vigorous reflow of blood into the digit, which causes it to become warm and reddened. This phenomenon is different and much more pronounced than the normal mottling or diffuse and persistent discoloration sometimes seen in hands and feet exposed to cold. Raynaud's phenomenon is usually symmetrical, involving both hands or both feet, and is usually apparent in sufferers by age 40 years. Because Raynaud's phenomenon can be associated with a number of underlying diseases or anatomic abnormalities, a first-time sufferer should seek medical evaluation. Prevention in the outdoors involves primarily protecting the hands and feet and keeping them warm, avoiding drugs that cause blood vessel constriction, and prohibiting tobacco use. Many drugs have been recommended to treat Raynaud's phenomenon, but at the current time the calcium-channel blockers (such as nifedipine) and drugs that block the sympathetic nervous system (which causes blood vessels to constrict) are most in favor as therapies for use outside of the hospital. Blood vessel dilators, such as nitroglycerin or niacin, have not been proved effective. Some sufferers have found that "windmilling" the arms and hands during an episode may help to reverse the vasospasm.

HIVES INDUCED BY EXPOSURE TO COLD

See page 220. Treatment is not as satisfactory as for hives due to an allergic reaction, in that antihistamines don't seem to be of great benefit.

SNOW BLINDNESS

See page 174.

INJURIES AND ILLNESSES DUE TO HEAT

BURN INJURIES

See page 108.

HEAT-RELATED ILLNESS (HYPERTHERMIA)

Human core temperature is maintained at 98.6° F (37° C), with little variation from individual to individual. Heat is generated by all of the metabolic processes that contribute to life, from the blink of an eyelid to the completion of a marathon, and must be shed constantly to avoid a condition of overheating. The resting person generates enough heat (60 to 80 kilocalories per hour) to raise body temperature by 1.8° F (1° C) per hour. A person exposed to the sun can absorb 150 kilocalories of energy an hour. Vigorous exercise can increase endogenous heat production 10-fold. As outlined in the section on hypothermia (see page 281), heat is lost to the environment through conduction, convection, radiation, and evaporation:

Conduction: Heat exchange between two surfaces in direct contact. Lying uninsulated on hot (or cold) ground can result in significant heat exchange. The same is true for immersion into hot or cold water.

Convection: Heat transferred from a surface to a gas or liquid, commonly air or water. When air temperature exceeds skin temperature, heat is gained by the body. Loose-fitting clothing allows air movement and assists conductive heat loss.

Radiation: Heat transfer between the body and the environment by electromagnetic waves. Clothing protects the body from radiant heat, and the skin radiates heat away from the body. Highly pigmented skin absorbs more heat than does nonpigmented skin.

Evaporation: Consumption of heat energy as liquid is converted to a gas. Evaporation of sweat is an effective cooling mechanism.

In the normal situation, skin is the largest heat-wasting organ, and radiates approximately 65% of the daily heat loss. The skin is also largely responsible for evaporation (of sweat). Extreme humidity impedes evaporation and greatly diminishes human temperature control. The National Weather Service heat index (Figure 211) roughly correlates air temperature and relative humidity

	AIR TEMPERATURE (°F)										
	70	75	80	85	90	95	100	105	110	115	120
RELATIVE HUMIDITY (%)	APPARENT TEMPERATURE (°F)										
0	64	69	73	78	83	87	91	95	99	103	107
10	65	70	75	80	85	90	95	100	105	111	116
20	66	72	77	82	87	93	99	105	112	120	130
30	67	73	78	84	90	96	104	113	123	135	148
40	68	74	79	86	93	101	110	122	137	151	
50	69	75	81	88	96	107	120	135	150		
60	70	76	82	90	100	114	132	149			
70	70	77	85	93	106	124	144				
80	71	78	86	97	113	136	157				
90	71	79	88	102	122	150	170				
100	72	80	91	108	133	166					

Figure 211. Heat index. Humidity contributes greatly to the accumulation of heat; when both air temperature and relative humidity are excessive, human temperature control is diminished.

to derive an "apparent temperature." At all temperatures, humidity makes the situation worse. For instance, at an air temperature of 85° F, if the relative humidity is 80%, the apparent temperature is 97° F.

To summarize these recommendations:

Apparent Temperature Range	Dangers/Precautions at This Range
80-90° F (27-32° C)	Exercise can be difficult; enforce rest and hydration
90-105° F (32-41° C)	Heat cramps and exhaustion; be extremely cautious; provide constant supervision
105-130° F (41-54° C)	Anticipate heat exhaustion; strictly limit activities
130° F and above (54° C and above)	Setting for heatstroke; seek cool shelter

When maximally effective, the complete evaporation of 1 quart (liter) of sweat from the skin removes 600 kilocalories of heat (equivalent to the total heat produced with strenuous exercise in 1 hour). The scalp, face, and torso are most important in terms of sweating. Sweat that drips from the skin without evaporating does not contribute to the cooling process, but may contribute to dehydration. World-class distance runners who are acclimated to the heat can sweat in excess of 3½ quarts per hour. Since the maximum rate of gastric emptying (a surrogate for fluid absorption) is only 1.2 quarts per hour, it's easy to see how a person can become dehydrated. Thus, a person should be able to tolerate a 1 quart per hour sweat rate and manage rehydration with oral fluids.

When heat-control mechanisms are overloaded, the body responds unfavorably. As opposed to hypothermia, in which moderate cooling may offer a protective effect, the syndromes of true hyperthermia (in which core body temperature is measurably elevated) can rapidly become life threatening as elevated temperature destroys vital organs and dismembers chemical systems essential to life. Fever in and of itself can set off a vicious cycle, because raising the body temperature by 1.8° F (1° C) can increase metabolism by approximately 13%, which hastens the generation of more heat. Dehydration may by itself raise body temperature. For all of these reasons, it's crucial to be familiar with heat illness, and to be prepared to respond promptly and decisively.

HEAT EXHAUSTION AND HEATSTROKE

Heat exhaustion and heatstroke are part of the same continuum, but of differing severity. Heat exhaustion is illness caused by an elevation of body temperature that does not result in permanent damage. Heatstroke is life threatening and can permanently disable the victim.

The signs and symptoms of heat exhaustion are minor confusion, irrational behavior, a rapid weak pulse, dizziness, nausea, diarrhea, headache, and temperature elevation (up to 104° F [40°C]). It's important to note that *sweating may be present or absent,* and that *the skin of the victim may feel cool to the touch.* It is the core temperature that is elevated and that must be measured (rectally).

The signs and symptoms of heatstroke are extreme confusion, weakness, dizziness, unconsciousness, low blood pressure or shock (see page 58), seizures, increased bleeding (bruising, vomiting blood, bloody urine), diarrhea, vomiting, shortness of breath, red skin rash (particularly over the chest, abdomen, and back), tea-colored to deeply darkened ("machine oil") urine (caused by breakdown of muscle tissue that releases pigment into the bloodstream), and major core body temperature elevation (up to 115.7° F [46.5° C] has been reported in a heatstroke survivor). Again, it's important to note that *sweating may be present or absent.* At the time of collapse, most victims of heatstroke are still sweating copiously. It's rare for someone to feel cool externally when his temperature exceeds 105° F (40.5° C), but it is not impossible.

The skin will usually be warm or hot to the touch when a victim suffers heat exhaustion or heatstroke, but, again, this is not absolutely constant. *Carry a rectal thermometer so you can take a temperature reading.* If no thermometer is available, and you're fairly certain that the victim is suffering from heat exhaustion or heatstroke, proceed with therapy.

The most important aspect of therapy is to *lower the temperature as quickly as possible.* The body may lose its ability to control its own temperature at 106° F (41.1° C), so from that point upward, temperature can skyrocket. Manage the airway (see page 22) and administer oxygen (see page 405) at a flow rate of 10 liters per minute by face mask. Don't give liquids by mouth unless the victim is awake and capable of purposeful swallowing. Cooled liquids don't assist the cooling process enough to risk choking the uncooperative or confused victim.

Cooling the Victim

1. Remove the victim from obvious sources of heat. Shield him from direct sunlight and remove his clothing. Stop him from exercising.
2. The most efficient method of cooling is to drench the victim with large quantities of crushed ice and water, accompanied by vigorous massage. If you have a limited amount of ice, place ice packs in the armpits, behind the neck, and in the groin. Note that chemical cold packs don't provide the same cooling power as do real ice packs, and rapidly lose their effectiveness.
3. Alternatively, you can cover the victim with ice water–soaked sheets or towels, keeping them continuously moist and cold. There are safety issues to consider with total body immersion in cold water to treat hyperthermia, including access to the victim and even the risk for drowning. However, in a life-threatening field situation, if the only method available for cooling is immersion in a cold mountain stream, do it! Be alert for the need to remove the victim from the water to accomplish resuscitative measures. Never leave the victim unattended. If you immerse someone in cold water for cooling, circulate the water as best possible to maximize the cooling effect. If it's impossible to immerse the victim, soak towels or spare clothing in the cold water and apply them to the victim.

4. If ice is not available, wet down the victim and begin to fan him vigorously. Evaporation is a very efficient method of heat removal. Use cool or tepid water; *don't sponge the victim with alcohol.* If electric fans are available, use them. Don't be concerned with shivering, so long as you continue to aggressively cool the victim.

5. There is a device (CoreControl) for athletes that increases circulation through the hand to allow a cooling mechanism to have its effect on this area of brisk heat transfer.

6. Recheck the temperature every 5 to 10 minutes, to avoid cooling much below 98.6° F (37° C). When you have cooled the victim to 99.5° F to 100° F (37.5° C to 37.8° C), taper the cooling effort. After the victim is cooled, recheck his temperature every 30 minutes for 3 to 4 hours, because there will often be a rebound temperature rise.

7. *Don't use aspirin or acetaminophen unless the victim has an infection.* These specific drugs are used to combat fever that is caused by the release of chemical compounds from infectious agents into the bloodstream. Such compounds affect the portion of the brain (hypothalamus) that serves as the body's thermostat, causing body temperature to rise. Aspirin or acetaminophen acts to block this chemical interaction in the brain, and thus eliminates the fever. If elevated body temperature is not caused by an infection, aspirin or acetaminophen will not work—and may in fact be harmful, leading to bleeding disorders or liver inflammation, respectively.

8. If the victim is alert, begin to correct dehydration (see page 194) using oral rehydration. This is particularly important if the urine is seen to be darkened in color. Be certain that the concentration of carbohydrates or sugar in the beverage does not exceed 6%, so as not to inhibit intestinal absorption. Try to get 1 to 2 quarts (liters) into the victim over the first few hours. For every pound (0.45 kg) of weight loss attributed to sweating, have the victim ingest a pint (473 mL or 2 cups) of fluid. Adequate rehydration may take up to 36 hours.

MUSCLE CRAMPS

Muscle cramps in a warm environment accompany overuse (see page 262) or water and salt losses in the individual who exerts strenuously. A well-trained athlete can lose 2 to 3 quarts (liters) of sweat per hour (a potential 20 g sodium loss each day). In most cases, these painful cramps are caused by replacement of water without adequate salt intake. Heat per se doesn't actually cause the cramps—they accompany exercise.

Treatment for cramps consists of gentle motion, massage, and stretching of the affected muscles, accompanied by fluid and salt replacement. This can be done by drinking water and balanced salt solutions or sports beverages before and during heavy exertion. One recommendation is to drink a solution that contains 3.5 g of sodium chloride and 1.5 g of potassium chloride in a quart (liter) of water. As a rough measure, ¼ to ½ teaspoon (1.3 to 2.5 mL) of table salt in water will suffice. With proper fluid and electrolyte replacement, salt tablets (which irritate the lining of the stomach) are usually unnecessary.

Sometimes rubbing the affected muscles with ice or ice packs for 5 to 10 minutes may hasten resolution of heat-related muscle cramps.

Muscle cramps that occur at night may have no identifiable cause. Some doctors treat these with quinine sulfate or with a glass of tonic water at bedtime.

HEAT SWELLING

In warmer climates, normal people, particularly elders, may suffer from swelling (sometimes called *edema*) of the feet and ankles. This is noted after prolonged periods of walking or sitting and is not necessarily indicative of heart failure. Often, the swelling will disappear as a person becomes adjusted to the warm environment over several days. The swelling is painless and there is no sign of infection (redness). Body temperature is not elevated.

Treatment for heat swelling is to minimize periods of walking and to use support stockings that rise at least to midthigh. The legs should be elevated whenever possible. There is no reason to use fluid pills (diuretics). If the sufferer is short of breath or otherwise ill in association with leg swelling, he should seek the advice of a physician.

FAINTING

Fainting has many causes (see page 154). Fainting due to heat exposure occurs when a person (particularly an elder) adapts by dilating blood vessels in the skin and superficial muscles to deliver warm blood to the surface of the body, where the excess heat energy can be delivered back to the environment. Expansion of the superficial blood vessels allows a greater-than-normal proportion of the circulating blood volume to be away from the central circulation, which supplies, among other organs, the brain. This lack of sufficient central pressure is worsened when a person is on his feet for a prolonged period of time, because gravity allows a significant blood volume to pool in his lower limbs. Combined with fatigue and mild dehydration, the diversion of blood leads to a fainting episode, because not enough blood (with oxygen and glucose) is pumped to the brain. Dehydration can also stimulate the vagus nerve, which causes the heart rate to slow ("vasovagal" or "vagal" episode). A person with anemia, fever, low blood sugar, or acute injury may be particularly prone to fainting. Other risk factors for fainting due to vagal stimulation include prolonged standing, vigorous exercise in a warm environment, fear, emotional distress, and severe pain.

A victim who has suffered a fainting episode in the heat should be examined for any head or neck injuries, as well as other possible breaks or cuts. Other causes of fainting (low blood sugar, abnormal heart rhythm, and so on) must be considered. If fainting is due to the heat, the victim will reawaken shortly, because assuming a horizontal position returns blood to the brain and solves the major problem. In general, body temperature is not elevated.

The victim of a fainting spell due to heat should be rested in a horizontal position for 15 to 30 minutes, and should not immediately assume a standing posture without first sitting for 5 minutes. Encourage him to consume a pint or two (½ to 1 liter) of cool sweetened liquid (such as Gatorade or Gatorade G2). To avoid further episodes, efforts should be made to avoid dehydration, missing meals, or standing in one position for a prolonged period. Support hose may help, as might regular leg muscle exercise. The victim should learn to recognize the warning signs of a fainting spell, which include episodes of dizziness, light-headedness, nausea, weakness, sweating, blurred vision, or seeing flashing lights. When a warning sign occurs, the victim should immediately assume a horizontal position or at least sit and lower his head to a position between his knees. If a person is wearing a tight collar and feels faint, loosen the collar. Any person over age 40 who suffers a fainting episode should eventually be examined by a doctor to be certain that the red blood count is normal and that there is no heart disease.

AVOIDING HEAT ILLNESS

1. Avoid dehydration. Drink 1 pint (473 mL) of liquid 10 to 15 minutes before beginning vigorous exercise. Drink at least 1 pint to 1 quart (½ to 1 liter) of liquid with adequate electrolyte supplementation (see later) each hour during heavy exercise with sweating in a hot climate. *Adequate water ingested during exercise is not harmful, does not cause cramps, and will prevent a large percentage of cases of heat illness.* Encourage rest and fluid breaks. DON'T WITHHOLD WATER FROM ATHLETES DURING PRACTICE AND COMPETITIONS. The temperature of the fluid ingested should be cool, to encourage it to empty from the stomach. It is a myth that ingesting cold fluid causes abdominal cramps, so long as the amount ingested is prudent. There is no evidence that "hyperhydrating" before heat exposure, or cooling the body before exercise, lessens the risk for heat-related illness.

A terrific method for carrying water is the CamelBak hydration system, or any similar setup, which allows you to sip continuously from an over-the-shoulder delivery tube.

If the urine becomes darkened or scant, fluid requirements aren't being met. ("Cloudy," or unclear, urine may indicate a different sort of problem, such as protein in the urine or a urinary tract infection.) As a general rule, people outdoors should consume at least 3 quarts (liters) of fluid each day to replenish that lost through urination, exhaled moisture, skin evaporation, and defecation. With moderate activity, this should be increased to at least 4 to 5 quarts (liters). Don't rely on thirst as an absolute guide to fluid requirements. In general, merely quenching thirst does not adequately replace fluid losses in heat stress or high-altitude conditions. It is possible to sweat up to 3 quarts (liters) per hour when exercising in extremely hot and humid conditions. During heavy exertion in hot weather, consider drinking at least a quart (liter) of liquid per hour.

With a normal diet, there is no need to take salt tablets. Electrolyte requirements can be met with food salted to taste. Electrolyte- and sugar-enriched drinks, such as Gatorade or Gatorade G2, should be used when normal meals cannot be eaten or when sweating is excessive (during athletic training or military forced marching, for example). A home brew (see page 194) may be used if a Gatorade-type beverage is not available. Accelerade is a sports beverage that contains 15 g of carbohydrate and 4 g of protein per 8 fluid oz. This combination may be muscle-sparing during periods of high exertion, in warm or cold weather.

The normal daily diet may be safely supplemented during times of extreme sweating (greater than $\frac{1}{4}$ to 1 quart, or liter, per hour) with 5 to 10 g of sodium (normal daily dietary intake is 4 to 6 g; most adults would be fine with 1 to 3 g) and 2 to 4 g of potassium. Supplemental salt is advised when weight loss from sweating exceeds 5 lb (2.3 kg) in a single session, particularly early in the acclimatization period when salt losses in sweat are great. Consume 0.5 g ($\frac{1}{10}$ teaspoon) sodium chloride (table salt) with a pint (473 mL) of water for each pound (0.45 kg) of weight loss over 5 lb (2.3 kg). If large quantities of electrolytes are lost and not replaced (e.g., if large quantities of water are consumed without salt, typically during an endurance athletic event), a person can become quite ill. Hyponatremia (low serum [in the blood] sodium) is a condition that occurs when excessive water drinking occurs without salt replenishment. Symptoms include nausea, vomiting, headache, weakness, fatigue, muscle weakness, difficulty with balance and walking, confusion, fluid in the lungs (shortness of breath and coughing, sometimes productive of frothy and/or blood-tinged sputum), and seizures. The condition may become fatal. Similarly, salt without water can be harmful. Salt tablets can be very irritating to the stomach and should not be used unless salt-containing solutions aren't available. Coffee, tea, and alcohol-containing beverages cause increased fluid loss through excessive urination (diuretic effect) and should be avoided.

2. Be watchful of the very young and very old. Their bodies don't regulate body temperature well and can rapidly become too hot or too cold. Don't bundle up infants in warm weather.

3. Stay in shape. Obesity, lack of conditioning, insufficient rest, and ingestion of alcohol and/or illicit drugs all contribute to an increased risk for heat illness. The herb ephedra contains ephedrine, which is reputed to enhance athletic performance; however, it increases metabolic rate and has caused many cases of heat illness and, on occasion, deaths.

4. Condition yourself for the environment. Gradual increased exposure to work in a hot environment for a minimum of an hour or two a day for 8 to 10 days will allow an adult to acclimatize. Children require 10 to 14 days. More time spent in the heat hastens the process. Acclimatization is manifested as increased sweat volume with a decreased

electrolyte concentration (more efficient sweating), greater peripheral blood vessel dilatation (more efficient heat loss), lowered heart rate, decreased skin and rectal temperatures during exercise, increased water and salt conservation by the kidneys, and enhanced metabolism of energy supplies. Eat potassium-rich vegetables and fruits, such as broccoli and bananas. Don't restrict fluid intake during acclimatization. On the contrary, it's necessary to increase fluid intake to accompany increased sweat volume.

5. Wet bulb globe temperature (WBGT), which is a fairly precise predictor of human physiologic heat strain, takes into account ambient temperature, wind, solar radiation, and humidity. It is measured with a sling psychrometer, which most people will not be carrying. WBGT temperature values used as a guide to recommend activity levels to avoid heat-related illnesses cannot be equated to simply measured ambient temperatures. Furthermore, WBGT can be too liberal a measure because it does not take into account exercise, clothing, and other factors. The following recommendations (based on WBGT measurements) thus need to take into account any restriction on sweating, ability to spend partial time in a cooler situation (e.g., shade), the presence of a cooling breeze or dip in a stream, and so forth.

   a. 60°F (15.5°C): No precautions

   b. 61-70°F (16.1-21.1°C): No precautions if adequate hydration

   c. 71-75°F (21.7-23.8°C): If not acclimatized, minimal exercise; if acclimatized, exercise with caution with rest and water breaks every 20 to 30 minutes

   d. 76-80°F (24.4-26.6°C): If not acclimatized, avoid hiking, vigorous sports, and sun exposure; if acclimatized, moderate to heavy work with caution

   e. 81-85°F (27.2-29.4°C): If not acclimatized, no significant exercise; if acclimatized and fit, limited brief exercise under close observation

   f. 88°F (31°C) and above: No exercise or sun exposure

     In general, curtail heavy exercise when it's hot, and particularly when it's humid. Above 75% humidity, you will have difficulty evaporating sweat, so your natural cooling mechanism is impeded.

6. Wear clothing appropriate for the environment. Dress in layers so that you can add or shed clothing as necessary. Clothing should be lightweight and absorbent. Wear a loose-fitting broad-brimmed hat to shield yourself from the sun, but don't wear a hat if you don't need protection from the sun. Don't wear plastic or rubber sweat suits in the heat. Don't try to lose water weight as part of any weight loss program.

7. Towel off your face and scalp frequently, because 50% of sweating occurs from these areas. Remove headgear when possible to allow evaporation from the head. Allow the scalp, face, and upper torso access to air circulation, since these are the major areas of sweating and therefore provide opportunity for sweat evaporation.

8. Keep out of the sun on a hot day. When you feel hot, seek a cooler location. Resting on hot ground increases heat stress; the sun can heat the ground by more than 40°F (22.2°C) above the air temperature. If you must lie on the ground, dig a shallow (a few inches, or centimeters) trench to get down to a cooler surface.

9. Avoid taking drugs that inhibit the sweating process (such as atropine, antispasmodics, anti–motion sickness), diminish cardiac output (beta-blockers), disrupt certain features of physiologic activity (antidepressants, antihistamines), increase muscle activity (hallucinogens, cocaine), or promote dehydration (diuretics).

10. To find water in the desert, look for green plants. Near the ocean shore, drinkable water may be found below a sandy or gravel surface at an elevation above seawater. Look for green plants. Water may be found at the foot of cliffs that have become waterfalls after a rainstorm or flood. Look under rocks, even if the surface appears dry.

11. If you are prone to fainting episodes, particularly of the ("vagal") type, learn to recognize the warning symptoms that occur before fainting, which include weakness, feeling light-headed, sweating, blurred vision, nausea, headache, warm or cold feeling, yawning, nervousness, and growing pale. You may also feel "out of body" or disoriented. If any of these occur and you recognize that you might faint, immediately try to lie face down on the ground, so that you don't fall, and allow gravity to assist in bringing blood from your limbs back to the central circulation and your brain.

WILDLAND FIRES

The wilderness adventurer or casual hiker in a forest or timbered park may find himself face to face with a wildland fire. This section will discuss high-risk situations, survival techniques, and medical considerations. Review the sections on burns (see page 108), lightning injuries (see page 340), heat illness (see page 296), and inhalation injuries (see page 112) as well.

HIGH-RISK SITUATIONS

The risk for a wildland fire is increased under certain environmental conditions. Pay heed to posted warnings of fire hazard, and don't venture into the woods unprepared to escape. Be particularly cautious when:

1. There are drought conditions. Low humidity, higher air temperatures, and gusty winds create dry fuel for a fire.
2. You are in an area rich with abundant fuel, such as dead grass, pine needles, shrubs, fallen trees, and the like.
3. You travel through gullies, in canyons, along steep slopes, or in other regions where wind and fuel are ideal for rapid advance of an established fire.
4. Fires have occurred recently in the vicinity.
5. You cannot see the main fire and are not in contact with anyone who can.
6. Terrain and fuels make escape to safety zones difficult.

STANDARD FIRE ENCOUNTER PRINCIPLES

1. Have advance knowledge of weather conditions and forecasts before undertaking an expedition. Don't travel in hazardous regions in times of high fire risk. Local ranger stations are the best source of information. *Never plan an extended journey without leaving an itinerary with the proper authorities.* In the event of a fire, try to maintain communication with firefighters or other rescuers.
2. At every campsite, take a few moments to prepare a plan for an evacuation, with at least two escape routes. Be certain that everyone understands the routes.
3. If a fire is in the area, pay attention to it, so that you will know what the fire is doing. Obtain current information on fire status. If there is any chance that it can involve your party, *get out early.*
4. If you see smoke or fire at a distance, post a lookout to watch for any changes that might indicate increased danger.
5. In all situations, stay calm and act with authority. Give orders concisely and be sure that they are understood. Base all of your actions on the current and expected behavior of the fire.
6. Don't attempt to fight the fire unless you have provided for safety first. Your first responsibility is to evacuate all potential victims and provide necessary first aid. In general, it's best to leave firefighting to professionals. If you become a fire fighter, provide for safety first. Determine safety zones and escape routes.

7. Don't sleep near a wildland fire. If the wind and fire direction change, you may be overcome with smoke and unable to escape.

WHAT TO DO WHEN CAUGHT IN A WILDLAND FIRE

A safe area is one with light or no fuels, such as a rocky surface, marshy area, large area of pavement, center of a sufficiently large body of water, or recently burned area. This option only works if the distance between the fire and entry into the safe area is short, the fire is advancing slowly, and it is easy to reach the safe area.

1. Try not to panic. This is difficult, but if anything will save your life, it will be a clear head.
2. Don't move downhill toward a fire, because fires have a tendency to run uphill.
3. Unless the path of escape is clear, don't start running. Conserve your strength, and seek the flank of the fire. Continually observe changes in speed and direction of the fire and smoke to choose travel away from fire hazards. Be alert, keep calm, and avoid injury from rolling or falling debris.
4. Enter a burned area, particularly one with little fuel (grass or low shrubs). Although there is a chance that the area might burn again, you're better off here than in an area of fresh fuel. If you have to cross the fire line, cover your skin as well as possible, take a couple of deep breaths, and dash through the lowest flames (less than 5 ft, or 1.5 m, tall and deep and where you can see through them). If smoke is dense, crawl along the ground for better air and visibility.
5. If you cannot enter a burned area, ignite grass or other fine fuels between you and the fire edge. Carry wind-resistant matches for this purpose. After this area burns, step into it and cover your exposed skin with clothing or dirt. This is not an effective technique in areas of heavier fuels.
6. Try to avoid breathing smoke. Hold a moistened cloth over your mouth. If the air is very hot, use a dry cloth (dry heat is less damaging to the lungs than is steam). If you have a choice of clothing, cover your skin with closed-toe shoes, a long-sleeved cotton or wool shirt, cotton or wool pants, a hat, and gloves.
7. Seek refuge from the radiant heat. Take shelter in a trench, in a pond, behind rocks, or in a stream, vehicle, or building. Don't climb into elevated water tanks, wells, caves, or any other place where you might be trapped or quickly use up the available oxygen.
8. If all else fails and you cannot escape the advancing flames, lie face down on the ground and cover your exposed skin as best possible to shield from radiant heat. This is better than standing or kneeling. If available, a fire-retardant blanket or shield is desirable. Radiant heat can kill a person long before the flames reaches him. When a fire passes over and around a person, heating of body tissues from thermal radiation can be unbearable. Staying calm and not getting up until the fire has substantially dissipated is critical.
9. If you are near a vehicle, and there is no route for escape, it's better to stay in the vehicle than to run from the fire. Try to position the vehicle in an area of little natural vegetation. Avoid driving through dense smoke. Turn off the headlights and ignition. Roll up the windows, close the air vents, and shield yourself from the radiant heat by covering up with floor mats or hiding under the dash. Stay in the vehicle as long as possible (it's rare for a gasoline tank to explode, and it takes a minute or two for the vehicle to catch on fire). Don't be overly alarmed if the vehicle rocks, or if smoke and sparks enter the vehicle. When the fire passes, cover your nose and mouth with a moistened cloth to avoid inhaling fumes from burning plastics and paint. Use urine if no other liquid is available.
10. If you are in a building and a fire is approaching, attach hoses to external water fixtures to achieve as much water spray coverage as possible. Place lawn sprinklers on the roof or use the hoses to soak down the roof. Put a ladder outside that will reach the roof. Locate

and position buckets, rakes, axes, and shovels. Soak down shrubs and combustible foliage within 20 ft (6 m) of the building. If you have time, also do the following:

- Close windows, vents, doors, and blinds. Remove combustible drapes and window dressings. Close doors inside the house to prevent drafts.
- Turn off the gas at the meter. Turn off all pilot lights (heater, range, oven, and so on). Turn off any propane tanks.
- Open the fireplace damper and close the fireplace screens.
- Place water in containers to fight the fire. A wet mop may be used to extinguish sparks and embers.
- Turn on a light in each room (for visibility if smoke accumulates).
- Move flammable furniture away from windows and sliding glass doors.
- Move flammable patio furniture indoors or far away from the building.
- Keep all of your pets in one room.
- If you have a car or truck, back it into the garage or park it in an open space facing the direction of escape. Shut the doors and roll up the windows. Leave the key in the ignition. Close the garage door(s) and windows, but leave them unlocked. Disconnect any automatic garage door opener.

HOW TO REPORT A FIRE

If you suspect a wildland fire, *immediately* report it to local fire protection authorities. You should be prepared to give your name and location, the location of the fire, a description of the fire (flames, color, smoke), and a list of any people in the area, with their most exact locations.

CREATING A DEFENSIBLE SPACE

Everyone now must consider how best to safeguard their homes and property against an encroaching wildfire. At the wildland-urban interface, human dwellings are juxtaposed against the wilderness. As opposed to the man-made fire breaks imposed by living in the city, there is often scant protection out "in the country." The recommendations that follow are applicable in an urban setting as well, but are much more important in a wildland setting:

1. Use fire-resistant external construction materials, particularly for the roof, where embers may fall. Wooden shakes are highly flammable. Keep the gutters clean of combustible materials.
2. Remove combustible materials from close proximity to the dwelling. This includes piles of wood, flammable refuse, leaf litter, dead limbs, and piles of slash. Dry underbrush within stands of trees close to a dwelling serves as tinder for a fire.
3. If landscaping is flammable, maintain it as far as possible from the dwelling, so that it does not provide an easy flame path to your home. The further that combustible landscaping is located from the at-risk buildings, the better. A recommended minimum distance is 30 to 50 feet. In addition, create paths and openings that allow firefighters easy access to the dwelling.
4. Keep all trees and shrubs pruned of dead limbs and leaves. Don't allow large trees, dead or alive, to overhang your home. Maintain a green lawn if the lawn is adjacent to your home. Don't allow grass to grow tall and become dry so that it can easily burn.
5. To block embers from entering your home, use metal screens over vents and other openings. Otherwise, they can enter and ignite the inside of the dwelling.

MEDICAL CONSIDERATIONS

The three most common medical problems in a wildland fire situation are burns (see page 108), smoke inhalation (see page 113), and dehydration (see page 194), followed by heat illness (see page 296) and poison ivy or oak exposure (see page 216). Anyone exposed to the constant and intense heat of a forest fire should consume at least a pint to a quart ($\frac{1}{2}$ to 1 liter) of fluid per hour.

CARBON MONOXIDE POISONING

In general, there is not a shortage of oxygen in the region of an outdoor fire, so long as there is adequate ventilation. However, in an enclosed space, oxygen may be rapidly depleted as toxic gases and smoke accumulate. This can occur when people cook inside a tent or snow cave, particularly with gasoline or kerosene as fuel. The most commonly inhaled toxin is carbon monoxide, which is the tasteless, odorless, and colorless product of incomplete combustion. Carbon monoxide binds to hemoglobin (the oxygen-carrying pigment in red blood cells) with 200 times the affinity of oxygen. Thus, a human victim suffers from markedly diminished delivery of oxygen to all organ systems. Symptoms of carbon monoxide intoxication include the following:

Mild (10% level measured in the blood): Decreased exercise tolerance, decreased ability to concentrate, headache, nausea.

Moderate (20% level): Severe headache, vomiting, poor coordination, decreased vision, decreased hearing, shortness of breath.

Severe (30% level): Confusion, lethargy.

Catastrophic (40% to 60% level): Fainting, unconsciousness, gasping respirations, seizures, shock, death.

If a person is suspected to have inhaled any toxic gas, he should be moved to fresh air as soon as possible and have oxygen (see page 405) administered at a flow rate of 5 to 10 liters per minute by face mask. Anyone overcome with smoke inhalation should be rapidly transported to a hospital. Be prepared to manage the airway (see page 22). The definitive treatment for severe carbon monoxide poisoning is treatment with oxygen in a hyperbaric chamber. If a person suffers from carbon monoxide poisoning and is allowed to breathe normal air, it takes 4 to 5 hours for half of the carbon monoxide in his system to be eliminated. This elimination time ("half-life") is decreased to 45 to 60 minutes if he breathes 100% oxygen through a face mask, and can be decreased to 15 to 20 minutes if oxygen is breathed under 3 atmospheres of pressure in a hyperbaric chamber.

Prevention of carbon monoxide poisoning in the outdoor setting can be accomplished by proper venting of all tents and snow caves, and considering the possibility of exposure when using camp stoves and any other device fueled by gasoline, propane, natural gas, or charcoal.

HIGH ALTITUDE–RELATED PROBLEMS

Altitudes of 8000 to 14,000 ft (2438 to 4267 m) are attained regularly by skiers, hikers, and climbers in the continental United States. Outside the United States, mountain climbers may reach altitudes of up to 29,029 ft (8848 m) (Mount Everest). Appendix 2 (see page 479) lists common conversion numbers from feet to meters and vice versa.

Most difficulties at high altitude are a direct result of the lowered concentration of oxygen in the atmosphere. Although the percentage of oxygen in the air is relatively constant at about 20%, the absolute amount of oxygen decreases with the declining barometric pressure. At 19,030 ft (5800 m) there is half the barometric pressure, and therefore half the oxygen, that is available at sea level. A person transported suddenly to this altitude without time to acclimatize or without the provision of supplemental oxygen would probably lose consciousness; sudden transport to the summit of Mount Everest (where the amount of inspired oxygen is 28% that at sea level) would cause rapid collapse and death. Although high-altitude illness is common with rapid ascent above 8202 ft (2500 m), the most common range for severe high-altitude illness is 11,483 to 18,045 ft (3500 to 5500 m). Above 18,045 ft (5500 m), altitude is considered extreme, and a human deteriorates rather than adapts. Commercial airplanes are pressurized to an atmospheric pressure equivalent to that at approximately 8000 ft (2438 m) above sea level.

Being at high altitude causes a generalized decreased tolerance for exercise and physical stress. However, to a certain extent, humans can adapt to high altitude and become more efficient in the oxygen-poor environment. The prevention of high altitude–related disorders is best accomplished by gradual acclimatization to the lowered oxygen content of atmospheric air. In this process, you increase the rate and depth of your breathing; this delivers more oxygen to and removes more carbon dioxide from your body. This, along with changes that occur in kidney function, causes your blood to become more alkaline, which allows it to take up and deliver more oxygen to your tissues. Resting heart rate gradually increases. Over time, red blood cell production is increased, and your heart and skeletal muscles become more efficient.

In addition to the effects of less oxygen available at high altitude, mountaineers are subjected to other environmental hazards, such as temperature. As one ascends, for each 3281 ft (1000 m) gain in altitude, temperature drops by 11.7° F (6.5° C). Cold temperatures may contribute to high-altitude illnesses by adding the complications of hypothermia (see page 281) or frostbite (see page 291). Also, for each 984 ft (300 m) gain in altitude, ultraviolet light (see page 174) increases its penetration through the atmosphere by 4%. This increases risks for sunburn, skin cancer, and snow blindness. Dehydration is also common at high altitude, because of exertion, low humidity, rapid breathing, and inadequate oral fluid intake. Sunlight reflecting off glaciers absent a cooling wind can transfer intense radiant heat.

PREVENTION OF HIGH ALTITUDE–RELATED DISORDERS

Avoid direct or sudden ascent to a sleeping altitude above 9843 ft (3000 m). Acclimatization requires gradual exposure to high altitude, with a rate of ascent not to exceed 1500 ft (457 m) per day at altitudes above 8000 ft (2438 m). Rest days at a constant altitude are essential at heights above 10,000 ft (3048 m). For acclimatization purposes, mild exercise is fine, but extreme exercise may be deleterious. Acclimatization is achieved by adhering to a schedule of ascent:

For any climb above 9843 ft (3000 m), spend an initial 2 to 3 nights at 8202 to 9843 ft (2500 to 3000 m) before proceeding higher. The first day should be a rest day. Don't sleep at an altitude more than 984 ft (300 m) above the previous night's sleeping altitude. If anyone shows signs of high altitude–related illness, spend additional time at this altitude. Don't ascend to sleep at a higher altitude if you have any symptoms of high-altitude illness.

For any climb above 13,000 ft (3962 m), all members of the party should add 2 to 4 days for acclimatization at 10,000 to 12,000 ft (3048 to 3658 m). Subsequent climbing should not exceed 1500 ft (457 m) per day. A rest day every 2 to 3 days is advised, along with an extra night for acclimatization with any ascent of 2000 ft (609 m) or more. The party should sleep at the lowest altitude that does not interfere with the purpose of the expedition, and should sleep no higher than 1312 to 1968 ft (400 to 600 m) above the sleeping altitude of the previous night. The mantra is "Climb high—sleep low." After a person has acclimatized by adhering to a schedule of slow ascent, it's important to remember that even a few days at low altitude may cause the adjustments to disappear, so that a person is once again susceptible to high-altitude illness, particularly high-altitude pulmonary edema (HAPE).

The drug acetazolamide (Diamox) has proved to be useful in stimulating breathing, diminishing the sleep disorder associated with acute mountain sickness (AMS; see page 312), facilitating the body's normal adjustment to high altitude, and thus improving nocturnal oxygenation. It is administered in a dose of 125 mg twice a day beginning 24 hours before ascent, and continued for a period of 2 days after the highest altitude to be attained; within this period, the initial physiologic acclimatization process should become operative. It may also be given as a

500 mg sustained-action capsule every 24 hours. Acetazolamide should be used if an ascent will be unavoidably rapid. *Don't use acetazolamide in persons with a history of a severe allergic reaction (including anaphylaxis—see page 64) to sulfa or penicillin-derivative drugs.* If you intend to use acetazolamide, take a trial dose of the medication at sea level well in advance of the high-altitude travel, to identify any adverse side effects. Be aware that acetazolamide commonly causes increased urination, altered (bitter) taste of carbonated beverages, numbness and tingling of hands and feet (particularly in cold weather or accompanying sudden temperature changes, such as washing in hot water), and sometimes bone marrow suppression or even impotence.

Ibuprofen has recently been shown to be somewhat effective in reducing the incidence of AMS. It was given to adults in a dose of 600 mg by mouth three times a day, beginning 6 hours before ascent. It has not yet been determined for how long after the maximum altitude is attained that the drug should be continued in order to maintain its beneficial effect. Furthermore, ibuprofen is a painkiller in and of itself, so if using it "masks" the hallmark headache symptom of AMS, that might be dangerous. Until more is known, if ibuprofen is used to prevent AMS, pay particularly close attention to the users.

Children who have previously suffered from acute mountain sickness may benefit from acetazolamide, which should be administered in a dose of 2.5 mg/kg (2.2 lb) of body weight every 12 hours, up to 125 mg twice per day.

Acetazolamide has a diuretic (increased urination) effect, so that it's extremely important to drink sufficient fluids to prevent dehydration. Begin administering acetazolamide a day before ascent in order to get past the diuretic (excessive urination) effect, which is maximal in the first 24 hours. Fluid losses are generally greater at high altitude, so don't rely on thirst as a gauge of adequate fluid intake. Drink enough to keep the urine clear and light colored. *Acetazolamide is no substitute for proper acclimatization!*

Using dexamethasone (Decadron), a steroid medication, to prevent AMS (and presumably, HACE [see page 311]), is controversial in the wilderness medicine community. Proponents note that it is effective; opponents argue that it encourages too-rapid ascents and removes a "rescue drug" that should be reserved for treatment and not used for prevention. If it is used to prevent AMS (such as for persons who are allergic to acetazolamide and who must make a rapid ascent), it can be administered to adults in a dose of 2 mg by mouth every 6 hours *or* 4 mg by mouth every 12 hours beginning 24 hours before ascent, and optimally continued for no more than 48 hours, at which time the recipient should return to an altitude at or below the origin of the ascent. It is not recommended for use in children as a preventive drug.

Other substances have been advocated for prevention of high-altitude illnesses. These include drugs to prevent high-altitude pulmonary edema (see later for these recommendations), *Gingko biloba* (inconsistent results, perhaps related to purity of the compound and/or dose), antioxidant "cocktails" (not yet proved effective), and other medications such as naproxen, antacids, and diuretics (none yet proved effective). *Gingko biloba* seems harmless, but should not yet be considered a substitute for acetazolamide. While adequate hydration is important, overhydration has never been shown to be of benefit to prevent or treat high-altitude illness.

When you're traveling at high altitudes, avoid the use of alcohol, stay warm, keep out of the wind, avoid exhaustion, and eat regularly to avoid weight loss. A diet relatively high in carbohydrates may be preferable to one high in fat and protein. Avoid the use of alcohol or any drugs for sleep during the first few days at high altitude. Disturbed (poor quality, interrupted) sleep is common at high altitude. Acetazolamide 62.5 to 125 mg by mouth at bedtime diminishes the "periodic breathing" that has traditionally been associated with sleep disturbance, but it may be the enhancement of oxygenation and acclimatization achieved by taking acetazolamide that improve sleep quality. If insomnia is severe *after the acclimatization process has occurred,* zolpidem (Ambien) 5 mg, temazepam (Restoril) 10 to 15 mg, or zaleplon (Sonata) 5 to 10 mg by mouth may be used with caution under the guidance of personnel extremely experienced with high-altitude medical syndromes. Impaired performance (e.g., driving) may be present the morning after using zolpidem, particularly extended-release forms of the medication. A sleeping aid drug may be used in combination with acetazolamide.

It is not known if sleep apnea contributes to AMS or HAPE. However, a person with sleep apnea should be extremely cautious when traveling at high altitude. Findings suggestive of sleep apnea include the following: daytime—excessive sleepiness, feeling tired on awakening, fatigue, irritability, difficulty with simple tasks, and shortness of breath; nighttime—loud snoring, witnessed episodes of diminished or absent breathing, poor sleep, frequent awakening, frequent urination at night, and bedwetting. Acetazolamide used in combination with an autoadjusted continuous positive airway pressure (auto-CPAP) device may be more effective than auto-CPAP alone in reducing breathing disturbances in persons with obstructive sleep apnea.

Since oxygen is transported in red blood cells, it's advisable to avoid being anemic at high altitude. Iron-deficiency anemia related to menstrual bleeding is common in women. If this is recognized, it should be corrected under the supervision of a physician with administration of ferrous sulfate 300 mg per day; note that a side effect is constipation.

A pregnant woman who wishes to travel to high altitude should be certain that she has a normal pregnancy (e.g., normal blood pressure, no abnormal bleeding, placenta in proper position as determined by ultrasound if necessary). There is a possible increased risk for dangerous hypertension associated with pregnancy (preeclampsia) at high altitude. Proper acclimatization is essential. Try to keep the sleeping altitude no higher than 10,000 ft (3048 m) and never above 12,000 ft (3658 m). If a woman has a complicated pregnancy in which her obstetrician has advised caution or restrictions beyond those associated with a normal pregnancy, she should not hike higher than an altitude of 12,000 ft (3658 m).

Regarding children at high altitude, don't bring children younger than 4 to 6 weeks of age to high altitude. Infants who required supplemental oxygen during the neonatal period are at particular risk for high-altitude illness. Avoid traveling to altitude with children who have suffered recent viral infection or situations associated with high pressure in the lungs' vascular system. Children with trisomy 21 are more prone to HAPE than are those with normal chromosomes. Physical fitness, while desirable for mountaineering, does not protect against high-altitude illness. It is, of course, good to be in excellent physical condition, but this does not substitute in any way for proper acclimatization.

In terms of preexisting conditions and the risk for high-altitude illness, here are some other general guidelines:

Probably no extra risk: Extremes of age, obesity, diabetes, stable condition (e.g., no ongoing angina) after coronary artery bypass surgery, mild chronic obstructive pulmonary disease (COPD), controlled asthma, normal (low-risk) pregnancy, controlled high blood pressure, controlled seizure disorder, psychiatric disorder, cancer, inflammatory diseases

Caution: Moderate COPD, congestive heart failure, sleep apnea, worrisome irregular heart rhythms, recurrent episodes of angina, sickle cell trait, cerebrovascular diseases, abnormal lung circulation, uncontrolled seizure disorder, radial keratotomy

High risk: Sickle cell anemia with history of crises, severe COPD, pulmonary hypertension, poorly controlled congestive heart failure

Persons with preexisting neurologic conditions may have stable or unstable (worsening or improving) situations. Persons with unstable conditions should not travel to high altitude, because resultant low blood oxygen levels may impair or prevent recovery from the condition.

Absolute contraindications to active (e.g., trekking or climbing) or passive (e.g., motorized vehicle transport) ascent are an unstable condition, high risk for a repeat stroke, or a transient ischemic attack (TIA, see page 136) within the past 90 days. Persons with a residual "central" neurologic deficit (e.g., from a stroke) or peripheral (e.g., from multiple sclerosis or severe diabetic neuropathy) deficit should not actively ascend, but they may passively ascend. Relative contraindications (speak to your physician for advice) include a severe narrowing or occlusion of a cerebral artery, space-occupying lesion (e.g., brain tumor), poorly controlled seizure disorder, or cerebral aneurysm (dilated blood vessel that might leak or burst). Any person who has suffered a stroke should consult with his physician to determine whether or not a high-altitude sojourn should be allowed, and if so, if antiplatelet (anti–blood clotting) therapy should be started. Persons with dementia should be watched very closely for increase in impairment. Preexisting headaches are not a contraindication for a trip to high altitude.

If a person suffers from any chronic condition, he should clear travel of an extreme nature (high altitude, cold, hot, exertion) with a physician and become educated on potential problems and solutions.

HIGH-ALTITUDE PULMONARY EDEMA

Pulmonary edema is excess fluid in the lungs, either in the lung tissue itself or in the space normally used for gas exchange (oxygen for carbon dioxide). Fluid in the lungs renders them unable to perform their normal task, and thus the victim cannot get enough oxygen.

High-altitude pulmonary edema (HAPE) usually occurs in an unacclimatized individual—typically a male—who rapidly ascends to an altitude that exceeds 8000 ft (2438 m), particularly if heavy exertion is involved. Prior traditional physical conditioning is not protective; many cases involve young, previously healthy individuals. If the victim exercises above 8000 ft (2438 m) but sleeps at a lower altitude (such as 6000 ft, or 1829 m), his risk for developing HAPE is much less.

Symptoms begin 1 to 3 days after arrival at high altitude. They include shortness of breath (very worrisome if it occurs at rest), cough, weakness, easy fatigue (especially when walking uphill), and difficulty sleeping. Signs of AMS (see page 312) are often present. As greater amounts of fluid accumulate in the lungs, the victim develops drowsiness, severe shortness of breath, and rapid heart rate; his initial dry and gentle ("soft") cough produces white phlegm and then blood (pink, frothy sputum—a late sign); he exhibits confusion and cyanosis (bluish discoloration of the skin, particularly noticeable in the nail beds and lips). If you place an ear to the victim's chest, you may hear crackling or gurgling noises. The symptoms worsen at night. Rapidly, the victim becomes extremely agitated, disoriented, and sweaty; he is in obvious extreme respiratory distress. Confusion, collapse, and coma follow. The victim may show a fever of up to 101.3° F (38.5° C).

As soon as the earliest signs of HAPE are present, the victim should be evacuated (carried, if necessary) to a lower altitude at which there were previously no symptoms. Such warning signs include rapid heart rate (greater than 90 to 100 beats per minute at rest), weakness, shortness of breath, cough, difficulty walking, inability to keep up, and poor judgment. Maximum rest is advised.

The definitive treatments are descent and administration of oxygen; if it is available, oxygen at a flow rate of 4 to 6 liters per minute should be administered by face mask (see page 405). Improvement is rarely noted until oxygen is administered or descent of at least 1000 to 2000 ft (305 to 610 m) is accomplished. Attempt to descend at least 3000 ft (914 m). If the victim improves, diminish the flow rate of oxygen to 2 to 4 liters per minute to conserve supplies.

In no case should a victim be left to descend by himself. Always have a healthy person accompany him. If the victim must be carried down, he should be kept in a sitting position, if possible. Keep him warm.

Have the victim inhale albuterol or salmeterol from a metered-dose inhaler according to the directions. Administration of fluid pills (diuretics) is controversial and should be done only under strict medical supervision, as should administration of morphine.

Some aid stations in high-altitude regions are equipped with an inflatable pressure bag (such as a "Gamow bag") large enough to enclose a human. This is used to simulate conditions at lower altitude and may be used to treat moderate or severe high-altitude illness. The cylinder-shaped Gamow container is a small, portable hyperbaric chamber that can be pressurized with a foot pump to 2 lb (0.9 kg) per square inch, which simulates a descent of approximately 5248 ft (1600 m); the exact equivalent of descent depends on the altitude at which the bag is deployed. The victim should be placed in the bag for 2 to 6 hours. In addition, oxygen from a tank can be administered to the victim by face mask (see page 405) within the bag. If a Gamow-type bag is used, note that foot pumping to keep it inflated must usually be continuous, so it's wise to recruit additional rescuers.

A drug that physicians are using successfully to treat HAPE is nifedipine, which lowers obstructive pressure in the pulmonary arterial circulation (which carries deoxygenated blood from the heart through the lungs). The first dose is 10 mg chewed and then swallowed. This is followed by 10 mg every 4 to 6 hours, or 30 mg sustained-release preparation every 12 hours (or 20 mg extended-release every 8 hours). The dose in children for HAPE is 0.5 mg/kg (2.2. lb) of body weight (to a maximum dose of 10 mg) by mouth every 8 hours. Since this drug is also used to treat high blood pressure, a side effect can be low blood pressure and dizziness, particularly if the victim is dehydrated. These particular side effects seem to be minimal when the sustained-release preparation is used. Sildenafil (Viagra) 50 mg by mouth every 8 hours, or tadalafil (Cialis) 10 mg by mouth every 12 hours, has been used to treat HAPE, because of its effect on lowering pressure in part of the circulation within the lungs. These drugs may also be used to prevent HAPE in persons with a history of this condition.

Nifedipine has also been used successfully to prevent HAPE in subjects with a history of repeated episodes. The dose for prevention is 20 mg of the sustained-release preparation every 8 hours or 30 mg of the sustained-release preparation every 12 hours. Other drugs that have been suggested for prevention include tadalafil 10 mg every 12 hours, sildenafil 50 mg every 8 hours, and inhaled salmeterol 125 µg by inhalation twice a day (in conjunction with oral medication; not to be used alone for prevention). Dexamethasone in a dose of 4 mg every 6 hours, or 8 mg twice a day, has been suggested to prevent HAPE, particularly in persons with a history of this condition, but this awaits further validation.

Once a victim has been judged to suffer from any degree of HAPE, he should no longer be a candidate for high-altitude travel until cleared by a physician. Such a precaution does not include routine jet airplane transportation.

HIGH-ALTITUDE CEREBRAL EDEMA

High-altitude cerebral edema (HACE) is the medical term for a disorder (theoretically linked to brain swelling) that involves an alteration of mental status seen at high altitude, related to diminished atmospheric oxygen. It may be present in someone who has worsened from acute mountain sickness (see below) or who is suffering from HAPE. When HACE occurs, it is often after two or more days at an altitude of 13,123 ft (4000 m) or more. Symptoms include headache (often throbbing), difficulty walking (loss of balance, inability to walk a straight line, staggering, or frank inability to walk), clumsiness, confusion, amnesia, difficulty in speaking, drowsiness, vomiting, mild fever, and, in severe cases, blurred vision, blindness, unconsciousness, paralysis, and/or coma. Other symptoms may include mood changes, hallucinations, paralysis of an arm and/or leg, and seizures (rare). Victims are often gray or pale in appearance. Imbalance or the inability to walk heel to toe in a straight line is a very worrisome sign and should prompt immediate action to treat the victim. An extremely drowsy person may slip rapidly into a coma. "High-altitude headache" is often the first noxious symptom noted on exposure to high altitude, and may be the harbinger of AMS (see later).

Treatment for HACE is immediate descent to an altitude below one at which the victim previously had no symptoms, and administration of oxygen at a flow rate of 5 to 10 liters per minute by face mask or nasal cannula (tube) (see page 405). Attempt to descend at least 3000 ft (914 m).

If the victim becomes severely ill, he should be brought (carried, if necessary, and preferably in the sitting position) to a lower altitude (below 5000 ft, or 1524 m). In addition, administration of the steroid drug dexamethasone (Decadron) 8 mg first dose, and then 4 mg every 6 hours until descent is accomplished, may be helpful. The pediatric dose of dexamethasone is 0.3 mg/kg (2.2 lb) of body weight for the first dose, followed by 0.15 mg/kg every 6 hours. Again, *never leave a potentially seriously ill person to fend for himself.* A victim of HACE or HAPE can deteriorate rapidly, and most will need to be transported down the mountain. As with HAPE, a Gamow bag can be used for treatment. Because the early symptoms of acute mountain sickness (see later) and HACE are similar, pay close attention to the condition of ill members of your climbing party.

ACUTE MOUNTAIN SICKNESS

Acute mountain sickness (AMS) is the most common high altitude–related disorder. It affects persons who ascend to altitudes above 8200 ft (2500 m) from below 4921 ft (1500 m) and are unable to keep pace with acclimatization. A person who is partially acclimatized may be stricken if he ascends rapidly to a higher altitude, overexerts, or uses sleep medication (which can be a respiratory depressant). Symptoms may start within 2 hours after arrival at altitude and rarely begin after 48 hours at a given altitude. They may be quite subtle in the beginning and are most commonly headache (in its mildest form sometimes called "high-altitude headache") of a throbbing nature, followed in incidence by fatigue, dizziness, and loss of appetite. The headache may be global, located on both sides of the head or in the back of the head; made worse by simultaneously straining and holding one's breath; or when bending over. Other symptoms include insomnia, poor appetite, nausea, vomiting, drowsiness, dizziness, lightheadedness, weakness, fatigue, poor sleep, and loss of motivation or apathy. Some people have described the suffering associated with AMS as similar to a hangover. Children are prone to nausea and vomiting as a manifestation of AMS, as well as fussiness, lack of playfulness, poor appetite, and poor sleep. The lips and fingernails may have a blue discoloration (cyanosis) if HAPE is present.

The most common and disabling symptom of AMS is headache that typically occurs on the second or third day at high altitude and may be complicated by difficulty in walking (particularly if HAPE is present) and impaired memory. The headache is mild to severe and as described earlier. Mild symptoms of HACE accompany AMS; they include decreased appetite, mood swings, and lack of interest in activity. Some victims complain of a deep inner chill. AMS is sometimes mistaken for a viral illness, such as the flu, or exhaustion or dehydration. Lassitude may be so severe that the victim is too apathetic to contribute to his or her own basic needs. The symptoms of AMS may be confused with dehydration, exhaustion, bacterial or viral infection, hypothermia, carbon monoxide poisoning, migraine headache, low blood sugar, transient ischemic attack or stroke, illicit drug ingestion, or psychiatric disease.

One hallmark of AMS, known as periodic breathing, is an alteration of the normal sleeping pattern. Sleep is fitful, with periods of wakefulness or disturbing dreams. The pattern of breathing becomes irregular, such that the sleeper has periods of rapid breathing (very deep breaths) alternated with periods of no breathing. The latter can be quite startling to the casual observer—intervals of 10 seconds may pass without a breath. Acetazolamide, 125 mg at bedtime, diminishes periodic breathing, improves oxygenation, and is safe to use as a sleeping aid. Insomnia from other causes may respond to short-acting drugs for sleep, such as zolpidem (Ambien) 5 to 10 mg, zaleplon (Sonata) 5 to 10 mg, triazolam (Halcion) 0.125 mg, or temazepam (Restoril) 10 to 15 mg. As mentioned previously, these medications must be used with extreme caution in a person who is suffering incipient AMS, because any amount of respiratory depression might lead to decreased oxygenation. Also, sleep medication may mask the symptoms of HACE.

Treatment for AMS includes rest, adequate fluid intake to avoid dehydration, and mild pain medicine for the headache. Oxygen administration (0.5 to 1.5 liters per minute by nasal cannula or simple open face mask) may be effective for the headache, as might be acetaminophen or an

NSAID. The victim may be led to a lower altitude, preferably at least 1640 to 3281 ft (500 to 1000 m) below that where symptoms began. This should be done particularly when the victim is felt to suffer from severe AMS. However, many victims of AMS will adjust to the current altitude in a period from 12 hours to 3 to 4 days, and therefore may remain at a stable altitude if symptoms are mild. *In no case should a person attempt to climb to (or, particularly, sleep at) a higher altitude until the symptoms of AMS have completely subsided.* If symptoms worsen appreciably while a person remains at rest at a constant altitude, descent is indicated. Attempt to descend at least 1500 ft (457 m). The goal is to descend to lowest reasonable possible altitude. With mild AMS, acetazolamide (Diamox) can be administered in a dose of 250 mg by mouth every 12 hours until symptoms diminish. The dose in children is 2.5 mg/kg (2.2 lb) of body weight every 12 hours, up to 250 mg per dose.

Prochlorperazine (Compazine) 10 mg by mouth or 25 mg by suppository can be given for nausea and vomiting, with the added benefit that it may stimulate the beneficial ventilatory (breathing) response that is triggered by a low oxygen content in the blood (associated with high altitude and called the "hypoxic ventilatory response"). The dose in children older than 2 years of age is 0.4 mg/kg (2.2 lb) of body weight per day, by mouth or by oral suppository, in three or four divided doses. Promethazine (Phenergan) is fine as an alternative for adults, in a dose of 25 to 50 mg by mouth or suppository. Another effective drug is ondansetron (Zofran) 4 mg oral dissolving tablet. Aspirin, acetaminophen, or ibuprofen may be given for headache. Avoid the use of alcohol or other respiratory depressants. Minimize physical exertion.

If an oxygen cylinder is available (see page 405), low-flow (0.5 to 2 liters per minute) oxygen by nasal cannula (tube) or face mask is particularly effective if used for sleep. This alone may be adequate to halt the progression of mild AMS and allow a victim to acclimatize without descent to a lower altitude. However, if this approach is taken, the victim should not be left alone until all symptoms of AMS have resolved. The victim who spends a few hours in a hyperbaric chamber, which simulates descent, will notice diminution of symptoms and benefit from hastened acclimatization. The "Gamow bag" hyperbaric bag, and other similar lightweight fabric pressure bags, are inflated by manual air pumps. Inflation at 2 lb per square inch is roughly equivalent to a descent of 5249 ft (1600 m). A few hours of pressurization may have noticeable beneficial effect lasting for many hours. To completely eliminate AMS, it's sometimes necessary to remain in the bag for 6 hours.

If AMS is moderate to severe and certainly if there is reason to suspect that HACE is developing (the victim wishes to be left alone or is becoming confused, cannot perform simple tasks such as eating and dressing, is vomiting, and cannot walk a straight line), administer dexamethasone as previously recommended for HACE. AMS can progress to HACE with coma in less than 24 hours.

As noted previously, dexamethasone is used by some climbers to prevent AMS. Dexamethasone should not be used for routine prevention, because it does not enhance acclimatization, but rather, masks symptoms. It may be useful for persons who are performing a rapid ascent and who cannot tolerate acetazolamide, but with extreme caution, as it does nothing to prevent HAPE and if descent is delayed and dexamethasone discontinued, the rebound effect can cause rapid onset of severe AMS or HACE. It may be used to treat AMS in an adult dose of 8 mg by mouth first dose, then 4 mg every 6 hours. It should optimally be used for no more than 48 hours, during which time descent should be undertaken, from where acclimatization may proceed. A person should not ascend until he or she is asymptomatic and not taking dexamethasone. At that point, if reascent is attempted, strong consideration should be given to using acetazolamide at an adult dose of 250 mg by mouth twice a day.

Ginkgo biloba administered in a dose of 80 to 100 mg by mouth twice a day has been suggested to reduce the incidence of AMS, and perhaps to be helpful as a therapy. Choose a commercial product that has a validated amount of active ingredient(s).

Untreated, AMS may resolve spontaneously within approximately 3 days. If symptoms of AMS worsen despite 24 hours of additional acclimatization and/or treatment, have the victim descend immediately to a lower altitude. A reasonable descent is a minimum of 1640 to 3281 ft (500 to 1000 m). The goal is to descend to lowest reasonable possible altitude.

OTHER DISORDERS OF HIGH ALTITUDE

High-Altitude Headache

The first unpleasant symptom of high-altitude exposure is often headache, which may or may not be a prelude to AMS (which would be accompanied by nausea, vomiting, fatigue, dizziness, or difficulty sleeping). It may be effectively treated with an NSAID, acetaminophen, or aspirin, and has been effectively treated with the drugs used to prevent AMS (acetazolamide and dexamethasone), or oxygen inhalation at low flow rates (0.5 to 2 L/min by nasal cannula). High-altitude headache may be confused with migraine headache (see page 160), which would be better treated with antimigraine medication (such as sumatriptan [Imitrex]). If headache is present at high altitude, it should be presumed to be a high-altitude headache and the victim not allowed to ascend further until the headache is completely gone.

Fluid Retention

Swelling of the face, hands, and feet may occur after 4 to 10 days at increased altitude. Women are more commonly affected than are men, and they note puffiness of the hands, feet, eyelids, and face, particularly in the morning after a night's sleep or just before a menstrual period. Ten or more pounds (4.5 kg) can be gained in fluid retention. The swelling persists for 1 to 3 days after return to lower altitude, and then spontaneously disappears (increased urination is noted at this time). The disorder is a nuisance, but of no real medical hazard. Salt intake should be controlled so as not to be excessive. Avoid fluid pills (diuretics), which promote dehydration and rarely reduce the swelling to any significant degree. These should be used only in the absence of AMS under the supervision of trained medical personnel. A person who retains fluid at high altitude should be examined for signs and symptoms of HACE and HAPE.

Visual Changes after Radial Keratotomy

Visual changes may occur at high altitude in persons who have undergone radial keratotomy, in which 4 to 8 incisions are made in the cornea to cure nearsightedness. Perhaps because the cornea is now not as strong, or for other reasons yet to be determined, there may be a significant farsighted shift and corneal flattening, which cause blurred vision. This does not appear to be the case following photorefractive keratectomy or laser-assisted in situ keratomileusis (LASIK). A person who has undergone radial keratotomy should consider carrying "plus" glasses or goggles to correct an unexpected condition of farsighted vision.

High-Altitude Flatus Expulsion

High-altitude flatus expulsion (HAFE) is the spontaneous and unwelcome passage of increased quantities of rectal gas noted at high altitude. It may become an embarrassment but is of no true medical concern. Avoid foods such as chili and beans that are known to induce flatulence at low altitudes, and show consideration for other members of the party in sleeping arrangements. If stricken, a traveler may benefit from chewable tablets of simethicone (Mylicon 80 mg) or simethicone 80 mg with activated charcoal 250 mg (Flatulex tablets) once or twice a day. Charcoal Plus is another simethicone-activated charcoal preparation.

Altitude Throat

Altitude throat (pharyngitis) is a sore throat caused by nasal congestion and mouth breathing during exertion at high altitudes. Because the air is dry and cold, the protective mucous coating of the throat is dried out and the throat becomes extremely irritated, with redness and pain. In general, this can be distinguished from a bacterial or viral infection (see page 181) by the absence of fever, swollen lymph glands in the neck, or systemic symptoms (fatigue, muscle aches, sweats, and the like). Prevention is difficult and treatment is only mildly satisfying. The victim should keep his throat moist by sipping liquids and sucking on throat lozenges or hard candies (Life Savers, for instance). As soon as convenient, nighttime breathing of warm humidified air should be instituted. Avoid anesthetic gargles, since they will mask the signs of a true infection. If the inside of the nose becomes dried out, this may be treated with topical ointment (e.g., bacitracin, mupirocin, or petroleum jelly).

High-Altitude Bronchitis and Cough

Most bronchitis has an infectious cause (see page 192). High-altitude bronchitis is more likely to be caused by relative hyperventilation of cold, dry air. This causes the secretions in the respiratory passages to thicken. The resulting airway irritation causes a persistent cough, which can cause coughing fits sufficiently severe to lead to broken ribs. Treatment consists of humidification of inspired air, which can be accomplished transiently by cautiously breathing steam, and over the longer term by breathing through a porous scarf or balaclava that allows retention of moisture and heat. High-altitude cough has been treated successfully empirically by inhalation of an inhaled fluticasone propionate–salmeterol (steroid-bronchodilator) combination drug (Advair Diskus).

Snow Blindness

See page 174.

SNAKEBITE

POISONOUS SNAKES

Two types of poisonous snakes are indigenous to the United States: pit vipers (rattlesnake, cottonmouth [water moccasin], copperhead) and coral snakes. Their distributions are as follows:

Northeast: Cottonmouth, copperhead, timber rattlesnake

Southeast: Cottonmouth, copperhead, eastern diamondback rattlesnake, pygmy rattlesnake, eastern coral snake

Central: Cottonmouth, copperhead, massasauga rattlesnake, timber rattlesnake, prairie rattlesnake

Southwest: Cottonmouth, copperhead, pygmy rattlesnake, massasauga rattlesnake, northern black-tailed rattlesnake, prairie rattlesnake, sidewinder, Mojave rattlesnake, western diamondback rattlesnake, red diamondback rattlesnake, Texas coral snake, Sonoran coral snake

Pacific Coast: Northern Pacific rattlesnake, southern Pacific rattlesnake, Great Basin rattlesnake, western diamondback rattlesnake, red diamondback rattlesnake, sidewinder, Mojave rattlesnake

In the United States, 98% of venomous bites are from pit vipers. In addition, many "nonvenomous" species, such as colubrid (rear-fanged) snakes (including the red-neck keelback), are capable of producing venomous bites. There are no indigenous venomous snakes in Hawaii or Alaska.

Pit vipers are typified by rattlesnakes, which have a characteristic triangular head, vertical elliptical pupils ("cat's eyes"), two elongated and hinged fangs in the front part of the jaw, heat-sensing (infrared-sensing) facial pits on the sides of the head midway between and below the level of the eyes and the nostrils, a single row of scales on the underbelly leading to the tail (not seen in nonpoisonous snakes, which have a double row of scales on the underbelly), and (often) rattles on the tail (Figure 212). The snake's age and potency of venom are not determined by the number of rattles, since molting may occur up to four times a year. Because fangs are replaced every 6 to 10 weeks in the adult rattlesnake, bites may demonstrate from one to four large puncture marks. An adult pit viper can strike at a speed of 8 ft (2.4 m) per second. The rattlesnake may strike without a preliminary warning rattle.

Coral snakes are characterized by their color pattern, with red, black, and yellow or white bands encircling the body (Figure 213). With the venomous species, the rings completely encircle the body, and every other mid-body ring is yellow (or white). A general rule is "red on yellow (or white)—kill a fellow (venomous); red on black—venom lack (nonvenomous)." This rule applies to coral snakes native to the United States, but does not apply to species in non-U.S. countries. The fangs are very short and fixed; the snakes have round pupils, and they bite with a chewing, rather than striking, action. They also may have a double row of scales on the underbelly.

A three-step identification method has been proposed to recognize dangerous snakes in the United States and Canada. The mid-dorsal (top) scales of native pit vipers have a longitudinal ridge like a keel; these ridged scales can be easily distinguished from smooth scales without

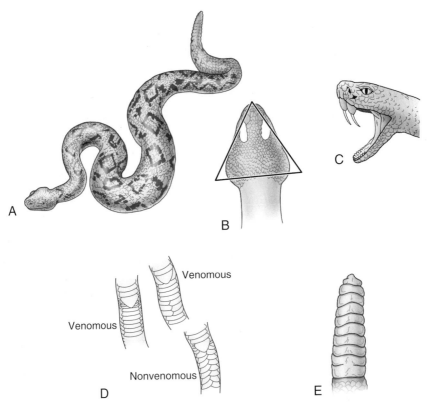

Figure 212. Rattlesnake. **A,** Typical rattlesnake appearance, with features of identification that include triangular head **(B),** hinged fangs **(C),** single row of underbelly scales leading up to the anal plate **(D),** and a rattle on the tail **(E).**

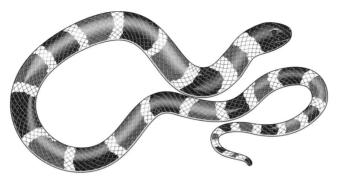

Figure 213. Coral snake.

ridges. As previously noted, all native pit vipers have a single row of scales on the underbelly, while harmless native snakes have a double row of scales on the underbelly. The tree snakes that are exceptions to this rule, in that they are harmless but have a single row of subcaudal scales, also have smooth dorsal scales, indicating that they are not venomous. So, to determine whether a snake is a venomous species, one first asks, "Are scales near the top surface midline keeled? If the answer is "no," then the snake is not dangerous. If the answer is "Yes," then the question is asked, "Are most of the underbelly scales in a single row?" If the answer is 'No,' then the snake is not dangerous. If the answer is "Yes," then the snake is dangerous. Rattlesnakes have both ridged dorsal scales and a single row of underbelly scales, but it is entirely reasonable to forego inspection when a rattle is obviously present.

For venomous coral snakes in the United States, the rings completely encircle the body, and every other mid-body ring is yellow or white. So, to determine a venomous species, one first asks, "Is every other mid-body ring yellow or white?" If the answer is "No," then the snake is not dangerous. If the answer is "Yes," then the question is asked, "Do all three colors completely encircle the body, including across the belly?" If the answer is "No," then the snake is not dangerous. If the answer is "Yes," then the snake is dangerous.

Signs of Envenomation

Most snakebites don't result in envenomation, because the snake does not release venom, the skin is not penetrated, or the venom is not potent. Therefore, it's important to recognize the signs of envenomation, in order to avoid needless worry, evacuation, and improper therapy.

The most common signs of envenomation are as follows:

Pit Vipers

1. One or more fang marks. Most snakebites (venomous and nonvenomous) will demonstrate rows of markings from the teeth. In the case of venomous snakes, there will be one to four larger distinct markings from the elongated fangs that inoculate the victim with venom (Figure 214). Venomous snakebite wounds tend to bleed more freely than bites from animals and insects.
2. Burning pain at the site of the bite. *This may not be present with the bite of the Mojave rattlesnake.*
3. Swelling at the site of the bite. This usually begins within 5 to 10 minutes of envenomation and may become quite severe. *This may not be present with the bite of the Mojave rattlesnake.*
4. Numbness and tingling of the lips, face, fingers, toes, and scalp 30 to 60 minutes after the bite. This can also be present if the victim hyperventilates with fear and excitement (see page 278). If a victim of a snakebite has immediate symptoms, these are likely to be due to hyperventilation.

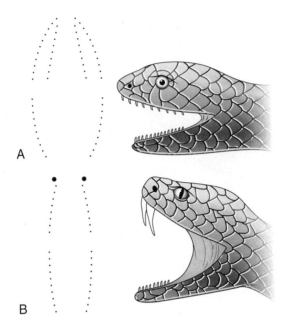

Figure 214. Snakebite patterns. **A,** Nonvenomous snake. **B,** Venomous snake.

5. Twitching of the mouth, face, neck, eye, and bitten extremity muscles 30 to 90 minutes after the bite.
6. Rubbery or metallic taste in the mouth 30 to 90 minutes after the bite.
7. Sweating, weakness, nausea, vomiting, and fainting 1 to 2 hours after the bite. Additional symptoms include chest tightness, rapid breathing rate (20 to 25 breaths per minute), rapid heart rate (125 to 175 beats per minute), palpitations, headache, chills, and confusion.
8. Bruising at the site of the bite. This usually begins within 2 to 3 hours. Large blood blisters may develop within 6 to 10 hours. The risk of developing bleeding after a rattlesnake bite is greater in persons who take anticoagulant medications ("blood thinners").
9. Difficulty breathing, increased bleeding (bruising, bloody urine, bloody bowel movements, vomiting blood), and collapse 6 to 12 hours after the bite.

Coral Snakes
1. Burning pain at the site of the bite may be present or absent. There is generally very little local swelling or bruising, and certainly much less than that seen with the bite of a pit viper.
2. Numbness and/or weakness of a bitten arm or leg within 90 minutes.
3. Twitching, nervousness, drowsiness, giddiness, increased salivation, and drooling in 1 to 3 hours. Vomiting may occur.
4. Slurred speech, double vision, difficulty talking and swallowing, and impaired breathing within 5 to 10 hours.
5. Death from heart and lung failure.

Treatment of Snakebite

If a person is bitten by a snake that could be poisonous, act swiftly. *The definitive treatment for serious snake venom poisoning is administration of antivenom. The most important aspect of therapy is to get the victim to an appropriate medical facility as quickly as possible.*

1. Don't panic. Most bites, even by venomous snakes, don't result in medically significant envenomations. Reassure the victim and keep him from acting in an energy-consuming,

purposeless fashion. If the victim has been envenomed, increased physical activity may increase his illness by hastening the spread of venom. If the victim is hyperventilating from fear, manage according to the instructions on page 278. For pit vipers, signs and symptoms that seem to portend more difficulty in initially diminishing the adverse clinical effects using antivenom (and therefore should encourage prompt evacuation to medical attention) are increased bleeding, neurologic symptoms, or a severe bite (as judged by the combination of progressive swelling and pain, and the presence of more than two other venom effects as listed previously.

2. Retreat out of the striking range of the snake, which for safety's sake should be considered to be the snake's body length (for pit vipers, it is actually approximately half the body length). A rattlesnake can strike at a speed of 8 ft (2.4 m) per second.

3. Locate the snake. If possible, identify the species. If you cannot do this with confidence (which is really only important for the Mojave rattlesnake and coral snake), photograph the snake using a digital camera. Don't attempt to capture or kill the snake, for fear of wasting time and perhaps provoking another bite. Never delay transport of the victim to capture a snake. If the snake is dead, take care to handle it with a very long stick or shovel, and to carry the dead animal in a container that will not allow the head of the snake to bite another victim (the jaws can bite in a reflex action for up to 90 minutes after death). If you aren't sure how to collect the snake, it's best just to get away from it.

4. If materials are readily available, a splint may be fashioned to fit the bitten body part, to avoid unnecessary motion. Allow room for swelling within the splint. Maintain the bitten arm or leg in a position of comfort. Remove tight clothing and in particular any jewelry, which could become an inadvertent tourniquet. If a person needs to walk to get to medical attention, then a splint on the leg may be impractical. Don't waste time making a fancy arm splint—a sling will suffice. Some snakebite authorities are ambivalent about splinting, so if it can't be done, it's probably not a big problem.

5. Transport the victim to the nearest hospital. If you are alone, walk—don't run—toward help. If you travel for a few hours and nothing happens other than a bit of pain and swelling, then the prognosis is probably good. If you are so far away from help that walking for a few hours isn't going to accomplish anything, you may wish to stay put and conserve your strength. If there is any chance that the envenomation is significant, seek medical attention as soon as possible, so that antivenom can be administered under the guidance of a qualified health professional.

6. *Don't apply ice directly to the wound or immerse the part in ice water.* An ice pack placed over the wound (as one would do for a sprain) is of no proven value to retard absorption of venom, but may be useful for pain control. Application of extreme cold can cause an injury similar to frostbite, and possibly lead to enough tissue loss to require amputation.

7. *The impression of most snakebite experts is that incision and suction are of no value and should be abandoned.* It appears that little venom can actually be removed from the bite site. Furthermore, the incision may set the stage for inoculation of bacteria, infection, and a poorly healing wound. Mouth contact with the incision may cause a nasty infection that leaves a noticeable scar; there is also the risk of transmission of blood-borne disease to the rescuer.

8. Application of the Sawyer Extractor Pump (Sawyer Products) is not recommended. There is no evidence that the device can remove venom, and there is reason to believe that by using the device for a rattlesnake bite, it might cause concentration of tissue-toxic venom under the suction cup, leading to a more severe local reaction.

9. If the victim is more than 2 hours from medical attention, and the bite is on an arm or leg, one may use the pressure immobilization technique (Figure 215): Place a 2 inch × 2 inch (5 cm × 5 cm) cloth pad (¼ inch, or 0.6 cm, thick) over the bite and apply an elastic wrap

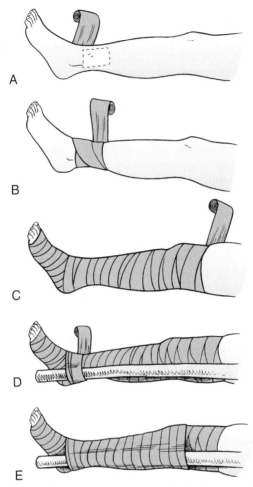

Figure 215. The pressure immobilization technique. **A,** Begin to wrap the limb directly over the bite site with an elastic bandage. The dotted square outlines a pad that may be placed over the bite site. **B,** Continue wrapping up the limb. **C,** Wrapped limb. **D,** Begin to apply a splint. **E,** Wrapped and splinted limb.

firmly around the involved limb directly over the padded bite site with a margin of at least 4 to 6 inches (10 to 15 cm) on either side of the wound, taking care to check for adequate circulation in the fingers and toes (normal pulses, feeling, and color). An alternative method is to simply wrap the entire limb at the described tightness with an elastic bandage. The wrap is meant to impede absorption of venom into the general circulation by containing it within the compressed tissue and microscopic blood and lymphatic vessels near the limb surface. You should then splint the limb to prevent motion. If the bite is on a hand or an arm, also apply a sling. Keep the bandage in place until the victim is at a medical facility and antivenom is being infused. Until that occurs, check at least once an hour to be certain that pulses are present. It should be noted that as is the case for splinting, use of the pressure immobilization technique is somewhat controversial, in that certain experts believe that it is not particularly helpful, and that localizing venom in a single area might even lead to an increased chance for tissue damage.

An alternative to the pressure immobilization technique is a constriction band (*not* a tourniquet) wrapped a few inches closer to the heart than the bite marks on the bitten limb. This should be applied tightly enough to only occlude the superficial veins and lymph passages. To gauge tightness, the rescuer should be able to slip one or two fingers under the band, and normal arterial pulses should be present. The band may be advanced periodically to stay ahead of the swelling. It is of questionable usefulness if 30 minutes have intervened between the time of the bite and application of the constriction band (or pressure immobilization technique). Again, this recommendation is controversial, for the reasons mentioned in the previous paragraph.

10. Have the victim drink liquids to encourage proper hydration. However, "snakebite medicine" (whiskey) is of no value and may actually be harmful if it increases circulation to the skin.
11. There is no scientific evidence that electrical shocks applied to snakebites are of any value. On the contrary, there are experiments that refute this concept.
12. The bite wound should be washed vigorously with soap and water. If medical care at a hospital will not occur for 5 or more hours, the victim should be treated with dicloxacillin, erythromycin, or cephalexin for 7 days.
13. If the victim is many hours or days from a hospital, assist him to walk out or arrange for a litter rescue, allowing frequent rest periods and adequate oral hydration. Splinting and positioning (e.g., elevating or lowering) the bitten part are secondary to any effort to reach a facility where antivenom can be administered.
14. Watch for an allergic reaction (see page 64) caused by the snakebite. This might cause the victim to be short of breath with or without an airway obstruction from swelling of the mouth, tongue, and throat. Once the victim is in the hospital, the severity of envenomation will be ascertained, and the victim treated with antivenom if necessary. The criteria that doctors in the United States use to treat with antivenom are worsening tissue injury, systemic symptoms (e.g., low blood pressure or difficulty breathing), or abnormal blood clotting tests. Antivenom therapy must be carried out under the supervision of a physician, because serious allergic reactions to antivenoms are possible, although with modern antivenom products, only about 10% of recipients suffer allergic (immediate or delayed) manifestations.

Dogs also may be bitten by poisonous snakes (see page 500).

Avoidance of Poisonous Snakes

1. Know the behavior and habitats of snakes in your area. Avoid the known habitats of poisonous snakes, such as rocky ledges and woodpiles.
2. Don't reach into areas that you cannot visually examine first. Walk on clearly marked trails, and use a walking stick to move suspicious objects. Don't reach blindly behind rocks. In flooded areas, avoid touching tree limbs and brush.
3. Wear adequate protective clothing, particularly loose-fitting bloused trousers and boots to cover your feet and lower legs. Even tightly worn pants, such as denim, may provide a certain amount of benefit in terms of the amount of venom injected by a snake into a victim.
4. Never hike alone in snake territory. Carry an elastic wrap and a SAM Splint (see page 70).
5. Avoid hiking at night in snake territory. Carry a flashlight and walking stick.
6. Don't handle snakes unless you know what you're doing. Some authorities mention that a defensive bite by a snake may release more venom than an offensive (feeding) bite. You can be bitten and envenomed by seemingly dead or nonvenomous snakes. Stay at least one body length away from a snake.

NONPOISONOUS SNAKES

Many snakes (e.g., the gopher snake and king snake) are nonvenomous and don't create serious medical problems with a bite. However, identifying a snake from the bite puncture wounds is often extremely difficult for the amateur. Unless the snake can be positively identified as a non-venomous species, the victim should be considered to have been bitten by a poisonous snake and managed appropriately. The snake may be very carefully captured or photographed for identification (see page 319). If the snake is absolutely known to be nonvenomous, the wound should be washed vigorously with soap and water, and the victim treated with dicloxacillin, erythromycin, or cephalexin.

Gila Monster and Mexican Beaded Lizard

The Gila monster *(Heloderma suspectum)* and Mexican beaded lizard *(H. horridum)*, which can grow to 14 inches (35 cm) long, are found in the Great Sonoran Desert area of southern Arizona and northwestern Mexico. They possess grooved teeth and venom glands. Most envenomations occur when an animal bites and holds on, or when a tooth is shed into the bite wound. If the Gila monster holds on, the grip may need to be loosened by mechanical means or incision of the jaw muscles.

Symptoms of an envenomation include burning pain at the site of the bite, swelling of the bite wound, red or blue discoloration, nausea and vomiting, weakness, anxiety, rapid heart rate, and sweating. Low blood pressure is the most serious complication. Intense pain from the bite may last for 3 to 5 hours, and then subside after 8 hours.

The wound should be washed vigorously and all pieces of teeth removed. The victim should have his arm or leg splinted and should be transported to a hospital. Severe reactions are unusual; most victims recover uneventfully. Be prepared to treat the victim for shock (see page 58). Don't administer alcohol, stimulants, or narcotic pain medicines. Don't apply ice directly to the wound or immerse a bitten limb in ice water.

If it will be more than 24 hours before you can reach medical care, administer an antibiotic (cephalexin, erythromycin, or amoxicillin-clavulanate).

INSECT AND ARTHROPOD BITES

BEES, SPIDERS, SCORPIONS, AND OTHER SMALL BITERS

Bees, Wasps, Hornets, and Ants

This group of insects includes honeybees, bumblebees, wasps, hornets, and yellow jackets; each possesses a stinger, which is used to introduce venom into the victim. Most stings occur on the head, neck, arms, and legs.

"Killer bees" are an Africanized race of honeybees created by interbreeding of the African honeybee *Apis mellifera scutellata* (originally brought for experiments into Brazil) with common European honeybees. The hazard from these bees is that they tend to be more irritable, sense threats at farther distances than do their European counterparts, swarm more readily, defend their nests more aggressively and stay agitated around the nest for days, and impose mass attacks on humans. The venom of an Africanized bee is not of greater volume or potency than that of a European honeybee. However, the personality of the Africanized bees is such that they may pursue a victim for up to ⅔ mile (1 km), and may recruit other attacking bees by up to the thousands. A victim may be stung from 50 to more than 1000 times; it is estimated that 500 stings achieves the lethal threshold. The bees are established in Arizona, New Mexico, and

California, and unfortunately appear to be increasing their habitat as they adapt to colder temperatures.

The sting mechanism for a honeybee is composed of a doubly barbed stinger attached to a venom sac that pumps venom into the victim. When the bee attempts to escape after a sting, the stinger and sac remain in the victim (this kills the bee) and continue to inject venom. Unless the stinger is removed within 30 seconds, the venom sac is usually emptied into the victim. The honeybee can sting only once, whereas a wasp, with a smooth stinger that does not become entrapped, can sting multiple times, as can yellow jackets, hornets, and bumblebees.

Pain from a bee, wasp, or hornet sting is immediate, with rapid swelling, redness, warmth, and itching at the sting site. Blisters may occur. Sometimes the victim will become nauseated, vomit, and/or suffer abdominal cramping and diarrhea. If the person is allergic to the venom, a dangerous reaction may follow within minutes, but occasionally may be delayed by up to several hours. This consists of hives, shortness of breath, difficulty breathing, tongue swelling, weakness, vomiting, low blood pressure, and collapse. People have swallowed bees (undetected in beverage bottles) and sustained stings of the esophagus, which are enormously painful.

A common diagnostic dilemma is whether or not a bee, wasp, or hornet sting has become infected. A sting commonly causes a skin reaction with redness (including streaking along the lines of the lymphatic vessels [see page 223]), swelling, itching, and pain. This is very similar to the appearance of skin that is inflamed by a bacterial infection (cellulitis, see page 222). A wasp sting may also cause blistering with or without "brawny" swelling, which is when the skin feels thickened, warm, and bumpy to the touch. Either a sting or an infection can cause lymph nodes ("glands") that service the affected tissue to become swollen and tender. Therefore, determination of an infection becomes a judgment call. Infection following a sting usually develops 48 to 72 hours after the sting, so if someone has suffered a sting, appears to be improving, and then has his condition deteriorate, infection should be suspected. Fever can be present with a sting or an infection, but is more common with an infection. If the area of skin initially affected by the sting seems to be stable for a few days, then the redness and swelling begins to spread, particularly if there is any reddish streaking traveling up an arm or leg toward the heart, increasing skin warmth, or increasing skin tenderness, an infection may be present. If any liquid leaks from the site of the sting, particularly if it is cloudy or thickened, like pus, suspect an infection.

A severe allergic reaction may follow the sting(s) of a fire (red) ant *Solenopsis invicta*, because it marches along the victim and leaves a trail of small, painful blisters. The fire ant hangs onto the victim's skin with pincers, and then uses a posterior stinger to deliver up to 8 stings while it pivots around. The bites and stings cause itching and swelling. A day or two after the ant bite, the fluid in the blister turns cloudy or white, and a small, sterile pseudo-pustule develops. This may continue to be painful and itch for a week or more. Harvester ants generally produce less severe reactions.

In rare cases, stings from killer bees, fire ants, and certain wasps, particularly if the stings are in large numbers, may cause breakdown of muscle tissue. If this is the case, then the urine will appear very darkened and the victim should be brought promptly to medical attention in order to receive treatments designed to protect the kidneys from pigment (myoglobin) released from the injured muscle cells. If you are in a remote location, keep the victim well hydrated (see page 194).

Treatment for Insect Sting

1. Be prepared to treat a severe allergic reaction (see page 64). If the victim develops hives, shortness of breath, and profound weakness, and appears to be deteriorating, *immediately* administer epinephrine. *Anyone known to have insect allergies who travels in the wilderness should carry epinephrine.* Epinephrine (adrenaline) is injected intramuscularly (see page 444) as an aqueous solution of 1:1000 concentration in a dose of 0.3 to 0.5 mL for an adult and 0.01 mL/kg of body weight for a child (not to exceed 0.3 mL). For weight

estimation, 1 kg equals 2.2 lb. It should be injected into the lateral thigh. If the thigh is obese, whether in an adult or a child, such that the needle might not reach into muscle, then inject into the lower thigh. If obesity is extreme, consider injecting into the mid-calf. The only reason to administer the drug subcutaneously (see page 446) is if the equipment is not available for an intramuscular injection. The drug is available in preloaded syringes in certain allergy kits, which include the EpiPen autoinjector and EpiPen Jr. autoinjector, the Auvi-Q "talking" autoinjector (0.3 mg or 0.15 mg dose), and the Adrenaclick (0.3 mg or 0.15 mg dose). Other devices worldwide are the Jext, Emerade, Allerject, and Anapen. Instructions for use accompany the kits. For dosing purposes, a 0.3 mg autoinjector should be used for adults and children over 66 lb (30 kg) in weight. Children 66 lb and under should be injected with a 0.15 mg autoinjector.

Take particular care to handle preloaded syringes properly, to avoid inadvertent injection into an unintended location, such as a finger or toe. Don't intentionally inject epinephrine into the buttocks or a vein. Epinephrine should not be exposed to heat or sun, but does not need to be kept refrigerated. If clear (liquid) epinephrine turns cloudy or discolored, it should be discarded. When administering an injection, *never* share needles between people.

2. Administer diphenhydramine (Benadryl) by mouth, 50 to 100 mg for an adult and 1 mg/kg (2.2 lb) of body weight for a child. This antihistamine drug may be used by itself for a milder allergic reaction. Topical antihistamine lotions or creams may be beneficial.

3. Stingers or pieces of stingers left in the skin should be removed as soon as possible (Figure 216). It used to be taught that pulling the stinger out with fingers or forceps squeezed more venom into the victim, but this is currently not believed to be true. So, it's better to flick or pull a stinger and venom sac out of the skin of the victim using tweezers or your fingers than to waste precious time searching for a straight-edged object, such as a knife or credit card, to scrape away the stinger. Furthermore, crude scraping runs the risk of breaking off the stinger and leaving it embedded in the skin. An alternative is to try to pull out the stinger, then apply the Extractor device (Figure 217), if it is available, immediately after the sting has occurred.

4. Apply ice packs to the site of the sting.

5. Home topical remedies, such as crushed aspirin, a 20% aluminum salt-containing preparation (including many household antiperspirants), or paste of baking soda or

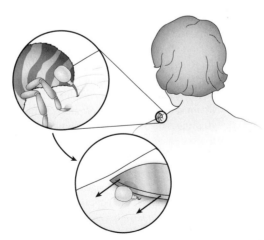

Figure 216. Honeybee sting. Because the venom sac is still attached to the stinger, both should be scraped or pulled free from the skin as soon as possible.

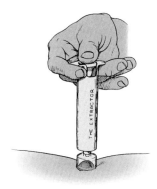

Figure 217. Application of the Extractor to a bee sting.

papain-containing meat tenderizer (such as Adolph's unseasoned meat tenderizer) and water applied directly to the wound (for no more than 15 minutes), are of unproven value. Don't apply mud. The commercial product After Bite (Tender Corporation), a mixture containing ammonia 3.5%, is moderately effective for relief of pain and itching following insect bites, but will not abort an allergic reaction. StingEze liquid (Wisconsin Pharmacal) is a mixture of camphor, phenol, benzocaine, and propylene glycol. StingEze MAX[2] contains twice the benzocaine. StingEze products are good to control itching and mild pain following any insect bite. Lidocaine 4% applied topically may help diminish discomfort.

6. If a person suffers an extensive skin and soft tissue reaction (swelling, itching, blisters), he may benefit from administration of a corticosteroid, such as prednisone (60 mg by mouth day 1, tapered by 10 mg per day over the next 5 days) or methylprednisolone (24 mg by mouth day one, tapered over the next 5 days).

7. If a person stung by an insect develops more than a mild to moderate local reaction, transport him to a hospital.

8. A bee sting in general does not pose a large risk for tetanus infection. Although deep punctures caused by other means deposit bacteria into the wound(s), where *C. tetani* can thrive in the absence of oxygen, a bee sting puncture isn't that deep. However, the stinger might transfer bacteria from the skin surface, wherein lies the greatest risk. To play it safe, if a person has been immunized within the past 5 years, it is unnecessary to get a Td (or Tdap) booster immunization. If it has been more than 5 years but less than 10 years since the last tetanus shot, a Td (or Tdap) booster is indicated. If it has been more than 10 years since the last tetanus shot, both a Td (or Tdap) booster and tetanus immune globulin are indicated, if you go by the book.

9. Fire ant pseudo-pustules should be kept clean and not be unroofed or otherwise disturbed, in order to avoid infection.

Avoidance of Stinging Insects

1. Store garbage, particularly fruit, at a distance from the campsite.

2. Remove *(carefully)* beehives and wasp nests from children's play areas.

3. Wear light-colored clothing. Dark- and bright-colored clothing is attractive to insects and may evoke a defensive (sting or bite) response. Keep shirt sleeves closed and tuck pants into boots. Wear light-colored socks. Be aware of nests near or on the ground.

4. Avoid wearing sweet fragrances that make you smell like a flower. Avoid carrying sweet-smelling soft drinks and fruit juices.

5. Avoid orchards in bloom, fields of clover, and areas with lots of flowers.

6. Don't anger bees or wasps. If confronted by a swarm, cover your face (eyes, nose, and mouth) and move rapidly from the area. If necessary, throw a blanket or towel over your head. Run if you must. Maneuver through bushes or weeds to confuse the bees. Don't jump into a pool—the bees may wait for you and a severe allergic reaction from a sting while in the water may be extremely dangerous. Don't poke sticks or throw rocks into bee holes.

7. Avoid rapid or jerky movements near bees. Don't swat at them. Remain calm.

SPIDERS

Although more than 20,000 different species of spiders live in the United States, only a few pose any real hazard to humans. The troublemakers are those that bite and deliver toxins from venom glands. The nature of the reaction depends on the type and quantity of venom. Most spiders only bite their victims one time in a defensive effort, so if there are multiple bites or lesions, you should suspect an insect like a flea or mite, or an infection.

To avoid spider bites, remove trash carefully and keep dwellings and sleeping areas clean. Shake out clothing and shoes before wearing them. Store equipment and apparel in sealed plastic bags when not in use for prolonged periods. Wear gloves for protection when handling wood, particularly that taken from piles.

Black Widow Spider

In the United States, the female black widow spider *(Latrodectus mactans)* is about ⅝ inch (15 mm) in body length, black or brown, and with a characteristic red (or orange or yellow) hourglass marking on the underside of the abdomen (Figure 218). The top side of the spider is shiny and features a fat abdomen that resembles a large black grape. The longest legs are directed toward the front. This species and other *Latrodectus* species are found scattered in rural regions, in barns, within harvested crops, and around outdoor stone walls. Some are arboreal.

The bite of the black widow spider is rarely very painful (usually more like a pinprick) and often causes little swelling or redness, although there can be a warm and reddened area around the bite. If much venom has been deposited, the victim develops a typical reaction within an hour. Symptoms include muscle cramps, particularly of the abdomen and back; muscle pain; muscle twitching; numbness and tingling of the palms of the hands and bottoms of the feet; headache; droopy eyelids; facial swelling; drooling; sweating; restlessness and anxiety; vomiting; chest muscle spasms that cause difficulty breathing; fever; and high blood pressure. A man may develop a persistent penile erection (priapism). A small child may cry persistently. A pregnant woman may develop uterine contractions and premature labor.

Untreated, most people recover without help over the course of 8 hours to 2 days. However, very small children and elderly victims may suffer greatly, with possible death. There is an antivenom available to medical practitioners for treating the bite of the black widow spider. It is used for severe, sometimes life-threatening, symptoms.

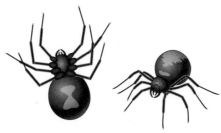

Figure 218. Female black widow spider with typical hourglass marking on the underside of the abdomen.

Treatment for a Black Widow Spider Bite

1. Apply ice packs to the bite.
2. *Immediately* transport the victim to a medical facility.
3. Once the victim is in the hospital, the doctor will have a number of therapies to use, which include intravenous calcium solutions and muscle relaxant medicines for muscle spasm; antihypertensive drugs for elevated blood pressure; pain medicine; and, in very severe cases, antivenom.
4. If you will be unable to reach a hospital within a few hours and the victim is suffering *severe* muscle spasms, you may administer an oral dose of diazepam (Valium) or lorazepam (Ativan), if you happen to be carrying it. The starting dose of diazepam for an adult who does not regularly take the drug is 5 mg, which can be augmented in 2.5 mg increments every 30 minutes up to a total dose of 10 mg, so long as the victim remains alert and is capable of normal, purposeful swallowing. The starting dose for a child age 2 to 5 years is 0.5 mg; for a child age 6 to 12 years the starting dose is 2 mg. Total dose for a child should not exceed 5 mg; *never* leave a sedated child unattended. The starting adult dose of lorazepam for an adult is 1 mg, which can be augmented in 0.5 mg increments every 30 minutes up to a total dose of 2 mg.

Recluse Spiders

At least eleven species of recluse spiders are found in the United States. The brown recluse spider *(Loxosceles reclusa)* is the best known and found most commonly in the South and southern Midwest. However, interstate commerce has created habitats in many other parts of the country for the brown recluse and related species. The spider is brown, with an average body length of just under ½ inch (10 mm). A characteristic dark violin-shaped marking ("fiddleback" or "violin" spider) is sometimes, but not always, found on the top of the upper section of the body (Figure 219). Recluse spiders have six equal-sized eyes arranged in three pairs. The brown recluse spider is found in dark, sheltered areas, such as under porches and in storage areas, in attics and woodpiles, and in crates of fruit. It is most active at night. It commonly bites when it is trapped, but is not otherwise aggressive toward humans.

The bite of the brown recluse spider may cause very little pain at first, or a sharp sting may be felt. The stinging subsides over 6 to 8 hours, and is replaced by aching and itching. Within 1 to 5 hours, a painful red or purplish blister sometimes appears, surrounded by a bull's-eye of whitish-blue (pale) discoloration, with occasional slight swelling. The red margin may spread into an irregular fried-egg pattern, with gravitational influence, such that the original blister remains near the uppermost part of the lesion. The victim may develop chills, fever, weakness, and a generalized red skin rash. Severe allergic reactions within 30 minutes of the bite occur infrequently. Over 5 to 7 days, the venom causes a violet discoloration and breakdown of the surrounding tissue, leading to an open ulcer that may take months to heal. If the reaction has been severe, the tissue in the center of the wound becomes destroyed, blackens, and dies.

A rare reaction is "systemic loxoscelism," in which the venom binds to red blood cells and induces severe symptoms within 24 to 72 hours. These include a flu-like presentation with fever,

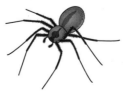

Figure 219. Brown recluse spider with typical violin-shaped marking on the top side of the cephalothorax.

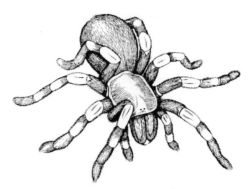

Figure 220. Tarantula.

chills, headache, fatigue, weakness, nausea, vomiting, muscle and joint aches, blood in the urine, yellow skin discoloration (jaundice), kidney failure, and even shock, seizures, coma, and rarely death. This is more common in children and requires intensive medical therapy.

Treatment for a Brown Recluse Spider Bite

Because the bite of the brown recluse spider typically causes severe tissue destruction, the victim should see a physician, who will prescribe medicine or another therapy as soon as possible. In the meantime, apply cold packs to the wound for as long as is practical and administer an antibiotic (erythromycin, azithromycin, or cephalexin). Don't apply a heating pad or hot packs. Depending on the severity of the reaction, the doctor may advise taking medicines. There are therapies that have been reported, but not been proven, effective. These include surgical excision of the bite; dapsone (a drug used to inhibit certain cells that are part of the inflammatory response); topical application of nitroglycerin; and hyperbaric oxygen therapy.

Until you receive other advice, treat the wound with a thin layer of mupirocin or bacitracin ointment, or mupirocin cream, underneath daily dressing changes. Don't apply topical steroids.

Other Spiders

Other spiders that may produce painful bites and a small amount of local tissue breakdown (ulcers) include the tarantula, wolf spider, jumping spider, yellow sac spider, orb weaver, and hobo spider *(Tegenaria agrestis)*. The bites should be treated with ice packs, pain medicine, and standard wound care.

Some tarantulas (Figure 220) carry hairs that can irritate the skin, eyes, and mucous membranes of humans. When the spider is threatened, it rubs its hind legs over its abdomen and flicks thousands of hairs at its foe. These hairs can penetrate human skin and cause swollen bumps, which can itch for weeks. If any hairs or hair fragments remain in the skin, they can be removed by applying and peeling off sticky tape. After that, treatment is with an oral antihistamine and topical medication such as StingEze liquid. A topical antihistamine or corticosteroid preparation may provide some relief.

SCORPIONS

Scorpions are hardy nocturnal creatures found in deserts and warm tropical climates, hidden under stones, fences, wood, shed tree bark, and garbage. They can survive easily in adverse environmental circumstances. In the United States, the most dangerous species is the bark scorpion *Centruroides exilicauda,* which is found almost exclusively in the southwestern states and can be up to 2 in (5 cm) long. This yellowish-brown (straw-colored), solid or striped species is distinguished from other scorpions by its slender body and a small tubercle (telson) at the base of its stinger (Figure 221). The sting is inflicted with the last segment of the tail, and it is

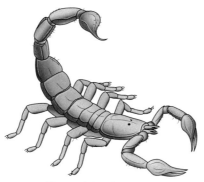

Figure 221. Scorpion.

immediately exquisitely painful; the pain is made much worse by tapping on the site of the injury. Other symptoms include excitement, increased salivation, sweating, numbness and tingling around the mouth, nausea, double vision, nervousness, muscle twitching and spasms, rapid breathing, rapid heart rate, shortness of breath, high blood pressure, seizures, paralysis, and collapse. Depending on the species of scorpion, sometimes sweating is noted only at the site of the sting. Extremely low blood pressure may follow the period of high blood pressure. Children under age 2 years are at particular risk for severe reactions. Stings by nonlethal scorpion species are similar to bee stings.

If someone is stung by a scorpion, immediately apply an ice pack to the wound and immobilize the affected body part. Seek immediate care, particularly for stings of *C. exilicauda*. If a health care professional has a local anesthetic that can be injected into the sting site, this may provide some relief from the pain. Antivenom (Anascorp) is sometimes available to physicians in Arizona and Nevada to treat victims of *C. exilicauda* scorpion sting.

To prevent scorpion stings, be careful when handling dead wood and working in piles of leaves. Clothing, shoes, bedrolls, and sleeping bags should be shaken out and inspected before use. The cuticle of *C. exilicauda* fluoresces under an ultraviolet light (Wood's lamp or "black light") and can be spotted glowing green at night in this manner. When traveling abroad in scorpion habitat, sleep under mosquito netting and don't sit on the floor in mud huts with your back against the wall.

MOSQUITOES

Female mosquitoes bite humans in quest of a blood meal, in order to lay eggs. Because they breed in water, they are most frequently found in marshy, wetland, or wooded areas. Although many tend to swarm at dusk, different species feed at different times. The insects are attracted to host odors (long-range), exhaled carbon dioxide (mid-range), and heat and moisture (short-range). During a bite, mosquito saliva is injected into the victim. This liquid contains the substances that cause the classic reaction—a small white or red bump that itches and then disappears. Persons who have been sensitized because of previous bites can have delayed (12 to 48 hours) reactions, which include intense swelling and itching. In addition, mosquitoes transmit diseases such as malaria (see page 137) and various types of encephalitis.

Therapy for mosquito bites is limited to cool compresses and skin hygiene to prevent infections. If someone is bitten intensely and suffers a severe delayed allergic reaction, he may benefit from a course of prednisone similar to that used to treat poison oak (see page 218). Oral antihistamines, such as cetirizine hydrochloride, given before mosquito exposure, may lessen the reaction to mosquito bites in highly sensitized persons.

Insect repellents are discussed on page 336.

BITING FLIES

A midge (also called a gnat or no-see-um) is a small biting fly that creates a painful red bump that seems out of proportion to the insect's size. After your immune system has become sensitized to these bites, your reactions may become worse with repeated bites, and you may develop blisters or small sores.

Blackflies, buffalo gnats, turkey gnats, and green-headed flies create larger punctures that may bleed. The immediate pain, swelling (welt), and redness are usually intense and persistent. The sores may last for weeks, and be accompanied by weakness and fever when there are multiple bites. Swollen lymph glands may occur, particularly in children. Horsefly, deerfly, mango fly, breeze fly, and sand fly bites are generally less noxious, but may on occasion be severe. In addition, they may transmit diseases, such as is the case with sand flies and leishmaniasis.

Treatment is symptomatic and similar to that applied under step 5 for the local reaction to an insect sting (see page 324).

FLEAS

Fleas are parasitic on mammals and birds. The wingless body enables the critters to run and jump with ease. They live on blood. They are more active in warmer climates, and are commonly associated with domestic animals. A flea bite usually is a small dark red or purplish dot surrounded by a circular area of lighter redness and swelling. Itching is common. Persons who have been sensitized may develop blisters or ulcers. Flea bites may appear in unpatterned clusters, most commonly on the legs, ankles, and feet.

Treatment is symptomatic and similar to that applied under step 5 for the local reaction to an insect sting (see page 324).

The female *Tunga penetrans* flea (burrowing flea, chigo, sand flea, jigger) causes tungiasis in Central and South America and in Africa, particularly in soil near cattle and pigs. The impregnated female flea burrows into a human's skin until only the flea's posterior end remains external. The insect sucks blood, becomes larger, and appears as a firm, itchy nodule the size of a small pea, which has a dark spot in the center (the hind end of the flea). The most common sites of infestation are the feet, buttocks, or perineum of humans who don't wear shoes or who squat on dusty soil. The burrowed flea can be killed with topical ether, cryotherapy (cold), or certain drugs, such as ivermectin. However, it then must then be surgically removed. To prevent tungiasis, don't walk barefoot or wear open-toed footwear. The insect repellent mixture of aloe, coconut oil, and jojoba oil applied at least twice daily may discourage fleas from entering the skin.

CHIGGERS

Chiggers (red bugs, harvest mites) are an enormous nuisance, particularly in the southeastern United States. The adult mites lay their eggs on vegetation (such as grass). The newly hatched larvae attach themselves to a human and inflict the bites; each is terribly itchy, and marked initially with a small red dot that becomes a red welt over the next 24 hours. Bites may number in the hundreds. Blisters, weeping, and severe swelling may appear. The feet and ankles are most commonly affected. The lesions resolve over 2 weeks, but not without flare-ups of intense itching and discomfort.

Treatment is symptomatic and similar to that applied under step 5 for the local reaction to an insect sting (see page 324). One percent phenol in calamine may be helpful. Home remedies for chigger bites are common and include application of dabs of clear nail polish or meat tenderizer. None are of proven benefit. If a person is bitten intensely and suffers a severe reaction, he may benefit from a course of prednisone similar to that used to treat poison oak (see page 218), or application of superpotent topical corticosteroid cream or ointment, such as 0.05% clobetasol applied thinly several times daily, but for only a few days' duration. Prevention is key; pretreatment of clothing with permethrin, similar to the approach taken to repel ticks, is beneficial.

CENTIPEDES AND MILLIPEDES

Centipedes bite their victims with their fangs, not with their feet or rear-end appendages. *Scolopendra* species bites have been reported to cause burning pain, swelling, redness, and swollen lymph glands. More severe reactions are rare. Treatment is symptomatic and similar to that applied under step 5 for the local reaction to an insect sting (see page 324), with the exception that the application of meat tenderizer has never been suggested to be of benefit for a centipede bite.

Millipedes don't bite their human victims; instead, they eject secretions that can cause skin irritation. In tropical regions, this has been reported to begin with brown skin staining, followed by a burning sensation with blisters. Millipede secretions that enter the eye may cause severe irritation similar to a corneal abrasion (see page 168). There is no specific treatment, other than to irrigate the affected area (particularly the eyes) promptly and thoroughly with disinfected water or saline solution, and then treat as a burn (see page 108) or, if the eye is injured, as a corneal abrasion (see page 168).

TICKS

Ticks (Figure 222) are blood-feeding arthropods. There are "hard ticks" and "soft ticks." Ticks are ubiquitous in wooded regions and fields, and readily attach to the skin of victims, most commonly on the legs, lower abdomen, genitals, back, and buttocks. They may also attach to the scalp, armpits, groin, and other cozy (for a tick) areas. They like shade and moist skin, and may wander for a while in search of a comfortable spot. Up to 20% of tick attachments are in locations that cannot be visualized by the victim. Once in place, ticks hang on with their mouthparts and feed on the victim's blood. The tick is the intermediate host for the vectors of many diseases, such as Rocky Mountain spotted fever (see page 145), Colorado tick fever (see page 145), relapsing fever (see page 142), ehrlichiosis (see page 147), babesiosis (see page 148), and Lyme disease (see page 146). Ticks are the most common insect vectors of disease in the United States.

A tick bite can cause a local reaction that ranges from the common small, itchy nodule to an extensive ulcer. It is common to see redness, swelling, and itching at the site of a tick bite. Some tick mouthparts are barbed, and there may also be a cement secreted by the tick to anchor it into the victim. With large or multiple bites, the victim may suffer fever, chills, and fatigue in the absence of infection. Normally, the bite wounds resolve over a week or two. A persistent lump may be a collection of reactive (to tick saliva) tissue that requires surgical excision.

Tick Paralysis

If a person (particularly a young child with long hair) is traveling in or has just returned from tick country and begins to complain of fatigue and weakness, you may have discovered a case of tick paralysis.

The disorder is most common in spring and summer when ticks are feeding. Certain female ticks (North American wood tick, common dog tick, and Australian marsupial tick) attach to

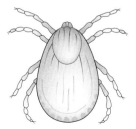

Figure 222. Tick.

the skin and slowly (over several days) release a neurotoxin that causes profound lethargy and muscle weakness in the victim. The disorder usually begins 5 to 7 days after tick attachment. At first the victim may be irritable and restless, and complain of numbness and tingling in his hands and feet. Over the next day or two (but occasionally as quickly as within a few hours), the victim becomes weak, with an ascending (beginning in the feet and advancing toward the head) paralysis, which can become total. Just a portion of the face can be paralyzed if a tick is lodged behind the ear.

Search the skin (particularly the hair-covered areas) thoroughly for ticks and remove them properly (see later). Improvement is usually noted within hours, and complete recovery occurs in 24 to 48 hours after removal of the tick. However, if the tick isn't removed, the victim can die.

Tick Avoidance

When traveling in forests and fields, it's a good idea to inspect the body (particularly the hairline, groin, underarms, navel, scalp, and other hair-covered areas) thoroughly for ticks each day. Have a companion check areas of your body that you cannot visualize. Don't forget to brush ticks out of the fur of all dogs and pack animals.

Wear proper clothing to prevent tick attachment. Ticks have a more difficult time attaching to smooth, tightly woven fabrics. Keep shirts tucked into pants and trouser cuffs tucked into socks. Light-colored clothing displays ticks. If clothing is worn loosely fitting, it will not be pulled close to the skin, and it will be more difficult for a tick or insect to bite through and reach the skin. If mesh clothing or a head net is deployed, the mesh size should be less than 0.3 mm. Wear a light-colored, broad-brimmed hat to protect the head and neck. If ticks are seen on clothing, they may be removed by trapping them on a piece of cellophane tape or using a sticky tape lint roller device. Unless a hot cycle in a clothing dryer is employed, washing clothing may not remove tick nymphs. The deer tick, which transmits the infectious agent of Lyme disease, is extremely small, particularly in juvenile stages. The best repellent is permethrin (Permanone) applied to clothing, *not to skin* (see page 336), but DEET is also effective. Insect Shield Repellent Apparel and Insect Shield Repellent Gear are impregnated with a proprietary permethrin formula. The clothing is claimed to withstand 70 launderings and retain repellency.

Here's more advice about how to avoid ticks. At home, keep grass trimmed short. Remove thick piles of grass and leaves. Remove brush from woodpiles and areas adjacent to dwellings. Keep the woodpiles distant. Don't tempt deer to approach your dwelling by landscaping with plants that are tasty. If you have pets (particularly dogs that can hide ticks in their fur), inspect them regularly, particularly if they have access to wooded areas or have been along with you on a hike. Use veterinarian-approved pesticide sprays, powders, treatments and tick collars. Wood chips, mulch, and gravel don't tend to harbor ticks, so can be used against wooden fences, under sandboxes and playgrounds, or to create borders adjacent to tick habitat. Apply a perimeter of pesticides around the perimeter of your property. Mice and chipmunks carry fleas, so discourage their presence.

Tick Removal

The proper way to remove a tick is to grasp it close to its mouthparts with tweezers or with the fingernails and pull it straight out with a slow and steady motion (Figure 223). Another excellent way to remove a tick is with a grooved or V-shaped device designed to slide between the tick and the skin to trap the tick and allow it to be pulled from the skin. Don't twist the tick. If you must remove it with your fingers, use tissue paper or cloth to prevent skin contact with infectious tick fluids. Don't touch the tick with a hot object (such as an extinguished match head) or cover it with mineral oil, alcohol, kerosene, camp stove fuel, or Vaseline; these remedies might cause the tick to struggle and regurgitate infectious fluid into the bite site. Viscous lidocaine 2% applied to a tick for 5 minutes will cause it to detach its grip, but it is not known if the tick regurgitates

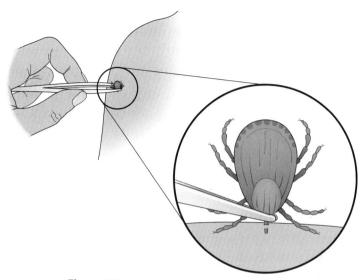

Figure 223. Removing a tick with tweezers.

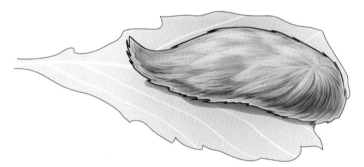

Figure 224. Puss caterpillar.

because of using this technique. If a tick head is buried in the skin, you can apply permethrin (Permanone insect repellent), using a cotton swab, to the upper and lower body surfaces of the tick. After 10 to 15 minutes, the tick will relax and you will be able to pull it free. After the tick is removed, carefully inspect the skin for remaining head parts, and gently scrape them away. Wash the bite site with soap and water or with an antiseptic, and also wash your hands.

CATERPILLARS

The puss caterpillar, *Megalopyge opercularis* (Figure 224), is found in the southern United States. The gypsy moth caterpillar, *Lymantria dispar* (Figure 225), and the flannel moth caterpillar, *Megalopyge crispata,* are found in the northeastern United States. The numerous bristles that cover the bodies of these species cause skin irritation when the caterpillar is directly touched, or when there is contact with detached bristles deposited on outdoor bedding or hung clothes. Shortly after exposure, the victim suffers a rash with redness, itching, burning discomfort, and hives. Blisters are rare. If a large area of skin is involved, the victim can become nauseated and weak and can suffer from high fever. If the small bristle hairs are inhaled, shortness of breath or asthma-like (see page 42) symptoms may follow. If the eyes come into contact with these hairs, symptoms include redness, itching, tearing, and swollen eyelids. Handling particularly venomous species can cause intense pain, headache, fever, vomiting, and swollen lymph glands.

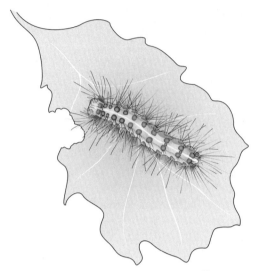

Figure 225. Gypsy moth caterpillar.

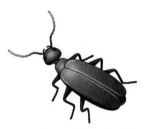

Figure 226. Blister beetle.

Treatment of the skin consists of applying adhesive tape (duct tape is best) to attempt removal of the bristles, followed by an application of calamine lotion. A good alternative is to apply a commercial facial peel or thin layer of rubber cement, allow it to dry, and then peel it off; the bristles will be carried with it. Management of an allergic reaction similar to that from poison oak is described on page 218. If the redness and swelling are prominent, the victim may be treated with an oral antihistamine, such as fexofenadine (60 mg twice a day) or loratadine (Claritin) 10 mg once a day, and an NSAID for 5 days. If the pain is severe, administer a potent pain medicine.

BEETLES

Beetles are the largest group of insects. Fortunately, no beetle has a bite or sting that can envenom a human, although some types produce toxic secretions that can be deposited on the skin.

Blister beetles of the *Epicauta* species (Figure 226) are found throughout the eastern and southern United States. These insects are usually about ½ inch (1.3 cm) long and extremely agile. When they make contact with the skin, they release a chemical substance (cantharidin) that's very irritating. Initial contact is painless. Within a few hours, blisters appear, which aren't particularly painful unless they are large and broken. If a blister beetle is squashed on the skin, an enormous blister follows.

The treatment is the same as for a second-degree burn (see page 108). If "beetle juice" enters the eye, the eye should be irrigated copiously and the injury managed as you would snow

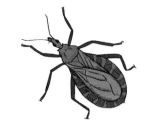

Figure 227. Triatomid "kissing bug."

blindness (see page 174). In general, it's a good idea to wash the skin with soap and water after any insect contact.

SUCKING BUGS

These insects have sucking mouthparts and are typified by the assassin bugs and their subset of triatomids ("kissing bugs," "wheel bugs," and Mexican bed bugs). Aquatic sucking bugs include the giant water bugs and "water scorpions."

Triatomids (Figure 227) usually bite humans during the night on exposed body parts, and feed for up to 30 minutes. The initial bite is painless, without any immediate reaction. However, a bite from a wheel bug, black corsair, or masked bed bug hunter may cause pain similar to that of a hornet sting.

A triatomid may continue to bite until there is a cluster or line of red, itchy bumps that may last for up to a week. If the reaction is more severe, there are large hives, swollen lymph glands, fever, and blisters.

The common bed bug and tropical bed bug are found worldwide. These tiny (about the size of an apple seed) creatures bite mostly at night in a painless fashion. Bed bug bites often create an itchy bump with a central red spot. After the bugs bite, they move on. If you believe that you have been bitten by bedbugs, wash all clothing and bedding in very hot water.

Treatment is symptomatic and similar to that applied under step 5 for the local reaction to an insect sting (see page 324).

SKIN INFESTATION BY FLY LARVAE

Skin infestation by fly larvae is called myiasis, and is most commonly noted in Mexico and Central and South America, the latter two involving the botfly *Dermatobia hominis*. The fly egg, which may actually be carried by another species of insect (such as a mosquito), is deposited onto human skin, where it hatches, allowing the emerging larva to burrow into the skin through the insect bite or another opening (such as a hair follicle or small scratch or nick). The Tumbu fly *Cordylobia anthropophaga* in sub-Saharan Africa is a blowfly that lays eggs in the ground or on clothing, from which they approach human skin.

The larva then develops within a dome-shaped cavity (swelling) that enlarges over 4 to 7 weeks. A central breathing pore drains clear or slightly bloody fluid. Drainage may begin within the first 2 weeks after penetration. There is often redness and itching. Movement may be felt under the skin as the larva wiggles. This may also feel like a crawling sensation or brief flash of sharp pain, because the larva has many parallel rows of bristly spines.

The mature larva will attempt to exit the skin through the breathing pore, and is noticed as a small white object "peeking" through the hole. To test to see if a larva is present, place a small amount of the victim's saliva over the hole—if it bubbles, the larva is likely there and breathing. You can force it to exit through the hole by suffocating it. Cover the breathing pore with bacon or pork fat, a strip of meat, chewing gum, wax, fingernail polish, paraffin, or a plug of grease. Usually, 12 hours of occlusion will cause the larva to exit the hole or die from asphyxiation.

Moistened tobacco leaves or nicotine drops will paralyze the larva. It is unwise to make an incision to remove the larva, because if the creature is ruptured, it will leak substances into the wound that cause inflammation and promote infection. It is sometimes possible to simply squeeze the lesion and force extrusion of the larva, but care must be taken not to rupture the larva. If nothing is done to force the larva to leave the skin, it will do so on its own in a few weeks, but this is generally not recommended because of the pain and potential for abscess (see page 224) formation.

Another way to remove the larva is to use the Extractor Pump. First, apply an occlusive layer of antiseptic cream covered by thin plastic wrap, or other occlusive method (see earlier), over the breathing hole for 30 minutes. Next, wipe the area clean with alcohol or soap and water. Then apply the Extractor with the suction cup selected to completely cover the skin bump and opening. Activate the Extractor. If the technique works, the larva will slide to the surface within a few minutes.

Other fly larvae that can invade humans and cause myiasis may "migrate," or travel under the skin, usually settling over the head or shoulders. They may emerge from the lesions or die where they are, in which case they don't need to be removed.

Wound myiasis describes the situation in which flies (including the green- or bluebottle fly, housefly, black blowfly, and flesh fly) have deposited eggs into a wound, where the larvae feed on the decaying tissue. This is seen most commonly in elderly victims with underlying chronic diseases. The "maggots" are unsightly, but don't harm the victim. Screwworms, on the other hand, which originate from outbreaks among livestock, may invade humans and cause destructive ulcers, particularly if they enter through the nose.

For wound myiasis confined to the skin, a mixture of 5% chloroform in olive oil kills the larvae, so that they can be removed manually. After the creature is extracted, rinse the wound with a solution of 5% povidone–iodine in water. In the absence of this mixture, simple irrigation and mechanical removal of the larvae will suffice.

INSECT REPELLENTS AND OTHER PROTECTION AGAINST INSECTS
Clothing
In insect-laden areas, where contact is inevitable, the traveler should wear proper clothing. Cover the head and neck with a full-brimmed hat (with or without netting) and scarf (temperature permitting). Shield the ankles and wrists. Tuck pant cuffs into socks. Light-colored clothing is less attractive than dark clothing to biting insects, and also makes it easier to spot any mosquitoes, ticks, and flies that have landed.

Nylon (particularly double layered) and sailcloth are more difficult for insects to hang on to or penetrate and are generally preferred over cotton or cloth with a loose weave. Loose-fitting clothing made with tightly woven fabric, along with a T-shirt underlayer, makes for reasonable upper body protection. Where clothing can be pulled tight against the skin, a mosquito can bite through.

Clothing needs to be checked regularly and brushed free of insects; this is best done with the sticky side of adhesive tape. Insect repellents applied to clothing are extremely effective and avoid skin irritation. It's a good idea to test the repellent on a small area of clothing before general application, to be certain that it will not blemish the fabric.

Screens, Bed Nets, Coils, Candles, and Traps
Portable insect screens and bed nets (insecticide-treated or untreated) should be deployed when necessary. Place screens over windows. Use screened enclosures, particularly on outhouses and other places where insects would tend to congregate. Don't use lights that attract insects unless necessary. Select a campsite that is dry, elevated, and not cluttered. Use bed nets, particularly in malaria-endemic areas. Insect coils (typically made from pyrethrum powder) and candles are

sometimes useful to lower the number of flying insects in a relatively confined area. In areas of dense flying insect populations, particularly at night, smoke is a weak deterrent. Repellent candles contain paraffin and substances such as citronella, linalool, or geraniol. In one test in which the repellent substance was present in an amount of 5% of the total candle, geraniol was more effective than linalool than was citronella, but none should be considered as effective as a potent insect repellent applied to skin.

If you use a bed net, be certain that it is free of holes and has its edges tucked in. The net needs to be woven to a tightness of 18 threads per inch (6 to 7 per cm). Tighter mesh may hinder ventilation and create an uncomfortable environment. A net that has been dipped in an insecticide, usually permethrin, is more effective. A head net may be invaluable during times of high mosquito infestation.

Electric-light traps with electrocution grids, ultrasound devices, and audible sound devices have not been shown scientifically to repel insects or to decrease the concentration of biting insects in their vicinity. Mosquito traps, such as The MegaCatch Premier Mosquito Trap or the Mosquito Magnet are advertised to be effective. They emit combinations of chemical attractants, carbon dioxide, heat, and moisture to draw mosquitoes and certain other biting insects close enough to a suction intake to be captured.

Repellents

Chemical insect repellents are mandatory when you travel through mosquito, sand fly, or tick territory. Different repellents work by different mechanisms, and therefore their effectiveness varies for different types of insects, but I can offer some general recommendations that will be applicable in most situations.

Effective repellents contain the chemicals DEET (N,N-diethyl-3-methylbenzamide), Indalone (butyl 3,4-dihydro-2,2-dimethyl-4-oxo-2H-pyran-6-carboxylate), Rutgers 612 (2-ethyl-1,3-hexanediol), and DMP (dimethyl phthalate). Picaridin (also known as KBR 3023; brand name Bayrepel) is a repellent that is odorless and nongreasy, and should be present in a concentration of 15%. Early anecdotal reports from users suggests that it is not as effective as DEET. Oil of lemon eucalyptus (Repel Lemon Eucalyptus Repellent) is another increasingly popular repellent that's thought to be as effective as 7.5% DEET. It is actually not from eucalyptus, but is a product from the lemon-scented gum tree *Corymbia citriodora*. The product is water-distilled from the leaves, and the repellent is found in the spent fraction as *para*-menthane-3,8-diol (PMD). Oil of lemon eucalyptus may be used on children ages 3 years and older. Along with isopulegol and citronellal, oil of lemon eucalyptus is contained in the product Mosi-guard Natural. Of particular note, true eucalyptus oil does not work as an insect repellent.

Di-n-propyl isocinchomeronate (R-326) has been promoted as useful against biting flies. IR3535 (ethyl butylacetylaminopropionate)-containing repellent is far less useful (1 hour maximum protection) than DEET. Mosbar soap is a product sold abroad that contains 20% DEET and 0.5% permethrin. N-octyl bicycloheptene dicarboximide synergist combined with DEET (Sawyer Products' Broad Spectrum; S. C. Johnson's Ticks OFF or Deep Woods OFF) is a tick repellent, also effective against biting flies and gnats, that can be applied directly to the skin. Neem *(Azadirachta indica),* used in India for millennia, reputedly has both insecticide and repellent properties. Soybean oil, sometimes used in combination with other repellent substances, may in and of itself have repellent properties.

Citronella and Avon Skin-So-Soft bath oil or skin stick are far less effective (15 minutes of protection versus 6 hours with 25% DEET). Other relatively ineffective (protection from a few minutes to [rarely] 2 hours) repellents include essential oils of cedar, peppermint, lemongrass, verbena, pennyroyal, lavender, pine, cinnamon, vanilla, rosemary, basil, thyme, allspice, garlic (topical or ingested), and geranium. Bite Blocker contains soybean, geranium, and coconut oils and has been claimed effective for up to 3.5 hours against mosquitoes. Bite Blocker for Kids (soybean oil, 2%) provides approximately 90 minutes of protection. Ingesting vitamin B_1 has not been proved to deter biting insects. It may decrease the skin irritation that follows an insect bite, but this would not diminish the transmission of infectious disease(s) via the bite.

2-Undecanone (BioUD) is a repellent derived from the wild tomato plant. A concentration of 7.5% provides repellency comparable to 25% DEET. It is particularly effective against ticks.

To be effective, a repellent should be applied to the skin (liquid) and clothing (spray). After you swim, bathe, or perspire excessively, reapply it. If you are being bitten by insects, reapply the repellent. In windy conditions, repellents evaporate quickly and may need to be reapplied. Children under 2 years of age should not have insect repellent applied to the skin more than once in 24 hours (it's more effective to apply it to the clothing anyhow). If you're applying both a sunscreen and an insect repellent, apply the sunscreen first, so that it can be absorbed; wait 30 minutes, and then apply the insect repellent. There are also sunscreen–insect repellent combinations, such as Coppertone Bug & Sun. Bug Guard contains Skin-So-Soft (mostly mineral oil) in combination with citronella, enhanced by a sunscreen.

With regard to DEET-containing products, don't use repeated applications or concentrations greater than 15% in children under age 6 (Skedaddle, Skintastic, and other preparations intended for use on children contain approximately 6.5% to 10% DEET). In adults, skin irritation and/or rare severe side effects may be seen following the use of concentrated (75% to 100%) products. Most authorities recommend avoidance of concentrated products, noting the effectiveness of a 50% concentration in jungle settings. A concentration not to exceed 30% to 50% for routine adult use seems reasonable. One recommended product is Ultrathon Insect Repellent (34% DEET). A product that may significantly decrease absorption through human skin of DEET is Sawyer Controlled Release DEET Formula, which uses a protein that encapsulates the DEET and allows slow (sustained) release of its 20% concentration. Sawyer Ultra 30 Insect Repellent Lotion is formulated in a liposome base for slow release.

Insect repellent containing DEET should be applied to skin, not clothing. Care should be taken to avoid contact of DEET with plastics (including contact lenses), rayon, spandex, leather, or painted and varnished surfaces, because DEET may cause damage to these.

The following recommendations are offered to avoid toxicity:

1. Apply repellent sparingly, and only to exposed skin or clothing. Keep it out of the eyes. Don't apply repellent underneath clothing.
2. Avoid high-concentration products on the skin, particularly with children.
3. Don't apply repellent to cuts, wounds, or irritated skin. Apply to face by dispensing into the palms of your hands, and then using these to apply a thin layer to the face. Then, wash your hands.
4. Don't inhale or ingest repellents. Don't spray aerosol or pump products directly onto your face. Spray your hands and then use them to rub the repellent onto the face, avoiding the eyes and mouth. Don't spray around food.
5. Use long-sleeved clothing and apply repellent to fabric rather than to skin.
6. Don't use repellent on children's hands, which may be rubbed in the eyes or placed in the mouth.
7. Repellent applied to a wristband is not sufficient protection—you must apply the repellent directly to all the skin areas to be protected.
8. Don't reapply repellent in normal weather conditions (unless it is a non-DEET repellent).
9. Wash repellent off the skin after the insect bite risk has ended.

Permethrin, a synthetic pyrethroid based on the naturally occurring pyrethroids that are extracted from the East African pyrethrum flower (a chrysanthemum), is actually an insecticide; that is, permethrin-containing products kill insects and ticks. Because *permethrin carries some potential toxicity to humans, it should be used only on clothing (or on shoes, certain camping gear, bed nets, etc.), not on skin.* For instance, permethrin is known to cause eye irritation if the chemical comes in contact with a person's eyes. Although permethrin in a 5% lotion or cream is sometimes prescribed by physicians for application to skin for treatment of mite (e.g., scabies) infestation, these medical dermatologic preparations aren't recommended for use as insect repellents. In the past, combination DEET-permethrin (the latter in very low concentration) soaps have been field tested for use as an insect repellent. While they have been acceptable to the persons who used them, a commercial product based on this concept has not yet come to market.

There is ongoing discussion about the toxicities possibly associated with permethrin. These include potential cancer-causing potential, and perhaps abnormalities of the immune system. Properly used (e.g., applied to clothing and not directly to skin), permethrin has not yet been directly linked with serious adverse effects on humans, so it remains an effective barrier against insect-borne infections, such as Lyme disease and West Nile virus. It is best used in combination in its application to clothing with an approved insect repellent (such as picaridin or DEET), when the latter is applied to skin.

There are sprays to treat clothing, and permethrin-treated clothing on the market. It's important to closely follow label instructions. Clothing that is sold pretreated with permethrin is often advertised to be effective (as a repellent) for up to 25 washings. Insect Shield Repellent Apparel and Insect Shield Repellent Gear are impregnated with a proprietary permethrin formula. The clothing is claimed to withstand 70 launderings and retain repellency. If you're going to be in a high-risk (for an insect or arthropod bite capable of transmitting a disease) situation, to play it safe, the effectiveness should be assumed to begin to decrease after half the advertised allowable number of washings. Also, it should not be assumed to protect skin adjacent to the clothing, only to keep insects from biting through the clothing.

If you decide to apply permethrin spray to clothing, be certain to do the following:

1. Follow the manufacturer's instructions closely. Don't exceed recommended spraying times.
2. Treat clothing only. Don't apply to skin.
3. Apply the permethrin in a well-ventilated outdoor area, protected from the wind.
4. Only spray the permethrin on the outer surface of clothing and shoes.
5. In a concentration of 0.5%, it can be sprayed on both sides of clothing to lightly moisten the outer surface of the clothing item; it's not necessary to have the clothing soaked through (saturated).
6. Be certain to apply completely over socks, trouser cuffs, and shirt cuffs, where insects may attempt to crawl or fly through openings to your skin.
7. Hang treated clothing outdoors and allow to dry for at least 2 to 4 hours in nonhumid conditions and for at least 4 hours in humid conditions.
8. Treat clothing no more often than every 2 weeks.
9. Launder treated clothing separately from other clothing at least once before retreating.
10. Assume that your treated clothing is effective for repellency for 2 weeks or more. Wear it only when you need to repel insects and arthropods. Store it in a separate impermeable (to permethrin) bag when not in use.

Permethrin (Permanone tick repellent; Duranon tick repellent) may be applied to clothing, netting, and footwear. A single application is usually good for 1 to 2 weeks, or 20 washings. To apply permethrin to clothing or netting, add 2 oz of permethrin to a quart of water in a plastic bag. The solution will turn milky white. Put the garment or netting in the bag, seal the bag, and let the item soak for 10 minutes. After the soak, allow the clothing or netting to effectively dry (in the sun or hung) for a few hours.

PermaKill 4 Week Tick Killer is a 13.3% permethrin liquid concentrate that is diluted ($\frac{1}{3}$ oz, or 10 mL, in 16 oz, or 473 mL, of water) to be sprayed from a pump bottle. It can also be diluted 2 oz (59 mL) in 1$\frac{1}{2}$ (355 mL) cups of water to soak a bed net, shirt, and pants, which are then air-dried.

Fleas, horseflies, blackflies, sand flies, deerflies, chiggers, gnats, and other assorted nuisances may not be repelled by insect repellents. Protective netting and a lot of swatting may be your only defenses.

LEECHES

Leeches are parasitic annelid worms that live on land or in water. They attach to human skin with a painless bite to extract blood through the skin. Some of them release a substance called hirudin, which is an anticoagulant (causes increased tendency to bleed). Aquatic leeches are found in fresh water and are considered more dangerous than those on land, because they can attach inside the mouth, throat, lungs, vagina, urethra, and other internal sites.

To remove a leech, don't pull it off—the residual sore may be larger. Instead, apply lemon juice, salt, vinegar, tobacco juice, menthol oil (peppermint or mint camphor), or insect repellent. Using a lighted or recently extinguished match or glowing ember may cause a skin burn. If the detached leech sticks to your fingers, roll it between them. If a leech is attached to someone's eye, shine a flashlight close to it; it may move toward the light and away from the eye. The medical considerations for a leech bite are persistent bleeding, itching, and secondary infection. Bleeding usually stops spontaneously or with pressure. If the oozing is continuous, apply a hemostatic (blood-stopping) dressing, such as QuikClot gauze, under pressure for 15 minutes. Insect repellents (see page 336), particularly DEET applied to clothing and skin, will discourage leech attachment. Slippery grease (such as petroleum jelly) applied to exposed skin may also help. Wear waterproof boots when wading in leech-infested water, and tuck in pant legs.

LIGHTNING STRIKE, TORNADO (CYCLONE), HURRICANE (TYPHOON), FLOOD, EARTHQUAKE, TIDAL WAVE (TSUNAMI), LANDSLIDE (MUDSLIDE), VOLCANO, AND SNOW AVALANCHE

Natural phenomena have medical considerations, such as broken bones, lacerations, crush wounds, hypothermia, drowning, and others discussed throughout this book. Because it can be life-saving, it's very important to know how to seek safety and behave during a severe weather event or natural disaster.

LIGHTNING STRIKE

Lightning strikes the earth at least 100 times per second during an estimated 3000 thunderstorms per day. Fortunately, the odds of being struck by lightning aren't very great. Still, approximately 50 persons per year are victims of fatal strikes in the United States. The wise traveler respects thunderstorms and seeks shelter at all times during a lightning storm.

Lightning is the direct-current electrical discharge associated with a thunderstorm; it releases an initial charge (the vast majority of which travels from ground [positive] to cloud [negative]) of average 30 million volts to neutralize a potential difference (within a hundredth to a ten-thousandth of a second) of 200 million to a billion volts. A lightning flash may be made up of multiple (up to 30) strokes, which causes lightning to seem to flicker. Each stroke lasts less than 500 milliseconds. The diameter of the main stroke is $2\frac{1}{2}$ to 3 inches (6 to 8 cm); the temperature has been estimated to be anywhere from 14,432° F to 90,032° F (8000° C to 50,000° C—four times as hot as the surface of the sun). Within milliseconds, the temperature falls to 3632° F to 5432° F (2000° C to 3000° C).

Thunder, which is always present with lightning, is attributed to the nearly explosive expansion of air heated and ionized by the stroke of lightning. To estimate the approximate distance in miles from your location to the lightning strike, time the difference in seconds between the flash of light and the onset of the thunder, and divide by five. Note that thunder is seldom heard if it is generated more than 10 miles (16 km) away.

Lightning can injure a person in many ways:
1. Direct hit, which most often occurs in the open.
2. Splash, which occurs when lightning hits another object (tree, fence, building). The current seeks the path of least resistance, and may jump to a human. Splashes may occur from person to person.
3. Contact, when a person is holding on to a conductive material that is hit or splashed by lightning.
4. Step (stride) voltage (or ground current), when lightning hits the ground or an object nearby. The current spreads like waves in a pond.
5. Ground current.
6. Surface arcing.
7. Upward streamer current.
8. Blunt injury, which occurs from the victim's own muscle contractions and/or from the explosive force of the shock wave produced by the lightning strike. These can combine to cause the victim to be thrown, sometimes a considerable distance.

When lightning strikes a person directly, splashes at him from a tree or building, or is conducted along the ground, it usually largely flows around the outside of the body (flashover phenomenon), which causes a unique constellation of signs and symptoms. The victim is frequently thrown, clothes may be burned or torn ("exploded" off by the instantaneous conversion of sweat to steam), metallic objects (such as belt buckles) may be heated, and shoes removed. The victim often undergoes severe muscle contractions—sufficient to dislocate limbs. In most cases, the person struck is confused and rendered temporarily blind and/or deaf. In some cases, there are linear (1½ to 2 inches [1.3 to 5 cm] wide, following areas of heavy sweat concentration), "feathered" (fernlike; keraunographism; Lichtenberg's flowers—cutaneous imprints from electron showers that track over the skin) (Figure 228, *A*), or

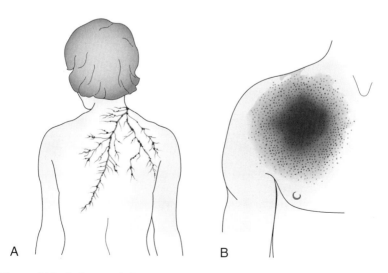

Figure 228. A, Ferning lightning burn. **B,** Punctate (starburst) lightning burn.

"sunburst" patterns of punctate burns over the skin (see Figure 228, B), loss of consciousness, ruptured eardrums, and inability to breathe. Occasionally, the victim ceases breathing and suffers cardiac arrest. Seizures or direct brain damage may occur. Eye injuries occur in half of victims.

A victim struck by lightning may not remember the flash or thunder, or even recognize that he has been hit. The confusion, muscle aches, body tingling, and amnesia can last for days. With a more severe case, the skin may be mottled, the legs and/or arms may be paralyzed, and it may be difficult to locate a pulse in the radial (wrist) artery (see page 30), because the muscles in the wall of the artery are in spasm. First-, second-, or third-degree skin burns may be present. Broken bones are not uncommon.

If a person is found confused, burned, or collapsed in the vicinity of a thunderstorm, consider the possibility that he was struck by lightning. The victim is not "electrified" or "charged"—you will not be jolted or stunned if you touch him.

1. Maintain the airway and assist breathing (see page 28). Continue to perform artificial respiration and cardiopulmonary resuscitation (CPR) (see page 30) until advanced help can be obtained. Victims of lightning strike may have paralysis of the breathing mechanism for a period of up to 30 minutes, and then make a remarkable recovery. A seemingly lifeless individual may be saved if you breathe for him promptly after the injury. Don't assume that dilated or nonreactive (to light—see page 34) pupils are a sign of death, because they may represent direct injury to the eye(s).
2. Assume that the victim has been thrown a considerable distance. Protect the cervical spine (see page 35).
3. Examine the victim for any other injuries and treat accordingly.
4. Transport the victim to a hospital.
5. If you are in the vicinity of a thunderstorm, seek shelter for the victim and yourself. Lightning *can* strike twice in the same place!

LIGHTNING AVOIDANCE AND HOW TO SEEK SAFETY

1. Know the weather patterns for your area. Don't travel in times of high thunderstorm risk. Avoid being outdoors during a thunderstorm. Carry a radio to monitor weather reports. Lightning can lash out from many miles in front of a storm cloud, in seemingly clear weather. If you calculate (see earlier) that a nearby lightning strike is within 3 miles (5 km) of your location, anticipate that the next strike will be in your immediate area. The "30-30 rule" specifies that if you see lightning and count less than 30 seconds before hearing thunder, seek shelter immediately. Since thunder is rarely heard from more than 10 miles (16 km) away, if you hear thunder, it's best to curtail activities and seek shelter from lightning. Don't resume activities outdoors for at least 30 minutes after the lightning is seen and the last thunder heard.
2. If a storm enters your area, immediately seek shelter. Enter a hard-roofed auto or large building. Tents and convertible autos offer essentially no protection from lightning. Tent poles are lightning rods. Metal sheds are dangerous because of the risk of side splashes. Indoors, stay away from windows, open doors, fireplaces, and large metal fixtures. Inside a building, avoid plumbing fixtures, telephones, and other appliances attached by metal to the outside of the building.
3. Don't carry a lightning rod, such as a fishing pole or golf club. Don't touch long conductors, such as wet ropes, metal fences, and handrails. Avoid tall objects, such as ski lifts and power lines. Avoid being near boat masts or flagpoles. Don't seek refuge near power lines or tall metal structures. Avoid being near metal pipes and fences. If you're in a boat, try to get out of the water. If you're swimming in the water, get out. Don't stand near a metal boat. Get off bicycles, motorcycles, and golf carts.

4. Move off ridges and summits. Thunderstorms tend to occur in the afternoon, so attempt to summit early and be heading back down by noon. In the woods, avoid the tallest trees (stay at a distance from the nearest tree that's at least equal to that tree's height) or hilltops. Shelter yourself in a thick stand of smaller trees (e.g., saplings). Don't shelter under an isolated tree. Avoid clearings—you become the tallest tree. If you are in a clearing, seek the lowest point, such as a valley or ravine. Don't stay at or near the top of a peak or ridge. Avoid cave entrances. If you are out in the open and cannot find shelter, then put your feet together and try to stand on insulation, such as a foam hiking pad. Crouch down and try to put your chest against your thighs or knees, and keep your head low. This may be an uncomfortable position to hold, but do your best. Never lie flat on the ground. Insulate yourself from ground current by crouching on a sleeping pad, backpack, jacket, or coiled rope.

5. Stay in your car and roll up the windows. The rubber tires are not protective. If it is a convertible, huddle on the ground at least 50 yards (46 m) from the vehicle.

6. If you are part of a group of people, spread the group out so that everyone isn't struck by a single discharge.

7. If your hair stands on end, you hear high-pitched or crackling noises, or see a blue halo (St. Elmo's fire) around objects, there is electrical activity near you that precedes a lightning strike. If you can't get away from the area immediately, crouch down on the balls of your feet and keep your head down. Don't touch the ground with your hands.

8. The StrikeAlert Personal Lightning Detector (Outdoor Technologies, Inc.) is the size and configuration of a pager and uses an audible warning and LED display to show the wearer how far away lightning is striking and if a storm is approaching or leaving. The StrikeAlert HD is larger and has additional features.

TORNADO AVOIDANCE AND HOW TO SEEK SAFETY

1. Be alert for a tornado if the weather conditions are rapidly changing, particularly if a stormy sky is dark gray or green and you see large hail or dark rotating clouds or hear a loud roaring noise. If you see revolving, funnel-shaped clouds, you're in danger.

2. As soon as you note an approaching storm, seek shelter. If a storm shelter is available, use it. The best location is an underground cave or concrete structure. Otherwise, go to the lowest floor of a sturdy building. Don't remain in a tent or camper. Mobile homes are not adequate protection.

3. If you are already indoors, go to a shelter area such as a storm cellar or basement; otherwise stay in the center of an interior room on the lowest level away from corners, windows, doors, and outside walls. Don't open windows. Get under a sturdy table and protect your head and neck.

4. If a tornado is in your vicinity and you are caught outside in open country, hunker down or lie flat in a depression, ditch, culvert, or ravine. Cover your head with your arms and hands. Don't get under an overpass or bridge—you're safer in a low, flat location.

5. Don't try to outrun a tornado. There is no way to predict when it will change direction. Flying debris is everywhere, and also be alert for flooding.

HURRICANE: HOW TO SEEK SAFETY

1. Listen to a National Oceanic and Atmospheric Administration (NOAA) weather radio, television, or Internet for weather updates.

2. Evacuate if so advised. Don't remain in a mobile home or temporary structure. Don't remain on the coast, on a floodplain, near a river, or on an inland waterway.

3. If you are not advised to evacuate, prepare any permanent dwelling for the storm. Close storm shutters, board the windows, brace external doors, and secure outdoor objects or bring them indoors.

4. If so instructed, turn off utilities. Turn off propane tanks. Anticipating power loss, turn the refrigerator and freezer settings to their coldest, and keep the doors to these appliances closed.

5. Moor all boats.

6. Fill toilets and tubs with water.

7. Don't stay in higher levels of high-rise structures unless a storm surge is possible (see Tidal Wave, later).

8. If caught in the storm, stay indoors away from doors and windows, close all interior doors, and keep the curtains and blinds closed. Shelter in an interior room or closet on the lowest level, or lie on the floor under a table or other sturdy object.

FLOOD: HOW TO SEEK SAFETY

1. Floods occur in streams, rivers, drainage channels, and canyons. It's possible that a storm many miles away can cause flooding in your vicinity with no warning other than a color change of the water, sudden appearance of debris in the flowing water, and sudden water level rise. Take care to camp far from flood zones during times of bad weather.

2. In flood conditions, avoid walking in moving water. Don't try to drive into flood waters. If your vehicle stalls or becomes trapped, abandon it quickly and seek dry ground.

3. When walking through water, use a walking stick for balance and to check your footing.

EARTHQUAKE: WHAT TO DO AND HOW TO SEEK SAFETY

If you are caught in an earthquake in a wilderness setting, do the following:

1. Seek a safe location, out of the path of rockfall, mudslides, or snow avalanches. If you can, move into a clearing away from buildings, trees, and power lines. If the ground shaking is extreme, position yourself on your hands and knees. Stay away from walls of buildings that might collapse.

2. If you are in a moving vehicle, drive to a clearing, set the parking break, and stay in it until the shaking stops. Some experts recommend leaving the car because if something collapses on it while you are inside, you may be crushed, and if you are outside the vehicle, it may compress and create a safe space adjacent to it. There is no absolute right or wrong about whether to stay in the car or exit it. In either case, don't stop near or under buildings, bridges, trees, overpasses, or utility wires.

3. If you're indoors, stay put until you are certain that it's safe to go outside. Move away from glass windows. Curl into a fetal position, and position yourself next to or under something that can compress, but not crush, and thereby protect you by leaving an adjacent void. If you're in a bed during an earthquake, roll off the bed and remain next to it. Don't remain in a doorway, and try to stay off stairs.

4. Near the ocean coast, move to higher ground at least 100 ft (30.5 m) or 2 miles (3.2 km) inland in anticipation of a tidal wave.

5. If you are trapped under debris, don't light a match or kick up dust. Cover your mouth and nose with a cloth, and if you have a whistle, blow on it to be located. Avoid shouting and taking deep breaths of dust-laden air.

6. Eliminate any obvious fire hazards. If you're in a cabin supplied with natural gas, turn it off at the source if there is any odor or you believe there might be a leak.

7. Be prepared for aftershocks.

8. Secure a supply of drinking water. Be certain that you're prepared for a period of time without electrical power.

9. Prepare a shelter, store sufficient food, and locate equipment necessary for survival. Keep first-aid supplies and a flashlight within easy reach.

TIDAL WAVE: HOW TO SEEK SAFETY

1. Heed all warnings and storm sirens.
2. Near the ocean coast, move to higher ground (at least 100 ft [30.5 m]) or 2 miles (3.2 km) inland in anticipation of a tidal wave. Remain there until you are instructed that it is safe to return.
3. If you see the surf water pulled far out as if it is low tide (or lower), then make haste to seek higher ground.
4. If you cannot move to higher ground, seek refuge at the highest level of a tall reinforced concrete building. If a life jacket is available, put it on.

LANDSLIDE: HOW TO SEEK SAFETY

1. During any storm in which a landslide might occur, remain awake and alert. Listen to a NOAA weather radio.
2. Have a pre-planned escape route.
3. Watch and listen for indications of moving debris. Examples are stones hitting against a building or trees cracking.
4. Try to move from the path of the flow or future flow.
5. If you can't escape, curl into a ball and protect your head and face.
6. Unless absolutely necessary to save a life, don't enter into a slide area. The ground may be unstable and there may be another slide.

VOLCANO

The eruption of a volcano can be a cataclysmic event. Since recorded time, pyroclastic flows (described later) have killed the greatest number of people, while flying solid objects (called "tephra" by volcanologists) thrown out by the volcano are the most frequent killers. Usually, when an explosive volcano erupts, a cloud of gas, ash, and lava fragments rises up into the atmosphere. If the eruption cloud becomes more dense than the surrounding air, it may fall back toward the ground, propelled by the forces of gravity. This can lead to formation of an incredibly hot (more than 1500° F [816° C]), high-speed (faster than 180 miles/hr [290 km/hr]) avalanche of ash, volcanic gases, lava fragments, and heated air, which is called a pyroclastic flow. Because of the forces and temperatures involved, no living being caught in this infernal river can survive. Most human victims die from suffocation, exposure to the heat, or burial under the volcanic debris. The extreme temperatures may also generate gale-force winds. Anyone who travels in the vicinity of an active volcano should be aware of the risks and have a realistic evacuation plan.

What to Do If Working or Traveling Near an Active Volcano

1. To learn the volcano's pattern of eruption, read about past eruptions and accidents.
2. Know the current volcano warning level. Obey local authorities.
3. Travel with an experienced guide.
4. Leave details about your itinerary with someone who can report you as delayed or missing.
5. Wear a hardhat and carry a gas mask.
6. Beware of rockfall, avalanche, and hazardous gases.
7. Observe for warning signs of an eruption. Leave immediately if the area becomes dangerous.
8. Don't approach lava that is flowing through vegetation.

SNOW AVALANCHE

Some of the factors that influence a buried victim's chances for survival are time buried, depth buried, clues on the surface (to facilitate location of the victim and rescue), rescue equipment, injury, ability to fight the avalanche, body position, snow density, presence of air (breathing) pocket and size of air pocket, and luck. A victim who is uninjured and able to fight on the downhill ride usually has a better chance of ending up only partly buried, or if completely buried, a better chance of creating an air pocket for breathing. A victim who is severely injured or knocked unconscious is like a rag doll being rolled, flipped, and twisted. Being trapped in an avalanche is a life-and-death struggle, with the upper hand going to those who fight the hardest.

Avalanches kill in two ways. First, serious injury is always possible in a tumble down an avalanche path. Trees, rocks, cliffs, and the wrenching action of snow in motion can do horrible things to the human body. Second, snow burial causes asphyxiation (either obstructed airway or exhausted oxygen supply). A very small percentage of avalanche victims succumb to hypothermia, probably because they succumb to injuries or asphyxia before they have a chance to become sufficiently hypothermic to expire.

The problem of breathing in an avalanche does not start with being buried. A victim swept down in the churning snow has an extraordinarily hard time breathing. Inhaled snow clogs the mouth and nose; asphyxiation occurs quickly if the victim is buried with the airway already blocked. Snow that was light and airy when a skier carved turns in it becomes viselike in its new form.

Snow sets up hard and solid after an avalanche. It is almost impossible for victims to dig themselves out, even if buried less than a foot deep. Hard debris makes recovery very difficult in the absence of a sturdy shovel. The pressure of the snow in a burial of several feet sometimes is so great that the victim is unable to expand his or her chest to draw a breath. Warm exhaled breath freezes on the snow around the face, eventually forming an ice lens that cuts off all airflow.

Another factor that affects survival is whether the victim is buried face up or face down. The most favorable position is face up. Data from a limited number of burials show that the victim is twice as likely to survive if buried face up rather than face down. If buried face up, an air pocket forms around the face as the back of the head melts into the snow; if buried face down, an air pocket cannot form as the face melts into the snow.

A completely buried victim has a poor chance of survival. Survival is interrelated with both time and depth of burial. Survival probabilities diminish with increasing burial depth. To date, no one in the United States who has been buried deeper than 7 ft (2.1 m) has been recovered alive.

Time is the true enemy of the buried victim. In the first 15 minutes, more persons are found alive than dead. At 30 minutes, an equal number are found dead and alive. After 30 minutes, more are found dead than alive, and from there the survival rate continues to diminish. In favorable circumstances, buried victims can live for several hours beneath the snow; therefore rescuers should never abandon a search prematurely. For instance, in 2003, two snowshoers caught near Washington's Mt. Baker survived burials of 22 and 24 hours.

To maximize your chance of not being caught in an avalanche and surviving should you be caught in an avalanche:

1. Carry and know how to use appropriate avalanche safety and rescue equipment. This may include a proper snow shovel, collapsible probe pole or ski pole probe, avalanche rescue beacon (transceiver), avalanche airbag system, AvaLung, and Recco Rescue System. Stay current on equipment advances and proper use techniques.
2. Never ski alone in dangerous conditions.
3. Know how to cross an avalanche-prone snow-covered slope:
   a. Tighten up clothing, fasten zippers, and wear hats, gloves, and goggles.
   b. Loosen or remove heavy backpacks.
   c. Remove ski pole straps and ski runaway straps.
   d. Check rescue beacon batteries and set the beacon to "transmit."
   e. Cross the slope at a high point, and try to stay on ridges.

   f. Cross far out from "runout zones."

   g. Cross slopes as quickly as possible.

   h. When climbing or descending a potential avalanche path, try to keep to the sides.

   i. Cross one person at a time.

   j. Try to move toward natural safety islands.

   k. Plan an escape route before crossing the slope.

4. Know how to survive an avalanche:

   a. Escape to the side.

   b. Shout and then close your mouth.

   c. If knocked off your feet, kick off your skis and discard your ski poles. Get your hands up to your face. Grab a jacket collar or pack strap.

   d. Snowmobile riders should try to stay on their vehicles.

   e. Try to grab onto a fixed object.

   f. If you sense you are near the surface, thrust an arm and hand up through the snow.

5. Rescue:

   a. Assess the danger. Avoid triggering a second avalanche.

   b. Assign a leader.

   c. Call for help.

   d. Safely access the avalanche debris and go to the spot where the victim was last seen.

   e. Spread searchers out to scan the debris.

   f. Turn all transceivers to "receive" to pick up signals.

   g. Make shallow probes at likely burial spots with an avalanche probe, ski pole, or tree limb. Likely burial spots include the uphill sides of trees, exposed rocks, and other fixed structures; bends in the direction of the debris; and at the toe of the debris.

   h. Shovel quickly and efficiently.

HAZARDOUS AQUATIC LIFE AND AQUATIC INFECTIONS

Anyone who gets an infection following a wound acquired in a natural aquatic environment should be treated with an antibiotic to cover *Staphylococcus* and *Streptococcus* species (use dicloxacillin, erythromycin, or cephalexin), and a second antibiotic to cover *Vibrio* or *Aeromonas* species (use ciprofloxacin, trimethoprim–sulfamethoxazole, or doxycycline). An infection from *Vibrio* or *Aeromonas* bacteria is more likely in deep puncture wounds, if there is a retained spine (such as from a stingray), and in people who suffer from an impaired immune system (diabetes, acquired immunodeficiency syndrome [AIDS], cancer, chronic liver disease, alcoholism, chronic corticosteroid therapy).

A very rare brain infection acquired from natural freshwater (lakes, rivers, and hot springs) is amebic meningoencephalitis caused by *Naegleria fowleri,* an ameba. This infects people by entering the nose, usually from swimming in or diving into natural freshwater or inadequately chlorinated pool water. It has occurred after using a neti pot with contaminated water (which may be tap water that was heated to less than 117°F [47°C]) to irrigate the sinuses. One to seven days after infection, symptoms of headache, fever, vomiting, and stiff neck occur. Death may follow rapidly. To avoid this infection, the Centers for Disease Control and Prevention recommends that persons avoid water-related activities in warm freshwater during periods of high water temperature and low water levels, hold the nose shut or use nose clips while taking part in water-related activities in bodies of warm freshwater, and avoid digging in or stirring up sediment while taking part in water-related activities in shallow warm freshwater areas. Irrigation of sinuses should only be undertaken using distilled or sterile (previously heated to at least 117°F [47°C]) or previously boiled water, and the irrigation device should be thoroughly rinsed and allowed to fully air dry after each use.

SHARKS

The jaws of the shark contain rows of razor-sharp teeth, which can bite down with extreme force. The result is a wound with loss of tissue that bleeds freely and can lead rapidly to shock (see page 58).

The basic management of a major bleeding wound is described on page 50. Even if a shark bite appears minor, the wound should be washed out and bandaged, and the victim taken to a doctor. Often, the wound will contain pieces of shark teeth, seaweed, or sand debris, which must be removed to avoid a nasty infection. Like other animal bites, shark bites should not be sewn or taped tightly shut, to allow drainage. This helps prevent serious infection. The victim should be started on an antibiotic to oppose *Vibrio* bacteria (ciprofloxacin, trimethoprim–sulfamethoxazole, or doxycycline).

The skin of many sharks is rough, like sandpaper, and can cause a bad scrape. If this occurs, it should be managed similar to a second-degree burn (see page 108).

Shark Avoidance

1. Seek the advice of locals before entering waters where shark attacks have occurred.
2. Obey lifeguards if they request you to leave the water. Do so slowly and quietly.
3. Avoid shark-infested waters, particularly at dusk and after dark. Don't dive in known shark feeding grounds. Avoid pinniped (e.g., sea lions and seals) rookeries and congregation areas.
4. Swim in groups. Sharks tend to attack single swimmers.
5. When diving or swimming, avoid deep drop-offs, sandbars, jetties, areas where birds are diving into the water, where there are leaping baitfish, murky water, river mouths, or areas near sewage outlets. Don't stray far from shore.
6. Don't swim with dogs or horses in the water.
7. Pods of dolphins or porpoises may indicate the presence of sharks. If they head inshore, exit the water.
8. Don't tether captured (speared, for example) fish to your body.
9. Don't corner or provoke sharks. Don't touch or harass any shark.
10. If a shark appears, leave the water with slow, purposeful movements. *Don't panic or splash.* If a shark approaches while you're diving in deep water, attempt to position yourself so that you are protected from the rear. If a shark moves in, attempt to strike a firm blow to the snout.
11. If you're stranded at sea and a rescue helicopter arrives to extract you from the water, exit the water at the earliest opportunity.

BARRACUDAS

Barracudas may bite victims and create nasty wounds with their long canine-like teeth. These wounds are managed similar to shark bites (see earlier). Because barracudas seem to be attracted to shiny objects, the swimmer, boater, or diver is advised to not wear bright metallic objects, particularly not a barrette in the hair or anklet dangled on a leg near the surface from a boat or dock.

MORAY EELS

Although they look quite ferocious, moray eels seldom attack humans, unless provoked. They have muscular jaws equipped with sharp fanglike teeth, which can inflict a nasty bite. The usual wound is one or more punctures, but can be a large and deep cut. A moray tends to bite and hold on.

A moray bite should be managed similar to a shark bite (see page 348). Even if the bite is very small, it should be examined by a physician to be sure that all tooth fragments have been removed. If the bite is more than superficial and on the hand, on the foot, or near a joint, the victim should be started on an antibiotic (ciprofloxacin, trimethoprim–sulfamethoxazole, or doxycycline) to oppose *Vibrio* bacteria. Avoid sewing or otherwise tightly closing a moray bite unless absolutely necessary.

SPONGES

Sponges handled directly from the ocean can cause two types of skin reaction. The first is an allergic type similar to that caused by poison oak (see page 218), with the difference that the reaction generally occurs within an hour after the sponge is handled. The skin becomes red, with burning, itching, and occasional blistering. The second type of reaction is caused by small spicules of silica from the sponges that are broken off and embedded in the outermost layers of the skin. This causes irritation, redness, and swelling. When large skin areas are involved, the victim may complain of fever, chills, fatigue, dizziness, nausea, and muscle cramps.

Because it's difficult to tell precisely which type of skin reaction has occurred, if a person develops a rash after handling a sponge, undertake the following therapy:

1. Soak the affected skin with white vinegar (5% acetic acid) for 15 minutes. This may be done by wetting a gauze pad or cloth with vinegar and laying it on the skin.
2. Dry the skin, and then apply the sticky side of adhesive tape to the skin and peel it off. This will remove most sponge spicules that are present. An alternative is to apply a thin layer of rubber cement or a commercial facial peel, let it dry and adhere to the skin, and then peel it off.
3. Repeat the vinegar soak for 15 minutes or apply rubbing (isopropyl 40%) alcohol for 1 minute.
4. Dry the skin, and then apply hydrocortisone lotion (0.5% to 1%) thinly twice a day until the irritation is gone. Don't use topical steroids before decontaminating with vinegar; this might worsen the reaction.
5. If the rash worsens (blistering, increasing redness or pain, swollen lymph glands), this may indicate an infection, and the victim should be started on an antibiotic to oppose *Vibrio* bacteria (ciprofloxacin, trimethoprim–sulfamethoxazole, or doxycycline). If the rash is persistent but there is no sign of infection, a 7-day course of oral prednisone in a tapering dose (for a 150 lb, or 68 kg, person, begin with 70 mg and decrease by 10 mg/day) may be helpful. Corticosteroids should always be taken with the understanding that a rare side effect is serious deterioration of the head ("ball" of the ball-and-socket joint) of the femur, the long bone of the thigh. Corticosteroids are interchangeable to a certain degree. If you must substitute, here is a rough measure of equivalence: 20 mg prednisone equals 16 mg methylprednisolone equals 3 mg dexamethasone.

JELLYFISH

Jellyfish is the term commonly used to describe an enormous number of marine animals that are capable of inflicting a painful, and occasionally life-threatening, sting. These include fire coral, hydroids, jellyfish (including sea wasps), and anemones. The stings occur when the victim comes into contact with the creature's tentacles or other appendages, which may carry millions of microscopic stinging cells (cnidocytes), each cell equipped with a toxin-laden microscopic stinging apparatus (nematocyst). Depending on the species, size, geographic location, time of year, and other natural factors, stings can range in severity from mild burning and skin redness to excruciating pain and severe blistering with generalized illness (nausea, vomiting, shortness of breath, muscle spasms, low blood pressure, and so on). Broken-off tentacles that are fragmented in the surf or washed up on the beach can retain their toxicity for months and should not be handled, even if they appear to be dried out and withered.

The dreaded box jellyfish *(Chironex fleckeri)* of northern Australia and the Indo-Pacific contains one of the most potent animal venoms known. A sting from one of these creatures can induce death in minutes from cessation of breathing, abnormal heart rhythms, and profound low blood pressure (shock). A sting from the Irukandji *(Carukia barnesi)* causes a syndrome of muscle spasm (back pain), sweating, nausea and vomiting, high blood pressure, and perhaps death.

Be prepared to treat an allergic reaction following a jellyfish sting (see page 64).

The following therapy is recommended for all unidentified jellyfish and other creatures with stinging cells, including the box jellyfish, Portuguese man-of-war ("bluebottle"), Irukandji, fire coral, stinging hydroid, sea nettle, and sea anemone:

1. If the sting is thought to be from the box jellyfish *(C. fleckeri),* immediately flood the wound with vinegar (5% acetic acid). Keep the victim as still as possible. Continually apply the vinegar until the victim can be brought to medical attention. If you are out at sea or on an isolated beach, allow the vinegar to soak the tentacles or stung skin for 10 minutes before you attempt to remove adherent tentacles or further treat the wound. In Australia, surf lifesavers (lifeguards) may carry antivenom, which is given as an intramuscular injection at the first-aid scene. The pressure immobilization technique is no longer recommended as a therapy for jellyfish stings.

2. For all other stings, if a topical decontaminant (vinegar or isopropyl [rubbing] alcohol) is available, pour it liberally over the skin or apply a soaked compress. Some authorities advise against the use of alcohol on the theoretical grounds that it has not been proved beyond a doubt to help. However, some clinical observations support its use. Since not all jellyfish are identical, it's extremely helpful to know ahead of time what works for the stingers in your specific geographic location. Vinegar may not work as well to treat sea bather's eruption (see page 219); a better agent may be a solution of papain (such as unseasoned meat tenderizer—see below for precaution about duration of therapy). For a fire coral sting, citrus (e.g., fresh lime) juice that contains citric, malic, or tartaric acid may be effective. Topical lidocaine 4% may effectively numb a jellyfish sting, and also perhaps lessen the envenomation.

3. Until the decontaminant is available, you can rinse the skin with seawater. Don't rinse the skin gently with fresh water or apply ice directly to the skin, as these may worsen the envenomation. A brisk freshwater stream (forceful shower) may have sufficient force to physically remove the microscopic stinging cells, but nonforceful application is more likely to cause the cells to fire, increasing the envenomation. A nonmoist ice or cold pack may be useful to diminish pain, but take care to wipe away any surface moisture (condensation) before the application. Observations from Australia suggest that hot (nonscalding) water application or immersion may diminish the sting of the Portuguese man-of-war from that part of the world. The generalization of this observation to treatment of other jellyfishes, particularly in North America, should not automatically be assumed, because of the fact that application of fresh water worsens certain envenomations.

4. Apply soaks of vinegar or lidocaine for 30 minutes or until pain is relieved. Baking soda powder or paste is recommended to detoxify the sting of certain sea nettles, such as the Chesapeake Bay sea nettle. A paste made from unseasoned meat tenderizer (don't exceed 15 minutes of application time, particularly not on the sensitive skin of small children) or papaya fruit may be helpful. These contain papain, which may also be quite useful to alleviate the sting from the thimble jellyfish that causes sea bather's eruption (see page 219). Don't apply any organic solvent, such as kerosene, turpentine, or gasoline.

While likely not harmful, urinating on a jellyfish, or any other marine, sting has never been proved to be effective.

5. After decontamination, apply a lather of shaving cream or soap and shave the affected area with a razor. In a pinch, you can use a paste of sand or mud in seawater and a clamshell. If a topical decontaminant (see numbers 1 and 2) is not available, simply applying a lather of shaving cream and shaving the affected area may lessen the pain from a sting.

6. Reapply the lidocaine, vinegar or rubbing alcohol soak for 15 minutes.

7. Apply a thin coating of hydrocortisone lotion (0.5% to 1%) twice a day. Anesthetic ointment (such as lidocaine hydrochloride 2.5% or a benzocaine-containing spray) may provide short-term pain relief.

8. If the victim has a large area involved (an entire arm or leg, face, or genitals), is very young or very old, or shows signs of generalized illness (nausea, vomiting, weakness, shortness of breath, chest pain, and the like), seek help from a doctor. If a child has placed tentacle fragments in his mouth, have him swish and spit whatever potable liquid is available. If there is already swelling in the mouth (muffled voice, difficulty swallowing, enlarged tongue and lips), don't give anything by mouth, protect the airway (see page 22), and rapidly transport the victim to a hospital.

To prevent jellyfish stings, an ocean bather or diver should wear, at a minimum, a synthetic nylon-rubber (Lycra [DuPont]) dive skin. Safe Sea Sunblock with Jellyfish Sting Protective Lotion (www.getsafesea.com), which is both a sunscreen and a jellyfish sting inhibitor, has been shown to be effective in preventing stings from many jellyfish species. Other prevention measures include being aware of surface jellyfish, not diving into water headfirst, checking snorkel and scuba mouthpieces carefully for tentacle fragments, watching out for stinging tentacles on ropes—anchor lines—fishing lines, and obeying posted warnings.

CORAL AND BARNACLE CUTS

Cuts and scrapes from sharp-edged coral and barnacles tend to fester and become infected wounds. Treatment for these cuts is as follows:

1. Scrub the cut vigorously with soap and water, and then flush the wound with large amounts of water.

2. Flush the wound with a half-strength solution of hydrogen peroxide in water. Rinse again with water.

3. Apply a thin layer of bacitracin or mupirocin ointment, or mupirocin cream, and cover with a dry, sterile, nonadherent dressing. If no ointment or dressing is available, the wound can be left open. Thereafter, it should be cleaned and redressed twice a day.

4. If the wound develops a poorly healing pus-laden crust, you can use wet-to-dry dressing changes to remove the upper nonhealing layer to expose healthy, healing tissue. This is done by putting a dry, sterile gauze pad over the wound (without any underlying ointment), soaking the gauze pad with saline or a dilute antiseptic solution (such as 1% to 5% povidone–iodine in disinfected water), allowing the liquid to dry, and then "brutally" ripping the bandage off the wound. The dead and dying tissue adheres to the gauze and is lifted free. The pink (hopefully), slightly bleeding tissue underneath should be healthy and healing. Dressings are changed once or twice a day. Use wet-to-dry dressings for a few days, or until they become nonadherent. At that point, switch back to the treatment in the previous paragraph.

If the wound shows signs of infection (extreme redness, pus, swollen lymph glands) within 24 to 48 hours after the injury, start the victim on an antibiotic to oppose *Vibrio* bacteria (e.g., ciprofloxacin, trimethoprim–sulfamethoxazole, or doxycycline), as well as an antibiotic to oppose *Staphylococcus* bacteria (e.g., dicloxacillin or cephalexin).

5. Coral poisoning occurs if coral cuts are extensive or the cuts are from a particularly toxic species. The symptoms include a coral cut that heals poorly or continues to drain pus or cloudy fluid, swelling around the cut, swollen lymph glands, fever, chills, and fatigue. An antibiotic (see step 4) should be started, and the victim seen by a physician, who may elect to treat the victim for a week or two with an oral corticosteroid.

SEA URCHINS

Some sea urchins are covered with sharp venom-filled spines (Figure 229) that can easily penetrate and break off into the skin, or with small pincer-like appendages (Figure 230) that grasp the victim and inoculate him with venom from a sac within the pincer. Sea urchin punctures or stings are painful wounds, most often of the hands or feet. If a person receives many wounds simultaneously, the reaction may be so severe as to cause difficulty in breathing, weakness, and collapse. The treatment for sea urchin wounds is as follows:

1. Immerse the wound in nonscalding hot water to tolerance (110°F to 113°F, or 43.3°C to 45°C). This frequently provides sufficient pain relief. Administer appropriate pain medicine.
2. Carefully remove any readily visible spines. Don't dig around in the skin to fish them out—this risks crushing the spines and making them more difficult to remove. Don't intentionally crush the spines. Purple or black markings in the skin immediately after a sea urchin encounter don't necessarily indicate the presence of a retained spine fragment. Such discoloration is more likely dye leached from the surface of a spine, commonly from a black urchin (*Diadema* spp.). The dye will be absorbed over 24 to 48 hours, and the discoloration will disappear. If there are still black markings after 48 to 72 hours, a spine fragment is likely present.

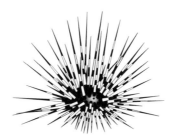

Figure 229. Spiny sea urchin.

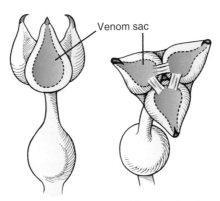

Figure 230. Sea urchin pincer with embedded venom sac.

3. If the sting is caused by a species with pincer organs, use hot-water immersion and then apply shaving cream or a soap paste and shave the area.
4. Seek the care of a physician if you feel that spines have been retained in the hand or foot, or near a joint. They may need to be removed surgically, in order to minimize infection, inflammation, and damage to nerves or important blood vessels.
5. If the wound shows signs of infection (extreme redness, pus, swollen lymph glands) within 24 to 48 hours after the injury, or if the spine is felt to have penetrated into a joint, start the victim on an antibiotic to oppose *Vibrio* bacteria (e.g., ciprofloxacin, trimethoprim–sulfamethoxazole, or doxycycline), as well as an antibiotic to oppose *Staphylococcus* bacteria (e.g., dicloxacillin or cephalexin).
6. If a spine puncture in the palm of the hand results in a persistent swollen finger without any sign of infection (fever, redness, swollen lymph glands in the elbow or armpit), it may become necessary to treat a 150 lb (68 kg) victim with a 7-day course of oral prednisone in a tapering dose (begin with 70 mg and decrease by 10 mg per day). Corticosteroids should always be taken with the understanding that a rare side effect is serious deterioration of the head ("ball" of the ball-and-socket joint) of the femur, the long bone of the thigh.

STARFISH

The crown of thorns starfish *(Acanthaster planci)* is a particularly venomous starfish found in tropical oceans worldwide. It carries sharp and rigid spines that may grow to 3 inches (7.5 cm) in length. The cutting edges easily penetrate a diver's glove and cause a very painful puncture wound with copious bleeding and slight swelling. Multiple puncture wounds may lead to vomiting, swollen lymph glands, and brief muscle paralysis.

The treatment is similar to that for a sea urchin puncture (see page 352). Immerse the wound in nonscalding hot water to tolerance (110° F to 113° F, or 43.3° C to 45° C) for 30 to 90 minutes. This frequently provides pain relief. Administer appropriate pain medicine. Carefully remove any readily visible spines. If there is a question of a retained spine or fragment, seek the assistance of a physician.

Other starfish, such as the rose star, can cause a skin rash. This may be treated with topical calamine lotion with 1% menthol or topical hydrocortisone 1% lotion.

CUCUMBERS

Sea cucumbers (Figure 231) are sausage-shaped creatures that produce a liquid called holothurin, which is a contact irritant to the skin and eyes. Because some sea cucumbers dine on jellyfish, they may excrete jellyfish stinging cells and venom as well. Therefore, anyone who sustains a skin irritation from handling a sea cucumber may benefit from the treatment for jellyfish stings described beginning on page 350. If the eyes are involved, they should be irrigated with at least a quart (liter) of water, and immediate medical attention should be sought. If the victim is out at sea, treat the eye injury as a corneal abrasion (see page 168).

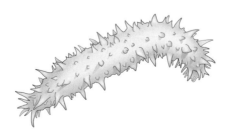

Figure 231. Sea cucumber.

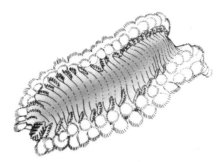

Figure 232. Bristleworm.

BRISTLEWORMS

Bristleworms are small, segmented marine worms covered with chitinous bristles arranged in soft rows around the body (Figure 232). When a worm is stimulated, its body contracts and the bristles are erected. Easily detached, they penetrate skin like cactus spines and are difficult to remove. Some marine worms are also able to inflict painful bites.

The bite or sting of a marine worm may induce intense inflammation typified by burning sensation with a raised, red, and itchy rash, most frequently on the hands and fingers. Untreated, the pain is generally self-limited over the course of a few hours, but the redness and itching may last for 2 to 3 days. With multiple punctures, there may be marked swelling.

Remove all large visible bristles with tweezers. Then gently dry the skin, taking care to avoid breaking or embedding the spines farther into it. Apply a layer of adhesive tape, rubber cement, or a facial peel to remove the residual smaller spines. If the residual inflammation is significant, the victim may benefit from administration of topical hydrocortisone 1% lotion.

CONE SNAILS (SHELLS)

Cone snails (shells) are beautiful, yet potentially lethal, cone-shaped mollusks that carry a highly developed venom apparatus, consisting of a rapid-acting poison that is injected by means of a dartlike, barbed tooth (Figure 233). The venom causes a mild sting (puncture wound) that initially is characterized by bee sting–like pain or, rarely, numbness and blanching. This is rapidly followed by numbness and tingling at the wound site, around the mouth and lips, and then all over the body. If the envenomation is severe, the victim is afflicted with muscle paralysis, blurred vision, and breathing failure. A sting can be fatal.

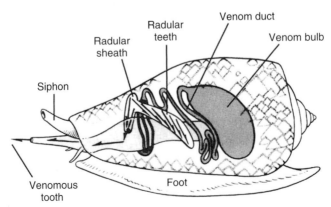

Figure 233. Cone snail, with a depiction of its venom apparatus.

There is no antivenom for a cone snail envenomation. While many first-aid remedies (such as hot-water immersion, surgical excision of the sting site, and injection of a local anesthetic) have been recommended, the one that makes the most sense is the pressure immobilization technique (see page 319) to contain the venom until the victim can be brought to advanced medical attention. Be prepared to offer the victim assistance for breathing (see page 28).

STINGRAYS

A stingray does its damage by lashing upward in self-defense with a muscular tail-like appendage, which carries up to four sharp, swordlike stings (Figure 234). The stings are supplied with venom, so that the injury created is both a deep puncture or laceration and an envenomation. The pain from a stingray wound can be excruciating and accompanied by bleeding, weakness, vomiting, headache, fainting, shortness of breath, paralysis, collapse, and occasionally, death. Most wounds involve the feet and legs, because unwary waders and swimmers tread on the creatures hidden in the sand. If a person is struck by a stingray, immediately do the following:

1. Rinse the wound with whatever clean water is available. Immediately immerse the wound in nonscalding hot water to tolerance (110°F to 113°F, or 43.3°C to 45°C). This may provide some pain relief. Generally, it's necessary to soak the wound for 30 to 90 minutes. Gently extract any obvious piece of stinger, unless it's felt to have penetrated into a location (e.g., chest, neck, abdomen, or groin) where it may have cut and is now occluding a large blood vessel, such as the heart or a major artery or vein. In such a case, leave the stinger in place, regardless of pain, and rush the victim to a hospital.
2. Scrub the wound with soap and water. Don't try to sew or tape it closed; doing so could support a serious infection.
3. Apply a dressing and seek medical help. If more than 12 hours will pass before a doctor can be reached, start the victim on an antibiotic (ciprofloxacin, trimethoprim–sulfamethoxazole, or doxycycline) to oppose *Vibrio* bacteria.
4. Administer appropriate pain medication.

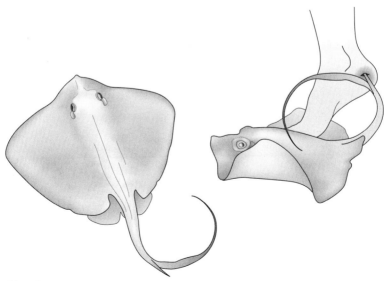

Figure 234. Stingray. The ray thrusts upward in self-defense with venom-laden spine(s) into the foot of an unwary victim.

Avoidance of Stingray Injuries

1. Always shuffle your feet when wading in stingray waters.
2. Always inspect the bottom before resting a limb in the sand.
3. Never handle a stingray unless you know what you're doing. Even seemingly "domesticated" stingrays, such as those at "Stingray City" off Grand Cayman Island in the British West Indies, have bitten victims with their grinding plate mouths, resulting in serious bite wounds, when handled.
4. Don't approach a stingray within striking distance of its barbed appendage.

CATFISH

Catfish sting their victims with dorsal and pectoral fin spines, which are charged with venom. When a fish is handled, the spines are extended and "locked" into position. The wound can be exceedingly painful, resembling the sting of a stingray. The treatment is the same as that for a stingray wound. Soaking the wound in nonscalding hot water to tolerance (110°F to 113°F, or 43.3°C to 45°C) may provide dramatic pain relief.

Tiny South American catfish of the genus *Vandellia* are known as "urethra fish" in English. They can swim up the human urethra or other urogenital openings and lodge within the victim, where they extend short spines on their gill covers. This can be extremely painful. Nonsurgical treatment is the ingestion of megadose (1 to 2 g per day) ascorbic acid (vitamin C); when excreted in the urine, this supposedly slowly softens the spines and allows the fish to be excreted as well. Surgical removal is generally required because the victim cannot tolerate the discomfort caused by a retained urethra fish.

SCORPIONFISH

Scorpionfish include zebrafish (lionfish, turkeyfish) (Figure 235), scorpionfish, and stonefish. They possess dorsal, anal, and pelvic spines that transport venom from venom glands into puncture wounds. Common reactions include redness or blanching, swelling, and blistering. The injuries can be extremely painful and occasionally life threatening. The treatment is the same as that for a stingray wound. Soaking the wound in nonscalding hot water to tolerance (110°F to 113°F, or 43.3°C to 45°C) may provide dramatic relief of pain from a lionfish sting, is less likely to be curative for a scorpionfish sting, and may have little effect on the pain from a stonefish sting, but it should be undertaken nonetheless, because the heat may perhaps destroy some of the harmful proteins contained in the venom. If the victim appears intoxicated or is weak, vomiting, short of breath, or unconscious, seek immediate advanced medical aid. Scorpionfish stings

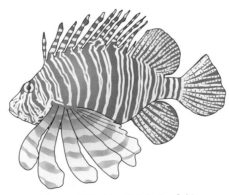

Figure 235. Lionfish (zebrafish).

frequently require weeks or months to heal, and therefore require the attention of a physician. There is an antivenom available to physicians to help manage the sting of the dreaded stonefish.

SURGEONFISH

Surgeonfish are tropical reef fish that carry one or more retractable jackknife-like skin append-ages on either side of the tail. When a fish is threatened, the appendage(s) is extended, where it serves as a blade to inflict a cut. The appendage may carry venom, which contributes to the pain.

Treatment is to soak the wound in nonscalding hot water to tolerance (110° F to 113° F, or 43.3° C to 45° C) for 30 to 90 minutes or until the pain is relieved, and then scrub vigorously to remove all foreign material. Watch closely for development of an infection.

OCTOPUSES

Octopus bites are rare. A nonvenomous octopus bite causes a local irritation that does not require any special therapy, other than wound cleansing and observation for infection. However, a bite from the Indo-Pacific blue-ringed or spotted octopus inoculates the victim with a sub-stance extremely similar to tetrodotoxin, one of the most potent poisons (also found in pufferfish—see page 358) found in nature.

Most victims are bitten on the hand or arm as they handle the creature or "give it a ride." The bite consists of one or two small puncture wounds and may go unnoticed. Otherwise, there is a small amount of discomfort, described as a minor ache, slight stinging, or pulsating sensation. Occasionally, the site is initially numb, followed in 5 to 10 minutes by discomfort that may spread to involve the entire limb. By far the most common local reaction is the absence of symptoms, a small spot of blood, or a tiny blanched area.

More serious symptoms develop within 15 minutes of the bite and include numbness of the mouth and face, followed by blurred vision, difficulty speaking, incoordination, weakness, vom-iting, muscle paralysis, and breathing failure. The victim may collapse quickly and die from inability to breathe.

First aid is the pressure immobilization technique (see page 319). Be prepared to provide artificial respiration (see page 28) until the victim can be brought to advanced medical attention. If oxygen (see page 405) is available, it should be administered by face mask at a flow rate of 10 liters per minute.

SEA SNAKES

Sea snakes are the most abundant reptiles on Earth, although they are found only in the Pacific and Indian Oceans. They can attain a length of 9 ft (2.7 m) and are equipped with a paddle-like tail that allows them to swim forward and backward with considerable speed and agility.

A sea snake can bite a victim with two to four fangs. The venom is extremely toxic, and causes paralysis, destruction of red blood cells, and widespread muscle damage.

The diagnosis of sea snake envenomation is determined as follows:

1. Unless you are handling a snake (commonly, fishermen emptying nets), you must be in the water to be bitten by a sea snake. The animals cannot move easily on land and don't survive very long there. However, you must be cautious when exploring regions of tidal variation, particularly in mangrove vegetation or near inlets where snakes breed.
2. Sea snake bites rarely cause much pain at the bite site.
3. Fang marks. These are like pinholes and may number from one to four (rarely, up to 20).
4. If symptoms don't occur within 6 to 8 hours of the bite, significant poisoning has not occurred. The symptoms include weakness, paralysis, lockjaw, drooping eyelids, difficulty speaking, and vomiting. Later, the victim will develop darkened urine and difficulty breathing.

5. If a person is bitten by a sea snake, seek *immediate* medical attention while you implement the pressure immobilization technique (see page 319). The definitive therapy is similar to that for a land snakebite—namely, administration in a hospital of the proper antivenom.

SKIN RASHES CAUSED BY AQUATIC PLANTS (SEAWEED DERMATITIS) OR CREATURES (SEA BATHER'S ERUPTION, SWIMMER'S ITCH)

See page 219.

POISONINGS FROM SEAFOOD

A number of fish and seafood products cause poisonings because they contain natural toxins or accumulated man-made toxins. For instance, in the past, the U.S. Food and Drug Administration has issued an advisory cautioning women who are or might be pregnant, small children, and nursing mothers to not eat shark, swordfish, king mackerel, or tilefish because of accumulations of methylmercury.

Scombroid Poisoning

Scombroid poisoning is caused by improper preservation (inadequate refrigeration or drying) of fish in the family Scombridae, which includes tuna, mackerel, bonito, skipjacks, and wahoo. Nonscombroid fish that can also cause this syndrome include mahi-mahi (dolphinfish), anchovies, sardines, and Australian ocean salmon. Most of these fish are dark fleshed. When they aren't preserved properly, bacteria break down chemicals in the flesh to produce the chemical histamine, which causes an allergic-type reaction in the victim. Although the fish may have a peppery or metallic taste and "dull" appearance, they may also have normal color, flavor, and appearance. Tuna burgers may be seasoned, which masks any abnormal taste.

Minutes after eating the fish, the victim becomes flushed, with itching, nausea and sometimes vomiting, diarrhea, low-grade fever, abdominal pain, and the development of hives (see page 220). Occasionally, a victim will develop low blood pressure and become weak and short of breath, sometimes with wheezing. The reaction is similar to that seen with monosodium glutamate (MSG) sensitivity ("Chinese food syndrome"). Treatment is the same as for an allergic reaction (see page 64). If the victim does not improve with diphenhydramine (Benadryl), he may benefit from cimetidine (Tagamet) 300 mg, fexofenadine (Allegra) 60 mg, or loratadine (Claritin) 10 mg by mouth. Administer cimetidine or fexofenadine every 6 to 8 hours, or loratadine once a day, until symptoms resolve—generally, within 12 to 24 hours.

Pufferfish Poisoning

Certain pufferfish (blowfish, globefish, swellfish, porcupinefish, and so on) contain tetrodotoxin or saxitoxin, among the most potent poisons in nature. These fish are prepared as a delicacy (fugu) in Japan by specially trained and licensed chefs. The toxin is found in the entire fish, with greatest concentration in the liver, intestines, reproductive organs, and skin. After the victim has eaten the fish, symptoms can occur as quickly as 10 minutes later or be delayed by a few hours. They may even be delayed by up to 20 hours. These include numbness and tingling around the mouth, light-headedness, drooling, sweating, vomiting, diarrhea, abdominal pain, weakness, difficulty walking, paralysis, difficulty breathing, and collapse. Many victims die.

If someone is suffering from pufferfish poisoning, immediately transport him to a hospital. Pay attention to his ability to breathe, and assist his breathing if necessary (see page 28). Unfortunately, there is no antidote, and the victim will need sophisticated medical management until he metabolizes the toxin. Eating pufferfish, unless they are prepared by the most skilled chefs, is dietary Russian roulette.

Ciguatera Fish Poisoning

Ciguatera fish poisoning involves a large number of tropical and semi-tropical bottom-feeding fish that dine on plants or smaller fish that have accumulated toxins from microscopic dinoflagellates, such as *Gambierdiscus toxicus*. Therefore, the larger the fish, the greater the toxicity. The ciguatoxin-carrying fish most commonly ingested include the barracuda, jack, grouper, and snapper. Ciguatoxin has recently been identified in lionfish caught in U.S. coastal waters. Symptoms, which usually begin 15 to 30 minutes after the victim eats the contaminated fish, include abdominal pain, nausea, vomiting, diarrhea, tongue and throat numbness, tooth pain, difficulty walking, blurred vision, skin rash, itching, tearing of the eyes, weakness, twitching muscles, incoordination, difficulty sleeping, and occasional difficulty in breathing. A classic sign of ciguatera intoxication is the reversal of hot and cold sensation (hot liquids seem cold and vice versa), which may reflect general hypersensitivity to temperature. Unfortunately, the symptoms persist in varying severity for weeks to months. Victims can become severely ill, with heart problems, low blood pressure, deficiencies of the central and peripheral nervous systems, and generalized collapse.

Treatment is for the most part supportive, although certain drugs are beginning to prove useful for aspects of the syndrome. An example is intravenous mannitol for abnormal nervous system behavior or abnormal heart rhythms. These therapies must be undertaken by a physician. Prochlorperazine may be useful for vomiting; hydroxyzine or cool showers may be useful for itching. There is not yet a specific antidote. Anyone who displays symptoms of ciguatera fish poisoning should be seen promptly by a physician.

During recovery from ciguatera poisoning, the victim should exclude the following from his diet: fish, fish sauces, shellfish, shellfish sauces, alcoholic beverages, nuts, and nut oils.

Paralytic Shellfish Poisoning

Paralytic shellfish poisoning is caused by eating shellfish that contain concentrated toxins produced originally by certain planktons and protozoans in the ocean. These same microorganisms are responsible for the "red" (blue, brown, white, black, and so on) tides that occur in warm summer months. The shellfish (such as California mussels, which are quarantined each year from May through October) dine on the microorganisms and concentrate the poison in their digestive organs and muscle tissues. Generally, crabs, shrimp, and abalone are safe to eat.

Minutes after eating contaminated shellfish, the victim complains of numbness and tingling inside and around his mouth, and of his tongue and gums. He soon becomes light-headed, weak, and incoherent, and begins to suffer from drooling, difficulty swallowing, incoordination, headache, thirst, diarrhea, abdominal pain, blurred vision, sweating, and rapid heartbeat. Even if a victim becomes paralyzed, he may continue to be aware of what is happening, unless he does not receive enough oxygen to the brain (because he stops breathing).

The victim of paralytic shellfish poisoning should be brought immediately to a hospital. If he is having trouble breathing, be prepared to assist him (see page 28).

Hallucinatory Fish Poisoning

Certain reef fish of the tropical Pacific and Indian Oceans carry heat-stable toxins in their head parts, brain, and spinal cords, and (to a lesser degree) in their muscles. Typical species include surgeonfish, goatfish, mullets, sergeants major, damselfish, and rudderfish. The toxicity of the fish can vary with the season.

Symptoms occur within 90 minutes of ingestion, and include dizziness, numbness and tingling around the mouth and lips, sweating, weakness, incoordination, auditory and visual hallucinations, nightmares, shortness of breath, brief paralysis, and sore throat. People don't die from this affliction. Treatment is supportive. The victim should be observed closely to see that he does not injure himself by exercising bad judgment.

Anisakidosis

Anisakidosis is caused by penetration of the nematode *Anisakis simplex* or *Pseudoterranova* worm larvae through the lining of the stomach. This occurs when someone eats raw or under-cooked fish, such as sushi. The most common carriers, which serve as intermediate hosts via sea mammals, are mackerel, Pacific herring and cod, coho salmon, hake, anchovies, squid, silvergray and yellowtail rockfish, bocaccio, and, in rare cases, tuna.

Symptoms begin within 1 hour of eating the fish and include severe pain in the upper abdomen, nausea, and vomiting. The victim may appear quite ill. Occasionally, he may have the symptoms of an allergic reaction.

If the worm(s) is not removed by a physician, who must do this physically through an endo-scope passed through the esophagus into the stomach, it dies within a few days. However, implantation can initiate an abscess. Some worms don't implant, but are coughed up, vomited up, or passed in the stool. If a worm crawls into the esophagus or throat, an unusual tingling feeling can develop.

A worm that passes through the stomach and implants in the intestine (up to 7 days after ingestion) causes abdominal pain, nausea, vomiting, diarrhea, and fever. It may penetrate com-pletely through the bowel. When this happens, an operation may be performed for suspected appendicitis or intestinal cancer, only to discover the true cause of the victim's symptoms.

Unfortunately, there is no drug or purgative treatment that will eliminate the parasite once it has been ingested. It's either regurgitated or passed in the stool, or has to be physically removed, which can be as complicated as surgically removing a section of intestine.

To prevent this problem, any fish should be cooked to a temperature above 140° F (60°C) or frozen for 24 hours to −4° F (−20°C) before it is eaten. Smoking, marinating, pickling, brining, and salting may not kill the worms. A fish should be gutted as soon as possible after it is caught to prevent migration of the worms from its internal organs into its muscle tissue. An allergic reaction may still occur from eating properly preserved or cooked, but parasitized, fish.

UNDERWATER DIVING ACCIDENTS

On land at sea level, the human body is constantly exposed to 14.7 lb (6.7 kg, or 1 atmosphere) of pressure from the weight of the atmosphere (an air column 165 miles [266 km] high). As a human descends underwater in the ocean, with every 33 ft (10 m) of depth an additional atmos-phere of pressure is exerted. With increasing pressure (P) that occurs on descent, the volume (V) of gas in an enclosed space is diminished, as determined by Boyle's law: $P_1V_1 = P_2V_2$. Con-versely, during ascent from the depths, the gas in an enclosed space expands. Underwater, the greatest relative volume changes with increasing and decreasing pressure occur near the surface (Figure 236).

Any diver who is recovered from the water in an unconscious, pulseless, and nonbreathing condi-tion should be treated as a drowning victim (see later), with rescue breathing and CPR as indicated for drowning.

AIR EMBOLISM

An air embolism occurs when there is a rupture in the barrier between the microscopic air space of a lung and its corresponding blood vessel, which carries oxygenated blood back to the heart (where it can be distributed to the body). With air embolism, bubbles of air are released into

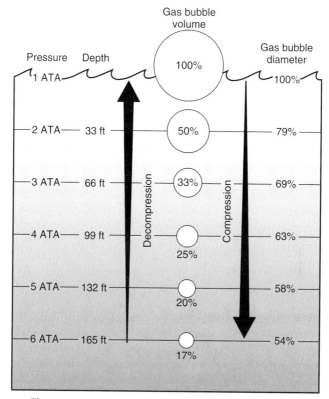

Figure 236. Volume changes with depth and pressure.

the arterial bloodstream, where they act as physical barriers to circulation, and can cause a stroke (see page 135), heart attack (see page 47), headache, spinal cord injury, and/or confusion. Typically, the victim is a scuba (self-contained underwater breathing apparatus) diver who ascends too rapidly without exhaling, thus allowing overexpansion of the lungs—and rupture of the tissue—as the external water pressure decreases with ascent. In other words, as a diver ascends from the depths, the air in his lungs (which was delivered from the scuba tank through a regulator at a pressure equal to the surrounding water pressure on the lungs, thereby allowing lung expansion) expands. If the rate of exhalation does not keep pace with this lung expansion, the increased pressure within the lungs causes air to be forced through the lung tissue, where it appears in the bloodstream in bubble form and travels directly to the heart. From the heart, the air circulates to and may occlude critical small blood vessels that supply the heart, brain, and spinal cord.

The most common symptoms are unconsciousness, confusion or disorientation, seizures, and/or chest pain immediately on surfacing. Others include dizziness, visual blurring, loss of vision, headache, abnormal personality, confusion, total or partial paralysis, and weakness. Any disorder that appears in a previously normal diver more than 10 minutes after surfacing is probably not due to air embolism.

Anyone suspected of having suffered an air embolism should be placed in a head-down position (with the body at a 15- to 30-degree tilt), turned onto his left side, assisted with breathing if necessary (see page 28), and *immediately transported to an emergency facility*. If oxygen (see page 405) is available, it should be administered by face mask at a flow rate of 10 liters per minute. The treatment for arterial gas embolism is recompression in a hyperbaric oxygen chamber, which pressurizes the victim's environment and shrinks the bubbles. This must be accomplished as rapidly as possible to save the victim's life and to minimize disability. A portable recompression chamber manned by trained personnel may be used to initiate field treatment. If the victim is capable of purposeful swallowing, administer one adult aspirin by mouth.

If the air that expands on ascent does not rupture into a blood vessel and become an air embolism, it can rupture into the actual lung tissues or into the pleural space between the lung and the inside of the chest wall, and cause a collapsed lung (pneumothorax) (see page 39). Other symptoms include air that escapes into the soft tissues, so that there is swelling of the chest and neck, and sometimes a "Rice Krispies" feel to the skin. If the air dissects into the neck, it can cause hoarseness, difficulty swallowing, and sore throat. In this case, oxygen administration is advised. Recompression in a hyperbaric chamber is not advised for a pneumothorax unless there are also severe symptoms associated with an air embolism.

When transporting a victim of air embolism, it's recommended that you use an aircraft that can be pressurized to 1 atmosphere or keep the flight altitude (in an unpressurized aircraft) below 1000 ft (305 m).

The Divers Alert Network (www.diversalertnetwork.org) maintains a 24-hour hotline (919-684-9111) to assist with care coordination and evacuation assistance for diving accidents.

DECOMPRESSION SICKNESS (THE "BENDS")

When a scuba diver descends in the water, nitrogen present in the compressed air he breathes is absorbed into the tissues of his body. This process is analogous to the introduction of carbon dioxide into a beverage for the purpose of carbonation. In the human case, there is a limit to the time and depth that a diver can tolerate before exceeding the amount of nitrogen he can absorb safely without a staged decompression (ascent). If this limit is exceeded, and/or if the diver ascends too rapidly, this nitrogen leaves his tissues and enters his bloodstream in the form of microscopic bubbles (like opening a bottle of soda pop).

The signs and symptoms caused by these bubbles in the body represent decompression sickness, also known as the "bends." Symptoms may begin immediately after ascent from a dive or may be delayed by a number of hours. These include deep boring joint pain without swelling/warmth/redness, numbness and tingling of the arms and legs, difficulty walking, back pain, fatigue, weakness, inability to control the bladder or bowels (spinal cord "hit"), paralysis, double vision, diminished vision, headache, confusion, dizziness, nausea, vomiting, difficulty speaking, itching, skin mottling ("marbling"), shortness of breath, cough, and collapse. A rapid, simplified neurologic examination (see page 136), such as administered to a suspected stroke victim, may identify a subtle abnormality.

If you suspect someone of suffering the bends, immediately have him begin to breathe oxygen (at a flow rate of 10 liters per minute by face mask) (see page 405) and begin rapid transport to an emergency facility. Oxygen breathing should occur for at least 30 minutes. The definitive treatment is recompression in a hyperbaric chamber. *Don't put the diver back into the water to attempt in-water recompression;* this can be very hazardous. If possible, have the victim lie down in a comfortable position, preferably on his side, but don't let him obstruct blood flow to a limb by resting his head on an arm or crossing his legs. A portable recompression chamber manned by trained personnel may be used to initiate field treatment.

Because the pressure inside a commercial jet aircraft flying at 30,000 ft (9150 m) is equivalent to an unpressurized environmental altitude of 8000 ft (2440 m), a diver should not fly for 24 hours following a scuba dive. When transporting a victim of decompression sickness, it is recommended that you use an aircraft that can be pressurized to 1 atmosphere or keep the flight altitude (in an unpressurized aircraft) below 1000 ft (305 m).

The Divers Alert Network (www.diversalertnetwork.org) maintains a 24-hour hotline (919-684-9111) to assist with care coordination and evacuation assistance for diving accidents.

NITROGEN NARCOSIS

When absorbed into the bloodstream in sufficient concentration, nitrogen acts as an anesthetic agent. Thus, at depths that exceed 90 ft (27 m), divers are at risk for euphoria, confusion, inappropriate judgment, and unconsciousness induced by nitrogen absorbed into the bloodstream from air breathed under pressure. The treatment is prompt (but cautious) ascent, to allow the absorbed levels of nitrogen to decrease. *No one should ever dive alone. Always pay attention to your dive buddy's behavior. If he acts in a strange manner, assist him to the surface.*

EAR SQUEEZE

As a diver descends in the water, the external water pressure on his eardrum increases rapidly. If he cannot equalize this pressure from within by forcing air into the eustachian tube (a small passageway that connects the middle ear and the throat) and into the middle ear, the eardrum stretches inward (extremely painful) and then ruptures (Figure 237). This rupture allows water to rush into the middle ear, with resultant severe pain, hearing loss, vertigo (see page 364), nausea, vomiting, and disorientation. If the diver cannot make his way to the surface, he may drown. If the eardrum is injured but not ruptured, the pain is similar to that of an ear infection. In this situation, the eardrum is intact, but tissue fluid and blood have collected in the middle ear, partially or completely filling it. In addition to pain, the victim notes decreased hearing and a sense of fullness in the ear. If this occurs, diving should be prohibited (see later) and the person treated with decongestants and, in a severe case, with prednisone (begin with 60 mg first dose for an adult and decrease by 10 mg each day for 5 days) to decrease inflammation.

Inability to "clear" the ears (equalize pressure from within) to prevent inward bulging and rupture of the eardrum should keep a diver out of the water. A person with an upper respiratory tract infection (and narrowed eustachian tube) should not dive, and should avoid travel in an unpressurized aircraft.

If a diver suddenly feels pain in his ear and is stricken with dizziness, nausea, or visual difficulty, he should remain calm and slowly ascend to the surface. The ear should be allowed to

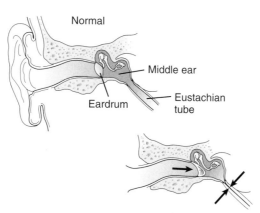

Figure 237. Middle ear squeeze. When a diver descends, air in the middle ear contracts, the eustachian tube collapses, and the eardrum bulges inward, causing pain. If the external water pressure is sufficient, the eardrum can rupture.

drain and dry on its own. Don't insert cotton swabs into the ear, because you may poke the eardrum and increase the damage. Don't instill any medicines into the ear, unless you are carrying ofloxacin otic solution 0.3% or Cortisporin solution (*not* "suspension"). Transport the victim to an ear specialist. Suspend all diving activities until the eardrum is healed or repaired. If dizziness is profound, administer a drug(s) for motion sickness (see page 411). The victim should be started on an antibiotic (ciprofloxacin [or another fluoroquinolone antibiotic], trimethoprim–sulfamethoxazole, or doxycycline) to oppose *Vibrio* bacteria. If one of these antibiotics is not available, use amoxicillin–clavulanate. An oral or topical nasal decongestant (such as 0.5% oxymetazoline) is useful for the first few days after the episode. Because sudden dizziness may also be due to an air embolism or the bends, the victim should be observed closely for worsening of his condition.

Alternobaric vertigo refers to a condition in which the pressure in the middle ear can be different between the two ears, usually on ascent. This may cause a person to suffer from vertigo of relatively short duration, ringing in the ears, and hearing loss. The treatment is patience until the pressures in the middle ears equalize; decongestants may help hasten the process.

SINUS SQUEEZE

Sinus squeeze occurs if pressurized air cannot be forced into the sinuses during descent. In such a case, the air within the sinus contracts, causing the walls of the sinus to bleed, accompanied by intense, sharp pain. Symptoms include pain over the affected sinus, in the upper teeth (when the maxillary, or cheek, sinus is involved), and nosebleed. A "reverse squeeze" occurs during ascent, when air expands in the sinus without being able to escape. This is also very painful, but fortunately self-limited, because the air will be absorbed slowly into the tissues that line the sinuses.

If a sinus squeeze occurs, slowly ascend to the surface. This generally alleviates most of the pain, but it may take a while for the bleeding to stop. Because the sinus may now be blood-filled, the victim is at high risk for developing sinusitis (see page 181) and should be placed on amoxicillin–clavulanate or azithromycin for 4 days, along with oral and nasal decongestants to promote drainage. If the pain is severe and persists for more than 12 hours after the initial incident, the victim may benefit from a short course of prednisone, 60 mg the first day, 40 mg the second, and 20 mg the third. This combats the inflammation, but should not be given if the victim has symptoms of a sinus infection (foul nasal discharge, fever, facial tenderness).

TOOTH SQUEEZE

Increasing pressure during descent into the water can cause entrapped gas in the interior of a tooth or in the structures surrounding a tooth to contract (tooth squeeze). In an extreme case, this can cause a tooth to crack or implode. Conversely, air under a filling or within a cavity or abscess can expand on ascent, causing a minor (and painful) "explosion." To minimize the risk of a tooth squeeze, don't enter the water for at least 24 hours after dental treatment.

DROWNING

One of the most common tragic accidents, particularly of children, is drowning. Drowning is defined as submersion or immersion into liquid that causes breathing impairment. If a person is rescued, it is considered a "nonfatal drowning." Drowning can occur in a variety of settings, but the medical problems encountered seldom vary:

1. Lack of oxygen. If death occurs during the drowning episode, it is most likely because of suffocation due to being submerged or immersed in water. Another factor is spasm of the

vocal cords, which blocks the passage of air through the windpipe (most commonly seen in cold-water drowning). If a drowning victim inhales forcefully against a closed airway, this in and of itself can create a lung injury. When submerged, the body is starved of oxygen, which is essential to survival. If the submersion lasts long enough, the victim loses consciousness and ultimately suffers a cardiac arrest. A person who has experienced a drowning episode and survived may have delayed complications related to aspiration of water and hypoxia.

2. Body chemistry abnormalities. Because of the lack of oxygen delivery to the organs and tissues of the body, there is rapid accumulation of waste products that cannot be effectively removed. This results in accumulation of acid and other chemicals that alter the function of the heart, brain, kidneys, liver, and other organ systems. There is no fundamental physiologic difference between drowning in freshwater and saltwater.

3. Accompanying problems, such as hypothermia (see page 281), injuries, and serious illnesses (e.g., heart attack or stroke). Sadly, alcohol figures prominently in adult boating and drowning accidents.

RECOGNIZING A VICTIM OF DROWNING

A person who is drowning may be obviously struggling, but sometimes it takes an astute observer to recognize that a person in the water is in trouble, because the victim may be not be strong or alert enough to call or signal for help. Less obvious indications of drowning include:

1. Bobbing up and down in the water with wide open mouth and rapid or gasping breaths
2. Head tilted back in the water with open mouth
3. Mouth at or below water level
4. Eyes "glassy" or closed; blank stare
5. Eyes and forehead covered with hair
6. Not using the legs at all to swim or remain afloat while remaining upright in the water
7. Purposeless swimming
8. Swimming hard without forward progress
9. Within earshot but not responding to your call for a response
10. Children who are quiet in the water

If a drowning incident occurs, do the following:

1. Remove the victim from the water, while ensuring that you and others remain safe. If immediate rescue is difficult or impossible, and at the earliest opportunity, send someone for help. In-water resuscitation is difficult at best. It should be attempted only by a trained rescuer. Administering a couple of rescue breaths to a nonbreathing victim while he or she is still in the water (see page 28) may be helpful; the chest compressions of CPR should not be attempted. If the victim is placed on the beach, keep him far enough from the water to avoid incoming waves.

2. After the victim is removed from the water, check for breathing by feeling over the mouth and nose while watching the chest rise. Open the mouth and sweep it clean with two fingers. Align the victim on the ground with his head at the level of his trunk (not head down). Begin mouth-to-mouth or mouth–to–mouth-and-nose (for a child) breathing, if necessary (see page 28). Administer 5 initial rescue breaths.

3. Check for pulses and begin chest compressions if necessary (see page 30). For drowning, use the "ABC" (airway, breathing, circulation/chest compressions) order for CPR, rather than the currently recommended CAB sequence). Chest compression–only CPR is not recommended for drowning. Administer 5 initial rescue breaths.

4. If the victim is unconscious but breathing, place him in the lateral lying rescue position (see page 25) with the head higher than the trunk.

5. If the victim is short of breath or worse, administer oxygen (see page 405) at a flow rate of 15 liters per minute by non-rebreathing face mask.

6. Suspect a broken neck in the appropriate circumstances. For instance, someone who has been seen to collapse in a swimming pool probably hasn't broken his neck. (If he dove into the pool, that's another story!) However, someone who tumbles into the waves off a surfboard and washes up unconscious onto the beach may well have a neck injury. However, even if you suspect a broken neck, if the victim is unconscious, CPR protocols are the priority. Don't delay resuscitation procedures in an attempt to address possible spinal injuries. Do what is necessary to aid the victim, then remember to protect his neck (see page 35) if dictated by the circumstances.

7. The Heimlich maneuver (see page 27) and other choking protocols (e.g., back slaps, chest hugs) are not recommended for use in the rescue of drowning victims, because they may cause the victim to regurgitate and inhale vomit.

8. Hypothermia (see page 281) is commonly associated with drowning. Cover the victim above and below with blankets. Gently remove all wet clothing. Because hypothermia may be protective for the heart and brain (with regard to lack of oxygen) to a considerable degree, if the victim is cold, continue the resuscitation until trained rescuers arrive or until you are fatigued. Remember, "no one is dead until he is warm and dead."

9. If the victim responds to your measures, the following guidelines for further medical assistance are recommended by the International Life Saving Federation:

   Persons who require further evaluation/assistance (likely at a hospital):
   Loss of consciousness (even if briefly) at any point; received rescue breathing; underwent CPR; serious condition (e.g., heart attack, spinal or other significant injury, asthma, marine animal sting, intoxication, altered mental status) suspected. A person who is already short of breath and coughing may deteriorate quickly.

   Persons who may be considered to be safely released from care at the scene:
   Victim should be observed for 15 minutes and seen to have *all* of the following: no coughing, normal rate of breathing, normal pulse (strength and rate), normal skin color and temperature, no shivering, fully awake and alert. These victims will nearly always do well. However, it should be noted that on occasion a person who has suffered a drowning event and appears well at first may develop cough, shortness of breath, or fever. If this happens, they should be brought promptly to medical attention.

PREVENTION OF DROWNING

1. Watch your children. Toddlers are at greatest risk for drowning. Children under the age of 14 years are at high risk for drowning. Additional risk factors are poor education, inadequate supervision, rural location, and risky behavior.

2. Completely fence in all pools and swimming areas to a height of at least 4 feet. Install a self-closing, self-latching gate. Maintain the water level in a pool as high as possible to allow a person who reaches the edge to pull himself out. Don't leave inflatable pools unattended if small children can gain access. Consider using effective pool covers and pool alarms. Don't leave floats, balls, and other toys in a pool or surrounding area unless an adult supervisor is present.

3. Don't leave large pails or buckets full of water near small children.

4. Children may become entrapped in pool or spa drains, either by inserting a foot or hand into an open drain pipe and becoming trapped by suction that causes tissue swelling or by hair entanglement. These incidents can be avoided by using special drain covers, safety vacuum-release systems, filter pumps with multiple drains, and other pressure-venting filter construction techniques.

5. Teach children to swim, but be advised that such teaching does not absolutely "drown-proof" a child. In other words, never let a small child out of your sight when he is near the water, even if he knows how to swim. In a drowning situation, children may not have the body strength, judgment, or emotional reserve to allow self-rescue. Furthermore, new swimmers and children may have a false sense of security and take undue risks after being taught how to swim. Swimming lessons in the 1- to 4-year-old age group may reduce drowning risk, but once again, small children should never be left unattended in potentially dangerous situations.

6. Never place nonswimmers in high-risk situations: small sailboats, whitewater rafts, inflatable kayaks, and the like.

7. Don't swim alone. Obey safety signs and warning flags.

8. Watch for dangerous water conditions (big waves, rip currents) and weather conditions (e.g., thunderstorm with lightning).

9. When boating or rafting, always wear a properly rated personal flotation device (PFD, commonly called a "life vest" or "life jacket") with a snug fit and a head flotation collar. Don't substitute air-filled swimming aids, such as "water wings," for properly fitted PFDs. In a kayak or raft traversing whitewater, wear a proper helmet.

10. Don't jump or dive headfirst into unknown water for the first entry.

11. Persons at risk for a seizure should not be left alone in the water.

12. Don't mix alcohol and water sports.

13. Know your limits. Feats of endurance and demonstrations of bravado in dangerous rapids or surf are for idiots.

14. Be prepared for a flash flood. In times of unusually heavy rainfall, stay away from natural streambeds, arroyos, and other drainage channels. Signs of an impending abrupt rise in water level include clear water turning muddy or the appearance of floating debris. Use a map to determine your elevation, and stay off low ground or the very bottom of a hill. Know where the high ground is and how to get there in a hurry. Absolutely avoid flooded areas and unnecessary stream and river crossings. Don't attempt to cross a flowing stream where the water is above your knees. Abandon a stalled vehicle in a flood area. If a vehicle plunges into the water and will sink below the surface, attempt to leave the vehicle (from a door or window) before the vehicle submerges, assuming that the hazard of entering the water is acceptable for the escaping person(s).

15. If you anticipate that you might need to rescue a drowning person, you should know how to swim, complete an in-water rescue, start rescue breathing and CPR, and summon help.

ANIMAL ATTACKS

Most animal attacks are from "man's best friend," the pet dog. Other animals that will attack humans, given provocation, include the cat, rat, raccoon, tiger, lion, skunk, squirrel, camel, cougar (mountain lion), elephant, bear, alligator, crocodile, bat, wolf, rhinoceros, and hippopotamus. Although there are unique variations to the nature of the wounds created by different animals (in most part related to the size of the animal, types of teeth and claws, and risk of infection), the basic out-of-hospital management of an animal bite or mauling is the same for all creatures.

GENERAL TREATMENT

1. If a person is bitten or mauled by an animal, apply pressure to stop any brisk bleeding, and follow the instructions for management of bleeding and cuts (see pages 50 and 240).

2. It's important to clean the wounds well. Flush any injury that has broken the skin with at least 2 quarts (liters) of disinfected water, scrub with mild soap, and flush again. If you're carrying povidone–iodine (Betadine) solution 10% (not soap or scrub); benzalkonium (Zephiran) liquid 1% antiseptic; or, in a pinch, Bactine antiseptic (benzalkonium 0.13%), rinse the wound with one of these for 1 minute (to help kill rabies virus), and then rinse away the solution until there is no discoloration of the wound.
3. Don't tightly sew or tape closed any animal bite, unless it's absolutely essential to allow rescue. If a large tear is present, the wound edges can be held together with tape and wraps (see page 246). Tight closure of a contaminated wound (all animal bites and scratches introduce bacteria into the wound) can lead to a devastating infection. Apply a thin layer of bacitracin or mupirocin ointment or mupirocin cream into the wound.
4. If the victim is more than 5 hours from a physician, administer amoxicillin–clavulanic acid. If a person no longer has a spleen, either because it is not present or not functioning properly (e.g., persons with sickle cell anemia), then be certain to administer an antibiotic as soon as possible after the bite occurs. Alternative antibiotics include cefuroxime axetil, dicloxacillin, azithromycin, cefixime, cephalexin, trimethoprim–sulfamethoxazole, or ciprofloxacin with clindamycin. If the victim is allergic to penicillin, and if the bite is from a dog, administer clindamycin with levofloxacin (or ciprofloxacin), or for children clindamycin with trimethoprim–sulfamethoxazole; if the bite is from a cat, use cefuroxime axetil or doxycycline; if the bite is from a raccoon or skunk, use doxycycline. If the bite is from a cat, domestic or wild, administer an antibiotic as soon as possible. Animal bite wounds of the hands and feet seem particularly prone to bacterial infection. If an animal bite becomes infected, the same antibiotics are recommended, with the exception that for cat (domestic and "big" cat) bites, dicloxacillin should be given with penicillin.

SPECIAL CONSIDERATIONS

High-Risk Wounds

Wounds at high risk for infection include bites to the hands and feet and all puncture wounds (see page 239). These should be rinsed copiously and never cinched shut by any method. Anyone who sustains such a wound should be given antibiotics for 4 days (see step 4 above). Cat, human, and primate bites are enormously prone to infection, and require prompt attention by a physician. In a typical human bite, which occurs when a closed fist strikes an opponent's teeth, the cut extends deeply into a knuckle and inoculates the underlying tendon sheath with saliva and bacteria. As the fist is opened, the wound becomes "closed," and an infection can develop quickly. If a human bite is incurred in this manner, splint the hand in the position of function (see Figure 49) and administer cefuroxime axetil, ciprofloxacin plus erythromycin, or dicloxacillin plus ampicillin for 7 days.

Cat-Scratch Disease

Cat-scratch disease is most commonly caused by bacteria of the genus *Bartonella*. After the victim is scratched by a cat (most often a kitten), commonly on the hand, wrist, or forearm, a reddened or purplish sore forms at the scratch site within a few days. The sore may blister and then settle into an ulcer that remains for days to weeks. Along with the sore, the victim typically complains of swollen lymph glands (nodes) directly upstream from the injury. In the case of a scratch on the hand, these would appear behind the elbow and in the armpit. The swollen nodes are often tender and sometimes matted together. On occasion, they may become severely inflamed, soften, and drain through the skin surface. The victim may also complain of fever and fatigue. Although the response to antibiotics is not consistent, the victim may benefit from azithromycin once a day for 5 days, or from a 5-day course of ciprofloxacin, trimethoprim-sulfamethoxazole, or clarithromycin.

Rabies

Rabies virus infection occurs more frequently in wild than in domestic animals. In some foreign countries where immunization of animals is infrequently practiced, the risk is great even in domesticated animals. The virus is carried in saliva and is transmitted by bite or lick (if the skin is broken). It has been transmitted by bats in caves either by aerosolized saliva or undetected bites. Raccoons, dogs, cats, foxes, coyotes, skunks, wolves, bats, woodchucks, and groundhogs are the most common carriers. Rabies has not been reported in bears. Although rabbits, hares, mice, squirrels, chipmunks, rats, guinea pigs, and ferrets may be rabid, they are rarely involved in the transmission of rabies to humans. Domestic animals such as cattle, horses, and sheep become infected in regions where skunk or raccoon rabies is found. In developing countries in Asia, Africa, and South and Central America, dogs are the most common carriers.

Animals with rabies show abnormal behavior. In the "furious" phase, they are hyperactive, may have a fever, are overtly aggressive, and salivate excessively. With "dumb" rabies, they appear tired, lack coordination, and may become paralyzed.

Because of rabies risk, all wild animal bites or scratches, and bites or scratches of unregistered or strangely behaving cats and dogs, should be reported to the appropriate public health authority. If the animal is a pet with otherwise normal behavior, it should be observed for 10 days. If the animal is rabid, it will become very ill or die during that time, and its brain tissue can be analyzed for the presence of rabies. If the animal is a pet with unusual behavior, or a captured high-risk wild animal, it should be killed and examined. *If it is a high-risk animal and cannot be captured, it must be presumed to be rabid.*

Immediately scrub an animal bite wound or a wound that has been licked by a potentially rabid animal vigorously with soap and water. If benzalkonium chloride 1% (Zephiran); 10% povidone–iodine (Betadine) solution (less effective); or, in a pinch, Bactine (benzalkonium 0.13%) antiseptic is available, one of these should be used to irrigate and deeply swab the wound, since they may kill rabies virus.

If rabies is a consideration, the victim should seek the assistance of a physician, who will determine the need for postexposure rabies vaccination (a series of five injections) and injection of antirabies serum (human rabies immune globulin; as much as possible is injected around the bite wound, and the remainder intramuscularly). A person who has been previously immunized against rabies still needs two booster doses of rabies vaccine after high-risk contact with a rabid animal. In countries (Africa, Asia) where rabies is very prevalent in dogs and cats, the vaccination status of the biting animal should be ignored, because the vaccination may not have occurred or may have been ineffective. Begin postexposure vaccination of the human victim and then discontinue after 10 days if the biting animal is observed to remain healthy during that time period.

Preexposure vaccination against rabies should be administered to people at high risk of exposure (animal handlers, cavers, hunters, and trappers in rabies-endemic areas, along with travelers to certain foreign countries). This is given as a series of three intramuscular injections over 28 days, although a more recently advised 1-week schedule for the injections appears to be quite effective. An intradermal regimen can be used for immunization, but this technique may result in lower antibody level.

The incubation period of rabies ranges from 9 days to more than 1 year, but is usually between 2 and 16 weeks. The first symptoms are fatigue, weakness, anxiety, irritability, fever, headache, nausea and vomiting, sore throat, abdominal pain, and loss of appetite. Some victims complain of numbness and tingling where they were initially bitten. After a few days to 2 weeks, the virus shows its devastating effect on the nervous system, with symptoms of increased agitation, hyperactivity, seizures, hallucinations, increased salivation, uncontrollable behavior, and inability to drink (hydrophobia: fear of swallowing liquids) because of muscle spasms in the throat. This constellation is called "furious rabies." Occasionally, a victim may suffer from aerophobia (fear of air), because these same spasms can be caused by air blowing across the face or traversing the airway. With "dumb" rabies, a person becomes progressively weak, uncoordinated, and paralyzed. Unfortunately, rabies is virtually always fatal, with the terminal events being one or more of coma, respiratory failure, seizures, abnormal heart rhythms, high blood pressure, paralysis, and pneumonia.

To avoid rabies, be certain that all pets and livestock are properly vaccinated, don't feed or handle wild animals, don't feed or touch stray animals, avoid sick or strange-acting animals, keep garbage and food (including feed for animals) covered and away from wild animals, don't keep wild animals as pets, don't touch or pick up dead animals, and don't handle bats.

Skunks

In addition to biting a person and inoculating him with rabies virus, a skunk can spray secretions from its anal sacs. The main component of skunk musk is butyl mercaptan, which carries a horrible odor and causes skin irritation, eye redness and temporary blindness, and occasional seizures or loss of consciousness. The odor can be neutralized by strong oxidizing agents, such as household bleach diluted 1 : 5 with water. This solution can then be washed away with tincture of green soap, followed by a more dilute bleach rinse. An alternative mixture is 1 quart of 3% hydrogen peroxide, ¼ cup of baking soda, and 1 teaspoon of liquid laundry detergent. An effective product to neutralize skunk spray odor is Summer's Eve douche (C.B. Fleet Company, Inc.). To "deskunk" an animal, such as a dog, the method is to apply this product directly to the fur and work it into the deeper layers by hand. It may take many bottles to accomplish the task. For the animal's face, use a washcloth with the solution to apply the product. Tomato juice has been recommended, but may not be very effective, to deodorize hair, which may need to be bleached or cut short. Two other methods that have been recommended (but which I have not personally attempted) are:

1. Fels Naphtha soap. Wet an affected dog with water and rub it down with the soap. Be sure to rinse the animal well.
2. One box of baking soda. Slightly moisten the animal and then and rub the fur thoroughly with the baking soda, using gloved hands. Then, take a bottle of white household vinegar—keeping vinegar far away from eyes, nose, and mouth of the animal—and pour it directly onto the baking soda impregnated coat. The immediate and violent effervescence (carbon dioxide) is supposed to lift out the musk and odor. Spray or otherwise rinse the animal thoroughly after allowing for full interaction between baking soda and vinegar. This process sometimes generates enough heat to frighten the animal.

Other effective products to use on the pet or fabric (not on human skin) are Neutroleum Alpha, Skunk-Off, and Odormute.

Bubonic Plague

Cases of bubonic plague are still reported in the United States. The disease is transmitted by the bites of fleas that have acquired the plague bacillus, *Yersinia pestis,* from infected squirrels, rats, prairie dogs, chipmunks, marmots, rabbits, and mice. Rarely, the disease can be contracted from direct contact with infected pets, particularly cats. It can also be contracted from skinning an infected wild animal, such as a coyote or bobcat.

The incubation period for bubonic plague is 2 to 6 days after exposure. At first, the victim complains of high fever, chills, severe fatigue, abdominal pain, vomiting, diarrhea, muscle aches, and headache. At the same time, he develops extremely enlarged and tender lymph nodes associated with the entry point for the disease, such as in the groin if an insect bite has occurred on the leg. Thereafter, as the bacteria overwhelm the victim, he may collapse and develop a skin rash with large dark patches of hemorrhage ("Black Death"). If pneumonia develops, the victim coughs bloody sputum.

Treatment should be initiated promptly, and requires intramuscular or intravenous antibiotics. If you're isolated away from a hospital, start the victim on tetracycline 1 g for the first dose, then 50 mg/kg (2.2 lb) of body weight in six divided doses every 4 hours for the first day, then 30 mg/kg of body weight in four divided doses every 6 hours for 14 days. This is extremely suboptimal therapy; the victim needs to get to a hospital as soon as possible. The best available drug is streptomycin, which is administered by intramuscular injection.

The disease is contagious. All adults in direct face-to-face contact with a victim suffering from plague pneumonia (cough productive of sputum) should take tetracycline 500 mg four times a day, or trimethoprim–sulfamethoxazole one double-strength tablet twice a day, for 8 days. Children should take a pediatric dose of trimethoprim–sulfamethoxazole for 8 days. All contact people should have their temperature measured twice a day. If anyone develops a fever greater than 100° F (37.7° C), he should begin taking an antibiotic and be taken immediately to a physician.

With regard to prevention, pay attention to local public health warnings and don't travel with pets in areas of plague infestation. Take care to spray or dust your canine and feline companions with flea repellent regularly (after each time they get wet) when traveling in wooded areas. Don't allow children to handle small dead animals.

Preexposure immunization against plague is available (see page 426). If you have not been immunized against plague and will be actively exposed to plague-infected animals, ingest tetracycline 500 mg four times a day during the period of exposure.

Anthrax

Anthrax is a communicable disease caused by the bacterium *Bacillus anthracis* transmitted by spores via inhalation, ingestion (contaminated meat), or inoculation into the skin. The spores can persist in the environment for years and are typically present in infected animals or contaminated animal products (e.g., hides, wool). Anthrax is not transmitted from person to person. It presents in humans in three forms: inhalation, cutaneous, and gastrointestinal. After exposure to the spores, the incubation period is typically 1 to 6 days, although it can be as long as 40 days. With inhalation anthrax, the victim initially has a nonspecific flu-like illness (fever, fatigue, muscle pains, dry cough, and chest or abdominal pain) for 1 to 2 days, followed by severe respiratory distress and overwhelming infection that leads to shock and death. There may be an intervening few days of improvement after the flu-like illness and before the serious illness. With cutaneous anthrax, there is often itching soon followed by the first lesion, which is usually a painless red raised area on the head, neck, or limb, usually at the site of a small cut or scrape through which the spore enters. In a day or two, a clear blister(s) forms, surrounded by swelling. The blister ruptures, and then turns into a sunken ulcer covered by a black crust in approximately a week. This disappears in a few weeks. With gastrointestinal anthrax, the victim suffers abdominal pain and swelling, nausea, vomiting, and bloody diarrhea 1 to 7 days after eating the undercooked spore-containing meat. He may also suffer from dizziness, fatigue, muscle aching, and fever. Anthrax may rarely cause primary infection of the lining of the brain, and cause a clinical presentation similar to that of meningitis (see page 162).

Any adult known to be exposed to anthrax or who is believed to be suffering from anthrax should be administered ciprofloxacin 500 or 750 mg by mouth or doxycycline 100 mg by mouth twice a day for 10 days, or until it is determined if the anthrax is susceptible to penicillin or amoxicillin, at which time the antibiotic therapy can be altered. Cephalosporin antibiotics and trimethoprim–sulfamethoxazole aren't effective. Although ciprofloxacin and doxycycline are usually avoided in children because of potential damage to teeth or bone growth, in the setting of anthrax exposure, the benefits probably outweigh the risks. The pediatric doses are ciprofloxacin 10 to 15 mg/kg of body weight or doxycycline 4.4 mg/kg of body weight daily in two divided doses. Anthrax vaccine can be administered in three doses—on the day of exposure, day 14, and day 28—so antibiotic therapy should be continued for 28 days if the vaccine is administered, and for 60 days if the vaccine is not available. A newly approved drug (that is stored in the Strategic National Stockpile) for treatment of inhalational anthrax is raxibacumab (Abthrax), which is an antibody that targets the toxins produced by the anthrax bacteria.

To avoid anthrax, avoid handling the carcasses of animals from areas known to harbor anthrax and don't eat meat from animals that were known to not be healthy when they were killed.

Hantavirus Pulmonary (Lung) Syndrome

Hantaviruses (such as the sin nombre virus) cause a syndrome characterized by a combination of fever, lung failure, kidney failure, shock, and bleeding. The viruses are spread in the excreta of rodents; in the United States, hantavirus pulmonary syndrome (HPS) has been linked to the deer mouse *(Peromyscus maniculatus)* and white-footed mouse *(Peromyscus leucopus)*, as well as to the cotton rat *(Sigmodon hispidus)* and rice rat *(Oryzomys palustris)*. The animals shed the virus in saliva, urine, and feces. Aerosols are the most likely route of transmission from rodents to humans. Insect bites have not yet been implicated in transmission.

HPS has now been reported in most states west of the Mississippi River, as well as in a few eastern states. In Louisiana and Florida, two hantavirus species, bayou virus and Black Creek virus, have been identified. A person infected by the virus has an incubation period of typically 2 to 4 weeks (range, a few days to 6 weeks) after exposure, and then suffers from any or all of fever, muscle aches, chills, headache, nonproductive cough, fatigue, lightheadedness, dizziness, abdominal pain, back pain, nausea and vomiting, and diarrhea for a few days; this is followed by difficulty breathing, mottled skin on the limbs, shock, and, sometimes, bleeding. In the early stage, rash is conspicuously not present. Up to 35% of victims may die.

Most victims have had an interaction with rodents, such as when cleaning a barn or capturing the animals. So far, the disease does not appear to transmit from human to human. Unfortunately, there is not yet any specific therapy beyond supportive care.

To avoid unnecessary exposure to hantavirus, it's recommended that wilderness enthusiasts observe the following precautions: keep food and water covered and stored in rodent-proof containers; dispose of food clutter; spray dead rodents, nests, and droppings with disinfectant or 10% household bleach solution before handling (wear gloves) for disposal in sealed bags; clean and disinfect cabins and other shelters thoroughly before using; seal holes and cracks in dwellings; don't make camp near rodent sites; don't sleep on bare ground; burn or bury garbage promptly; and use only bottled or disinfected water for campsite purposes.

AVOIDANCE OF HAZARDOUS ANIMALS

Most wild animal encounters can be avoided with caution and a little common sense. Follow these rules:

1. Don't surprise or otherwise provoke animals. Unless they are apex predators, starving, senile, or ill, most animals will not attack humans without provocation. Don't corner or provoke a carnivore. Don't tease animals. Don't approach an animal when it is with young or during breeding season. If you're a photographer approaching a wild animal that may become provoked and charge, don't come any closer to the animal than 100 yards distance. Some experts say that you should attempt to stay even further away from a bear.
2. Don't leave young children alone with wild or potentially biting animals, regardless of the animal's demeanor.
3. Dogs, even though not necessarily "wild," are the most common biters of travelers abroad and in most outdoor settings. In addition to the general precautions for how to avoid hazardous animals, never pet an unfamiliar dog, particularly if it is confined or tied up. Don't feed an unfamiliar animal by hand.

4. Don't disturb a feeding or nursing animal. Don't explore into its feeding territory, approach during rut, or disrupt mating patterns. Avoid sudden movements around animals.

5. Don't separate fighting animals using your bare hands. If possible, drive animals apart using a long stick or club, or a strong stream of water or dousing with a bucketful of water.

6. After eating, wash hands before touching a hungry animal. Don't pet or feed stray animals, particularly dogs and monkeys.

7. In bear country, make your presence known by calling out, clapping your hands, or otherwise making noise, particularly when approaching streams and blind spots on the trail. Hang all food off the ground in trees away from the campsite. Sleep in a tent and have a flashlight handy. Keep sleeping bags unzipped or partially unzipped to allow a fast exit. Never keep food or captured game inside a tent. Use proper food storage to keep food away from bears. Cook at a site away from the sleeping area. Don't leave garbage or food buried or poured into the ground. Don't sleep in clothes worn while cooking or eating. Make noise when hiking, particularly on narrow paths or through tall grass. An "upwind bear" is more likely to be surprised than one that's "downwind," so be alert ahead of you, or if you're in a heavy forest, along a noisy river, or in the rain or fog. Bears frequent berry patches, streams with spawning fish, and elk calving grounds, so avoid these areas.

8. If you confront a brown (grizzly) bear, avoid eye contact and try to slowly back away. If you confront a black bear, shout, yell, throw rocks or sticks, or do whatever you can to frighten off the animal. If attacked by a bear, don't try to outrun it; you can't. Bears can climb trees.

9. If you're carrying pepper spray (at least 1% capsaicin or capsaicinoids) in a canister intended for use against a bear ("bear spray" or "bear pepper spray" that meets EPA standards; a spray distance of 25 feet under optimum conditions, minimum spray duration of 6 seconds, minimum net content of 7.9 oz or 2.25 g; there should be rapid intensive coverages of the attack area), use it if you have time. One product is UDAP 12HP Bear Spray. Personal defensive spray, such as Mace, will likely not work because the canister shoots a relatively thin stream and the substance is not sufficiently potent. Carry the spray where it is prominently visible and can be immediately deployed. It should be on a holster on your waist or chest, not in the bottom of your pack. Show your companions its location.

    If you're carrying pepper spray and discharge the canister in such a way that it burns your skin, applying the antacid Mylanta, which contains magnesium and aluminum hydroxide, promptly to the affected skin may lessen the pain. If the spray gets into your eyes, rinse them with a copious amount of fresh water (see page 168).

10. If you're not carrying bear pepper spray, cover your head and the back of your neck with your arms and curl into a fetal position or lay flat on the ground, face down, to protect your abdomen (Figure 238). If you're wearing a backpack, keep it on for additional protection. Use your elbows to cover your face if a bear turns you over. After a bear attack, remain on the ground until you're certain that the bear has left the area. More than one victim has successfully protected himself during the initial attack, only to arise too soon (before the bear has lost interest and left the area) and be mauled during the second attack.

11. In cougar (mountain lion) country, be aware that these animals hunt like a domestic cat: crouching, slinking, sprinting, pouncing, and then breaking the prey's neck. Like many potentially dangerous wild animals, the cougar can often be scared off by the victim's aggressive behavior, even after the attack has begun.

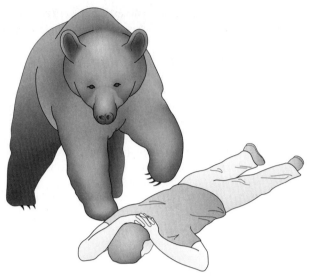

Figure 238. Protective position when confronted by an attacking bear.

WILD PLANT AND MUSHROOM POISONING

Toxic plants and mushrooms may be eaten by curious children, or by hikers and amateur herbalists who mistake their selections for edible species. *Never eat wild plants, mushrooms, roots, or berries unless you know what you're doing.* Bees that are bred to intentionally collect nectar from poisonous plants may manufacture poisonous honey.

MEDICAL HISTORY

Although the narrative description of the ingestion will have little bearing on the immediate management of a toxic ingestion, it's important to gather as much information as possible for the benefit of the physician who will ultimately care for the victim:

1. When was the plant eaten?
2. What parts of the plant were eaten? How many different plants were eaten?
3. What symptoms does the victim have? What were the initial symptoms (sweating, hallucinations, vomiting, abdominal pain)? What was the time interval between the ingestion and the onset of symptoms? Did anyone who did not eat the plant(s) develop similar symptoms? Did everyone who ate the plant(s) become ill?
4. Was the plant eaten raw, or was it cooked? How was it cooked? Was alcohol consumed within 72 hours of the plant ingestion?

It is also important to obtain as much of the original plant as possible for identification. If the patient vomits, save his vomitus, because it may contain part of the plant or spores that can be identified by an expert.

There are few specific antidotes for toxic plant ingestions, so most victims are managed according to their symptoms, which may include sweating, nausea, vomiting, diarrhea, shortness of breath, slow or rapid heartbeat, pinpoint or dilated pupils, salivation, increased frequency of urination, weakness, difficulty breathing, hallucinations, and many others.

TREATMENT FOR POISONINGS

If it is known that someone has eaten or handled a toxic plant or mushroom, remove plant parts from the mouth and hands, and wash any affected skin with soap and water. Encouraging a victim who has eaten a plant to vomit has largely fallen out of favor with toxicology experts, so is no longer advised. However, if someone has eaten a known poisonous plant or mushroom within the last 2 hours, he can be encouraged to vomit, so long as he is awake and alert and the airway is not compromised. Inducing vomiting may not be easy. Gagging the victim with his fingers is the safest method. Drinking mustard solution, salt solution, egg whites, okra slime, or dishwashing soap is usually ineffective and may be dangerous. Syrup of ipecac is no longer recommended by poison centers. *If the victim is drowsy or having difficulty breathing, regardless of when the ingestion occurred, don't induce vomiting.* Whether or not vomiting occurs, immediately seek the attention of a physician. Don't wait for symptoms, because early treatment is sometimes very important. Bring the plant or part of the plant with you for identification.

Children will eat just about anything. Nontoxic ingestions include stones, dirt, sand, candles, sunscreen, shampoo, and single doses of birth control pills, antacids, laxatives, and vitamins (without iron). Keep all toxic substances, particularly camp stove fuel, kerosene, iodine crystals (for water disinfection), and prescription drugs, out of the reach of small children.

COMMONLY INGESTED TOXIC PLANTS AND MUSHROOMS

1. Oleander (Figure 239) is a shrub, up to 20 ft (6 m) tall, commonly found along highways and in gardens. It carries attractive clusters of red, pink, or white flowers. The entire plant is toxic, including smoke from burning cuttings and water in which the flowers are placed. There have been deaths from use of the branches as skewers for roasting hot dogs. Symptoms begin 1 to 2 hours after ingestion and include nausea, vomiting, abdominal cramps, diarrhea, confusion, and blurred vision. In serious ingestions, the heart's rhythm may be disturbed.

2. Foxglove (Figure 240) is a European import that has toxic leaves and toxic tubular pink or purple flowers. Poisonings occur from ingestion of the plant parts or from foxglove tea. The symptoms are the same as those of oleander ingestion.

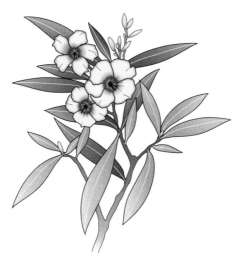

Figure 239. Oleander.

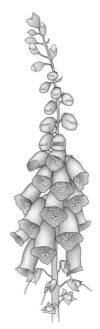

Figure 240. Foxglove.

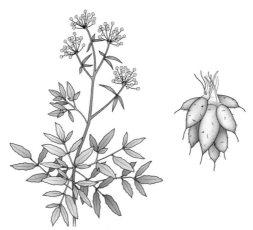

Figure 241. Water hemlock, with tuberous roots.

3. Water hemlock ("beaver poison") (Figure 241) is found in saltwater and freshwater marshes and along riverbanks. A member of the carrot family, the plant grows to 6 ft (1.8 m) and has clusters of whitish, heavily scented flowers, along with a bundle of tuberous roots. It is easily confused with wild parsnip, celery, or sweet anise. When injured, the stem and trunk exude a yellow oil that smells like celery or raw parsnip. The entire plant is toxic. Symptoms begin 15 to 60 minutes after ingestion and include excessive salivation, abdominal pain, diarrhea, and vomiting. In a serious ingestion, the victim may suffer seizures and collapse, while having difficulty breathing. Death may occur.

4. Castor bean (Figure 242) is a treelike shrub that may grow to 15 ft (4.6 m) with clusters of spiny seedpods, which contain seeds with coats that resemble pinto beans. The seeds contain a potent toxin (ricin) that causes immediate mouth burning and abdominal pain, followed by vomiting, diarrhea, abnormal heart rhythms, and collapse.

5. Monkshood (Figure 243) is a flowering plant with tuberous roots and blue helmet-shaped flowers. The leaves and roots are particularly toxic. Ingestion causes immediate mouth and throat burning, followed by vomiting, diarrhea, headache, muscle cramps, sweating, drooling, blurred vision, and confusion. In a serious ingestion, there may be abnormal heart rhythms and collapse.

6. Poison hemlock (Figure 244) is a marsh plant that grows to 9 ft (2.7 m) with leaves that resemble a carrot top. The white flowers are clustered and smell like urine if they are crushed. The seeds and white unbranched tuberous roots are also toxic. The symptoms are similar to those of water hemlock ingestion, without significant abdominal pain or diarrhea. Death may follow seizures or paralysis with breathing failure.

7. Pokeweed (Figure 245) is a widely distributed plant with clusters of white flowers and plentiful round purple berries. Ingestion of the root (commonly mistaken for

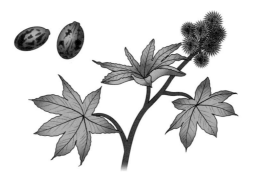

Figure 242. Castor bean.

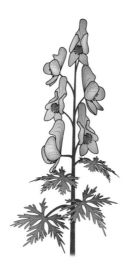

Figure 243. Monkshood.

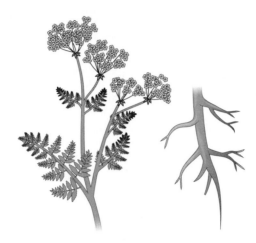

Figure 244. Poison hemlock.

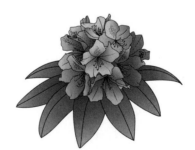

Figure 245. Pokeweed.

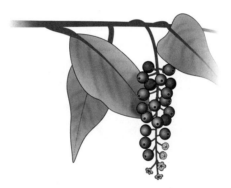

Figure 246. Rhododendron.

horseradish) or the berries (a favorite of children) causes the intoxication. Symptoms include sore mouth, tongue, and throat (delayed by 2 to 3 hours); thirst; nausea; vomiting; abdominal cramps; and diarrhea, which may become bloody. The illness can be severe and last for up to 2 days, particularly if the roots were ingested.

8. Rhododendrons (Figure 246) are common flowering plants that contain a number of toxins. Poisoning has occurred following ingestion of honey made from the flower nectar. Symptoms include mouth burning, followed by drooling, vomiting, diarrhea, headache,

and numbness and tingling. Serious ingestions cause weakness, blurred vision, seizures, fainting, low blood pressure, and collapse. "Mad honey poisoning" refers to ingestion of honey produced from toxic nectar from the rhododendron plant *Rhododendron ponticum*.

9. Jimsonweed (Figure 247) has white or purple flowers, with prickly seedpods. Adults sometimes ingest a tea made from the leaves or flowers. The entire plant is toxic. Symptoms include dry mouth, rapid heartbeat, hot and dry skin, weakness, difficulty walking, dilated pupils, and inability to urinate. Severe poisonings cause fever and collapse.

10. Skunk cabbage (Figure 248) is a marsh and forest plant that grows to 6 ft (1.8 m) and has broad pleated leaves. The entire plant is toxic and causes symptoms similar to those that follow ingestion of monkshood, but generally much less severe.

11. Pyracantha (Figure 249) is a thorned shrub with white flowers and clusters of small red berries. Ingestion of the berries in large quantities causes nausea and diarrhea. Birds

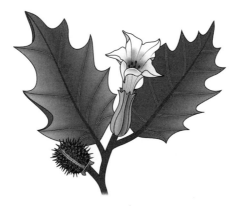

Figure 247. Jimsonweed.

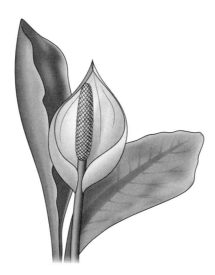

Figure 248. Skunk cabbage.

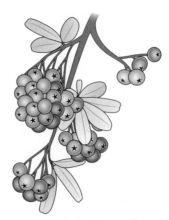

Figure 249. Pyracantha.

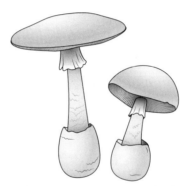

Figure 250. *Amanita phalloides* (death cap).

sometimes eat fermented pyracantha berries and become intoxicated. Scratches from the thorns may cause a burning skin irritation.

12. *Amanita phalloides* (death cap) is a gilled mushroom (Figure 250) with a shiny yellow to greenish cap found in the western United States. The entire mushroom is toxic and cannot be detoxified by cooking. Symptoms occur 6 to 12 hours after ingestion and include abdominal pain; persistent nausea, vomiting, or diarrhea; low blood pressure; and rapid heartbeat. The victim may appear normal for the next few days, but then rapidly shows signs of massive liver inflammation and destruction, which include jaundice (yellow skin and eyeballs, darkened urine), easy bleeding, and altered mental status. Fatalities are frequent with this species, as well as with *Galerina autumnalis*.

13. Most nonfatal mushroom toxins act rapidly, producing symptoms of nausea, vomiting, diarrhea, and headache within 1 to 4 hours. Severe abdominal pain and headache approximately 6 hours after ingestion are likely due to *Gyromitra esculenta*. Typically, diarrhea and vomiting caused by ingestion of *Amanita phalloides* are delayed by 6 to 12 hours. However, because most unknowledgeable mushroom foragers eat a mixture of species, a rapid onset of symptoms does not rule out a potentially disastrous ingestion. Approximately 10 species of the several thousand varieties of wild mushrooms in the United States can cause death by ingestion.

14. *Amanita muscaria* (fly agaric) is a gilled mushroom (Figure 251) with a variably colored (yellow, red, warty, and so on) cap. Most poisonings are intentional, because people brew

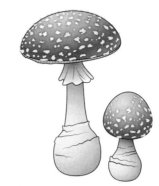

Figure 251. *Amanita muscaria* (fly agaric).

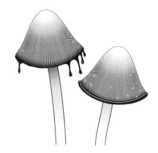

Figure 252. *Coprinus atramentarius* (inky cap).

and drink *Amanita* tea for its hallucinogenic effects. Symptoms occur 30 minutes to 2 hours after ingestion and include euphoria, difficulty walking, dizziness, hallucinations, and blurred vision. Severe ingestions can result in seizures and death.

15. *Coprinus atramentarius* (inky cap) is a gilled fungus (Figure 252) with a conical cap that liquefies and turns black when picked. If alcohol is consumed within 24 to 72 hours after ingestion of the fungus, the victim suffers abdominal pain, vomiting, sweating, facial flushing, and headaches. *Cortinarius rainierensis* may cause the victim to have enormous thirst and increased urination 3 to 17 days after ingestion, due to a toxic effect on the kidneys.

16. Many other plants (wild and houseplants) can cause illnesses if consumed in sufficient quantities (one apple seed will not poison you). When in doubt as to the identity of a plant ingested, its quantity, or its potential toxicity, it's wise to immediately consult a certified poison (control) center or a physician.

TOXICITY OF COMMON PLANTS

It is very important to know that the common (familiar) name of two or more different plant species (as designated by the precise Latin or common scientific name) can be identical or similar. So, to know if a particular plant is toxic to humans, it is essential to precisely identify the plant.

A fairly comprehensive list of toxic and nontoxic plants with both the common and Latin or common scientific names is maintained at "KNOW YOUR PLANTS!", which can be found at www.calpoison.org. That list classifies common plants as toxic or nontoxic, according to how they affect humans, and in certain cases, dogs and cats. For identification in the field, it would be best to also be able to compare the plant to a picture, if that resource is available to you.

The following list contains nontoxic and toxic plants, and is adapted from "KNOW YOUR PLANTS!"

TOXIC PLANTS BY COMMON NAME, LATIN OR COMMON SCIENTIFIC NAME—TYPE OF TOXICITY

Type of Toxicity

1. Skin contact with these plants can cause symptoms ranging from redness, itching, and rash to painful blisters.
2a. Contain oxalates with immediate adverse reaction. The juice or sap of these plants contains tiny oxalate crystals that are shaped like tiny needles. Chewing on these plants can cause immediate pain and irritation to the lips, mouth, and tongue. In severe cases, they may cause breathing problems by causing swelling in the mouth and throat.
2b. Contain oxalates with slower onset of toxic reaction. These plants contain oxalate crystals but they do not cause immediate problems. These oxalate crystals can lodge in the kidneys, where they cause injury as well as nausea, vomiting, and diarrhea.
3. Ingestion of these plants is expected to cause nausea, vomiting, diarrhea, and/or other symptoms that may cause illness, but are not life-threatening.
4. Ingestion of these plants, especially in large amounts, is expected to cause serious effects to the heart, liver, kidneys, or brain. If one or more of these plants is eaten in any amount, contact a poison center immediately.

spp: species

A

Absinth, *Artemisia absinthium*—4
Acacia, black, *Robinia pseudoacacia*—4
Acacia, false, *Robinia pseudoacacia*—4
Acacia palida, *Leucaena leucocephala*—4
Aconite, *Aconitium napellus*—4
Acorn, *Quercus* spp—1, 3
Adam-and-Eve, *Arum maculatum*—1, 2a
African lily, *Agapanthus* spp—1
Agapanthus, *Agapanthus* spp—1
Agapanthus, pink, *Nerine bowdenii*—3
Alder tree, *Alnus* spp—1
Allamanda, pink or purple, *Cryptostegia grandiflora*—4
Allamanda, wild, *Urechites* spp—4
Allium, *Allium sativum*—1, 3
Alocasia, *Alocasia* spp—2a
Aloe vera, *Aloe barbadensis*—1, 3
Alstroemeria, *Alstroemeria aurantiaca*—1, 3
Amaryllis, *Amaryllis* spp—3
Amaryllis, *Hippeastrum* spp—3
Amaryllis belladonna, *Amaryllis belladonna*—3
American valerian, *Cypripedium calceolus*—1
Amethyst flower, *Browallia* spp—1
Anemone, *Anemone* spp—1, 3
Angel wings, *Caladium*—2a

Angelica, *Angelica archangelica*—1, 4
Angel's tears, *Narcissus triandrus*—1, 3
Angel's trumpet, *Datura* spp—4
Anthurium, *Anthurium* spp—2a
Apple (chewed seeds), *Malus* spp—4
Apple (chewed seeds), *Pyrus sylvestris*—4
Apple, balsam, *Momordica balsamina*—3
Apple of Peru, *Datura stramonium*—4
Apricot (chewed pits), *Prunus armeniaca*—4
Apricot vine, *Passiflora incarnata*—4
Archangel, *Angelica archangelica*—1, 4
Arnica, *Arnica* spp—1, 4
Arrowhead vine, *Syngonium podophyllum*—2a
Arum, *Arum* spp—1, 2a
Ash, American, *Fraxinus americana*—1
Ash, European, *Fraxinus excelsior*—1
Asthma plant or weed, *Chamaesyce hirta*—1
Asthma plant or weed, *Euphorbia hirta*—1
Asthma weed, *Lobelia inflata*—1, 4
Atamasco lily, *Zephyranthes atamasco*—1, 3
Avocado (leaves, stems, seeds), *Persea americana*—4
Azalea, *Rhododendron* genus—4

B

Baltic ivy, *Hedera helix*—1, 3
Baneberry, *Actaea rubra*—1, 4

Barbados flower, *Caesalpinia pulcherrima*—3
Barbados pride, *Caesalpinia* spp—3
Barbados pride, *Poinciana gilliesii*—3
Barberry, *Berberis* spp—4
Basket flower, *Centaurea americana*—1, 3
Basket lily, *Hymenocallis americana*—3
Be still tree, *Thevetia peruviana*—4
Bean tree, *Cytisus laburnum*—4
Bean tree, *Laburnum* spp—4
Beech, European, *Fagus sylvatica*—3
Beech, Japanese, *Fagus crenata*—3
Beech, ornamental, *Fagus sylvatica*—3
Belladonna, *Atropa belladonna*—4
Belladonna lily, *Amaryllis belladonna*—3
Bindweed, *Calystegia sepium*—1, 3
Bird of paradise, *Caesalpinia gilliesii*—3
Bird of paradise, *Poinciana gilliesii*—3
Birdsfoot ivy, *Hedera helix*—1, 3
Bishop's weed, *Ammi majus*—1
Bitter almond, *Prunus dulcis*—4
Bitter orange, *Citrus aurantium*—1
Black cohosh, *Cimicifuga racemosa*—4
Black-eyed Susan, *Abrus precatorius*—4
Black-eyed Susan, *Rudbeckia hirta*—1
Black henbane, *Hyoscyamus niger*—4
Black oak, *Quercus velutina*—1, 3
Bleeding heart, *Dicentra formosa*—1, 4
Blood flower or blood lily, *Haemanthus coccineus*—3
Bloodroot, *Sanguinaria canadensis*—3
Blue bonnet, *Lupinus* spp—4
Blue buttons, *Vinca major*—4
Blue cohosh, *Caulophyllum thalictroides*—1, 4
Blue gum tree, *Eucalyptus globulus*—3
Boston ivy, *Parthenocissus tricuspidata*—2a, 2b
Bougainvillea, *Bougainvillea* spp—1
Box thorn, *Lycium halimifolium*—4
Boxwood, *Buxus sempervirens*—1, 4
Bracken fern, *Pteridium aquilinum*—4
Bradford pear, *Pyrus calleryana*—1
Breadfruit vine, *Monstera deliciosa*—2a
Bridesmaid, *Chrysanthemum* spp—1, 3
Broom bush, *Retama raetam*—4
Buckeye, *Aesculus* spp—3
Buckhorn, *Osmunda cinnamomea*—3
Buckthorn, *Karwinskia humboldtiana*—4
Buckthorn, *Rhamnus cathartica*—4
Burning bush, *Dictamnus albus*—1
Burning bush, *Euonymus atropurpurea*—3

Burning bush, *Kochia scoparia*—1, 2a, 2b
Buttercup, *Ranunculus* spp—1, 3
Butterfly iris, *Iris spuria*—1, 3
Butterfly weed, *Asclepias tuberosa*—4
Butternut, *Juglans cinerea*—1

C

Caffre lily, *Clivia miniata*—3
Caladium, *Caladium*—2a
Caladium, *Colocasia esculenta*—2a
Calico flower, *Aristolochia elegans*—4
California buckeye, *Aesculus californica*—3
California live oak, *Quercus agrifolia*—1, 3
Calla lily, *Zantedeschia* spp—2a
Calycanthus (seeds), *Calycanthus* spp—4
Camomile, *Anthemis cotula*—1
Camphor tree, *Cinnamomum camphora*—4
Camus, white, *Zigadenus elegans*—4
Candle berry tree, *Aleurites moluccana*—1, 3
Candle plant, *Senecio articulatus*—4
Candleberry, *Myrica cerifera*—1
Candleberry tree, *Jatropha moluccana*—1, 3
Candlenut oil tree, *Jatropha moluccana*—1, 3
Candlenut oil tree, *Aleurites moluccana*—1, 3
Cape belladonna, *Amaryllis belladonna*—3
Cardinal flower, *Lobelia cardinalis*—1, 4
Carnation, *Dianthus* spp—1
Carolina allspice (seeds), *Calycanthus* spp—4
Carolina jasmine, *Gelsemium sempervirens*—1, 4
Carolina jessamine, *Gelsemium sempervirens*—1, 4
Carolina moonseed, *Cocculus carolinus*—4
Carolina pink, *Spigelia marilandica*—4
Carolina wild woodbine, *Gelsemium sempervirens*—1, 4
Caroline yellow jessamine, *Gelsemium sempervirens*—1, 4
Cascara, *Rhamnus purshiana*—4
Cassava, *Jatropha manihot*—4
Castor bean, *Ricinus communis*—4
Catnip, *Nepeta cataria*—3
Cat's claw, *Pithecellobium unguis-cati*—1
Caustic weed, *Euphorbia drummondii*—1, 3
Cayenne pepper, *Capsicum* spp—1, 3
Cedar, *Juniperus virginiana*—1, 3
Century plant, *Agave americana*—1, 3
Cestrum, day blooming, *Cestrum diurnum*—4
Chalice vine, *Solandra longiflora*—4
Chamomile, *Anthemis cotula*—1

Chapparal leaf, *Larrea tridentata*—4

Chenille plant, *Acalypha hispida*—1, 3

Cherry (chewed pits), *Prunus* spp—4

Cherry laurel, *Laurocerasus officinalis*—4

Cherry laurel, *Prunus laurocerasus*—4

Cherry pepper, *Capsicum* spp—1, 3

Cherry tomato (green parts), *Lycopersicon lycopersicum*—4

Cherry tomato (green parts), *Physalis peruviana*—4

Cherry, bitter (chewed seeds), *Prunus emarginata*—4

Cherry, wild (chewed seeds), *Prunus serotina*—4

Chicken weed, *Euphorbia thymifolia*—1

Chili pepper, *Capsicum* spp—1, 3

Chinaberry, *Melia azedarach*—4

Chinese lantern, *Abutilon hybridum*—1

Chinese lantern plant, *Physalis alkekengi*—4

Chinese tallow tree, *Sapium sebiferum*—1, 3

Chokecherry (chewed seeds), *Prunus virginiana*—4

Christmas berry (leaves), *Photinia arbutifolia*—4

Christmas berry tree, *Schinus terebinthifolius*—1

Christmas candle, *Euphorbia tithymaloides* (formerly *Pedilanthus* spp)—1, 3

Christmas orange, *Solanum capsicastrum*—4

Christmas rose, *Helleborus niger*—4

Chrysanthemum, *Chrysanthemum* spp—1, 3

Cinnamonwood, *Sassafras* spp—4

Citronella grass, *Cymbopogon nardus*—1

Clematis, *Clematis* spp—1, 3

Clover, pink, *Dianthus caryophyllus*—1

Clover, sweet white, *Melilotus alba*—4

Clover, sweet yellow, *Melilotus officinalis*—4

Cocklebur, *Xanthium* spp—1, 3

Coffee bean, *Sesbania vesicaria*—4

Coffee tree, *Polyscias guilfoyei*—1, 3

Coffeeberry, *Rhamnus californica*—3

Cohosh, *Actaea spicata*—1, 4

Cola nut, *Cola nitida*—4

Colchicine, *Colchicum autumnale*—4

Colocasia, *Colocasia esculenta*—2a

Comfrey, *Symphytum officinale*—4

Coral beads, *Cocculus carolinus*—4

Coral bean, *Erythrina* spp—4

Coral berry, *Rivina humilis*—3

Coral berry, *Symphoricarpus* spp—3

Coral plant, *Jatropha multifida*—4

Coralberry, *Actaea spicata*—1, 4

Coriaria, *Coriaria* spp—4

Corn lily, *Veratrum* spp—4

Cotoneaster, *Cotoneaster* spp—4

Cow parsley, *Heracleum sphondylium*—1

Cow parsnip, *Heracleum sphondylium*—1

Cowbane, *Cicuta maculata*—4

Cowslip, *Caltha palustris*—1, 3

Cowslip, *Primula veris*—1

Crabapple (chewed seeds), *Malus baccata*—4

Crabapple (chewed seeds), *Pyrus sylvestris*—4

Crabapple, flowering, *Malus ioensis*—4

Crabapple, ornamental (chewed seeds), *Pyrus floribunda*—4

Creeping Charlie, *Glechoma hederacea*—3

Creeping Charlie, *Nepeta hederacea*—3

Creosote bush, *Larrea tridentate*—4

Crocus, autumn, *Colchicum autumnale*—4

Crocus, fall, *Colchicum autumnale*—4

Crotalaria, *Crotalaria spectabilis*—4

Croton, *Codiaeum* spp—1

Croton, *Croton tiglium*—1, 4

Crown of thorns, *Euphorbia milii*—1, 3

Crown plant, *Calotropis gigantea*—4

Crown vetch, *Coronilla varia*—1

Cruel plant, *Araujia sericifera*—1, 3

Cultivated tobacco, *Nicotiana tabacum*—4

Curly dock, *Rumex crispus*—1, 2b

Cycads, Cycadaceae family—4

Cycads, *Zamia* spp—4

Cycas, *Cycas* spp—4

Cycas, *Zamia* spp—4

Cyclamen, *Cyclamen* spp—3

Cyperus, *Cyperus* spp—4

D

Daffodil (bulb), *Narcissus* spp—1, 3

Daisy, *Chrysanthemum* spp—1, 3

Daphne, *Daphne mezereum*—1, 4

Datura, *Datura* spp—4

Day blooming cestrum, *Cestrum diurnum*—4

Day blooming jessamine, *Cestrum diurnum*—4

Dead man fingers, *Oenantha crocata*—4

Deadly hemlock, *Conium maculatum*—4

Deadly nightshade, *Atropa belladonna*—4

Deadly nightshade, *Solanum* spp—4

Death camus, *Zigadenus* or *Zygadenus* spp—4

Delphinium, *Delphinium* spp—4

Desert rose, *Adenium obesum*—4

Devil weed, *Datura stamonium*—4

Devil's backbone, *Kalanchoe daigremontiana*—4

Devil's backbone, *Pedilanthus tithymaloides*—1, 3

Devil's bit, *Chamaelirium luteum*—3

Devil's darning needle, *Clematis virginiana*—1, 3

Devil's ivy, *Epipremnum aureum*—2a

Devil's ivy, *Scindapsus aureus*—2a

Devil's tongue, *Amorphophallus rivieri*—1, 2a

Devil's apple, *Datura stramonium*—4

Devil's apple, *Solanum dulcamara*—4

Devil's backbone, *Euphorbia tithymaloides*—3

Devil's tobacco, *Lobelia tupa*—4

Devil's tomato, *Solanum eleagnifolium*—4

Devil's trumpet, *Datura stramonium*—4

Devil's ear, *Arisaema triphyllum*—1, 2a

Dieffenbachia, *Dieffenbachia* spp—2a

Dock, *Rumex* spp—2b

Dog fennel, *Anthemis cotula*—1

Dogwood, bloodtwig, *Cornus sanguinea*—1

Dolls-eyes, *Actaea spicata*—1,4

Donkeytail, *Euphorbia myrsinites*—1,3

Dragon lily or dragon plant, *Dracunculus vulgaris*—2a

Dragon root, *Arisaema* spp—2a

Dragon tail, *Arisaema dracontium*—2a

Dumb plant, *Dieffenbachia* spp—2a

Dumbcane, *Dieffenbachia* spp—2a

Dusty miller, *Senecio* spp—4

E

Easter flower, *Anemone patens*—1, 3

Easter rose, *Helleborus niger*—4

Eastern poison oak, *Rhus quercifolium*—1

Eastern poison oak, *Toxicodendron quercifolium*—1

Elderberry (all but ripe berries), *Sambucus* spp—3

Elephant garlic, *Allium ampeloprasum*—1, 3

Elephant's ear philodendron, *Philodendron hastatum*—2a

Elephant's foot, *Elephantopus scaber*—4

Elephant's ear, *Alocasia*—1, 2a

Elephant's ear, *Caladium*—2a

Elephant's ear, *Colocasia esculenta*—2a

English holly, *Ilex* spp—3

English laurel, *Laurocerasus officinalis*—4

English laurel, *Prunus laurocerasus*—4

English yew, *Taxus baccata*—4

Eucalyptus, *Eucalyptus globulus*—3

Euonymus, *Euonymus* spp—3

F

False Jerusalem cherry, *Solanum capsicastrum*—4

False parsley, *Aethusa cynapium*—4

False parsley, *Cicuta maculata*—4

False poinciana, *Daubentonia punicea*—4

False poinciana, *Sesbania punicea*—4

False Queen Anne's lace, *Ammi majus*—1

Fiddle flower, *Euphorbia tithymaloides*—3

Fiddleflower, *Pedilanthus tithymaloides*—1, 3

Fiddleheads, *Osmunda cinnamonea*—3

Fiddleleaf philodendron, *Philodendron bipennifolium*—2a

Filbert, *Corylus* spp—1

Fire cracker plant, *Aesculus pavia*—3

Fire fern, *Oxalis* spp—2b

Fire lily, *Hippeastrum amaryllis*—3

Fireball or firebush, *Kochia scoparia*—1, 2a, 2b

Fire-dragon, *Acalypha wilkesiana*—3

Fishtail palm, *Solanum aculeatissimum*—4

Flag, *Iris* spp—1, 3

Flag lily, *Iris versicolor*—1,3

Flamingo flower, *Anthurium scherzeranum*—2a

Flax, *Linium* spp—4

Fleur-de-lis, *Iris germanica*—1, 3

Flowering almond, *Prunus* spp—4

Flowering cherry, *Prunus* spp—4

Flowering crabapple (chewed seeds), *Malus ioensis*—4

Flowering crabapple (chewed seeds), *Pyrus ioensis*—4

Flowering maple, *Abutilon hybridum*—1

Flowering plum, *Prunus cerasifera* "atropurpurea"—4

Flying saucers, *Ipomoea tricolor*—4

Fool's parsley, *Aethusa cynapium*—4

Four o'clock (seeds), *Mirabilis jalapa*—1, 3

Foxglove, *Digitalis purpurea*—4

Foxtail, *Acalypha hispida*—1, 3

Foxtail, *Equisetum* spp—4

Fragrance of the night, *Cestrum nocturnum*—4
Fraxinella, *Dictamnus albus*—1
Fruit salad plant, *Monstera deliciosa*—2a

G

Garland flower, *Dapne cneorum*—1, 4
Garlic, *Allium sativum*—1, 3
Gelsemium, *Gelsemium sempervirens*—1, 4
Geranium, California, *Senecio petasitis*—4
Geranium, velvet, *Senecio petasitis*—4
Ginkgo, *Ginkgo biloba*—1, 4
Ginkgo biloba, *Ginkgo biloba*—1, 4
Ginseng, *Panax pseudoginseng*—4
Glacier lily, *Erythronium grandiflorum*—1, 3
Gladiola, *Gladiola*—3
Gloriosa lily, *Gloriosa superba*—4
Glory lily, *Gloriosa superba*—4
Golden buttons, *Tanacetum vulgare*—1, 3
Golden pothos, *Epipremnum aureum*—2a
Golden pothos, *Scindapsus aureus*—2a
Golden ragwort, *Senecio aureus*—4
Golden rain, *Cassia* spp—3
Golden seal, *Hydrastis canadensis*—4
Good luckleaf or plant, *Oxalis deppei*—2b
Gopher plant, *Euphorbia lathyrus*—1, 3
Gordoloba, *Achillea millefolium*—1, 3
Gotu kola, *Hydrocotyle* spp—1, 4
Green dragon, *Arisaema dracontium*—2a
Green dragon, *Datura stramonium*—4
Green hellebore, *Veratrum viride*—4
Green ripples, *Hedera helix*—1, 3

H

Habanero pepper, *Capsicum* spp—1, 3
Hawaiian baby woodrose (seeds), *Argyreia nervosa*—4
Hawaiian poppy, *Argemone glauca*—4
Hawaiian prickly poppy, *Argemone glauca*—4
Hawaiian woodrose, *Merremia tuberose*—4
Hazelnut, *Corylus* spp—1
Healing onion, *Ornithogalum caudatum*—1, 4
Heart-of-Jesus, *Caladium bicolor*—2a
Hearts and honey vine, *Ipomoea × multifida*—4
Heath/heather, *Calluna vulgaris*—4
Heavenly blue, *Ipomoea* spp—4
Heliotrope, *Heliotropium* spp—4
Hellebore, *Helleborus niger*—4
Hellebore, *Veratrum viride*—4
Hells bells, *Datura stramonium*—4

Helmet flower, *Aconitium napellus*—4
Hemlock, *Conium maculatum*—4
Hemlock, poison, *Conium maculatum*—4
Hemlock, spotted, *Cicuta maculata*—4
Hemlock, spotted, *Conium maculatum*—4
Hemlock, water, *Cicuta maculata*—4
Henbane, *Hyoscyamus* spp—4
Holly (berry), *Ilex* spp—3
Hop, common, *Humulus lupulus*—1
Hop, European, *Humulus lupulus*—1
Hops, wild, *Bryonia* spp—3
Horn-of-plenty, *Datura* spp—4
Horse chestnut, *Aesculus* spp—3
Horse poison, *Hippobroma longiflora*—4
Horse willow, *Equisetum* spp—4
Horseradish, *Armoracia rusticana*—3
Horsetail, *Equisetum* spp—4
Hyacinth (bulb), *Hyacinthus orientalis*—1, 3
Hydrangea, *Hydrangea* spp—4
Hypericum, *Hypericum perforatum*—1, 3

I

Incense cedar, *Calocedrus decurrens*—1
Indian aloe, *Aloe barbadensis*—1, 3
Indian apple, *Datura inoxia*—4
Indian bead or bean, *Abrus precatorius*—4
Indian bean, *Erythrina* spp—4
Indian currant, *Symphoricarpos* spp—3
Indian dye, *Hydrastis canadensis*—4
Indian hemp, *Apocynum cannabinum*—possibly 4
Indian paint, *Chenopodium capitatum*—1
Indian paint, *Hydrastis canadensis*—4
Indian paint brush, *Asclepias* spp—4
Indian pink, *Dianthus chinensis*—1
Indian pink, *Lobelia cardinalis*—1, 4
Indian pink, *Spigelia marilandica*—4
Indian poke, *Phytolacca acinosa*—3
Indian poke, *Veratrum viride*—4
Indian rubber vine, *Cryptostegia grandiflora*—4
Indian tobacco, *Lobelia inflata*—1, 4
Inkberry (pokeweed), *Phytolacca americana*—3
Ipomea, *Exogonium purga*—3
Iris, *Iris* spp—1, 3
Irish shamrock, *Oxalis acetosella*—2b
Irish tops, *Cytisus scoparius*—3
Irish tops, *Spartium scoparium*—4
Iron wood, *Cassia siamea*—4
Italian arum, *Arum italicum*—2a

Ivy, *Hedera* spp—1, 3

Ivy bush, *Kalmia latifolia*—4

Ivy, Algerian, *Hedera canariensis*—1

Ivy, Baltic, *Hedera helix*—1, 3

Ivy, California, *Hedera helix*—1, 3

Ivy, Canary, *Hedera canariensis*—1

Ivy, common, *Philodendron scandens*—2a

Ivy, English, *Hedera helix*—1, 3

Ivy, Madeira, *Hedera canariensis*—1

Ivy, parlor, *Philodendron scandens*—2a

Ivy, water, *Senecio mikanioides*—4

J

Jack-in-the-pulpit, *Arisaema triphyllum*—1, 2a

Jaggery palm, *Caryota urens*—1, 2a

Jalapeno peppers, *Capsicum* spp—1, 3

Japanese apricot, *Prunus mume*—4

Japanese aucuba, *Aucuba japonica*—3

Japanese bead tree, *Melia azedarach*—4

Japanese flowering apricot, *Prunus mume*—4

Japanese flowering cherry, *Prunus* spp—4

Japanese lantern, *Physalis alkekengi*—4

Japanese laurel, *Aucuba japonica*—3

Japanese pagoda tree, *Sophora japonica*—4

Japanese plum (seeds), *Eriobotrya japonica*—4

Jasmine, French, *Calotropis procera*—4

Jasmine, night blooming, *Cestrum nocturnum*—4

Jasmine, poet's, *Jasminum officinale*—1

Jasmine, yellow, *Gelsemium sempervirens*—4

Jequirity bean, *Abrus precatorius*—4

Jerusalem cherry, *Solanum pseudocapsicum*—3

Jessamine, day, *Cestrum diurnum*—4

Jessamine, day blooming, *Cestrum diurnum*—4

Jessamine, night blooming, *Cestrum nocturnum*—4

Jessamine, poet's, *Jasminum officinale*—1

Jessamine, yellow, *Gelsemium sempervirens*—1, 4

Jimson weed, *Datura stramonium*—4

Johnny jump up (seeds only), *Viola cornuta*—3

Juniper, *Juniperus* spp—1, 3

K

Kaffir lily, *Clivia miniata*—3

Kaffir-boom, *Erythrina* spp—4

Kalo nut, *Aleurites fordii*—1, 3

Klamath weed, *Hypericum perforatum*—1, 3

Kola nut, *Cola nitida*—4

L

Laburnum, *Laburnum* spp—4

Lacquer tree, *Rhus verniciflua*—1

Lacquer tree, *Toxicodendron vernicifluum*—1

Lady slipper, *Cypripedium* spp—1

Lady-of-the-night, *Brunfelsia americana*—4

Lady's fingers, *Abelmoschus esculentus*—1

Lady's lace, *Ammi majus*—1

Lady's slipper, *Cypripedium* spp—1

Lady's slipper, *Pedilanthus tithymaloides*—1, 3

Lady's sorrel, *Oxalis* spp—2b

Lamb's quarters, *Chenopodium album*—1

Lantana, *Lantana camara*—4

Larkspur, *Delphinium* spp—4

Laurel, *Kalmia angustifolia*—4

Laurel, great, *Rhododendron maximum*—4

Laurel, Indian (seed kernel), *Calophyllum inophyllum*—3

Laurelwood (seed kernel), *Calophyllum inophyllum*—3

Leather flower, *Clematis* spp—1, 3

Lemon (peels and thorns), *Citrus limon*—1

Lemon, wild, *Podophyllum peltatum*—1, 4

Lenten rose, *Helleborus* spp—4

Leopard lily, *Dieffenbachia* spp—2a

Leopard palm, *Amorphophallus rivieri*—1, 2a

Leopard's bane, *Arnica montana*—1, 4

Licorice, *Glycyrrhiza glabra*—4

Licorice vine, *Abrus precatorius*—4

Licorice, Indian, *Abrus precatorius*—4

Licorice, wild, *Abrus precatorius*—4

Lily of the Incas, *Alstroemeria aurantiaca*—1, 3

Lily of the Nile, *Agapanthus* spp—1

Lily of the palace, *Hippeastrum aulicum*—3

Lily, arum, *Zantedeschia aethiopica*—2a

Lily, black, *Dracunculus vulgaris*—2a

Lily, pig, *Zantedeschia aethiopica*—2a

Lily, trumpet, *Zantedeschia aethiopica*—2q

Lily-of-the-valley, *Convallaria majalis*—4

Lily-of-the-valley bush or shrub, *Pieris japonica*—4

Lily-of-the-valley bush or shrub, *Andromeda japonica*—4

Lime (peels and thorns), *Citrus aurantiifolia*—1

Linseed, *Linium* spp—4

Lion's beard, *Anemone nuttalliana*—1, 3

Liquorice, *Glycyrrhiza glabra*—4
Live oak, *Quercus virginiana*—1, 3
Lobelia, *Lobelia* spp—1, 4
Loco weed, *Datura stramonium*—4
Locoweed, *Astragalus* spp—4
Locoweed, *Cannabis sativa*—4
Locoweed, purple, *Oxytropis lambertii*—4
Locoweed, stemless, *Oxytropis lambertii*—4
Locoweed, white, *Oxytropis lambertii*—4
Locust, black or yellow, *Robinia pseudoacacia*—4
Loquat (seeds), *Eriobotrya japonica*—4
Lord and ladies, *Arum maculatum*—1, 2a
Love apple (green parts), *Lycopersicon lycopersicum*—4
Love bean, *Abrus precatorius*—4
Love-in-a-mist, *Nigella damascena*—3
Lucky bean, *Abrus precatorius*—4
Lucky seed, *Thevetia peruviana*—4
Lupine, *Lupinus* spp—4
M
Ma Huang, *Ephedra* spp—4
Mace, *Myristica fragrans*—4
Maidenhair tree, *Ginkgo biloba*—1, 4
Malabar tree, *Euphorbia tirucalli*—1, 3
Mandarin orange (peels and thorns), *Citrus nobilis*—1
Mandrake, *Podophyllum peltatum*—1, 4
Marble queen pothos, *Epipremnum aureum*—2a
Marble queen pothos, *Scindapsus aureus*—2a
Marguerite, *Chrysanthemum frutescens*—1, 3
Marigold, big, *Tagetes erecta*—1
Marmalade bush, *Streptosolen jamesonii*—4
Marsh horsetail, *Equisetum palustre*—4
Marsh marigold, *Caltha palustris*—1, 3
Match-me-if-you-can, *Acalypha wilkesiana*—1
Mate, *Ilex paraguariensis*—3
Matrimony vine, *Lycium halimifolium*—4
Mauna loa, *Spathiphyllum* spp—2a
Mayapple, *Podophyllum peltatum*—1, 4
Meadow crocus, *Colchicum autumnale*—4
Meadow saffron, *Colchicum autumnale*—4
Medicinal aloe, *Aloe barbadensis*—1, 3
Medicine plant, *Aloe* spp—1, 3
Mescal, *Lophophora williamsii*—4
Mescal (do not confuse with *Lophophora williamsii*—Peyote), *Agave uthaensis*—1, 3
Mescal bean, *Sophora secundiflora*—4
Mescal button, *Lophophora williamsii*—4

Mesquite, *Prosopis glandulosa*—1
Mexican bird of paradise, *Caesalpinia mexicana*—3
Mexican breadfruit, *Monstera deliciosa*—2a
Mexican breadfruit, *Philodendron pertusum*—2a
Mexican fireweed, *Kochia scoparia*—1, 2a, 2b
Mexican flame vine, *Senecio confusus*—1
Mexican horsetail, *Equisetum* spp—4
Mexican prickle poppy, *Argemone mexicana*—4
Mexican tea, *Chenopodium ambrosioides*—3
Mexican tea, *Ephedra* spp—4
Meyer lemon (peels and thorns), *Citrus meyeri*—1
Milk barrel, *Euphorbia* spp—1, 3
Milk bush, *Euphorbia tirucalli*—1, 3
Milk purslane, *Chamaesyce maculata*—1
Milk purslane, *Euphorbia maculata*—1
Milk weed, *Chamaesyce drummondii*—1
Milkweed, *Asclepias* spp—4
Milkweed, *Euphorbia drummondii*—1, 3
Miner's tea, *Ephedra* spp—4
Mistletoe, American, *Phoradendron flavescens*—3
Mistletoe, European, *Viscum album*—3
Moccasin flower, *Cypripedium* spp—1
Mock orange, *Citrus trifoliata*—3
Mock orange, *Laurocerasus caroliniana*—4
Mock orange, *Poncirus trifoliata*—3
Mock orange, *Prunus caroliniana*—4
Mole bean, *Ricinus communis*—4
Mole plant, *Euphorbia lathyris*—1, 3
Mona Lisa, *Codiaeum* spp—1
Monkshood, *Aconitum napellus*—4
Moon, *Lophophora williamsii*—4
Moon weed, *Datura stramonium*—4
Moonflower, *Datura inoxia*—4
Moonflower, *Ipomoea alba*—1
Moonflower, purple, *Ipomoea muricata*—4
Moonseed, *Menispermum* spp—1, 4
Mormon tea, *Ephedra* spp—4
Morning glory (seeds), *Ipomoea* spp—4
Morning-noon-and-night, *Brunfelsia* spp—4
Mother-in-law plant, *Caladium*—2a
Mother-in-law plant, *Dieffenbachia seguine*—2a
Mother-in-law's tongue, *Dieffenbachia* spp—2a

Mountain ivy, *Kalmia latifolia*—4
Mountain laurel, *Kalmia latifolia*—4
Mountain tobacco, *Arnica montana*—1, 4
Mum, *Chrysanthemum* spp—1, 3
Mustard tree, *Nicotiana glauca*—4
Myrtle, *Vinca minor*—4
Mysterious plant, *Daphne mezereum*—1, 4
N
Naked boys, *Colchicum autumnale*—4
Naked lady, *Amaryllis belladonna*—3
Narcissus, *Narcissus* spp—1, 3
Nectar of the gods, *Allium sativum*—1, 3
Nectarine (chewed pits), *Prunus persica*—4
Needlepoint ivy, *Hedera helix*—1, 3
Nephthytis, *Syngonium podophyllum*—2a
Nerve root, *Cypripedium* spp—1
Nettle, *Laportea canadensis*—1
Nettle, stinging, *Urtica* spp—1
Nicotiana, *Nicotiana* spp—4
Night blooming jasmine, *Cestrum nocturnum*—4
Night blooming jessamine, *Cestrum nocturnum*—4
Nightshade, American, *Phytolacca americana*—3
Nightshade, black, *Solanum nigrum*—4
Nightshade, blue, *Solanum dulcamara*—4
Nightshade, climbing, *Solanum dulcamara*—4
Nightshade, common, *Solanum nigrum*—4
Nightshade, deadly, *Solanum dulcamara*—4
Nightshade, poisonous, *Solanum dulcamara*—4
Nightshade, stinking, *Hyoscyamus niger*—4
Nightshade, woody, *Solanum dulcamara*—4
Nighshade, yellow, *Urechites* spp—4
Noah's ark, *Cypripedium* spp—1
Nutmeg, *Myristica fragrans*—4
Nutmeg flower, *Nigella sativa*—3
O
Oak, *Quercus* spp—1, 3
Ohio buckeye, *Aesculus glabra*—3
Oleander, *Nerium oleander*—4
Oleander, yellow, *Thevetia peruviana*—4
Onion (large quantities), *Allium cepa*—1, 3
Onion, wild, *Allium cernuum*—1, 3
Orange (peels and thorns), *Citrus sinensis*—1
Orange root, *Hydrastis canadensis*—4
Orchid, lady slipper, *Cypripedium* spp—1
Oregon crabapple (chewed seeds), *Malus fusca*—4
Oregon holly, *Ilex* spp—3

Oriental plum tree, *Ginkgo biloba*—1, 4
Oriental poppy, *Papaver orientale*—3
Ornamental cherry (chewed seeds), *Prunus* spp—4
Ornamental crabapple (chewed seeds), *Malus floribunda*—4
Ornamental crabapple (chewed seeds), *Pyrus floribunda*—4
Ornamental flowering plum, *Prunus cerasifera "atropurpurea"*—4
Ornamental nicotiana, *Nicotiana longiflora*—4
Ornamental pear, *Pyrus* spp—1
Ornamental pepper, *Capsicum* spp—1, 3
Ornamental pepper, *Solanum pseudocapsicum*—3
Ornamental plum (chewed seeds), *Prunus* spp—4
Oxalis, *Oxalis* spp—2b
P
Palm, fishtail, *Caryota mitis*—1, 2a
Palma Christi, *Ricinus communis*—4
Panda plant, *Philodendron bipennifolium*—2a
Pansy (seeds only), *Viola tricolor*—3
Paper flower, *Bougainvillea* spp—1
Paper plant, *Cyperus papyrus*—4
Paper white narcissus, *Narcissus tazetta*—1, 3
Paperbark tree, *Melaleuca* spp—1
Papyrus, *Cyperus papyrus*—4
Paradise plant, *Daphne mezereum*—1, 4
Paradise tree, *Melia azedarach*—4
Paraguay tea, *Ilex paraguariensis*—3
Parlor ivy, *Senecio mikanioides*—4
Parsley, *Petroselinum crispum*—1
Parsley, spotted, *Cicuta maculata*—4
Parsnip (all but root), *Pastinaca sativa*—1
Parsnip, poison, *Cicuta maculata*—4
Parsnip, wild, *Cicuta maculata*—4
Pasque flower, *Anemone patens*—1, 3
Passion flower, *Passiflora caerulea*—4
Passion fruit, *Passiflora edulis*—4
Passion vine, *Passiflora* spp—4
Passionaria, *Passiflora* spp—4
Pea, everlasting, *Lathyrus* spp—4
Pea, grass, *Lathyrus sativus*—4
Pea, seaside, *Lathyrus japonicus*—4
Peace lily, *Spathiphyllum* spp—2a
Peach (chewed pits), *Prunus persica*—4
Peacock flower, *Caesalpinia pulcherrima*—3
Pear (chewed seeds), *Pyrus communis*—1,4
Pearly gates, *Ipomoea* spp—4

Pecan (pollen and nut oil), *Carya illinoinensis*—1

Pencil cactus or pencil tree, *Euphorbia tirucalli*—1, 3

Pennyroyal, *Mentha pulegium*—4

Pennywort, *Hydrocotyle* spp—1, 4

Peony, *Paeonia officinalis*—1, 4

Peony, tree, *Paeonia suffruticosa*—1, 4

Pepper bush, *Croton humilis*—1

Pepper tree, *Schinus molle*—1, 3

Pepper, bell, *Capsicum* spp—1, 3

Pepper, sweet, *Capsicum* spp—1, 3

Pepper, tobasco, *Capsicum* spp—1, 3

Periwinkle, *Vinca rosea*—4

Periwinkle, Madagascar, *Cantharanthus roseus*—4

Periwinkle, rose, *Catharanthus roseus*—4

Persian lilac, *Melia azedarach*—4

Peruvian lily, *Hymenocallis americana*—3

Peyote, *Lophophora williamsii*—3

Philodendron, *Philodendron* spp—2a

Philodendron, giant, *Philodendron giganteum*—2a

Philodendron, heart leaf, *Philodendron scandens*—2a

Philodendron, split leaf, *Philodendron pertusum*—2a

Photinia arbutifolia (leaves), *Photinia arbutifolia*—4

Pie plant (leaves), *Rheum* spp—1, 2b

Pigeon berry, *Duranta repens*—1, 4

Pigeon berry, *Phytolacca americana*—3

Pigeonberry, *Rivina humilis*—3

Pimento, *Capsicum* spp—1, 3

Pinkroot, *Spigelia marilandica*—4

Pinks, *Dianthus* spp—1

Plum (chewed seeds), *Prunus domestica*—4

Podocarpus (do not confuse with *Taxus* spp), *Podocarpus macrophyllus*—3

Poinciana, *Caesalpinia* spp—3

Poinciana, *Poinciana gilliesii*—3

Poison berry, *Solanum nigrum*—4

Poison bush, *Acokanthera* spp—4

Poison camus, *Zigadenus nuttallii*—4

Poison creeper, *Toxicodendron* spp—1

Poison dogwood, *Toxicodendron vernix*—1

Poison elder, *Toxicodendron vernix*—1

Poison flag, *Iris versicolor*—1, 3

Poison hemlock, *Conium maculatum*—4

Poison ivy, *Rhus* spp—1

Poison ivy, *Toxicodendron radicans*—1

Poison nut, *Strychnos nux-vomica*—4

Poison oak, *Toxicodendron* spp—1

Poison parsley, *Conium maculatum*—4

Poison parsnip, *Cicuta maculata*—4

Poison sumac, *Toxicodendron vernix*—1

Poison tobacco, *Hyoscyamus niger*—4

Poison vine, *Rhus* spp—1

Poison vine, *Toxicodendron radicans*—1

Poison water hemlock, *Cicuta douglasii*—4

Poke berry, *Phytolacca americana*—3

Poke salad plant, *Phytolacca* spp—3

Pokeweed, *Phytolacca americana*—3

Polecat weed, *Symplocarpus foetidus*—2a

Polyscias, *Polyscias guilfoyei*—1, 3

Poppy, common, *Papaver somniferum*—3

Poppy, garden, *Papaver orientale*—3

Poppy, opium, *Papaver somniferum*—3

Poppy, Oriental, *Papaver orientale*—3

Potato (all green parts), *Solanum tuberosum*—4

Potato vine, *Solanum jasminoides*—4

Pothos, *Epipremnum aureum*—2a

Pothos, *Scindapsus aureus*—2a

Prarie crocus, *Anemone patens*—1, 3

Prayer bead or bean, *Abrus precatorius*—4

Precatory pea or bean, *Abrus precatorius*—4

Pregnant onion, *Ornithogalum caudatum*—1, 4

Prickly poppy, *Argemone mexicana*—4

Pride of Barbados, *Caesalpinia pulcherrima*—3

Pride of China, *Melia azedarach*—4

Pride of India, *Melia azedarach*—4

Pride of Madeira, *Echium* spp—4

Primrose, *Primula vulgaris*—1

Primula, *Primula* spp—1

Privet, *Ligustrum vulgare*—3

Privet, California, *Ligustrum californicum*—3

Privet, California, *Ligustrum ovalifolium*—3

Purple leaf plum, *Prunus cerasifera "atropurpurea"*—4

Pussy foot, *Eupatorium conyzoides*—3

Q

Queen Anne's lace, *Daucus carota*—1

Queen's delight, *Stillingia* spp—1

Queen's lace, *Daucus carota*—1

Queen's root, *Stillingia sylvatica*—1

R

Radish, Chinese (leaves), *Raphanus sativus*—1

Ragweed, *Ambrosia artemisiifolia*—1

Ragwort, tansy, *Senecio jacobaea*—4

Rain flower, *Grevillea banksii*—1

Rain lily, *Zephyranthes atamasco*—1, 3

Rain tree, *Brunfelsia undulata*—4

Rain tree, *Pithecellobium saman*—3

Rain tree, *Samanea saman*—3

Rainbow pink, *Dianthus chinensis*—1

Ranunculus, *Ranunculus* spp—1, 3

Rattlebox, *Crotalaria spectabilis*—4

Rattlebox, *Daubentonia punicea*—4

Rattlebox, *Sesbania punicea*—4

Red hot cat tail, *Acalypha hispida*—1, 3

Red hot poker tree, *Erythrina abyssinica*—4

Red ink, *Phytolacca americana*—3

Red root, *Ceanothus americanus*—3

Red root, *Sanguinaria canadensis*—3

Red spurge, *Euphorbia cotinifolia*—1, 3

Red squill, *Urginea maritima*—4

Redberry, *Arctostaphylos uva-ursi*—1, 4

Redberry, *Panax quinquefolius*—4

Redbird cactus or flower, *Euphorbia tithymaloides*—3

Redbird cactus or flower, *Pedilanthus tithymaloides*—1, 3

Rhododendron, *Rhododendron* genus—4

Rhubarb (leaves), *Rheum* spp—1, 2b, 3

Rock poppy, *Chelidonium majus*—1,4

Rocket larkspur, *Delphinium* spp—4

Rosary beads (not to be confused with Rosary vine), *Senecio* spp—4

Rosary bean or pea, *Abrus precatorius*—4

Rosary pearls, *Senecio* spp—4

Rose periwinkle, *Catharanthus roseus*—4

Rosebay, *Rhododendron maximum*—4

Rose-bay, *Nerium oleander*—4

Rosewood, *Dalbergia retusa*—1

Rubber tree, *Hevea brasiliensis*—1

Rubber vine, *Cryptostegia grandiflora*—4

Rush, *Equisetum* spp—4

S

Sacred datura, *Datura inoxia*—4

Saffron, *Crocus sativus*—4

Saffron crocus, *Crocus sativus*—4

Sagebrush, *Artemisia* spp—4

Sago cycas, *Cycas* spp—4

Sago cycas, *Zamia* spp—4

Sago palm, *Cycas* spp—4

Sambucus (all but ripe berries), *Sambucus caerulea*—3

Sand begonia, *Rumex venosus*—2b, 3

Sandberry, *Arctostaphylos uva-ursi*—1, 4

Sapphire flower, *Browallia* spp—1

Sassafras, *Sassafras* spp—4

Sassafras tea, *Sassafras* spp—4

Scorpion weed, *Heliotropium indicum*—4

Scorpion's tail, *Heliotropium angiospermum*—4

Scotch broom, *Cytisus scoparius*—3

Scotch broom, *Spartium scoparium*—4

Scotch heather, *Calluna vulgaris*—4

Scouring rush, *Equisetum hyemale*—4

Scrub oak, *Quercus utahensis*—1, 3

Sea onion, *Scilla verna*—4

Sea onion, *Urginea maritima*—4

Sea onion, false, *Ornithogalum caudatum*—1, 4

Seminole bead, *Abrus precatorius*—4

Sesbania, *Daubentonia punicea*—4

Shamrock, *Oxalis* spp—2b

Shasta daisy, *Chrysanthemum* spp—1, 3

Shell flower, *Pistia stratiotes*—2a

Silk weed, *Asclepias syriaca*—4

Silvercup, *Solandra grandiflora*—4

Singletary pea, *Lathyrus* spp—4

Skunk cabbage, *Symplocarpus foetidus*—2a

Skunk cabbage, *Veratrum* spp—4

Skunkweed, *Symplocarpus foetidus*—2a

Slipper flower or plant, *Euphorbia tithymaloides*—3

Slipper flower or plant, *Pedilanthus tithymaloides*—1, 3

Slipper orchid, *Cypripedium* spp—1

Slippery elm, *Ulmus fulva*—1

Slippery root, *Symphytum officinale*—4

Smoke plant, bush or tree, *Rhus cotinus*—1

Snake flower, *Echium vulgare*—4

Snake lily, *Iris* spp—1, 3

Snakeberry, *Actaea spicata*—1, 4

Snakeroot, *Aristolochia serpentaria*—4

Snakeroot, *Cicuta maculata*—4

Snakeroot, *Eupatorium rugosum*—4

Snakeroot, black, *Zigadenus* or *Zygadenus venenosus*—4

Snakeroot, black, *Cimicifuga racemosa*—4

Snakeweed, *Eupatorium adenophorum*—3

Snakewood, *Brosimum guianense*—1

Snow lily, *Erythronium grandiflorum*—1, 3

Snow on the mountain, *Euphorbia marginata*—1, 3

Snowberry, *Symphoricarpos* spp—3

Snowdrop, *Galanthus nivalis*—3

Snowflake, *Leucojum vernum*—3

Snowflower, *Spathiphyllum* spp—2a

Solandra, *Solandra* spp—4

Sorrel, *Oxalis* spp—2b

Sorrel, *Rumex* spp—2b

Southern mock orange, *Laurocerasus caroliniana*—4

Southern mock orange, *Prunus caroliniana*—4

Spanish broom, *Spartium junceum*—3

Spathe flower, *Spathiphyllum* spp—2a

Spathiphyllum, *Spathiphyllum* spp—2a

Spider flower, *Hymenocallis americana*—3

Spider lily, *Hymenocallis americana*—3

Spider mum, *Chrysanthemum* spp—1, 3

Spindle tree, *Euonymus europaea*—3

Split leaf philodendron, *Monstera deliciosa*—2a

Split leaf philodendron, *Philodendron pertusum*—2a

Spoonwood, *Kalmia latifolia*—4

Spring onion, *Scilla verna*—4

Spurdock, *Rumex crispus*—1, 2b

Spurge, *Euphorbia myrsinites*—1, 3

Spurge flax, *Daphne mezereum*—1, 4

Squaw tea, *Ephedra* spp—4

Squill, *Urginea maritima*—4

St. John's wort, *Hypericum perforatum*—1, 3

Star potato vine, *Solanum seaforthianum*—3

Star-of-Bethlehem, *Hippobroma longiflora*—4

Star-of-Bethlehem, *Laurentia longiflora*—4

Star-of-Bethlehem, *Ornithogalum* spp—4

Stink weed, *Datura stramonium*—4

Stinking hellebore, *Helleborus foetidus*—4

Stinking rose, *Allium sativum*—1, 3

Strawberry shrub (seeds), *Calycanthus* spp—4

String of beads, *Senecio* spp—4

String of pearls, *Senecio* spp—4

Sweet flag, *Acorus calamus*—1

Sweet pea, *Lathyrus odoratus*—4

Sweet William, *Dianthus barbatus*—1

Swiss cheese plant, *Monstera deliciosa*—2a

T

Tallow tree, *Sapium sebiferum*—1, 3

Tansy, *Chrysanthemum* spp—1, 3

Tansy, *Tanacetum vulgare*—1, 3

Taro, *Alocasia macrorrhiza*—2a

Taro, *Colocasia esculenta*—2a

Taxus, *Taxus sieboldii*—4

Tea tree, *Melaleuca quinquenervia*—1

Tea tree, *Sassafras* spp—4

Texas umbrella tree, *Melia azedarach*—4

Thistle, yellow star, *Centaurea solstitialis*—1, 3

Thornapple, *Argemone mexicana*—4

Thornapple, *Datura stramonium*—4

Tobacco, *Nicotiana* spp—4

Tobacco, cultivated, *Nicotiana tabacum*—4

Tobacco, tree, *Nicotiana glauca*—4

Tobacco, wild, *Lobelia inflata*—1, 4

Tobacco, wild, *Nicotiana attenuata*—4

Tomatillo (green parts), *Physalis ixocarpa*—4

Tomato (green parts), *Lycopersicon lycopersicum*—4

Tomato, devil's, *Solanum elaeagnifolium*—4

Toyon (leaves), *Photinia arbutifolia*—4

Tread-softly, *Cnidoscolus stimulosus*—1

Trumpet flower or trumpet plant, *Solandra* spp—4

Trumpet lily, *Datura stramonium*—4

Trumpet lily, *Zantedeschia aethiopica*—2a

Trumpet tree, *Tabebuia* spp—1, 3

Trumpet vine, *Campsis radicans*—1

Tuberose, *Polianthes tuberosa*—4

Tulip, *Tulipa* spp—1, 3

U

Umbrella leaf, *Podophyllum peltatum*—1, 4

Umbrella plant, *Cyperus alternifolius*—4

V

Valerian, *Valeriana officinalis*—4

Varnish tree, *Aleurites moluccana*—1, 3

Veratrum, *Veratrum* spp—4

Verbena, *Verbena* spp—1

Vinca major, *Vinca major*—4

Vinca minor, *Vinca minor*—4

Vinca rosea, *Catharanthus roseus*—4

Vinca rosea, *Vinca rosea*—4

Viola (seeds only), *Viola odorata*—3

Violet (seeds only), *Viola odorata*—3

Virginia creeper, *Parthenocissus quinquefolia*—2a, 2b

NONTOXIC PLANTS (COMMON NAME, LATIN OR COMMON SCIENTIFIC NAME)

NOTE: This list of nontoxic plants is NOT a recommendation that any of them be eaten. Unless you are extremely knowledgeable about plant identification, toxicity, and natural plant-derived foods, you should not eat wild plants (or mushrooms).

A

Abelia, *Abelia* spp
Abutilon hemp, *Abutilon theophrasti*
Acacia, *Albizia julibrissin*
Acanthus, *Acanthus* spp
African daisy, *Dimorphotheca pluvialis*
African daisy, *Gerbera jamesonii*
African iris, *Dietes* spp
African violet, *Saintpaulia ionantha*
Aglaonema, *Aglaonema* spp
Air plant, *Kalanchoe pinnata*
Ajuga, *Ajuga remota* or *Ajuga reptans*
Albizia, *Albizia*
Alder, black, *Viburnum* spp
Alpine goldflower or alpine sunflower, *Hymenoxys grandiflora*
Althea, *Hibiscus* spp
Aluminum plant, *Pilea cadierei*
Alumroot, *Heuchera sanguinea*
Alyssum, *Alyssum* spp
Alyssum, sweet, *Lobularia maritima*
American chestnut, *Castanea* spp
American olive, *Osmanthus americanus*
American sweet gum, *Liquidambar styraciflua*
Amylum, *Maranta* spp
Angel wing begonia, *Begonia coccinea*
Angel's tears, *Soleirolia soleirolii*
Anise, *Myrrhis odorata*
Anise root, *Osmorhiza longistylis*
Aphelandra, *Aphelandra* spp
Aralia, *Dizygotheca elegantissima*
Arbutus, *Arbutus unedo*
Areca palm, *Chrysalidocarpus lutescens*
Aregelia, *Neoregelia* spp
Arrowroot, *Maranta* spp
Artillery plant, *Pilea* spp
Artist's acanthus, *Acanthus* spp
Ash, mountain, *Sorbus* spp
Asparagus fern, *Asparagus densiflorus cv sprengeri*
Asparagus fern, *Asparagus setaceus*
Aspen, *Populus* spp

Aspidistra, *Aspidistra* spp
Aster, annual, *Callistephus chinensis*
Aster, giant, *Townsendia sericea*
Astilbe, *Astilbe japonica*
Australian laurel, *Pittosporum tobira*
Australian nut, *Macadamia* spp
Australian umbrella tree, *Brassaia actinophylla*
Australian umbrella tree, *Schefflera actinophylla*

B

Baby jade, *Crassula argentea*
Baby sun rose, *Aptenia cordifolia*
Baby sun rose, *Mesembryanthemum cordifolium*
Baby's breath, *Gypsophila paniculata*
Baby's tears, *Hypoestes phyllostachya*
Baby's tears, *Soleirolia soleirolii*
Baby's toes, *Fenestraria rhopalophylla*
Bachelor buttons, *Centaurea cyanus*
Balloon flower, *Platycodon grandiflorus*
Balloon vine, *Cardiospermum halicacabum*
Balm, *Molucella* spp
Balsam, *Impatiens* spp
Balsam tree, *Abies balsamea*
Bamboo bush, *Nandina domestica*
Bamboo palm, *Chamaedorea* spp
Bamboo, common, *Phyllostachys aurea*
Basket lily, *Hemerocallis* spp
Basket plant or vine, *Aeschynanthus* spp
Bayberry, *Aeschynanthus* spp
Bayberry, *Myrica pensylvanica*
Bead vine, *Crassula rupestris*
Bear's breech, *Acanthus* spp
Beautyberry, *Callicarpa* spp
Beauty bush, *Kolkwitzia amabilis*
Beech, American, *Fagus* spp
Begonia cissus, *Cissus* spp
Begonia, iron cross, *Begonia goegoensis*
Bell flower, *Platycodon grandiflorus*
Bellflower, *Campanula* spp
Bells of Ireland, *Moluccella* spp
Bigleaf palm, *Fatsia japonica*

Billbergia, *Aechmea marmorata*
Billbergia, *Quesnelia* spp
Birch tree, *Betula* spp
Bird's nest fern, *Asplenium nidus*
Bishop's cap or bishop's hood, *Astrophytum* spp
Bishop's elder or bishop's weed, *Aegopodium podagraria*
Bitter pecan, *Carya* spp
Bitternut, *Carya* spp
Black beech, *Nothofagus* spp
Black-eyed Susan vine, *Thunbergia alata*
Blazing star, *Liatris* spp
Bleeding heart, *Clerodendrum* spp
Bleeding heart vine, *Clerodendrum* spp
Bloodleaf plant, *Iresine* spp
Blue bottle, *Centaurea cyanus*
Blushing bromeliad, *Aregelia* spp
Blushing bromeliad, *Neoregelia* spp
Border grass, *Liriope muscari*
Boston fern, *Nephrolepis* spp
Bottle gourd, *Lagenaria siceraria*
Bottle palm, *Beaucarnea recurvata*
Bottle tree, *Brachychiton* spp
Bottlebrush, *Callistemon* spp
Brain plant, *Calathea makoyana*
Brassaia, *Brassaia actinophylla*
Breath of spring, *Lonicera fragrantissima*
Breath-of-heaven, *Coleonema ericoides*
Breath-of-heaven, *Diosma ericoides*
Bride's flower, *Stephanotis floribunda*
Bride's bonnet, *Clintonia uniflora*
Bright eyes, *Sinningia speciosa*
Brodiaea, *Dichelostemma pulchellum*
Bromeliad king, *Vriesea hieroglyphica*
Broom palm, *Coccothrinax argentea*
Buddleia, *Buddleia davidii*
Bunchberry, *Cornus canadensis*
Burro's tail, *Sedum morganianum*
Busy Lizzie, *Impatiens* spp
Butterfly bush, *Buddleia davidii*
Butterfly flower, *Schizanthus* spp
Butterfly ginger, *Hedychium coronarium*
Butterfly iris, *Spuria* spp
Butterfly lily, *Hedychium coronarium*
Butterfly palm, *Chrysalidocarpus lutescens*
Butterfly pea, *Centrosema virginianum*
Button fern, *Pellaea rotundifolia*
Buttons on a string, *Crassula rupestris*
Buzy Lizzie, *Impatiens* spp

C

Cabbage kale, *Brassica oleracea*
Cabbage tree, *Cordyline australis*
Cactus (except for thorns), Cactaceae family
Calathea, *Calathea* spp
Calendula, *Calendula officinalis*
California bayberry, *Myrica californica*
California bluebell, *Phacelia sericea*
California poppy, *Eschscholzia californica*
California wax myrtle, *Myrica californica*
Callistemon, *Callistemon* spp
Camellia, *Camellia japonica*
Camellia, *Thea japonica*
Campanula, *Campanula* spp
Campion, *Silene acaulis*
Campion, moss or mossy, *Silene acaulis*
Canary date palm, *Phoenix canariensis*
Candle plant, *Plectranthus oertendahlii*
Candleberry, *Myrica pensylvanica*
Cane apple, *Arbutus unedo*
Cane palm, *Chrysalidocarpus lutescens*
Canna lily, *Canna generalis*
Canterbury bell, *Campanula* spp
Canterbury-bell gloxinia, *Gloxinia perennis*
Cape honeysuckle, *Tecomaria capensis*
Cape jasmine, *Gardenia jasminoides*
Cape marigold, *Dimorphotheca pluvialis*
Cape primrose, *Streptocarpus* spp
Cardinal flower, *Gesneria* spp
Cardinal flower, *Rechsteineria cardinalis*
Cardinal flower, *Sinningia cardinalis*
Carob, *Ceratonia siliqua*
Carob tree, *Ceratonia siliqua*
Carob tree, *Jacaranda procera*
Carpet bugle, *Ajuga* spp
Casa blanca lily, *Lilium* spp
Cast iron plant, *Aspidistra elatior*
Cat tail, *Typha latifolia*
Catalpa, *Catalpa* spp
Cathedral bells, *Cobaea scandens*
Cathedral windows, *Calathea makoyana*
Cedar pine, *Pinus glabra*
Celosia, *Celosia* spp
Chain of love, *Antigonon leptopus*
Chain plant, *Tradescantia navicularis*
Checker lily, *Fritillaria* spp
Chenille plant, maroon, *Echeveria* spp
Chestnut, sweet, *Castanea* spp
Chia, *Salvia columbariae*

Chickens and hens or chicks and hens, *Echeveria* spp

Chicks and hens, *Sempervivum tectorum*

China doll, *Leea* spp

China doll, *Radermachera sinica*

China rose, *Hibiscus* spp

Chinese evergreen, *Aglaonema modestum*

Chinese hackberry, *Celtis sinensis*

Chinese hibiscus, *Hibiscus* spp

Chinese holly, *Osmanthus heterophyllus*

Chinese tulip tree, *Liriodendron chinense*

Chocolate soldier, *Episcia cupreata*

Chokeberry, *Aronia* spp

Christmas cactus, *Schlumbergera bridgesii*

Christmas dagger fern, *Polystichum* spp

Christmas flower, *Euphorbia pulcherrima*

Christmas kalanchoe, *Kalanchoe blossfeldiana*

Christmas star, *Euphorbia pulcherrima*

Cinderella slippers, *Sinningia pusilla*

Cinquefoil, *Potentilla* spp

Clarkia, *Clarkia* spp

Cleome, *Cleome* spp

Clianthus, *Clianthus* spp

Climbing begonia, *Cissus discolor*

Cloche, *Campanula* spp

Clustered wax flower, *Stephanotis floribunda*

Cobra lily or cobra plant, *Darlingtonia californica*

Cockscomb, *Celosia* spp

Coleus, *Coleus* spp

Columbine, *Aquilegia* spp

Column of pearls, *Haworthia chalwinii*

Common balm, *Melissa officinalis*

Common myrtle, *Myrtus communis*

Compass flower, *Hymenoxys grandiflora*

Cone flower, purple, *Rudbeckia purpurea*

Coneflower, *Echinacea* spp

Coral beads, *Sedum stahlii*

Coral bells, *Heuchera sanguinea*

Coral bells, *Kalanchoe uniflora*

Coral berry, *Ardisia* spp

Coral vine, *Antigonon leptopus*

Cordyline, *Cordyline* spp

Coreopsis, *Coreopsis californica*

Corn lily, *Clintonia borealis*

Cornflower, *Centaurea cyanus*

Cornplant, *Dracaena fragrans*

Cornstalk plant, *Dracaena fragrans*

Cosmos, *Cosmos* spp

Cottongum tree, *Nyssa aquatica*

Cottonwood, *Populus* spp

Coxcomb, *Celosia* spp

Crape myrtle or crepe myrtle, *Lagerstroemia indica*

Crassula, *Crassula* spp

Crataegus, *Crataegus* spp

Creeping Charlie, *Pilea nummulariifolia*

Creeping Charlie, *Plectranthus australis*

Creeping fig, *Ficus* spp

Creeping gloxinia, *Maurandia* spp

Creeping Jenny or creeping Joan, *Lysimachia nummularia*

Creeping nettle, *Soleirolia soleirolii*

Creeping zinnia, *Sanvitalia* spp

Crimson cup, *Aregelia* spp

Crimson cup, *Neoregelia* spp

Crocus, spring blooming, ONLY *Crocus* spp

Crossandra, *Crossandra* spp

Crotolaria, *Crotolaria ramosissima*

Cruel plant, *Cynanchum* spp

Cup and saucer plant, *Gilia* spp

Cup-and-saucer vine, *Cobaeae scandens*

Curiosity plant, *Tolmiea menziesii*

Cushion pink, *Silene acaulis*

D

Dagger plant, *Yucca* spp

Dahlia, *Dahlia* spp

Dandelion, *Taraxacum officinale*

Daphne, October, *Sedum sieboldii*

Day lily, *Hermocallis* spp

Deer's tongue, *Liatris* spp

Dipper gourd, *Lagenaria siceraria*

Dogwood, flowering, *Cornus florida*

Donkey's tail, *Sedum morganianum*

Double rose of China, *Hibiscus* spp

Dracaena, *Cordyline* spp

Dracaena, *Dracaena* spp

Dracaena queen, *Dracaena goldieana*

Dracaena, blue, *Cordyline* spp

Dracaena, blue, *Dracaena* spp

Dracaena, fountain, *Cordyline* spp

Dracaena, giant, *Cordyline* spp

Dracaena, giant, *Dracaena australis*

Dracaena, lance, *Pleomele thaliodes*

Dracaena, Malaysian, *Pleomele reflexa*

Dracaena, striped, *Dracaena deremensis*

Dragon lily, painted *Dracaena fragrans*

Dragon tree, *Dracaena draco*

Dusty miller, *Lychnis coronaria*

Dusty miller, *Senecio cineraria*

Dutch crocus, spring blooming, ONLY *Crocus* spp
Dwarf palm, *Chamaedorea elegans*
Dwarf royal palm, *Veitchia merrillii*
Dwarf schefflera, *Schefflera arboricola*
E
Easter flower, *Euphorbia pulcherrima*
Easter lily, *Lilium longiflorum*
Echeveria, *Echeveria* spp
Echinacea, *Echinacea* spp
Elephant's ear, *Bergenia cordifolia*
Elephant's ear, *Enterolobium cyclocarpum*
Elephant's ear fern, *Platycerium angolense*
Elephant's foot, *Dioscorea elephantipes*
Elephant's ear, *Saxifraga cordifolia*
Elk's horn, *Platycerium* spp
Emerald feather or emerald fern, *Asparagus densiflorus cv sprengeri*
English bluebell, *Endymion non-scriptus*
English lavender, *Lavandula* spp
Escallonia, *Escallonia* spp
Eugenia, *Eugenia cyanocarpa*
Eugenia, *Syzygium cuminii*
European grape, *Vitis vinifera*
Euryops, *Euryops* spp
Evening primrose, *Oenothera* spp
Evergreen plant, *Radermachera sinica*
Evergreen woodfern, *Dryopteris marginalis*
Exacum, *Exacum affine*
F
Fairwell-to-spring, *Clarkia amoena*
Fairy duster, *Calliandra eriophylla*
False aralia, *Dizygotheca elegantissima*
False heather, *Cuphea hyssopifolia*
False holly, *Osmanthus heterophyllus*
False hop, *Beloperone guttata*
False lily of the valley, *Maianthemum kamtschaticum*
Fan palm, *Coccothrinax alta*
Fan palm, *Livistona chinensis*
Farewell to spring, *Clarkia* spp
Fatsia, *Fatsia japonica*
Fern, bird's nest, *Asplenium nidus*
Fern, deer's foot, *Davallia canariensis*
Fern, hare, *Davallia fejeensis*
Fern, hen and chickens, *Asplenium bulbiferum*
Fern, iron, *Rumohra adiantiformis*
Fern, king and queen, *Asplenium* spp
Fern, leather, *Rumohra adiantiformis*

Fern, leatherleaf, *Rumohra adiantiformis*
Fern, mother, *Asplenium* spp
Fern, rabbit's foot, *Davallia fejeensis*
Fern, squirrel's foot, *Davallia fejeensis*
Ficus, *Ficus benjamina*
Fiddle leaf fig, *Ficus* spp
Fiddle leaf rubber plant, *Ficus* spp
Fiery spike, *Aphelandra* spp
Fig, *Ficus carica*
Fig, climbing, *Ficus* spp
Fig, weeping, *Ficus benjamina*
Fingernail plant, *Aregelia* spp
Fingernail plant, *Neoregelia* spp
Fir tree, *Abies* spp
Fir tree, *Pseudotsuga* spp
Fire ball plant, *Kalanchoe* spp
Fire lily, *Cyrtanthus* spp
Firebird, *Heliconia* spp
Firecracker, *Gesneria* spp
Firecracker flower, *Crossandra* spp
Firecracker plant, *Cuphea* spp
Firecracker plant or vine, *Manettia bicolor*
Firethorn (except for thorns), *Pyracantha* spp
Fireweed, *Epilobium angustifolium*
Fittonia, *Fittonia* spp
Flame violet, *Episcia reptans*
Flaming sword, *Vriesea splendens*
Flamingo plant, *Hypoestes phyllostachya*
Flocks, *Phlox* spp
Florida beauty, *Dracaena* spp
Flower of the Nativity, *Euphorbia pulcherrima*
Flowering flax, *Linum grandiflorum*
Flox, *Phlox* spp
Forget-me-not, *Myosotis* spp
Forsythia, *Forsythia* spp
Forsythia, white, *Abeliophyllum distichum*
Fort knight lily, *Dietes* spp
Fountain dracaena, *Dracaena australis*
Freckle face, *Hypoestes phyllostachya*
Freesia, *Freesia* spp
French lavender, *Lavandula* spp
French mulberry, *Callicarpa americana*
Friendship plant, *Billbergia* spp
Friendship plant, *Pilea involucrata*
Fritillaria, *Fritillaria* spp
Fruitless mulberry, *Morus* spp
Fuchsia, *Fuchsia* spp
G
Gardenia, *Gardenia jasminoides*
Gazania, *Gazania* spp

Geranium, *Pelargonium* spp
Gerbera daisy, *Gerbera jamesonii*
German violet, *Exacum affine*
Ghost plant, *Sedum weinbergii*
Giant bird's nest, *Pterospora andromedea*
Giant dracaena, *Dracaena australis*
Ginger lily, *Hedychium coronarium*
Ginger, white, *Hedychium coronarium*
Glory bush, *Pleroma* spp
Glory bush, *Tibouchina* spp
Gloxinia, *Gloxinia perennis*
Gloxinia, *Sinningia speciosa*
Gloxinia, hardy, *Incarvillea* spp
Godetia, *Clarkia amoena*
Godetia, *Godetia* spp
Gold bloom, *Calendula officinalis*
Gold dust dracaena, *Dracaena* spp
Gold dust plant, *Alyssum* spp
Gold dust plant, *Aucuba japonica*
Golden bells, *Forsythia* spp
Golden feather palm, *Chrysalidocarpus lutescens*
Golden stars, *Mammillaria elongata*
Goldfish plant, *Hypocyrta* spp
Good luck leaf, *Kalanchoe* spp
Good luck palm, *Chamaedorea elegans*
Good luck plant, *Cordyline terminalis*
Good luck plant, *Dracaena terminalis*
Good luck plant, *Kalanchoe daigremontiana*
Gourd, *Cucurbitaceae* spp
Grape, *Vitis vinifera*
Grape hyacinth, *Muscari* spp
Grape, wild, *Vitis californica*
Grecian vase, *Aechmea marmorata*
Ground elder, *Aegopodium podagraria*

H

Hackberry, common, *Celtis* spp
Hare's tail, *Lagurus ovatus*
Hawaiian good luck plant, *Cordyline terminalis*
Hawaiian good luck plant, *Dracaena terminalis*
Hawaiian hibiscus, *Hibiscus* spp
Hawaiian tree fern, *Cibotium* spp
Hawthorn, *Crataegus* spp
Heart of flame, *Bromelia balansae*
Heart pea, *Cardiospermum halicacabum*
Heart vine, *Ceropegia woodii*
Hearts entangled, *Ceropegia woodii*
Hearts-on-a-string, *Ceropegia woodii*

Heather, Mexican, *Cuphea hyssopifolia*
Heavenly bamboo, *Nandina domestica*
Helmet flower, *Gesneria* spp
Helmet flower, *Sinningia cardinalis*
Hemlock tree, *Tsuga* spp (do NOT confuse with toxic *Conium* or *Cicuta* spp)
Hen and chickens fern, *Asplenium* spp
Hen and chicks, *Echeveria* spp
Hen and chicks, *Sempervivum tectorum*
Hens and chickens, *Echeveria* spp
Heuchera, *Heuchera sanguinea*
Hibiscus, *Hibiscus* spp
Hickory, *Carya* spp
Hip berries, *Rosa* spp (except for *Rosa rugose*)
Hollyhock, *Althaea rosea*
Honesty plant, *Lunaria annua*
Honey flower, *Protea mellifera*
Honey plant, *Hoya* spp
Honeyberry, *Celtis australis*
Honeysuckle, *Lonicera fragrantissima*
Hoop pine, *Araucaria cunninghamii*
Horse's tail, *Sedum morganianum*
Hosta, *Hosta* spp
Hoya plant, *Hoya* spp
Hyacinth, summer, *Galtonia* spp

I

Ice plant, *Aptenia cordifolia*
Ice plant, *Lampranthus* spp
Ice plant, *Mesembryanthemum cordifolium*
Icicle plant, *Carpobrotus* spp
Impatiens, *Impatiens* spp
Inch plant, *Callisia* spp
Inch plant, *Zebrina pendula*
Indian hawthorn, *Rhaphiolepis indica*
Indian kale, *Xanthosoma lindenii*
Indian strawberry, *Duchesnea indica*
Indian tobacco, *Eriogonum umbellatum*
Irish moss, *Soleirolia soleirolii*
Iron plant, *Aspidistra* spp
Italian cypress, *Cupressus sempervirens*

J

Jacaranda tree, *Jacaranda procera*
Jade plant, *Portulacaria afra*
Jade plant/jade tree, *Crassula* spp
Jade vine, *Strongylodon macrobotrys*
Janet Craig plant, *Dracaena deremensis*
Japanese aralia, *Fatsia japonica*
Japanese fatsia, *Fatsia japonica*
Japanese lantern, *Hibiscus schizopetalus*
Japanese photina, *Photinia glabra*

Japanese privet, *Ligustrum japonica*
Japanese snowbell, *Styrax japonica*
Jasmine, *Jasminum rex*
Jelly beans, *Sedum pachyphyllum*
Jodetia, *Clarkia* spp
Johnny jump up (except for seeds), *Viola cornuta*
Joshua tree, *Sedum multiceps*
Joshua tree, *Yucca brevifolia*
June berry, *Rubus* spp
June grass, *Poa pratensis*

K

Kalanchoe, *Kalanchoe* spp
Kale, *Brassica oleracea*
Kentucky bluegrass, *Poa pratensis*
King and queen fern, *Asplenium* spp
Kohleria, *Kohleria lindeniana*

L

Lace flower vine, *Episcia dianthiflora*
Lady palm, *Rhapis* spp
Lady slipper, *Impatiens* spp
Lady's ear drops, *Fuchsia* spp
Lamb's ears, *Stachy* spp
Lamb's tail, *Sedum morganianum*
Lamb's lettuce, *Valerianella locusta*
Lantana, wild, *Abronia fragrans*
Lasiandra, *Pleroma* spp
Lasiandra, *Tibouchina* spp
Lavender, *Lavandula officinalis*
Leather leaf woodfern, *Dryopteris marginalis*
Lemon balm, *Melissa officinalis*
Leopard lily, *Lachenalia lilacina*
Liatris, *Liatris* spp
Licorice plant, *Helichrysum petiolatum*
Lilac, *Syringa* spp
Lily, Asiatic, *Lilium asiatic*
Lily, Casa Blanca, *Lilium* spp
Lily, cascade, *Lilium* spp
Lily, coral, *Lilium* spp
Lily, Easter, *Lilium longiflorum*
Lily, filmy, *Hermocallis* spp
Lily, Formosa, *Lilium* spp
Lily, Japanese, *Lilium* spp
Lily, Japanese showy, *Lilium* spp
Lily, Marco Polo, *Lilium* spp
Lily, Mariposa, *Calochortus* spp
Lily, Oriental, *Lilium* spp
Lily, Peruvian, *Hermocallis* spp
Lily, regal, *Lilium* spp
Lily, spider, *Hermocallis* spp

Lily, stargazer, *Lilium* spp
Lily, tiger, *Lilium* spp
Lily, torch, *Kniphofia* spp
Lily, western, *Lilium* spp
Lily, wood, *Lilium* spp
Linden tree, *Tilia americana*
Lion's tooth, *Taraxacum officinale*
Lipstick plant or vine, *Aeschynanthus* spp
Liquidambar tree, *Liquidambar styraciflua*
Lithops, *Lithops* spp
Live forever, *Sedum telephium*
Living plant, *Kalanchoe* spp
Living rock, *Ariocarpus fissuratus*
Living rock, *Mammillaria fissurata*
Living stone, *Lithops* spp
Living stone, *Pleiospilos* spp
Living stones, *Dinteranthus vanzylii*
Living vase, *Aechmea* spp
Lobster claw, *Heliconia humilis*
Lobster claws, *Vriesea carinata*
Lobster plant, *Euphorbia pulcherrima*
Locust pods, *Ceratonia siliqua*
London plane tree, *Platanus acerifolia*
London pride, *Lychnis chalcedonica*
Love vine, *Antigonon leptopus*
Lucky bamboo, *Dracaena sanderiana*

M

Macadamia nut, *Macadamia* spp
Madagascar dragon tree, *Dracaena marginata*
Madagascar lace plant, *Aponogeton fenetralis*
Madeira vine, *Anredera cordifolia*
Madrone, *Arbutus menziesil*
Magic flower, *Achimenes* spp
Magnolia, *Magnolia* spp
Magnolia bush, *Magnolia stellata*
Mahonia, *Mahonia* spp
Maid fern, *Adiantum decorum*
Maiden's tears, *Silene acaulis*
Maidenhair fern, *Adiantum decorum*
Maidenhair vine, *Muehlenbeckia complexa*
Mandevilla vine, *Mandevilla* spp
Manzanita, *Arbutus* spp
Manzanita, woolly, *Arctostaphylos tomentosa*
Maple tree, *Acer* spp
Maranta, *Calathea* spp
Maranta, *Maranta* spp
Marble plant, *Lithops* spp
Marbled rainbow plant, *Billbergia* spp
Marigold, *Calendula* spp
Mariposa lily, *Calochortus* spp

Maternity plant, *Kalanchoe* spp
Matilija poppy, *Romneya coulteri*
May bush, *Crataegus* spp
May flowers, *Leucocrinum montanum*
Merry Christmas, *Begonia rex*
Mexican apple, *Casimiroa edulis*
Mexican creeper, *Antigonon leptopus*
Mexican evening primrose, *Oenothera* spp
Mexican fan palm, *Washingtonia* spp
Mexican firecracker, *Echeveria* spp
Mexican flame tree or Mexican flameleaf,
    Euphorbia pulcherrima
Mexican hat, *Ratibida columnaris*
Mexican heather, *Cuphea hyssopifolia*
Mexican ivy, *Cobaea scandens*
Mexican love plant, *Kalanchoe* spp
Mexican orange, *Choisya ternata*
Mexican pincushion cactus, *Mammillaria*
    compressa
Mexican rosettes, *Echeveria* spp
Mexican shrimp plant, *Beloperone guttata*
Mexican shrimp plant, *Justicia brandegeana*
Mexican snowball, *Echeveria* spp
Mexican sunflower, *Tithonia* spp
Mexican tree fern, *Cibotium schiedei*
Mimicry plant, *Pleiospilos* spp
Mimosa, *Albizia julibrissin*
Miner's lettuce, *Montia perfoliata*
Miracle leaf, *Kalanchoe* spp
Mock orange, *Philadelphus* spp
Mock orange, *Pittosporum tobira*
Mock plane, *Acer pseudoplantanas*
Mock strawberry, *Duchesnea indica*
Mondo grass, *Liriope japonica*
Money plant, *Lunaria annua*
Monkey plant, *Kalanchoe daigremontiana*
Monkshood (NOT to be confused with
    Aconitum spp), *Astrophytum myriostigma*
Mosquito fern or mosquito plant, *Azolla*
    caroliniana
Mosquito plant, *Cynanchum* spp
Mosquito plant, *Pelargonium citrosum*
Moss agate, *Episcia reptans*
Moss rose, *Portulaca grandiflora*
Moss, club, *Lycopodium* spp
Mother fern, *Asplenium* spp
Mother hen and chicks, *Echeveria* spp
Mother of hundreds, *Mammillaria compressa*
Mother of millions, *Kalanchoe pinnata*
Mother of thousands, *Kalanchoe pinnata*

Mother of thousands, *Saxifraga stolonifera*
Mother of thousands, *Tolmiea menziesii*
Mother-in-law plant, *Kalanchoe pinnata* (not
    the *Sansevieria* spp)
Mother-of-pearl plant, *Graptopetalum*
    paraguayense
Mother-of-pearl plant, *Sedum weinbergii*
Mountain acanthus, *Acanthus* spp
Mountain dogwood, *Cornus nuttallii*
Mountain gum, *Eucalyptus dalrympleana*
Mountain ribbonwood, *Hoheria glabrata*
Mountain rose, *Antigonon leptopus*
Mountain sunflower, *Hymenoxys grandiflora*
Mountain sunflower, *Rudbergia grandiflora*
Mulberry tree or bush, *Morus* spp
Mulberry, French, *Callicarpa americana*
Mulberry, fruitless, *Morus* spp
Mullein, *Erysimum* spp
Mullein, *Verbascum* spp
Multiplication plant, *Kalanchoe* spp
Muscari, *Muscari* spp

N

Naegelia, *Smithiantha multiflora*
Nandina bush, *Nandina domestica*
Nasturtium, *Tropaeolum* spp
Neanthebella, *Chamaedorea elegans*
Necklace vine, *Crassula rupestris*
Necklace vine, *Muehlenbeckia complexa*
Nerve plant, *Fittonia* spp
Night jasmine, *Nyctanthes arbor-tristis*
Norfolk Island pine, *Araucaria heterophylla*
Norfolk pine, *Araucaria heterophylla*

O

October plant, *Sedum sieboldii*
Octopus tree, *Brassaia actinophylla*
Octopus tree, *Schefflera actinophylla*
Old man of the mountains, *Hymenoxys*
    grandiflora
Olive, wild, *Halesia* spp
Orange cup, *Lilium* spp
Orchid, *Cattleya* spp
Orchid, *Cymbidium* spp
Orchid, *Epidendrum* spp
Orchid, *Oncidium* spp
Orchid ginger, *Alpinia mutica*
Oregon grape or Oregon holly, *Mahonia*
    aquifolium
Ornamental cabbage, *Brassica oleracea*
Ornamental kale, *Brassica oleracea*
Ostrich fern, *Matteuccia struthiopteris*

P

Pacific dogwood, *Cornus nuttallii*
Pagoda flower, *Clerodendrum* spp
Paint brush, *Castilleja* spp
Painted cup, *Castilleja* spp
Painted dragon lily, *Dracaena fragrans*
Painted feather, *Vriesea carinata*
Painted lady, *Echeveria* spp
Painted leaf, *Euphorbia pulcherrima*
Palm lily, *Cordyline australis*
Palm, bigleaf, *Fatsia japonica*
Palm, date (except for thorns), *Phoenix* spp
Palm, desert fan, *Washingtonia* spp
Palm, tufted fan, *Rhapis* spp
Palo verde, *Cercidium microphyllum*
Pampas grass, *Cortaderia selloana*
Panda bear plant, *Kalanchoe tomentosa*
Panda plant, *Kalanchoe tomentosa*
Pansy (except for seeds), *Viola tricolor*
Paper plant, *Fatsia japonica*
Parakeet flower, *Heliconia psittacorum*
Parlor palm, *Chamaedorea elegans*
Parrot's flower, *Heliconia psittacorum*
Patience plant, *Impatiens* spp
Patient Lucy, *Impatiens* spp
Peace in the home, *Soleirolia soleirolii*
Peacock plant, *Calathea makoyana*
Peacock plant, *Kaempferia* spp
Pearl plant, *Haworthia margaritifera*
Peperomia, *Peperomia* spp
Perfume plant, *Matthiola longipetala*
Persian violet, *Exacum affine*
Petunia, *Petunia* spp
Phlox, *Phlox* spp
Photina, *Photina* spp (except *arbutifolia*, which is toxic)
Photinia, Japanese, *Photinia glabra*
Piggyback plant, *Tolmiea menziesii*
Pikake, *Jasminum sambac*
Pilea, *Pilea* spp
Pincushion flower, *Scabiosa* spp
Pine tree, *Pinus* spp
Pink dot, *Hypoestes phyllostachya*
Pink polka dot, *Hypoestes phyllostachya*
Pink porcelain lily, *Alpinia nutans*
Pink splash plant, *Hypoestes phyllostachya*
Pink vine, *Antigonon leptopus*
Pipe plant, *Aeschnanthus* spp
Pitcher plant, *Darlingtonia californica*

Pittosporum, *Pittosporum* spp
Plane tree, *Platanus occidentalis*
Plantago, *Plantago major*
Plantain, *Musa acuminata*
Plantain lily, *Hosta* spp
Plantain, broad-leaved, *Plantago major*
Plantain, false, *Heliconia* spp
Plantain, wild, *Heliconia bihai*
Plectranthus, *Plectranthus oertendahlii*
Plush plant, *Echeveria* spp
Plush plant, *Kalanchoe* spp
Plush vine, *Mikania apiifolia*
Poinsettia, *Euphorbia pulcherrima*
Poker plant, *Kniphofia* spp
Polka dot plant, *Hypoestes phyllostachya*
Pond lily, *Nymphaea odorata*
Porcelain flower, *Hoya* spp
Portulaca, *Portulaca oleracea*
Potentilla, *Potentilla* spp
Prayer plant, *Maranta leuconeura*
Privet, Chinese, *Ligustrum lucidum*
Privet, glossy, *Ligustrum lucidum*
Privet, tree, *Ligustrum lucidum*
Privet, wax-leaf, *Ligustrum lucidum*
Protea, *Protea* spp
Purple passion vine, *Gynura aurantiaca*
Purslane, *Portulaca oleracea*
Pussy willow, *Salix discolor*
Pyracantha (except for thorns), *Pyracantha* spp

Q

Quaking grass, big, *Briza maxima* or *Briza major*
Queen elkhorn, *Platycerium* spp
Queen of dracaenas, *Dracaena goldieana*
Queen's jewels, *Antigonon leptopus*
Queen's tears, *Billbergia* spp
Queen's spiderwort, *Tradescantia reginae*
Queen's umbrella tree, *Brassaia actinophylla*
Queen's umbrella tree, *Schefflera actinophylla*
Queensland nut, *Macademia* spp
Queensland umbrella tree, *Schefflera actinophylla*
Quince, common, *Cydonia oblonga*
Quince, flowering, *Chaenomeles* spp

R

Rabbit's foot, *Maranta leuconeura*
Rabbit's tail grass, *Lagurus ovatus*
Raffia, *Raphia farinifera*
Rainbow plant, *Billbergia* spp

Raphiolepsis, *Rhaphiolepsis indica*
Rattan cane, *Calamus rotang*
Rattlesnake plant, *Calathea* spp
Red bud, *Cercis canadensis*
Red gum, *Liquidambar styraciflua*
Red hot poker, *Kniphofia* spp
Resurrection lily, *Kaempferia* spp
Resurrection plant, *Selaginella lepidophylla*
Rex-begonia vine, *Cissus discolor*
Ribbon plant, *Chlorophytum comosum*
Ribbon plant, *Dracaena sanderiana*
Rock rose, *Cistus* spp
Rock rose, *Oenothera* spp
Rocket, *Barbarea vulgaris*
Rocket, *Eruca sativa*
Rosary bead plant, *Ceropegia woodii*
Rosary plant, *Crassula rupestris*
Rosary vine, *Ceropegia woodii*
Rosary vine, *Crassula rupestris*
Rose (except for thorns), *Rosa* spp (except for *Rosa rugosa*)
Rose of China, *Hibiscus sinensis*
Rose of Mexico, *Oenothera* spp
Rose of Sharon, *Hibiscus syriacus*
Rosehips (berries), *Rosa* spp (except for *Rosa rugosa*)
Roselle, *Hibiscus sabdariffa*
Rubber plant, *Ficus elastica*
Rubber tree plant, *Ficus elastica*
Rudbeckia, *Echinacea* spp
Rudbeckia, *Rudbeckia* spp
Rush rose, *Helianthemum scoparium*
Russian olive, *Elaeagnus* spp
S
Sacred bamboo, *Nandina domestica*
Safflower, *Carthamus tinctorius*
Saffron spike, *Aphelandra* spp
Sage, *Salvia* spp
Sage tree, *Vitex* spp
Sago, *Raphia farinifera*
Sago fern, *Sphaeropteris medullaris*
Salvia, *Salvia* spp
Sarsaparilla, wild, *Smilax glauca*
Saucer magnolia, *Magnolia x soulangiana*
Saxifraga, *Saxifraga* spp
Scabiosa, *Scabiosa* spp
Schefflera, *Brassaia actinophylla*
Schefflera, *Schefflera* spp
Scorpion weed, *Phacelia sericea*
Scotch thistle, *Onopordum acanthium*

Sedum, *Sedum* spp
Sego lily, *Calochortus* spp
Sensitive fern, *Onoclea sensibilis*
Sensitive plant, *Mimosa pudica*
Shell flower, *Alpinia nutans*
Shell flower, *Molucella* spp
Shell ginger, *Alpinia nutans*
Shrimp bush or shrimp plant, *Beloperone guttata*
Shrimp bush, *Justicia brandegeana*
Shrimp plant, *Beloperone guttata*
Silk grass, *Oryzopsis hymenoides*
Silk tree, *Albizia julibrissin*
Silver bell, *Halesia* spp
Silver berry, *Elaeagnus* spp
Silver calathea, *Calathea argyraea*
Silver dollar, *Astrophytum asterias*
Silver dollar, *Crassula arborescens*
Silver evergreen, *Aglaonema* spp
Silver gum, *Eucalyptus cordata*
Silver king, *Aglaonema* spp
Silver nerve, *Fittonia* spp
Silver palm, *Coccothrinax argentata*
Silver queen, *Aglaonema* spp
Silver star, *Cryptanthus lacerdae*
Silver thatch, *Coccothrinax argentea*
Silver thistle, *Onopordum acanthium*
Silver threads, *Fittonia* spp
Silver vine, *Actinidia polygama*
Silver weed, *Potentilla* spp
Slipper plant, *Calceolaria* spp
Smoke tree, American, *Cotinus* spp
Smoke tree, American, *Rhus cotinoides*
Smooth bouvardia, *Bouvardia glaberrima*
Snapdragon, *Antirrhinum majus*
Snow bush, *Breynia disticha*
Snowball, *Alternanthera* spp
Snowball bush, *Viburnum* spp
Snowball, Chinese, *Viburnum macrocephalum*
Snowball, Japanese, *Viburnum plicatum*
Snowball, prarie, *Abronia fragrans*
Snowbell tree, *Halesia* spp
Snowberry, mountain, *Symphoricarpos* spp
Snowberry, western, *Symphoricarpos* spp
Society garlic, *Tulbaghia violacea*
Spanish bayonet, *Yucca* spp
Spanish bluebell, *Endymion hispanicus*
Spanish moss, *Tillandsia usneoides*
Sparaxis, *Sparaxis tricolor*

Speargrass, *Poa pratensis*
Spice berry, *Ardisia* spp
Spider aralia, *Dizygotheca elegantissima*
Spider flower, *Cleome* spp
Spider flower, *Hermocallis* spp
Spider flower, *Tibouchina* spp
Spider ivy, *Chlorophytum comosum*
Spider lily, *Hermocallis* spp
Spider plant, *Chlorophytum comosum*
Spiraea, *Astilbe japonica*
Spiraea, blue, *Caryopteris* spp
Spirea, *Spirea* spp
Split rock, *Dinteranthus wilmotianus*
Spotted dracaena, *Dracaena* spp
Spotted laurel, *Aucuba japonica* variegated
Spruce pine, *Pinus glabra*
Spruce tree, *Picea* spp
Squaw bush, *Viburnum* spp
Squill, Italain, *Endymion italicus*
Staghorn fern, *Platycerium* spp
Star jasmine, *Trachelospermum jasminoides*
Star magnolia, *Magnolia stellata*
Star of Bethlehem, *Euphorbia pulcherrima*
Star rock, *Ariocarpus fissuratus*
Star rock, *Mammillaria fissurata*
Stargazer lily, *Lilium* spp
Statice, *Limonium* spp
Stephanotis, *Stephanotis floribunda*
Stock, *Matthiola incana*
Stone face, *Lithops* spp
Stone plant, *Lithops* spp
Stonecrop, *Sedum rubrotinctum*
Strawberry begonia, *Saxifraga* spp
Strawberry geranium, *Saxifraga* spp
Strawberry tree, *Arbutus unedo*
Strawflower, *Helichrysum bracteatum*
String of buttons, *Crassula rupestris*
String of hearts, *Ceropegia woodii*
Striped inch plant, *Callisia* spp
Sugar-pods, *Ceratonia siliqua*
Sun god, *Hymenoxys grandiflora*
Sundew, *Drosera* or *Droserae* spp
Sunflower, *Helianthus annuus*
Sunflower, alpine, *Hymenoxys grandiflora*
Sunflower, mountain, *Hymenoxys grandiflora*
Swedish ivy, *Plectranthus australis*
Sweet alyssum, *Alyssum* spp
Sweet gum, *Liquidambar styraciflua*
Sweet rocket, *Hesperis* spp
Sweet viburnum, *Viburnum odoratissimum*

Sweet William phlox, *Phlox diuaricata*
Sweetberry, *Viburnum lentago*
Sword fern, *Polystichum munitum*
Sycamore, *Acer pseudoplatanus*
Sycamore tree, *Platanus* spp

T
Tahitian bridal veil, *Tradescantia multiflora*
Tea plant, *Viburnum* spp
Tea-berry, *Viburnum cassinoides*
Teddy bear plant or vine, *Cyanotis kewensis*
Temple bells, *Smithiantha cinnabarina*
Thatch palm, *Coccothrinax crinita*
Thorn apple, *Crataegus* spp
Thread palm, *Washingtonia* spp
Ti plant, *Cordyline terminalis*
Ti plant, *Dracaena terminalis*
Tiger lily, *Lilium* spp
Tomato tree, *Cyphomandra betacea*
Touch-me-not, *Impateins* spp
Touch-me-not, *Mimosa pudica*
Trailing begonia, *Cissus discolor*
Transvaal daisy, *Gerbera jamesoni*
Tree of kings, *Dracaena terminalis*
Trumpet vine, *Distictis buccinatoria*
Tulip tree, *Liriodendron tulipifera*
Tulip tree, *Spathodea campanulata*

U
Umbrella plant, *Eriogonum umbellatum*
Umbrella tree, *Brassaia actinophylla*
Umbrella tree, *Magnolia tripetala*
Umbrella tree, *Schefflera actinophylla*
Urn plant, *Aechmea* spp

V
Valerian, red, *Centranthus ruber*
Velvet leaf, *Abutilon theophrasti*
Velvet leaf, *Kalanchoe beharensis*
Velvet plant, *Gynura aurantiaca*
Venus's hair *Adiantum capillus*
Venus's hair fern, *Adiantum capillus*
Verbena, *Verbena* spp (except *Verbena hastata*)
Veronica, *Hebe* spp
Veronica, *Veronica* spp
Vervain, *Verbena* spp (except *Verbena hastata*)
Vetch, common, *Vicia sativa*
Viburnum, *Viburnum* spp
Violas (except for seeds), *Viola* spp
Violets (except for seeds), *Viola odorata*

W

Wand flower, *Sparaxis tricolor*

Wandering Jenny, *Lysimachia nummularia*

Wandering Jew, *Zebrina pendula*

Water hyacinth, *Eichhornia crassipes*

Water lily, *Nymphaea* spp

Watsonia, *Watsonia* spp

Wax flower, *Stephanotis floribunda*

Wax plant, *Hoya* spp

Wax rosette, *Echeveria* spp

Wax-leaf privet, *Ligustrum japonicum*

Weeping fig, *Ficus benjamina*

Weigela, *Weigela* spp

White ash, *Aegopodium podagraria*

White wax tree, *Ligustrum lucidum*

Wild grape, *Vitis californica*

Wild hyacinth, *Camassia* spp

Wild hyacinth, *Dichelostemma pulchellum*

Wild lantana, *Abronia* spp

Wild mustard, *Brassica* spp

Wild olive, *Halesia* spp

Wild olive, *Nyssa aquatica*

Wild olive, *Osmanthus americanus*

Wild pepper, *Vitex* spp

Wild strawberry, *Fragaria* spp

Willow, *Salix* spp

Window plant, *Haworthia* spp

Wine grape, *Vitis vinifera*

Winter begonia, *Saxifraga ciliata*

Wintercress, *Barbarea* spp

Wood hyacinth, *Endymion* spp

X

Xylosma, *Xylosma* spp

Y

Yellow evening primrose, *Oenothera* spp

Yucca, *Yucca* spp

Z

Zebra plant, *Aphelandra squarrosa*

Zebra plant, *Calathea zebrina*

Zebra plant, *Cryptanthus zonatus*

Zinnia, *Zinnia* spp

Zygocactus, *Schlumbergera bridgesii*

PART FIVE

Miscellaneous Information

OXYGEN ADMINISTRATION

It may be advisable or necessary under certain circumstances to administer supplemental oxygen gas (O_2) to a person who would benefit from such therapy. Examples include those stricken with severe high-altitude pulmonary edema, acute severe congestive heart failure, carbon monoxide poisoning, decompression sickness (the bends), and so forth. Anyone who may be called on to use oxygen delivery equipment should be properly trained in its use ahead of time.

The equipment required to deliver oxygen includes a medical oxygen cylinder (tank), pressure gauge, pressure-reducing valve, flowmeter, tubing, and nasal cannula (tube) or face mask (with or without a reservoir bag).

Oxygen cylinders (aluminum or steel) in the United States are usually painted green or have distinctive green markings. They come in two practical field sizes: D (20 inches [50.8 cm] in length; carries 360 liters of oxygen) and E (30 inches [76.2 cm] in length; carries 625 liters of oxygen). The length of time that oxygen can be delivered is calculated by dividing the tank capacity by the flow rate. For instance, a D cylinder can deliver 10 liters per minute for 36 minutes. To make the oxygen last longer, keep the flow rate to the lowest effective number.

The pressure gauge reading indicates how much oxygen remains in the cylinder. At full capacity, an oxygen tank is pressurized to 2015 lb per square inch (psi). Thus, when the gauge indicates a pressure of 500 psi, one fourth of the tank's capacity for oxygen remains. At a reading of 200 psi, a tank is near empty.

The pressure gauge, pressure-reducing valve, and flowmeter combine to create the regulator, which reduces the pressure of the oxygen from that inside the tank to approximately 50 psi. This allows delivery to the victim at flow rates between 1 and 15 liters per minute.

The delivery device attached to the victim is either a two-pronged (one for each nostril) nasal cannula, or a face mask, the latter with or without a reservoir bag. A nonrebreathing face mask ("nonrebreather") is a face mask with a reservoir bag attached by a one-way valve such that the victim can breathe oxygen that is delivered into the bag, but cannot exhale carbon dioxide back into the bag (he cannot "rebreathe" from the bag). The nonrebreather is used to deliver high concentrations (as a percent of inspired air, 80% to 90% oxygen at flow rates of 10 to 15 liters per minute) of oxygen. The reservoir bag should be kept at least half full of oxygen. This can be accomplished with flow rates of 6 liters per minute or greater.

If lesser concentrations of oxygen are adequate or desired, as with a patient who has chronic obstructive pulmonary disease (see page 45), a nasal cannula can be used. The cannula will deliver 25% to 40% oxygen at flow rates of 1 to 6 liters per minute. The nasal cannula is less confining in that the victim can speak, drink, and eat without having to remove a face mask.

Since O_2 is dry, it is often desirable to interpose a humidifying device when O_2 delivery will be prolonged.

To administer oxygen:
1. Place the cylinder upright. Open and close the tank valve slowly ("crack the tank") with a wrench to clean debris from the outlet.

2. Close the regulator flow valve and attach the regulator to the tank. Tighten securely by hand. Never use a regulator without the proper O-ring fitting. *Never use tape to hold a loose regulator in place.*
3. Open the tank valve slowly one full turn, and then a half a turn beyond where the regulator becomes pressurized and there is a maximum reading on the pressure gauge.
4. Attach the plastic delivery tubing to the regulator outflow nipple. Attach the breathing face mask or nasal cannula to the other end of the tubing, if it is not already attached.
5. Open the regulator flow valve to the desired flow rate in liters per minute (LPM). A regulator marking of "low" indicates 2 to 4 LPM, "medium" is 4 to 8 LPM, and "high" is 10 to 15 LPM. Use 1 to 6 LPM for a nasal cannula. The flow rate for a nonrebreather face mask should not be less than 6 LPM and is more commonly 10 to 15 LPM.
6. Position the face mask or cannula on the victim's face. Adjust for comfort. Observe the victim to be certain that the device is tolerated, and that the reservoir bag fills properly.
7. When transporting the victim, be sure to secure the tank in a position where it can be reached and monitored.

PRECAUTIONS

1. Never allow an open flame near an oxygen-delivery system.
2. Where feasible, don't expose an oxygen tank to excessive heat (above 125° F [52° C]) or freezing cold.
3. Don't position any part of a person directly over a tank valve—a loose regulator can be blown off the top of the cylinder with tremendous force.
4. Don't drop a cylinder; don't roll a cylinder.
5. Close all valves when the cylinder is not in use.
6. Service the oxygen delivery mechanism every 2 years or as recommended by the manufacturer.

WATER DISINFECTION

Water *purification* is the removal of chemical pollutants by filtration through activated charcoal or active resin compounds. This usually improves the taste, but does not decrease the incidence of infectious disease, because microorganisms are not removed. Water *disinfection* is the treatment of water with chemicals, boiling, or filtration to remove agents of infectious disease, such as bacteria and cysts. Water *sterilization* is the removal of all life forms.

If at all possible, carry disinfected water with you. If you must drink water from a stream or lake that you cannot disinfect, try to use small tributaries that descend at right angles to the main direction of valley drainage. Clean melted snow is of less risk than ice taken from the surface of a lake or stream. Most bacteria that cause diarrhea can survive for months in ice.

The principal offending agents in contaminated water or on unwashed food that cause illness and diarrhea are the bacteria *Escherichia coli, Salmonella, Shigella,* and *Campylobacter,* and the flagellate protozoan *Giardia lamblia* (see page 193). Drinking nondisinfected water in parts of Africa, India, and Pakistan can cause dracunculiasis (guinea worm disease). In countries where water is improperly disinfected, stick to bottled or canned carbonated beverages, beer, and wine. However, be advised that bottled water in developing countries can be contaminated with bacteria that cause diarrhea, so even bottled water should probably be boiled or disinfected with chemicals or ultraviolet (UV) light before drinking. All containers should be wiped clean to remove external moisture and dirt. All ice should be considered contaminated. For purposes of preserving the environment, it's preferable to carry a reusable water container that is filled with disinfected water than to discard multiple plastic or glass containers.

Don't urinate or defecate (inadvertently) into or near your water supply. Build a latrine 8 to 10 inches (20 to 25 cm) deep into the ground at least 100 ft (31 m) and downhill from the water supply. Try to keep the latrine away from a gully or other formation that might become a runoff stream during a thaw or after heavy rainfall.

"Raw" drinking water should be allowed to rest for several hours in order for large particles to settle to the bottom. The top portion can be poured off, if possible, through a filter or fine cloth. Coagulation and flocculation techniques remove smaller suspended particles. Add a pinch of alum (an aluminum salt) to a gallon (3.8 liters) of water and mix well, then stir occasionally for 60 minutes. Allow the water to rest while the aggregated particles settle, and then pour off the upper (hopefully clearer) part through a paper filter (such as a laboratory-grade filter with a pore size of 20 to 30 microns).

Water may be disinfected by any of the following methods:

1. The usual advice—to boil water for 5 to 10 minutes plus 1 minute for each 1000 ft (305 m) of altitude above sea level—is probably overkill. Sterilization (killing of all microorganisms) occurs after 5 to 10 minutes of boiling at sea level. *Giardia* cysts are instantly killed in water heated to 158° F (70° C). To play it safe, bacteria and most viruses require a few minutes at this temperature. Hepatitis A virus requires a full minute of boiling to ensure inactivation.

   Time and temperature have an inverse relationship with respect to water disinfection. The higher the temperature, the less time is required, and vice versa. For instance, pasteurization of food products can occur at a lower temperature (158° F [70° C]) if 30 minutes at this temperature is allowed.

   The temperature at which water boils varies with altitude because of the surrounding barometric pressure. Barometric pressure is expressed in terms of the height (in inches or millimeters) of a column of mercury (Hg) that exerts a pressure equal to that of a column of air with the same size base. At sea level (barometric pressure 760 mm Hg), water boils at 212° F (100° C); at 5000 ft, or 1525 m (632 mm Hg), 203° F (95° C); at 10,000 ft, or 3050 m (522 mm Hg), 194° F (90° C); at 14,000 ft, or 4270 m (446 mm Hg), 187° F (86° C).

   Thus, boiling water is effective for disinfection at any altitude below 18,000 ft (5490 m) likely to be attained by a wilderness enthusiast. The time required to heat the water to boiling contributes to the disinfection process. To provide a wide margin of safety, boil the water for 3 minutes.

2. Halogens, such as iodine and chlorine, are effective chemical disinfectants. The rate at which they kill microorganisms depends on the concentration (measured in milligrams per liter, or parts per million [ppm], which are equivalent) of halogen and time allowed for disinfection. At a given water temperature and pH, contact time is inversely related to concentration. Thus, you double the contact time if half the concentration of halogen is present. Decreased (cold) water temperature or cloudy (more organic material) water requires a longer contact time or higher halogen concentration. Halogens can create an unpleasant taste if the concentration exceeds 4 mg/liter. They can lose effectiveness after prolonged exposure to moisture, heat, or air and may be corrosive or stain clothing. In general, to improve taste, use a lower concentration of halogen for a longer contact time. Eight mg/liter (or ppm) is considered the concentration of iodine effective for water disinfection in room-temperature, clear water. A pregnant woman or a person with thyroid disease or iodine allergy should consult a physician before using any iodine compound for water disinfection.

   Water disinfection tablets, such as Potable Aqua (see later) and other iodine- and chlorine-based products, may be used inside plastic hydration bladders, such as those found in the CamelBak. While they may discolor the plastic, they don't degrade it.

3. Add one tablet of fresh tetraglycine hydroperiodide (e.g., Potable Aqua) to 1 quart (liter) of water and allow the water to stand for 15 minutes. If the water is cloudy, use two tablets. If the water is cold, allow 1 hour after adding the tablets before drinking. Each tablet releases approximately 8 mg/liter of iodine. Don't leave an open bottle exposed to high heat and/or humidity.

Add to 1 Quart (Liter) of Water:

Water	Clear	Cloudy
Warm (>15° C, 59° F)	1 tablet for 15 minutes	2 tablets for 30 minutes
Cold	1 tablet for 60 minutes	2 tablets for 60 minutes

After adequate time for disinfection has elapsed, add a few grains of sodium thiosulfate per quart (liter) of water; this kills the iodine taste. Ascorbic acid (vitamin C) is also effective. Any fruit flavorings that contain vitamin C should be mixed in after full time for disinfection has elapsed. Potable Aqua Plus treatment includes an oxidizing tablet to remove the iodine taste. Granular activated charcoal removes organic material, chemicals, and radioactive particles by adsorption, but does not remove all microorganisms, and thus cannot be relied on to disinfect water. Rather, it should be used to improve taste and clarity. Use it after water has been properly disinfected.

Zinc metal reduces free chlorine or iodine in solution through a chemical reaction. A wand of zinc bristles stirred into a quart (liter) of water for 4 minutes will remove 10 mg/liter of residual chlorine.

Because a 50-tablet bottle of tetraglycine hydroperiodide contains only 0.4 g of iodine (1/50 the lethal dose), the tablet method is very safe. If you use military surplus iodine tablets, they should be steel gray in color and not crumble when pinched by two fingers; discard older, crumbled tablets. Also, no matter what chemical disinfection system you use, allow disinfected water to seep around the cap and threads of your canteen or water bottle, to disinfect them.

4. Add 8 to 10 drops (0.5 mL in each drop) of standard 2% iodine tincture per quart (liter) of water and allow it to stand for 15 minutes. Use a dropper for measurement. If the water is not at least 68° F (20° C), this technique may not eliminate *Giardia*. If the water is cold, allow it to stand for 1 hour before drinking. If you have extra time and don't like the iodine taste, use four to five drops of iodine and allow the water to stand for 8 hours or overnight. Five drops of tincture of iodine disperses to approximately 4 mg/liter.

Add to 1 Quart (Liter) of Water:

Water	Clear	Cloudy
Warm (>15° C, 59° F)	5 drops for 15 minutes	10 drops for 30 minutes
Cold	5 drops for 60 minutes	10 drops for 60 minutes

Another iodine product that can be used to disinfect water, but has not definitively been proved effective for this purpose, is 10% povidone-iodine (Betadine) solution (not "scrub").

Add to 1 Quart (Liter) of Water:

Water	Clear	Cloudy
Warm (>15° C, 59° F)	8 drops for 15 minutes	16 drops for 30 minutes
Cold	8 drops for 60 minutes	16 drops for 60 minutes

5. Fill a 1 oz (30 mL) glass bottle with iodine crystals (U.S. Pharmacopeia [USP] grade, resublimed: 2 to 8 g), and then fill the bottle with water. The bottle should have a

paper-lined Bakelite cap. Warm the water to 68° F to 77° F (20° C to 25° C). Shake vigorously, and then allow the crystals to settle to the bottom for 1 hour. This will create a saturated solution of iodine. As a crude measure, pour at least half of this liquid (not the remaining crystals), or approximately 12.5 to 15 mL, through a fine filter (such as Teflon) into a quart (liter) of water and allow it to stand for 30 minutes. If the water temperature is not at least 68° F (20° C), this technique may not eliminate *Giardia*. The crystals may be reused up to 1000 times. Two grams (0.07 oz) of iodine represents a potentially lethal dose if ingested, so it is absolutely essential to keep the iodine crystals out of the hands of children.

If one capful from a 2 oz (59 mL) bottle equals approximately 2.5 mL, then using a saturated solution prepared from iodine crystals in water:

Add to 1 Quart (Liter) of Water:

Water	Clear	Cloudy
Warm (>15° C, 59° F)	5 capfuls for 15 minutes	10 capfuls for 30 minutes
Cold	5 capfuls for 60 minutes	10 capfuls for 60 minutes

An alcohol-iodine solution can be prepared by adding 8 g of iodine crystals to 100 mL of 95% ethanol. The resulting supernatant yields 8 mg iodine per 0.1 mL. To add to water, measure with an eyedropper:

Add to 1 Quart (Liter) of Water:

Water	Clear	Cloudy
Warm (>15° C, 59° F)	0.1 mL for 15 minutes	0.2 mL for 30 minutes
Cold	0.1 mL for 60 minutes	0.2 mL for 60 minutes

6. Filter the water through a category-three (as set for purification by the Environmental Protection Agency) water treatment device. A few manufacturers that sell filtration devices are Mountain Safety Research, Katadyn, General Ecology Inc., Timberline, Aquamira Technologies Inc., Vestergaard Frandsen, and Sawyer Products. The Sawyer Point Zero Two water filter, with a 0.02 micron filter, is rated to remove viruses. This product is available with a bucket adapter kit, or can be fitted to 4-liter bags or a special water bottle. The Sawyer Mini Water Filtration System, with a 0.01 micron filter, is rated to remove bacteria and protozoa.

   If the filter doesn't come with a "prefilter" (nylon mesh or screen) to remove large particles, pour the water through filter paper (see later) or fine cheesecloth. This helps keep your expensive water filter from clogging, allows it to work more efficiently, and will improve the appearance and taste of the water.

7. Maximum filter pore sizes (in material or microns) for removing microorganisms are as follows: dracunculus (guinea worm) larvae—coffee filter or fine cloth; schistosome cercariae—coffee filter or fine cloth; parasitic eggs and larvae—20; *G. lamblia* cyst, *Entamoeba histolytica* cyst, *Cyclospora*—3 to 5; *Cryptosporidium* oocyst—1; enteric bacteria (such as *E. coli*)—0.2 to 0.4; and viruses—0.004 to 0.01.

8. Halazone (a mixture of monochloraminobenzoic and dichloraminobenzoic acids) and other chlorine (bleach) products have been considered less effective for field water disinfection. Halazone has been characterized as losing 75% of activity after 2 days' continuous exposure to air with high heat and humidity; having a shelf life of 6 months; and decreasing potency by 50% after storage above 104° F (40° C). Therefore, you should obtain a new bottle every 3 to 6 months.

   Each Halazone tablet releases 2.3 to 2.5 mg/liter of chlorine. To disinfect water:

Add to 1 Quart (Liter) of Water:

Water	Clear	Cloudy
Warm (>15° C, 59° F)	5 tablets for 15 minutes	7 tablets for 15 minutes
	2.5 tablets for 30 minutes	5 tablets for 30 minutes
Cold	5 tablets for 60 minutes	7 tablets for 60 minutes

Liquid bleach (hypochlorite solution; household bleach, usually 5.25%) can be used to disinfect water via chlorination. There should be a faint smell or taste of chlorine before drinking.

For 5.25% Bleach, Add to 1 Quart (Liter) of Water:

Water	Clear	Cloudy
Warm (>15° C, 59° F)	2 drops (0.1 mL) for 30 minutes	4 drops (0.2 mL) for 30 minutes
Cold	2 drops (0.1 mL) for 60 minutes	4 drops (0.2 mL) for 60 minutes

For 1% Bleach, Add to 1 Quart (Liter) of Water:

Water	Clear	Cloudy
Warm (>15° C, 59° F)	10 drops (0.5 mL) for 30 minutes	20 drops (1 mL) for 30 minutes
Cold	10 drops (0.5 mL) for 60 minutes	20 drops (1 mL) for 60 minutes

9. Superchlorination followed by dechlorination is an effective technique. This is a more complicated method. Add 27 g or more of calcium hypochlorite crystals to a gallon (3.8 liters) of water to attain a chlorine concentration of 27 to 30 parts per million. After the requisite disinfection time (10 to 30 minutes), add six drops of concentrated (30%, caustic) hydrogen peroxide to dechlorinate the water. The chemical reaction produces calcium chloride (which remains in solution), water, and oxygen.

10. Chlorination can be combined with flocculation. WATERMAKER sachets contain alum and sodium dichloroisocyanurate. This moves solids to the bottom of the container and also allows disinfection.

11. Aquamira water treatment uses stabilized 2% chlorine dioxide combined with an activator (5% food grade phosphoric acid) to improve the taste of water. One kit can be used to treat more than 120 liters of water. Mix seven drops of the two bottles together, let sit for 5 minutes, and then pour the contents into 1 quart of water. Oxygen is released in a highly active form to kill odor-causing bacteria. The process takes approximately 20 minutes.

12. The SteriPEN carries the promotional byline of "safe drinking water anywhere." This unique handheld water purifier that uses UV light is advertised to fit into most plastic consumer water bottles, as well as other types of containers up to 32 oz (1 liter). It operates on four AA batteries, with nickel-metal-hydride or lithium batteries recommended. According to the distributor, only 48 seconds of exposure to the UV light is required to disinfect 16 oz (½ liter) of water and 90 seconds for 32 oz (1 liter). The claim is that the device is effective against common outdoor and household pathogens, as well as less common microorganisms, to include bacteria, viruses, and protozoa. The test results are found at an Internet link provided by the company. According to the product literature, the SteriPEN meets U.S. Environmental Protection Agency standards for microbiologic water purifiers. A filter can be used to remove particulates from the water before UV treatment.

UV light works for water disinfection by destroying the DNA of microbes. This keeps the germs from reproducing, which is necessary in order for them to make a person ill. The light emitted by the SteriPEN device is in the UV-C range, of wavelength 254 nanometers. This wavelength is germicidal (kills germs) by causing adjacent thymine base nucleotides in DNA to bond together, which prevents them from being properly recognized ("read") in the replication process, which is necessary for DNA to allow a microorganism to reproduce. Thus, the germ(s) is rendered harmless. Used as directed, the UV light exposure is of no consequence, as this wavelength of UV light does not pass through most materials (e.g., glass, metal, ceramic, and nearly all plastics). Furthermore, the underside of the air/water surface in a water container acts as a reflector for UV-C. So, if the SteriPEN lamp is completely immersed in water and used according to the instructions, the UV-C is contained and does not pose any health risk to the user. For additional safety, the SteriPEN is equipped with water sensors and will not operate unless the lamp is under water. The SteriPEN contains a microcomputer that controls operation time, according to information it receives from integrated temperature sensors and user indication of the volume of water to be disinfected. During use, the device should be used to gently stir the water. It is intended for use in clear water, so cloudy water must be filtered or otherwise made clear before using the SteriPEN. Disposable lithium or rechargeable AA nickel metal hydride batteries will provide many more disinfection cycles than will alkaline batteries. The latter are better in a cold weather situation.

Another device that uses UV light to disinfect water is the CamelBak All Clear. This integrates the light-emitting source with a drinking bottle.

MOTION SICKNESS

Motion sickness (seasickness, or "mal de mer") is a common, annoying, and sometimes disabling problem for boaters and divers. Motion sickness is a complex phenomenon that involves the cerebellum (the part of the brain that controls, among other things, balance), vestibular system (labyrinth of the inner ear that plays a major role in the control of equilibrium), the nerve connections between the eyes and the inner ear, and the gastrointestinal tract. It is made worse by alcohol ingestion, emotional upset, noxious odors (e.g., boat exhaust fumes), and inner ear injury or infection. Most persons adapt to real motion after a few days, but may require treatment until they are adjusted to the environment.

Signs and symptoms of motion sickness include a sensation of dizziness or spinning, a sensation of falling, pale skin color, sweating, nausea, headache, drowsiness, weakness, yawning, and increased salivation. Vomiting may provide temporary relief, but prolonged salvation doesn't occur until the inner ear labyrinth acclimatizes to motion or you are able to intervene with an anti–motion-sickness device or medication. Persons who suffer from prolonged vomiting become dehydrated and exhausted.

To manage motion sickness:

1. Keep your eyes fixed on a steady point in the distance. If on board a ship, stay on deck. Splash your face with cold water. If the seas are rough, be careful to not slip or fall overboard. If you can have someone next to you who is not suffering, that is better than leaning over the rail by yourself to vomit when you're dizzy.
2. Use the ReliefBand device. This is advertised to relieve nausea and vomiting with gentle, noninvasive electrical stimulation on the underside of the wrist. It can be used before or after symptoms begin; carries no restrictions on food, beverages, or the use of medications; and has no drug-like side effects. The device looks like a wristwatch. The Adventurer

model contains a battery-powered electrical stimulator that's easily adjustable for five different stimulation levels. The device is positioned over the P6 acupuncture site (the Neiguan, or Nei Kuan, point on the pericardial meridian). This is located two fingerbreadths toward the heart from the wrist joint between the two prominent finger flexor tendons. When the device is turned on, a pulse is generated every 4 seconds and the user feels the episodic tingling sensation. It's theorized that the electrical signal transmitted via the median nerve in the wrist interrupts the nausea and vomiting messages that are transmitted between the brain and the stomach. The only side effect noted so far with the device is rare irritation where the electrodes make contact with the skin. This is easily managed by moving the device to the other wrist.

3. Some persons report that wearing a "sea band" is helpful. This is a knitted, elastic stretch band with a button(s) that applies pressure to an acupuncture point(s). This would not be expected to be nearly as effective as the ReliefBand device, but might help out in a pinch.

4. Ingest meclizine (Antivert, Bonine) 25 mg, cyclizine (Marezine) 50 mg, or dimenhydrinate (Dramamine) 50 mg orally every 4 to 6 hours, or cinnarizine (Stugeron) 15 mg every 8 hours as necessary to prevent and control motion sickness. These are adult doses. Children ages 2 to 12 years may be given dimenhydrinate 1 mg/kg (2.2 lb) body weight 1 hour before travel and then every 6 hours during the period of risk for motion sickness. An alternative drug is diphenhydramine (Benadryl) 0.5 mg/kg body weight, up to 25 mg. It's possible for children to have "paradoxical" hyperactivity instead of sedation with these medications. Therefore, a test dose should be given before travel. To be most effective, the first dose of medication should precede the environmental change by 1 hour. Medication given after the onset of seasickness will often be ineffective. Obviously, if you're vomiting so severely that you cannot keep any medication down, you may need to use a suppository, such as prochlorperazine (Compazine) 25 mg or promethazine (Phenergan) 25 mg, noting that these drugs won't cure the motion sickness—they might control vomiting, but have the side effect of drowsiness. Scopolamine 0.4 to 0.8 mg (1 or 2 tablets) taken 1 hour before anticipated seasickness and then every 8 hours is effective.

5. Place a transdermal scopolamine patch (Transderm Scōp 1.5 mg) on the skin behind the ear. This patch releases the drug slowly through the skin and can be very effective against motion sickness for up to 3 days. Side effects include drowsiness, blurred vision (sometimes with a dilated pupil in the eye on the side of the patch), decreased sweating, difficulty with urination (particularly in elderly males with enlarged prostate glands), dry mouth, and a propensity to be susceptible to heat illness during times of heat exposure. Persons with glaucoma should not use the patch. On a rare occasion, a person who uses a patch can become delirious or even psychotic as a side effect. Normal behavior returns within a few hours after the patch is removed.

   The patch should be positioned at least 3 hours before rough seas are encountered. If you touch the medicated (sticky) side of the patch with a finger and then let that finger come in contact with your eye, your pupil will almost certainly dilate and stay that way for up to 8 hours. *Be sure to wash your hands thoroughly with soap and water immediately after handling the patch, so that any drug that might get on your hands will not come in contact with your eyes.* Also, local absorption of the drug through the skin can dilate the pupil of the eye on the same side of the patch, causing difficulty with focusing of vision.

6. Reduce head movement. If you're on a large boat that is rocking bow to stern, seek the middle (equilibrium) of the vessel, so that motion is minimized. Look out from the boat and find a broad view of the horizon. Sit in the front seat of an automobile and bus, and prefer the seat adjacent to the wing of an airplane. Don't do close-focused visual tasks such as reading, writing, and navigation. If you're becoming motion sick and can't control your

symptoms, you might find some relief by lying face up in a well-secured and ventilated bunk. Close your eyes and try to sleep.

7. Some people recommend "keeping something in your stomach" during a bout of motion sickness. You can put something in there, but if you are truly sick, it won't stay there for long. Try to maintain your fluid intake with sips of something like an electrolyte-containing sports beverage (e.g., Gatorade or Gatorade G2). If you're known to suffer from motion sickness, take particular care to be well hydrated before your journey, because you will at a minimum have decreased appetite and fluid intake, and in the worst case, lose a fair bit of fluid by vomiting. While some persons recommend a light diet with predominantly carbohydrates, there is no evidence that any particular food or diet is beneficial. Don't consume alcoholic beverages, because these make you more prone to vertigo. Ginger (*Zingiber officinale*) is sometimes recommended to curb nausea. It is taken as 1000 mg (two 500 mg capsules) every 6 hours, supplemented by gingersnap cookies, ginger ale, and candied ginger. Another formulation is ginger extract 125 to 250 mg by mouth every 6 to 8 hours.

8. Headache, ringing in the ears, weakness in an arm or leg, difficulty with speech, difficulty swallowing, decreased vision, and palpitations are not features of motion sickness and should raise suspicion for another cause of dizziness. If any of these occur, especially if the seas are not particularly rough and no one else is suffering, the victim should seek medical attention. Similarly, if the symptoms occur after a dive, one must consider the possibility of central nervous system decompression sickness (bends) or arterial gas embolism.

9. Finally, don't try to cure serious motion sickness by putting on your dive gear and heading underwater. Mild nausea attributable to seasickness may disappear when you get under the surface (and the objectionable motion ceases), but if you are ready to vomit, you shouldn't put yourself and your companions in a situation in which you throw up underwater. It's not easy to vomit underwater and coordinate breathing through your regulator in order to avoid inhaling water or vomitus, and getting sick when you are in the water can lead to panic and a serious diving accident. Don't dive until you're feeling well.

JET LAG

Wilderness medicine and outdoor persons are commonly world travelers. Jet lag is a sleep disorder that results from crossing time zones too rapidly for the human biologic circadian "clock," which is synchronized to the sun's cycle of light and darkness, to keep pace. It has been estimated that the circadian clock resets an average of approximately 90 minutes later each day after a westward flight and approximately 60 minutes earlier each day after an eastward flight. Many people notice that it's more difficult from a jet lag perspective when traveling from west to east. Diet and exercise don't have any known effect on jet lag, but when optimized may make a person feel better and therefore be conducive to restful sleep.

Here are strategies recommended by sleep experts for managing jet lag:

1. Reset the circadian clock by using appropriately timed exposure to light. One shifts the clock to a later time by exposure to light in the evening, and shifts it to an earlier time by exposure to light in the morning. To keep it simple, when traveling eastward across up to eight time zones, one should seek exposure to bright light in the morning. When traveling westward across up to eight time zones, one should seek exposure to bright light in the evening. An additional recommendation is to stay indoors (e.g., avoid sunlight) for the first few hours of daylight after long eastward flights or for a few hours before dusk after long westward flights.

2. Take the hormone melatonin, which is normally secreted by the body for roughly 10 to 12 hours at night. It can be considered to be a darkness signal, with effects opposite those of exposure to light. Therefore, if melatonin is taken in the evening before it would normally be secreted, it resets the body clock to an earlier time, and when it is taken in the morning, it resets the clock to a later time. To promote shifting of the body clock to a later time (when you're traveling westward), take 0.5 mg (a short-acting dose) during the second half of the night until you have become adapted to local time. To promote shifting of the body clock to an earlier time (when you're traveling eastward), take 0.5 to 3 mg at local bedtime nightly until you have become adapted to local time.

Most people simply try to power through jet lag, but there is a science to it. To make a coordinated effort to minimize jet lag, here are additional recommendations, depending on whether a person is traveling westward or eastward:

For Traveling Westward
Before Travel
1. Shift the timing of sleep to 1 to 2 hours later for a few days before the trip; seek exposure to bright light in the evening.
2. Try to get an adequate amount of sleep.
3. Eat a healthful diet and get adequate rest.

In Flight
1. Try to be comfortable.
2. Drink plenty of water to stay hydrated. Don't drink caffeine if you wish to sleep. Don't mix alcohol with any sleep medication. Avoid alcohol in general.
3. Consider taking a short-acting sleep medication. Don't take sleep medication combined with alcohol, or if there is a risk for deep-vein thrombosis (blood clot formation in the legs or pelvis).
4. Take measures to avoid deep vein thrombosis (see page 269). These include staying well hydrated, wearing support stockings, changing positions frequently, and walking around when possible. Wear comfortable clothing and shoes.

On Arrival
1. Expect to have trouble sleeping until you become adjusted to local time.
2. If you are sleep deprived, it's OK to take a nap after arrival. Continue to take daytime naps if you're sleepy, particularly if you need to be alert for driving and technical activities, but keep the naps as brief as possible to avoid ruining bedtime sleep.
3. Consider using sleep medication at bedtime for a few nights until you're adjusted to local time.
4. Take melatonin as noted earlier.
5. Seek exposure to bright light in the evening.
6. For the first 2 days after arrival, avoid bright light for 2 to 3 hours before dusk. Starting on the third day, seek exposure to bright light in the evening.
7. If caffeine keeps you awake, then avoid it after mid-day because it may interfere with sleep at night.

For Traveling Eastward
Before Travel
1. Shift the timing of sleep to 1 to 2 hours earlier for a few days before the trip. Seek exposure to bright light in the evening.
2. Try to get an adequate amount of sleep.
3. Eat a healthful diet and get adequate rest.

In Flight

1. Try to be comfortable.
2. Drink plenty of water to stay hydrated. Don't drink caffeine if you wish to sleep. Don't mix alcohol with any sleep medication. Avoid alcohol in general.
3. Consider taking a short-acting sleep medication. Don't take sleep medication combined with alcohol, or if there is a risk for deep-vein thrombosis (blood clot formation in the legs or pelvis).
4. Take measures to avoid deep vein thrombosis (see page 269). These include staying well hydrated, wearing support stockings, changing positions frequently, and walking around when possible. Wear comfortable clothing and shoes.

On Arrival

1. Expect to have trouble sleeping until you become adjusted to local time.
2. If you're sleep deprived, it's OK to take a nap after arrival. Continue to take daytime naps if you are sleepy, particularly if you need to be alert for driving and technical activities, but keep the naps as brief as possible to avoid ruining bedtime sleep.
3. Consider using sleep medication at bedtime for a few nights until you're adjusted to local time.
4. Take melatonin as noted earlier.
5. Seek exposure to bright light in the morning.
6. For the first 2 days after arrival, avoid bright light for 2 to 3 hours after dawn. Starting on the third day, seek exposure to bright light in the morning.
7. If caffeine keeps you awake, avoid it after mid-day because it may interfere with sleep at bedtime.

FIRST-AID KITS

First-aid kits should be designed according to the environment to be encountered, number of travelers, medical training of the party leaders, and distance from advanced medical care. The following lists include items that could be included to deal effectively with the most common problems. They are not camping lists (shelter, food, toiletries, and the like). Basic survival supplies must be adequate. The more multipurpose your selections, the less the weight of your pack.

In all cases, what you should carry depends on your predetermined needs. Select the items that make sense for your group or expedition. As you review the sections of this book, you will be able to decide what to carry. For instance, a day hiker need not carry a portable traction splint, but a rock climber on a lengthy expedition should consider bringing one along. A scuba diver in Australia should carry a bottle of vinegar to pour on a box jellyfish sting. Carry a realistic quantity of supplies; you should be prepared to treat more than one person at a time. Specific medications to choose from are described in Appendix 1 and throughout the book. Remember to bring along pediatric doses (in liquid form, if necessary) when traveling with children.

First-aid supplies should be packed to be readily accessible, and marked clearly to allow rapid identification. *Before the trip, show all members of the expedition where the medical supplies are stored and explain how they are to be used.*

The supplies must be carried in a container(s) that can withstand physical abuse, extremes of temperature, and exposure to water. Conterra offers many options for medical carry packs and backpacks. On boating, rafting, or diving adventures, carry medical supplies in a plastic (a Pelican Case or OtterBox, for example) or metal container equipped with a rubber O-ring gasket for a tight, waterproof seal, or store the supplies in a "dry bag." Use Ziploc-type bags within the kit for extra material and to sort your supplies. For instance, it's helpful to partition supplies into modules "for wound care," "for an allergic reaction," and so forth.

Carry a small notepad and waterproof writing instrument. A preprinted first-aid report form, designed for use on mountain or backcountry expeditions, is a convenient way to record a victim's medical condition and treatment, while serving as a good checklist for proper evaluation. Space is usually provided for a written rescue request to be carried by a messenger in an emergency.

An excellent selection of first-aid kits is available in stores or by mail order from companies like Chinook Medical Gear, Inc. (www.chinookmed.com).

BASIC SUPPLIES

Brand names are shown to indicate representative products, not to indicate that these are the best or only products that may be used. Quality, availability, cost, and preference will influence which specific products you choose. Before you embark on an outdoor expedition, go through the relevant sections of this book and this list carefully and make a decision to include or exclude these items from your medical kit.

GENERAL SUPPLIES

- Medical guidebook
- First-aid report form
- Hand sanitizer
- Duct tape
- Pencil or pen with small notepad
- Steel sewing needle
- Paper clip
- Safety pins
- Needle-nose pliers with wire cutter
- Sharp folding knife
- Disposable scalpels (#11 and/or #12 blades)
- Paramedic or emergency medical technician (EMT) or trauma shears (scissors)
- Swiss Army knife or Leatherman-type tool
- Seam ripper
- Sharp-pointed surgical scissors
- Bandage scissors
- Splinter (sharp tip) forceps (tweezers)
- Standard oral thermometer: digital, mercury, or alcohol
- Low-reading hypothermia thermometer
- Wooden tongue depressors ("tongue blades")
- Rolled duct tape (3 inches × 1 yd, or 91 cm)
- $\frac{1}{8}$ to $\frac{1}{4}$ inch diameter braided nylon cord (minimum 10 ft, or 3 m)
- Water bottle (such as Nalgene $\frac{1}{2}$ to 1 liter)
- Blue "baby bulb" or "turkey baster" suction device
- Waterproof flashlight (such as Pelican MityLite)
- Headlamp (and spare batteries), preferably with floodlight and flash settings, and able to withstand moisture and temperature extremes
- Cyalume fluorescent light sticks
- Cardiopulmonary resuscitation (CPR) mouth barrier or pocket face mask (such as a Microshield X-L Mouth Barrier or NuMask CPR Kit)
- Sterile and nonsterile nitrile surgical gloves; because some people are allergic to latex, do not carry only latex gloves

- Signal mirror
- Magnifier
- Eyeglasses for protection and to allow close-up inspection; bring spares
- Ziplock plastic bags, assorted sizes
- Waterproof pill containers for distributing medication
- Waterproof matches
- Fine-mesh head net, mosquito bed net (insecticide-treated or untreated), or travel tent to repel insects
- Quick-dry travel towel
- Oral rehydration salts (ORS) or CeraLyte 70 oral electrolyte powder
- Rubber cement
- Urine pregnancy test
- Condoms
- Nonlatex (e.g., nitrile) surgical gloves
- Blood glucose (sugar) testing kit and supplies
- Mobile telephone with solar charger (adequate for the task)
- Whistle
- Superglue

WOUND CARE: PREPARATIONS AND DRESSINGS

- Elastic bandages (Band-Aid or Coverlet), assorted sizes (strip, knuckle, and broad); cloth with adhesive is preferable
- Band-Aid Liquid Bandage
- Butterfly bandages
- Adhesive strips for wound closure (Steri-Strip or Cover-Strip II), assorted sizes (such as $\frac{1}{4}$ inch × 4 inches, $\frac{1}{8}$ inch × 3 inches, $\frac{1}{2}$ inch × 4 inches), reinforced (plain or impregnated with an antimicrobial) or elastic
- Blood stopper bandage
- Hemostatic gauze
- 3 inch × 3 inch or 4 inch × 4 inch sterile gauze pads (packets of two to five) (such as Nu-Gauze highly absorbent)
- 5 inch × 9 inch or 8 inch × 10 inch sterile gauze ("trauma") pads (packets of two to five)
- 2 inch and 4 inch Army Battle Dressing (ABD) pads
- Nonstick sterile bandages (Telfa), assorted sizes
- 1 inch, 2 inch, 3 inch, and 4 inch rolled conforming gauze (C-wrap or Elastomull)
- 1 inch × 10 yd (9.1 m) rolled cloth adhesive tape
- 1 inch × 10 yd (9.1 m) rolled paper or silk (hypoallergenic) adhesive tape
- 1 inch × 10 yd (9.1 m) rolled waterproof adhesive tape
- $\frac{1}{2}$ inch × 10 yd (9.1 m) rolled waterproof adhesive tape
- Blist-O-Ban blister bandages (assorted sizes)
- Molefoam ($4\frac{1}{8}$ inches × $3\frac{3}{8}$ inches)
- Moleskin Plus ($4\frac{1}{8}$ inches × $3\frac{3}{8}$ inches)
- Spenco 2nd Skin (1.5 inch × 2 inches, 3 inches × 4 inches, 3 inches × 6.5 inches) and Spenco Adhesive Knit Bandage (3 inches × 5 inches)
- Aquaphor moist nonadherent (petrolatum-impregnated) dressing (3 inches × 3 inches)
- Hydrogel occlusive absorbent dressing (4 inches × 4 inches × $\frac{1}{4}$ inch)
- Tegaderm transparent wound dressing (also comes in combination with a Steri-Strip in a Wound Closure System)
- Liquid soap
- Sterile disposable surgical scrub brush

- Cotton-tipped swabs or applicators, sterile, two per package
- Safety razor
- Syringe (10 to 60 mL) and 18-gauge intravenous catheter (plastic portion) for wound irrigation. Don't use plastic disposable syringes to administer oral medications, because the small caps can dislodge and inadvertently eject into the patient's throat.
- Zerowet Splashield or Supershield (two)
- Tincture of benzoin, bottle or swabsticks
- Mastisol Liquid Adhesive
- Benzalkonium chloride 1:750 solution (Zephiran)
- Povidone-iodine 10% solution (Betadine), 1 oz bottle or swabsticks
- Suture material (nonabsorbable monofilament nylon on curved needle, suture sizes #3-0 and #4-0; consider sizes #2-0 (thicker) and #5-0 (finer)
- Stainless-steel needle driver
- Disposable skin stapler (15 staples)
- Disposable staple remover
- Tissue glue, such as DERMABOND ADVANCED Topical Skin Adhesive

SPLINTING AND SLING MATERIAL

- Cravat cloth (triangular bandage)
- 2 inch, 3 inch, and 4 inch elastic wrap (ACE)
- $4\frac{1}{4}$ inch × 36 inch SAM Splints (two)—consider other sizes
- Aluminum finger splints
- Kendrick femur traction device

EYE MEDICATIONS AND DRESSINGS

- Prepackaged individual sterile oval eye pads
- Prepackaged eye bandages (Coverlet Eye Occlusor)
- Metal or plastic (rigid) eye shield
- Sterile eyewash, 1 oz (30 mL)
- Contact lens remover (or mini-marshmallows)
- Ofloxacin, moxifloxacin, or gatifloxacin eye drops
- Oxymetazoline hydrochloride 0.025% eye drops

DENTAL SUPPLIES

- Oil of cloves (eugenol), 3.5 mL
- Cavit, 7 g tube
- Intermediate Restorative Material (IRM)
- Express Putty
- TempBond NE unidose packets
- Zinc oxide powder
- Dental floss
- Mouth mirror
- Paraffin (dental wax) stick
- Wooden spatulas
- Cotton (rolls and pellets)
- Dry tea bags

TOPICAL SKIN PREPARATIONS

- Hydrocortisone cream, ointment, or lotion (0.5% to 1%)
- Potent corticosteroid ointment

- Bacitracin ointment
- Mupirocin ointment
- Mupirocin calcium 2% cream
- Bacitracin-neomycin polymyxin B sulfate ointment
- Miconazole nitrate 2% antifungal cream
- Silver sulfadiazine 1% (Silvadene) cream
- Insect repellent
- Sunscreen lotion or cream
- Lip balm or sunscreen
- Sunblock
- Adolph's meat tenderizer (unseasoned)
- Kenalog in Orabase (oral adhesive steroid for canker [mouth] sores), 5 g container
- Aloe vera gel
- Hemorrhoidal ointment with pramoxine 1%

NONPRESCRIPTION MEDICATIONS

- Buffered aspirin, 325 mg tablets
- Ibuprofen, 200 mg tablets
- Acetaminophen, 325 mg tablets
- Antacid
- Decongestant (such as pseudoephedrine) tablets
- Decongestant (such as oxymetazoline) nasal spray
- Loperamide (Imodium A-D), 2 mg caplets
- Glutose (liquid glucose) paste tube
- Stool softener (such as docusate calcium, 240 mg gel caps)
- Polyethylene glycol powder (MiraLAX) to promote bowel movement
- Caffeine, 200 mg tablets (to stay awake for survival purposes, such as during a rescue). The average cup of coffee contains 135 mg of caffeine; a 12-oz can of soda contains approximately 50 mg of caffeine. There are caffeine-laden food products, such as JAVA Mallows, FOOSH Energy Mints, and Turbo Truffles.

PRESCRIPTION MEDICATIONS (SELECT FROM THIS LIST, AND FROM INFORMATION THROUGHOUT THIS BOOK, WHAT YOU FEEL YOU MIGHT NEED; THE DRUGS LISTED ARE "FOR EXAMPLE")

- Pain medication(s): e.g., hydrocodone 5 mg with acetaminophen 500 mg
- Asthma medication(s): e.g., metered-dose bronchodilator (albuterol)
- Allergy medication(s): e.g., epinephrine (injectable) and prednisone, 10 mg tablets
- Antibiotics: e.g.,
  - Penicillin V potassium, 250 mg tablets
  - Azithromycin, 250 mg tablets
  - Dicloxacillin, 250 mg tablets
  - Ampicillin, 250 mg tablets
  - Amoxicillin–clavulanate, 500 mg tablets
  - Erythromycin, 250 mg tablets
  - Cephalexin, 250 mg tablets
  - Ciprofloxacin, 500 mg tablets
  - Tetracycline, 500 mg tablets; or doxycycline, 100 mg tablets
  - Trimethoprim–sulfamethoxazole, double-strength tablets

- Antinausea medication(s): e.g.,
  - Prochlorperazine (Compazine) suppositories, 25 mg
  - Promethazine (Phenergan) suppositories, 25 mg
  - Ondansetron (Zofran ODT) oral disintegrating tablet, 4 or 8 mg

ALLERGY KIT

- Allergy kit with injectable epinephrine (EpiPen autoinjector [0.3 mg] and EpiPen Jr. autoinjector [0.15 mg]; the Auvi-Q "talking" autoinjector (0.3 or 0.15 mg dose), or Adrenaclick 0.3 or 0.15 mg autoinjector). Other devices worldwide are the Jext, Emerade, Allerject, and Anapen.
- Diphenhydramine, 25 mg capsules

FOREST AND MOUNTAIN ENVIRONMENTS

- Water disinfection equipment (filter; ultraviolet light) or chemicals (such as Potable Aqua tablets or iodine crystals)
- Calamine lotion
- SPACE Emergency Blanket (2 oz, 56 inches × 84 inches) (alternatives include Pro-Tech Extreme bag or vest, SPACE brand emergency bag, SPACE brand all-weather blanket)
- Hypothermia thermometer
- Hyperthermia thermometer
- Pulse oximeter
- Acetazolamide (Diamox), 250 mg tablets
- Dexamethasone (Decadron), 4 mg tablets
- Nifedipine (Adalat CC), extended-release 30 preparation
- Powdered electrolyte beverage mix (Oral Rehydration Salts)
- Instant chemical cold pack(s)
- Hand warmer (mechanical or chemical)
- Kendrick Traction Device (leg splint)

AQUATIC ENVIRONMENTS

- Waterproof dry bag or hard case (such as Pelican or Storm), to carry first-aid supplies
- Anti–motion sickness medicine
- Acetic acid (vinegar) 5%
- Isopropyl alcohol 40%
- Lidocaine-based jellyfish sting spray
- Hydrogen peroxide
- VōSoL otic solution
- Ofloxacin 0.3% ear drops
- Safe Sea Sunblock with Jellyfish Sting Protective Lotion

IMMUNIZATIONS

Because the spectrum of infectious diseases changes with time and location, travelers to or between foreign countries should be aware of the necessity for immunizations (also known as vaccinations). The Centers for Disease Control and Prevention (CDC) has a comprehensive traveler's health website at www.cdc.gov/travel. A detailed, updated list of required immunizations by country can be obtained in the publication *Health Information for International Travel* (CDC), also known as the "Yellow Book." A link to this publication is found at the CDC traveler's health website noted previously. The Advisory Committee on Immunization Practices (www.cdc.gov/vaccines/acip) annually reviews the recommended Adult Immunization Schedule to ensure that the schedule reflects current recommendations for licensed vaccines. Recommended adult and pediatric routine immunization schedules, by vaccine and age group, are also published by the CDC and updated regularly. The relevant website is www.cdc.gov/vaccines.

Vaccinations may be given under the supervision of any licensed physician. All travelers should carry a completed International Certificate of Vaccination with proper signature and validation for all vaccinations administered. Yellow fever and cholera vaccinations must be officially recorded and stamped. Failure to secure validation at an authorized city, county, or state health department renders the certificate invalid, and may force you to be revaccinated or quarantined.

It's extremely important to plan immunizations as far in advance of an expedition as possible, since some vaccines interact in ways that diminish effectiveness. For instance, yellow fever and cholera vaccines need to be given either on the same day or at least 3 weeks apart. Vaccine recommendations may be altered on a vaccine-by-vaccine basis for persons with medical conditions, such as pregnancy, immunocompromise, human immunodeficiency virus (HIV) infection (sometimes according to CD4$^+$ T lymphocyte count), diabetes, heart disease, chronic lung disease, chronic alcoholism, lack of a spleen, chronic liver disease, kidney failure, end-stage kidney disease, and need for hemodialysis. For instance, varicella (chickenpox) vaccine is not recommended during pregnancy, or for persons who are immunocompromised or who have HIV infection with CD4$^+$ T lymphocyte count less than 200 cells/microliter.

TETANUS

Everyone should be properly immunized against tetanus, which is caused by the bacterium *Clostridium tetani*. In the United States, diphtheria-tetanus-acellular pertussis (DTaP) vaccine is given as an intramuscular injection at ages 2, 4, 6, and 15 to 18 months, followed by a booster at age 4 to 6 years, usually before entry into school. These shots provide immunity from tetanus, as well as from diphtheria and pertussis (whooping cough), for about 10 years. The first booster shot is usually given at age 11 or 12 years in the form of Tdap vaccine. It should be given before the age of 18 years. Any adult 19 years through 64 years of age who has not received a dose of Tdap should get one as soon as is practical. For all adults, at a minimum, after the primary immunization series, one Td booster should be replaced by the Tdap vaccine in order to maintain immunity against pertussis ("whooping cough"). Thereafter, Td (tetanus and diphtheria) vaccine is recommended at 10-year intervals, although there is no reason why Tdap vaccine cannot be used (it may cause a greater local skin reaction). Following immunization against tetanus, immunity in any individual is unknown, and can be determined by measuring antibodies in blood. This is particularly important in elders, in whom the immune response to vaccination may be suppressed by a general lower level of the immune system associated with age. Ideally, women should receive the Tdap vaccine before becoming pregnant. However, if that has not occurred, pregnant women should receive the Tdap booster, preferably after 20 weeks of gestation, to protect infants from pertussis by transfer of protective maternal antibodies.

Here are the vaccines that are licensed as of this writing for different age groups:
1. DTaP (diphtheria, tetanus, pertussis): Daptacel (Sanofi Pasteur) ages 6 weeks to 7 years; Tripedia (Sanofi Pasteur) ages 6 weeks to 7 years; Infanrix (GlaxoSmithKline) ages 6 weeks to 7 years; Pediarix (GlaxoSmithKline) ages 6 weeks to 7 years
2. Tdap (tetanus, diphtheria, pertussis): Adacel (Sanofi Pasteur) ages 11 to 64 years; Boostrix (GlaxoSmithKline) ages 10 to 18 years
3. Td (tetanus, diphtheria): Td (Sanofi Pasteur) ages 7 years and older
4. One obvious question is, "Which vaccine should be used for children between ages 7 years and 10 years?" It's probably best to use the DTaP vaccine for this age group, even though

no vaccine is licensed for this age group, and either Tdap or DTaP would likely induce the proper immunities.

The current practice is to take a booster shot (Td) if one sustains a "dirty" wound, deep puncture, serious burn, significant crush injury, or similar injury and has not had a tetanus shot in the preceding 5 years. If a wound is believed to be at particularly high risk for infection with *C. tetani* (e.g., if it is a very deep puncture or contaminated by soil or animal feces), it may also be recommended to have an injection of tetanus immune globulin, as well as a tetanus booster immunization. Whether or not to administer tetanus immune globulin is generally a judgment call by the treating health care professional. The immune globulin contains actual antibodies against the bacteria, so that the recipient carries protective antibodies against the bacteria until his or her body has a chance to manufacture its own antibodies in response to the Td booster shot.

Any traveler who will be away from medical care for more than 48 hours should have adequate tetanus immunization. The recommendations are as follows:

1. A person previously immunized should receive a booster dose of tetanus toxoid if his last dose was not administered within the past 10 years. A dose of Tdap vaccine (tetanus, diphtheria, and pertussis) may be administered if pertussis is a concern. Diphtheria immunization is usually boosted simultaneously. If there is a good chance that the traveler will suffer an injury during the trip, he should take a booster if the last dose was not administered within the past 5 years.

2. Nonimmunized individuals should become immunized with a series of three injections (this requires 3 to 6 months).

Low-risk (for tetanus infection) wounds are those that are recent (less than 6 hours old), simple (linear), superficial (less than $\frac{1}{2}$ in [1.3 cm] deep), cut with a sharp edge (knife or glass), without signs of infection, and free of contamination with dirt, soil, or body secretions. High-risk wounds are those that are old (greater than 6 hours), crushed or gouged, deep (greater than $\frac{1}{2}$ in deep), burns, frostbite, with signs of infection, and contaminated. If someone suffers a wound, here are standard recommendations:

Victim	Low-Risk Wound (Not Heavily Contaminated)	Contaminated Wound (Tetanus-prone)
Never Immunized	*Tetanus toxoid*	*Tetanus toxoid*
	Tetanus immune globulin	*Tetanus immune globulin*
Immunized		
Last booster within 5 yr	*No shot*	*No shot*
Last booster within 10 yr	*No shot*	*Tetanus toxoid*
		Tetanus immune globulin
Last booster over 10 yr	*Tetanus toxoid*	*Tetanus toxoid*
		Tetanus immune globulin

POLIOVIRUS; DIPHTHERIA; PERTUSSIS (WHOOPING COUGH); MEASLES, MUMPS, RUBELLA (GERMAN MEASLES); CHICKENPOX; *HAEMOPHILUS* B; ROTAVIRUS

Immunization against poliomyelitis, diphtheria, pertussis, measles, mumps, and rubella should be obtained before travel. In the United States, these are routinely administered during childhood. Because of the incidence of these infectious diseases in developing countries, such immunizations are mandatory before travel. Immunizations against *Haemophilus* type b (which causes middle ear infections and meningitis) and the varicella virus (which causes chickenpox) are available, and should be considered under recommendation from your physician. The varicella vaccine is recommended by many medical professionals because chickenpox can be fatal to people of any age because of its complications, which include pneumonia and inflammation of the brain. Measles vaccine should be given to any person born in 1957 or later who has not received a prior booster dose. Mumps (a viral infection) is making a comeback in the United States and other countries because of failure to vaccinate. It is not a trivial disease, particularly in adults, and is highly communicable. In children, mumps typically causes fever, headache, muscle aching, fatigue, loss of appetite, and swelling of salivary glands, in particular the parotid glands, which are located in the cheeks directly in front of the ears. In adults, complications of mumps may include inflammation of brain, meningitis, swollen and painful inflamed testicles, ovarian or breast inflammation, miscarriage, and deafness. At the time of this writing, the two combination vaccines licensed and available in the United States to prevent these diseases are trivalent MMR (measles-mumps-rubella) vaccine and quadrivalent MMRV (measles-mumps-rubella-varicella) vaccine.

Polio is still present in developing nations (e.g., sub-Saharan Africa, India, Nepal, Indonesia, Pakistan). Unimmunized adults (older than 18 years of age) should receive a series of three injections of the inactivated (virus) Salk vaccine, not the oral (Sabin) vaccine, which is recommended for children. Persons under age 18 years who have never been immunized should receive three doses of oral polio vaccine 1 month apart. People who travel to high-risk areas (e.g., outside the Western Hemisphere) who were immunized as children should receive one booster dose of oral polio vaccine or an injection of e-IPV polio vaccine.

Two adolescent/adult formulations of pertussis vaccine are combined with diphtheria and tetanus toxoids (Tdap): Boostrix (approved for ages 10 to 18 years) and Adacel (approved for ages 11 to 64 years). One of these should be given instead of standard tetanus-diphtheria vaccine if pertussis is a concern (see page 157).

RotaTeq is an oral vaccine given in a three-dose series recommended for infants to prevent the gastrointestinal illness caused by rotavirus. Rotarix is given in two doses. It is advised that children who have had an episode of intussusception not receive these vaccines.

SMALLPOX

The last reported case of endemic smallpox (caused by the *Variola* virus) was in Somalia in 1977. Therefore, smallpox immunization is no longer required for international travel, and the vaccine is not commercially available. However, there is a chance that isolated cases still occur (without reporting) in India, the Himalayas, and equatorial Africa. Travelers to these areas should inquire about the latest recommendations from the CDC in Atlanta.

Because smallpox has been suggested as an agent of bioterrorism, a brief description of infection for the purpose of recognition follows. The virus enters a human through the respiratory tract. It incubates and multiplies for 7 to 17 days, after which the victim abruptly develops severe headache, backache, and fever. The mouth, tongue, and throat may show lesions before the onset of the rash on the skin, which begins as small red spots and bumps that become blisters over a few days. Usually, the rash appears first on the face and limbs, and then appears on the torso. The blisters may appear pus-filled with depressed centers and take a week to dry and form a crust. As opposed to chickenpox, in which the skin lesions are in various stages of development, all the lesions of smallpox are in the same stage of development. With chickenpox, the fever accompanies the onset of the rash, and the rash is more concentrated on the torso rather than the limbs.

Smallpox vaccine can be effective if administered before exposure or early enough in the incubation period.

Monkeypox, which along with smallpox is an "orthopox," is endemic to forested areas of western and central Africa, but does not as yet pose a significant public health risk; there is no vaccine against the causative agent. It has been reported to be present in southern Sudan.

CHOLERA

Cholera is an intestinal infection caused by two serogroups (O1 or O139) of the microorganism *Vibrio cholerae*, either of which induces painful diarrhea and extreme fluid losses through the gastrointestinal tract. Cholera can reach epidemic proportions. It's estimated that 4 out of every 100 persons who acquire the illness die. A person whose stomach contains normal gastric acid is not at much risk for acquiring cholera. No country currently requires immunization, and the CDC does not recommend cholera vaccination for travel. No cholera vaccine is currently available in the United States. The vaccine products Dukoral and Shanchol are available outside the United States. Some localities require proof of cholera immunization for travelers entering from a territory that still reports the disease. For this purpose, documentation of a single dose of oral vaccine generally is sufficient.

YELLOW FEVER

Yellow fever is acquired in tropical (sub-Saharan) Africa and tropical South America, where victims may suffer the bite of the *Aedes aegypti* mosquito (urban environment) or other mosquitoes (jungle environment). Immunization is effective in preventing the disease; a single 0.5 mL subcutaneous injection of 17-D-204 strain YF-VAX (Aventis) is administered, and immunity is acquired after a 10-day waiting period. The vaccine promotes immunity for 10 years, after which time a booster is recommended for many categories of individuals to maintain immunity. Check current recommendations regarding the duration of immunity and for whom booster doses are recommended. Infants younger than 9 months and pregnant women should not be routinely immunized, unless they are at high risk for contracting the disease. It is also contraindicated in people with immunosuppression (such as HIV infection) or with an allergy to eggs. Yellow fever vaccinations must be given at an officially designated Yellow Fever Vaccination Center, and the certificate validated at the same center. The vaccine is not required for travel from the United States into Canada, Mexico, Europe, or Caribbean countries, but should be considered for travel into the province of Darien in Panama. An exemption (from vaccination) letter from a doctor acceptable to the customs officials of a destination country may allow a person to skip the immunization requirement. The CDC travel Internet site should be consulted for the latest information on recommendations. To be maximally effective, cholera and yellow fever vaccines should be administered either at the same time or at least 3 weeks apart. A rare side effect of yellow fever vaccination is a severe reaction with symptoms similar to those of yellow fever. This may occur in 1 in 50,000 elderly (older than 65 years) recipients.

The current yellow fever vaccine is a live attenuated virus vaccine. An inactivated cell-culture vaccine is being developed and appears to be a safer alternative.

MENINGOCOCCUS

The meningococcus is a bacterium *(Neisseria meningitidis)* that can cause meningitis, particularly in children and young adults. Vaccination against meningococcal disease is not a requirement for travel to any country except Saudi Arabia, where travelers to Mecca during the annual Hajj and Umrah pilgrimage must have proof of vaccination. It's a wise idea for travelers to Nepal—particularly hikers and backpackers—to be immunized. Certain areas of sub-Saharan Africa are also considered high risk from December to June. Menactra and Menveo, tetravalent meningococcal polysaccharide-protein conjugate vaccines (MenACWY), provide protection against serogroups A, C, Y, and W-135 of the bacteria, and are given in one subcutaneous injection; protection for 5 years is achieved 1 to 2 weeks after administration. Menveo is approved for persons ages 2 months to 55 years; Menactra is approved for persons ages 9 months to 55 years. MenACWY is now recommended for children aged 11 to 12 years in the United States at their regular health care visit, and a booster dose at age 16 years—certainly before entry into college. The vaccine previously recommended by the CDC is Menomune, a tetravalent meningococcal polysaccharide vaccine (MPSV4) that's still available and is believed to be somewhat less effective. It is recommended for persons older than 55 years, or at any age if MenACWY is not available. If someone has not been immunized and comes in close contact with a person known to have meningococcal disease, oral antibiotics can be prescribed within 14 days of exposure for 2 days to prevent or minimize the spread of the disease. The recommended antibiotics are oral rifampin for children (dose for age less than 1 month is 5 mg/kg of body weight every 12 hours; age 1 month or older is 10 mg/kg of body weight every 12 hours) and adults (600 mg every 12 hours) or ciprofloxacin (500 mg once a day) for adults. An alternative is for a health care provider to administer a one-time intramuscular injection of ceftriaxone for children (dose 125 mg if age 15 years or younger; 250 mg otherwise) and adults (250 mg). Azithromycin in a single 500 mg dose for adults is also likely effective.

HERPES ZOSTER

Zostavax is a vaccine to reduce the risk for herpes zoster ("shingles") in adults ages 60 years and older. It is given in a dose of 0.65 mL one time subcutaneously. Because it contains live attenuated virus, it should not be given to anyone who is immunosuppressed for any reason. It appears to be quite effective in preventing shingles in persons who have never before suffered from this condition.

HUMAN PAPILLOMAVIRUS

Either of a bivalent or quadrivalent vaccine is approved to prevent infection with human papillomavirus in females ages 11 to 26 years. The vaccine is administered in three doses at 0, 2, and 6 months, intended to prevent infection that might lead to later development of cervical cancer. Males ages 11 to 21 years should also receive routine vaccination with the quadrivalent vaccine.

HEPATITIS

A recombinant DNA vaccine (Recombivax, not derived from human plasma) for immunization against viral hepatitis type B is recommended for travelers to underdeveloped countries. A series of three injections requires 6 months to complete. Another recombinant vaccine is Engerix-B, which can be given on an accelerated schedule over 2 months. If a person has not been immunized against hepatitis type B and is exposed to the virus (e.g., by a needlestick), he may require an injection of hepatitis B immune globulin to provide short-term protection until immunity can be acquired from the vaccine. Hepatitis B vaccination is now recommended routinely for adults with diabetes who are younger than age 60 years. Persons with diabetes who are age 60 years or older may be vaccinated at their physician's discretion.

Hepatitis A virus is spread through contamination of water and food and is often encountered in developing nations and areas of poor hygiene. Hepatitis A vaccine (Vaqta), inactivated, is available. It is administered intramuscularly to persons age 2 years or older at least 2 weeks before exposure to hepatitis A virus. The dose is 0.5 mL (25 units) up to age of 18 years, and 1 mL (50 units) in people older than 18 years. It is given in a series of two injections. Havrix is a similar vaccine. Twinrix is a combination vaccine (hepatitis A and B) given to persons age 18 years and older in a 1 mL dose in a three-injection series at 0, 1, and 6 months. In an alternative dosing regimen, it can be given at day 0, day 7, a day chosen between days 21 to 28, and at 1 year (booster).

Pooled immune serum globulin (ISG, or γ-globulin) can be administered to prevent or diminish the effects of viral hepatitis type A in unimmunized people. Administration of ISG interferes with the antibody response stimulated by other live-virus vaccines, so it should be administered 2 to 4 weeks after any other vaccines. Because the effects of ISG disappear after 6 months, it should be administered just before the trip, and at appropriate booster intervals during prolonged travel in endemic areas. It should be administered in the event that someone has been given his or her first dose of hepatitis A vaccine, but a period of less than 2 weeks has elapsed after injection and before risky travel.

BUBONIC PLAGUE

A preexposure vaccine is available for immunization against bubonic plague caused by *Yersinia pestis*. This is administered only to people whose travels or occupations place them at high risk. In most countries where plague is reported, the risk is greatest in rural mountain or upland regions. Vaccination is generally considered for those who will reside in regions where plague is endemic, and where avoidance of rodents and fleas is impossible. The vaccine is injected in two doses 1 month apart, followed by a booster dose after 6 months.

RABIES

Preexposure and postexposure rabies vaccinations are discussed on page 369.

MALARIA

Malaria is discussed on page 137.

TYPHOID FEVER

Typhim Vi polysaccharide vaccine is available for immunization against typhoid fever caused by *Salmonella typhi*. Immunization is recommended for travelers who visit countries (e.g., Cambodia, Nepal, South Africa, Indonesia, and many others) known to harbor the disease, and for persons with adventurous dietary habits. A single intramuscular injection is required, followed by booster injection at 2-year intervals, depending on the local disease risk. An oral vaccine (Vivotif Typhoid Vaccine Live Oral Ty21a, Berna Products) is given as one capsule every other day for four doses in people age 6 years or older. A booster series is necessary every 5 years. The oral vaccine regimen should be completed at least 7 days before travel. Capsules, which should be kept refrigerated, should be swallowed (not chewed) with cool or lukewarm water on an empty stomach and without concomitant alcohol within 2 hours of ingestion. Side effects, which include fever, headache, and flu-like symptoms, are more commonly associated with the injections. Gastroenteric symptoms may be associated with the oral vaccine.

TYPHUS FEVER

Typhus vaccine is no longer available in the United States and is not recommended for the foreign traveler.

INFLUENZA

There are three types of influenza virus—A, B, and C—of which the first two cause annual human epidemics. Proteins on the surface of the virus, namely hemagglutinin (H) and neuraminidase (N), may vary because of genetic mutations. At any time, a new strain can arise that can be transmitted from animals (e.g., birds or pigs) to humans, and then between humans. Each year, the manufacturers of influenza vaccine try to create a vaccine that will most effectively provide protection against influenza A strains H3N2 and H1N1 and the influenza B strains most likely to be prevalent during the upcoming flu season.

Influenza vaccine is optimally administered in one or two injections (see later) to children and adults in October and November (in the Northern Hemisphere) before the flu season (December through March), with a maximum duration of effect of 6 months. It is approved for use in persons ages 6 months and older. Persons 3 years of age or older should receive a single intramuscular injection of 0.5 mL. Children 6 to 35 months of age should receive only 0.25 mL.

Children younger than 9 years of age who have never been immunized should receive two doses spaced at least 4 weeks apart.

Vaccination of high-risk people (older than 65 years or with chronic illness) before flu season is essential. Persons for whom annual vaccination is especially recommended include the following:

- All persons (ages 6 months and older) who wish to reduce the risk of becoming ill with influenza or transmitting the disease to others
- Children ages 6 months to 4 years
- All persons ages 50 years or greater
- Children and adolescents ages 6 months to 18 years receiving long-term aspirin therapy who might be at risk for experiencing Reye syndrome
- Women who will be pregnant during influenza season
- Adults and children who have immunosuppression caused by medications or HIV
- Adults and children who have chronic pulmonary (including asthma), cardiovascular (except hypertension), kidney, liver, blood, or metabolic (including diabetes) disorders
- Adults and children with any condition that might compromise respiratory function
- Health care personnel

Each year, the vaccine contains the influenza virus strains that are believed to be most prevalent in the United States. Adults should continue to receive influenza vaccination, even if they are allergic to eggs. However, adults with egg allergy should receive inactivated (killed-virus) influenza vaccine, because safety data are available for this vaccination in this population. "Whole" vaccines should not be given to children under 13 years of age. Children should be given "split" vaccines, which have been chemically treated to reduce adverse reactions. An intradermal influenza vaccine, administered with a microinjector apparatus and ultrafine needle, is an option for adults ages 18 through 64 years.

Flublok is a trivalent influenza vaccine that is made using an insect virus expression system and is approved for use in persons ages 18 to 49 years. It does not use influenza virus or eggs in the production process. Flucelvax is a vaccine produced using cultured animal cells, instead of fertilized chicken eggs. It is approved for persons ages 18 years and older. Newer influenza vaccines may become "quadrivalent" if they contain activity against more than one influenza B strain.

A live, attenuated nasal spray vaccine (FluMist) is at least as effective as injected vaccine, and is approved for persons ages 2 to 49 years who are free of chronic illnesses. It is administered as a spray of 0.25 mL into each nostril (0.5 mL total dose). Children ages 2 to 8 years old who have not been previously immunized should receive two doses spaced at least 6 weeks apart. FluMist should not be administered to family members or close contacts of immunosuppressed persons requiring a protected environment.

Amantadine hydrochloride (Symmetrel) and rimantadine are prescription oral drugs that interfere with viral uncoating within living cells and are moderately effective in preventing influenza A. However, because they confer no protection against influenza B, they aren't considered substitutes for appropriate immunization. They are no longer routinely used in the United States because of influenza virus drug resistance to these drugs.

Oseltamivir phosphate (Tamiflu) is an antiflu pill given in a dose of 75 mg twice a day for adults. Zanamivir (Relenza) is a similar drug administered in a dose of two inhalations twice daily. These drugs (see page 191) interfere with the release of newly formed influenza virus from host cells and can be used to both prevent and treat influenza A and B. According to the CDC, persons at high risk for a severe case of influenza, and who would presumably benefit to a significant degree by taking oseltamivir or zanamivir, are:

1. Children younger than 2 years of age
2. Adults 65 years of age or older
3. Persons with chronic lung, heart, kidney, liver, blood, endocrine, or neurologic diseases

4. Immunosuppressed persons
5. Women who are pregnant or within 2 weeks after childbirth
6. Persons younger than 19 years of age who are taking long-term aspirin therapy
7. American Indians and Alaska Natives
8. Morbidly obese persons
9. Residents of nursing homes and other long-term care facilities

It should be noted that some experts have called into question the true benefit of treating influenza with oseltamivir or zanamivir, doubting whether the minimal reduction in duration of illness justifies the side effects and expense. So, recommendations for use of these drugs may change.

PNEUMOCOCCAL PNEUMONIA

A 13-valent pneumococcal polysaccharide vaccine (Prevnar 13) is available against pneumonia caused by *Streptococcus pneumoniae* (pneumococcus). In general, this vaccine is administered to infants as a routine vaccination. For persons who have not previously been immunized, it is particularly recommended for persons age 50 years and older; immunocompromised persons age 19 years and older; otherwise infirm persons (those with cancer or with chronic heart, kidney, liver, or lung disease; people without a spleen; alcoholics; diabetics; those with sickle cell anemia); and travelers who would be debilitated by a bout of pneumonia. A 23-valent vaccine (Pneumovax 23) is recommended to be given in addition to the 13-valent vaccine for adults ages 65 years and older, and for persons ages 2 to 64 years at high risk (e.g., they have significant underlying medical conditions) for invasive pneumococcal disease.

JAPANESE ENCEPHALITIS

Japanese encephalitis is caused by a virus of genus *Flavivirus* transmitted predominantly by *Culex* mosquitoes in South Asia, Southeast Asia, and the Asian Pacific Rim. Wind-blown mosquitoes have perhaps spread the virus from Papua New Guinea to the Australian mainland. The victim first suffers a mild, nonspecific viral illness accompanied by fever and headache. Most infections remain mild. However, in an extremely small number of cases, the victim goes on to develop severe meningoencephalitis, characterized by headache, weakness, fatigue, fever, confusion, seizures, symptoms similar to those of Parkinson's disease, paralysis, and altered mental status. There is no specific therapy beyond supportive care. From 20% to 30% of victims die, and many survivors have prolonged neurologic medical problems.

Travelers for more than 1 month to tropical Asia, particularly into rural rice-growing settings during Japanese encephalitis transmission season, are candidates for a Japanese B encephalitis vaccine, which depending on the vaccine chosen, is given in a series of two or three injections over 1 month. A booster dose may be given after 1 or 2 years, depending on the vaccine chosen. The current vaccines may cause side effects that may not occur until a week after the final injection, so it's recommended that travel not occur until at least that time has elapsed. Persons who will spend less than a month in an endemic area should consider becoming immunized if they will spend significant time outdoors (e.g., biking, hiking, trekking).

LYME DISEASE

See page 146.

PHYSICIANS ABROAD

A traveler to a foreign country may become ill enough to require the services of a physician. The International Association for Medical Assistance to Travellers (IAMAT) is a nonprofit organization that provides a list of approved doctors who adhere to international standards, which include standard fees. IAMAT (www.iamat.org) also distributes, free of charge, updated material on immunization requirements, malaria and other tropical diseases, and sanitary (food and water) and climatic conditions around the world. The directory of affiliated institutions can be obtained by calling or writing to IAMAT in Ontario, Canada. Other international medical assistance and rescue programs include the following (since specific street addresses, web addresses, and phone numbers are constantly changing, check for up-to-date information):

- Air Ambulance Network
- Divers Alert Network
- Global Rescue
- International SOS
- FrontierMEDEX
- Travel Assistance International
- Ripcord Travel Protection

TRANSPORT OF THE INJURED VICTIM

1. Never move a victim unless you know where you are going. If you're lost and caring for an injured victim (or yourself), prepare a shelter. Try to position yourself so that visual distress signals can be fashioned in an open field, in the snow, or near a visible riverbank. Keep the victim covered and warm. Assume that the victim is frightened and needs frequent reassurance. If he cannot walk, you must attend to his bodily functions. A urinal can be constructed from a wide-mouthed water bottle. Defecation is more complicated, but may be assisted by cutting a hole in a blanket or sleeping pad placed over a small pit dug in the ground.
2. Unless you are in danger, never leave a victim who is unconscious or confused.
3. If possible, send someone for help and wait with the victim, rather than perform an exhausting and time-consuming solo or duo extrication. If someone is to be sent for help, choose a strong traveler and provide him with a written request that details your situation (number of victims, injuries, need for supplies, specific evacuation method required). While you certainly don't want to underestimate the seriousness of the situation, don't request a helicopter evacuation for someone with a broken ankle who can easily be carried out in a litter. Anyone sent to obtain assistance should contact the closest law enforcement agency, which will seek the appropriate rescue agency.
4. Conserve your strength. Don't create additional victims with heroic attempts at communication or feats of strength and exertion.
5. Attempt to transport a victim only if waiting for a rescue party will be of greater risk than immediate movement, if there are sufficient helpers to carry the victim (as a general rule, it takes six to eight adults to carry one injured victim), and if the distance is reasonable (under 5 miles [8 km]). A victim who is carried on an improvised stretcher over difficult terrain usually gets a rough ride. Always test your carrying system on a noninjured person before you use it on the victim.

LIFTING AND MOVING TECHNIQUES
Straight Lift
If a person is seriously injured, profoundly weak, or unconscious, he should be lifted so that he remains motionless and with his spine in as straight an alignment as possible. This can be accomplished by five rescuers. The first kneels at the head, controls the victim's head and neck, and calls out commands. The other four rescuers kneel at the victim's sides, one at chest level and one at hip level on one side, and the others at lower back level and leg level on the opposite

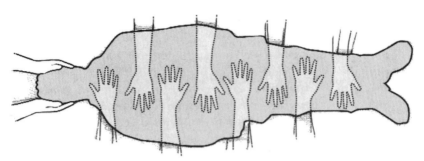

Figure 253. Proper hand positioning for straight lift.

side (Figure 253). In this way, they can slide their hands under the victim in a staggered fashion to provide a continuous chain of support. If necessary, the rescuer closest to the legs can free a hand to position a pad, backboard, or litter underneath the victim. The rescuers should lift the victim straight up into the air, taking care not to injure *their* backs.

Logrolling the Victim (see Figure 26)

The best way to carry and immobilize a person who may have an injured spine is to use a scoop stretcher or to slide a backboard underneath the victim. However, when these aren't available and a spine-injured person must be turned, logrolling is the best alternative. It is also the preferred method to turn a victim on his side in order to slide a pad, board, or litter underneath him.

1. The first rescuer approaches the victim from the head and keeps the head and shoulders in a fixed position (no neck movement).
2. The second rescuer extends the victim's arm (on the side over which the victim is to be rolled) above the victim's head. The first rescuer takes this arm and uses it to help support the head in proper position. If the arm is injured, it is maintained at the victim's side.
3. All rescuers work together to roll the victim, without moving his neck.

CARRIES AND LITTERS

The method of evacuation used to transport a victim will depend on the degree of disablement and what is available to the rescuer(s). To conserve the energy of all party members, victims of minor injuries should travel under their own power as much as possible, but should never travel unattended. One healthy and strong person should accompany anyone who must leave the group for medical reasons.

When lifting and carrying, take care to not injure yourself. This is best accomplished by handling a manageable load, using a safe grip, keeping the back straight and lifting with the legs, maintaining a wide stance to enhance balance, avoiding twisting, lifting slowly, and properly following commands when lifting as part of a group.

Carries

If the victim has suffered an injury that does not allow him to walk out, mechanical transport must be improvised. A single person who cannot walk but who does not need to be on a litter (one with, for example, a broken ankle, mild exhaustion, or acute mountain sickness) may be carried on the back of a strong rescuer using a rope seat. This is fashioned by passing a long 1 inch (2.5 cm) rope or strap across the victim's back and under his arms, then crossing the rope in front of his chest. The victim is loaded piggyback onto the rescuer's back, and the rope ends are passed forward over the shoulders of the rescuer, under his arms, and around to the rescuer's back, then between and through the victim's legs from the front, and around the outside of the victim's legs just under the buttocks, to be tied snugly in front of the rescuer's waist (Figure 254). Such a rope seat is far preferable to a standard fireman's carry, which is very fatiguing (Figure 255). A shoulder drag (Figure 256), fireman's drag (Figure 257), or blanket drag (Figure 258) is only good for very short distances, such as to pull a person quickly away from an immediate hazard. Piggyback (Figure 259) and cradle (Figure 260) carries are also quickly exhausting.

Other simple ways to carry a victim include the four-hand seat, limb carry, backpack carry, ski pole or tree limb backpack carry, three-person wheelbarrow carry, and coiled rope seat. In the first method, two rescuers interlock hands. Each rescuer first grasps his right wrist with his

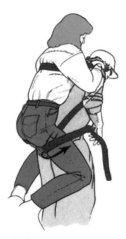

Figure 254. Fashioning a rope (webbing) seat.

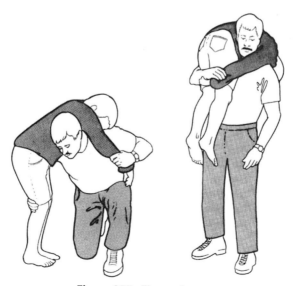

Figure 255. Fireman's carry.

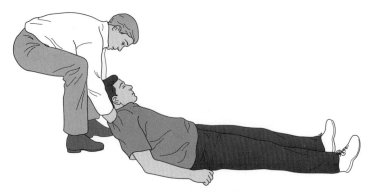

Figure 256. Shoulder drag.

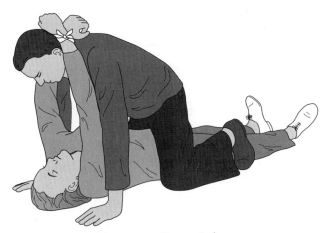

Figure 257. Fireman's drag.

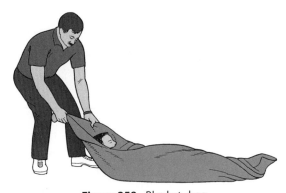

Figure 258. Blanket drag.

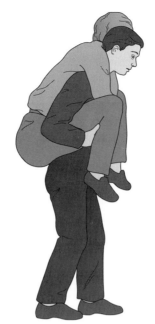

Figure 259. Piggyback carry.

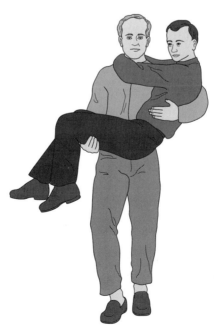

Figure 260. Cradle carry.

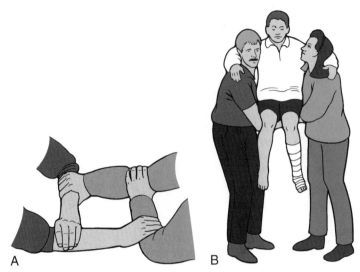

Figure 261. A, Overlapping hands to create a four-hand seat. **B,** Carrying the victim.

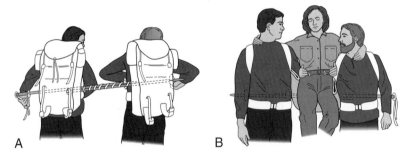

Figure 262. Fashioning a ski pole seat. **A,** The poles are slung between rescuers wearing backpacks. **B,** A victim can sit comfortably on the padded ski poles.

left hand. Holding the palms down, each rescuer then firmly grasps the left wrist or forearm of the other rescuer with his right hand, interlocking all four hands (Figure 261). The victim sits on the four-hand seat. In the limb carry, one person holds the victim's legs while another carries the victim under the arms. In the third method, leg holes can be cut into a large backpack, so that a victim can sit in it like a small child would in a baby carrier. In the fourth method, two rescuers with sturdy backpacks stand side by side. Pack straps are looped down from each pack, and ski poles or tree limbs are slung across through the loops, or the poles are placed to rest on the padded hip belts. The poles should be padded so that the victim can sit on the rigid seat, steadying himself by draping his arms around the shoulders of his rescuers (Figure 262). The three-person wheelbarrow carry (Figure 263) is an efficient method that can be used for long periods on fairly rough terrain. The split-coil rope seat is created by coiling a rope, then fixing the coil at one segment. The coil's loops are split and used to position the victim on the rescuer's back (Figure 264). A two-rescuer split-coil technique is also useful (Figure 265).

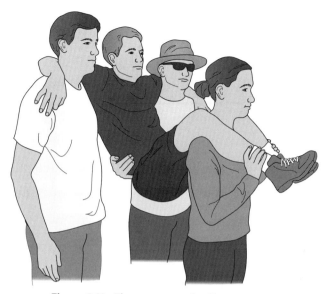

Figure 263. Three-person wheelbarrow carry.

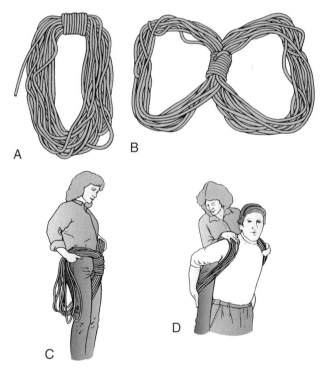

Figure 264. Creating a coiled rope seat. **A,** The rope is coiled and the loops secured. **B,** The loops of the coil are divided into equal sections at the point of fixation. **C** and **D,** The victim can step through the split loops, so that a single rescuer can carry the victim.

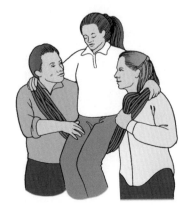

Figure 265. Two-rescuer split-coil rope seat.

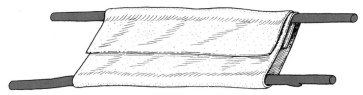

Figure 266. Blanket-pole litter.

Litters

The safest anatomic position for an injured victim (from a transport perspective) is supine with his back straight, eyes forward, and arms and legs straight with his hands at his sides. If the victim might vomit or is unconscious, he should be on his side, cushioned to protect against undue motion and to ensure an open airway.

If a specialized litter or stretcher (such as a Stokes basket or split scoop frame) is not available, an improvised litter can be constructed from a blanket or sturdy drop cloth and two 6 to 7 ft (1.8 to 2.1 m) poles or sturdy tree limbs (saplings). Separate the poles by slightly more than the width necessary to carry the victim. Fold the blanket over one pole, then fold the edges over the other pole sequentially and back again over the first pole (Figure 266). Secure the outside blanket flap with safety pins or stitches of cord. Test it to be sure that it can support the victim. Carry the victim so that his body secures the outside (free) blanket flap. Be sure to immobilize the victim on the litter, and cushion his head and neck.

Litters resembling ladders can be fashioned from tree limbs or ski poles fastened with twine, rope, clothing, or pack straps. Two backpack frames can be fastened together with tape or rope (Figure 267) to form a ladder-like platform for a sleeping bag or pads and blankets. A "parka litter" can be created by running two skis or long tree limbs through zipped jackets that are aligned bottom-to-bottom (Figure 268).

A rope stretcher is constructed by stretching a 150 to 200 ft (46 to 61 m) rope on the ground and determining its midpoint. At the midpoint, fold the rope back on itself. Measure 3 ft (91 cm) from the bend, and fold each half of the rope back again to the outside. This creates the central "rungs" of a "ladder" that will be 3 ft wide. Repeat the process of folding the rope back on itself in 3 ft segments, moving away from the central rungs in each direction and laying out a series

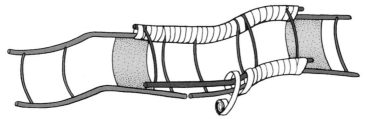

Figure 267. Construction of a backpack frame litter. Pads or a sleeping bag are placed on the litter.

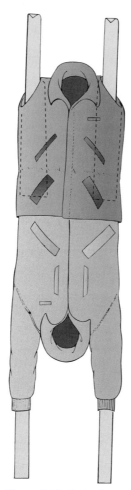

Figure 268. Parka litter.

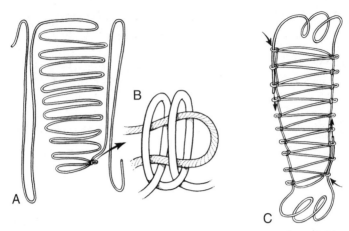

Figure 269. Making a rope stretcher. **A,** Having created a series of parallel loops, lay the lengthwise segments perpendicularly alongside. **B,** Use a clove hitch to secure the loop ends. **C,** The remaining long ends of the rope are passed through the outside loops to form the perimeter of the stretcher, and are tied off to complete the process.

of evenly spaced parallel loops. About 16 or 18 loops (rungs) should create a ladder approximately the same length as the victim. Take the two remaining long ends of the rope and lay them perpendicular to the rungs, alongside the bends in the rope (Figure 269). Use the long ends to secure the loops together (completing the long sides of the ladder) by tying a clove hitch (see Figure 286) or other secure knot onto each consecutive bend in the rope 2 to 3 inches (5 to 7.5 cm) inside the bend, so that a small loop remains to the outside of the knot. Each pair of knots should be separated by 3 to 4 inches (7.5 to 10 cm). After all the knots are tied, the rope ends are threaded through the small outside loops as the remaining lengths are circled around the outside of the stretcher and finally tied off.

A mummy litter (also called a daisy chain or cocoon wrap) can be constructed of a long climbing rope, large tarp, sleeping pads, blankets or a sleeping bag, and stiffeners (skis, poles, tree limbs, or the like). The rope is laid out with even U-shaped loops (Figure 270) that are roughly twice the victim's width. Tie a small loop at the foot end of the rope. Lay a tarp on the rope. On the tarp, lay down foam pads, then lengthwise stiffening rods, then another layer of pads. Lay the victim on the pads, and cover with the sleeping bag or blankets. Pull the sides of the tarp up to wrap the victim. To secure him, bring the first untied loop above the tied end (foot) loop through the tied loop, and pull it toward the center. Moving toward the head, feed the next loop through the preceding loop, and so on until the armpits are reached. At this point, bring a loop up over one shoulder and tie the rope off in front of the victim after bringing the rope end over the opposite shoulder.

Test any litter on an uninjured person before trusting it to bear the weight of the victim. Be certain to fasten the victim securely into the stretcher or litter, so that he doesn't fall out. Pad all injuries, and the head and neck in particular, to make the victim as comfortable as possible. Positioning on a litter is very important. In general, keep the injury uphill, to keep extra weight (pressure) and jostling from causing pain. If the chest is injured, keep the victim lying on his side with the wounded side (lung) down, to allow the good lung to expand more fully. If the victim has altered consciousness, is nauseated, or is vomiting, he should be kept on his side, to protect the airway (see page 22). If the victim has suffered a face, head, or neck injury, he should be transported with his head slightly elevated. Victims suffering from shock (see page 58),

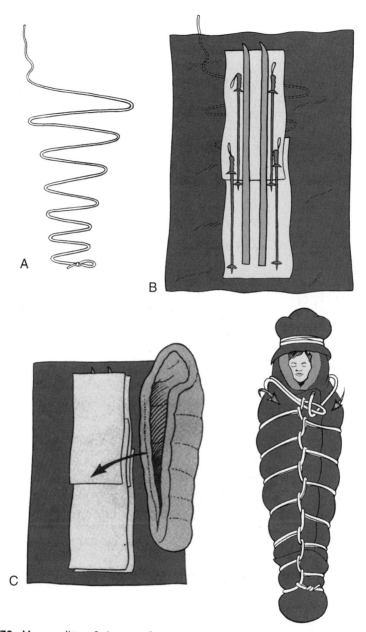

Figure 270. Mummy litter. **A,** Lay out the rope in even loops. **B,** Lay blankets or tarps over the loops, then long, rigid objects for stability. **C,** Place a sleeping bag or blanket in the center to hold the victim. **D,** Pass the first nontied loop through the tied loop and work your way to the top. Bring the finishing loops over the shoulders, and tie off.

bleeding, or hypothermia (see page 281) should be carried with the head down and feet elevated. Victims with chest pain and/or difficulty breathing, which might indicate a heart attack or heart failure (see page 44), should be carried with the upper body elevated.

All victims should be covered above and below with blankets, clothing, sleeping bags, or whatever else is available for warmth. Handle all suspected hypothermics gently. A victim secured to a stretcher should never be left unattended. Constantly reassure the victim. If the terrain is steep, keep his feet pointed downhill. Litter transport is exhausting for the rescuers and should not be entertained if the distance to be covered is more than a few miles.

If possible, position at least one rescuer at the head of the victim, one at each shoulder, one at each hip, and one at the legs. This allows a litter to be carried and facilitates a quick action to turn the victim, should that be necessary. A leader should call out all activities of the team.

A victim on a backboard must be securely tied down so that he cannot roll or slide off the board. This will involve straps and padding around the legs, waist and hips, chest, and head and neck. Carriers should be in a position to turn the board so that a victim may vomit without choking or falling off the board.

HELICOPTERS

Most helicopters used for medical evacuation can safely land at altitudes of up to 10,000 ft (3050 m) and are limited by visibility, landing space, and weather conditions. Rescue helicopters may operate under visual flight rules (VFR), which means that flight conditions must be free of clouds and airspeed can be slow enough for the pilot to see far enough to avoid a collision. Larger military and search and rescue helicopters can fly under instrument flight rules (IFR), using special navigational instruments, and can land at higher altitudes.

When calling for a helicopter, provide the following information: number of victims and their weights, injuries, and level of consciousness; reason why you need a helicopter; location of the landing zone; and the current and expected weather conditions (temperature, visibility, distance ["ceiling"] from ground to clouds, and wind speed/direction). People on the ground should be aware of the limitations of maneuverability, and should obey certain rules when involved with a helicopter rescue:

1. Prepare and brightly mark a proper landing zone (site). The ideal location is on level ground (bare rock is best; snow is worst) with no more than 10 degrees of incline and access from all sides. If possible, choose a site where the helicopter will be able to drop off during takeoff, rather than having to climb up. Ideally, there will be 360-degree access so that the helicopter can take off in any direction, depending on wind conditions. Clear an area a minimum of 100 ft (31 m) long by 100 ft wide of all debris that could interfere with landing or be scattered by gusts from the propellers. Colored lights may be placed to mark the perimeter or corners of the landing site. Any obstacles that cannot be removed, such as cables, wires or antennas, should be clearly marked. At night, if you have lights, shine them on objects that will alert the pilot to unseen danger (such as the poles of power lines). If the landing site can be marked with an "H" or "Y," that will be helpful to the pilot. Although the absolute minimum ground dimensions for a "safety square" can, under ideal weather and visibility conditions, be somewhat less than this, you should clear the full area (or even up to 100 ft [31 m] × 300 ft [93 m]), as a helicopter can rarely take off or land strictly vertically, particularly in the thinner air of high altitude. A smoky fire or smoke signal should be placed near the landing site so that the pilot can judge the wind (pilots prefer takeoffs and landings to be directed into the prevailing wind to increase lift). If this is not possible, stand away from the landing site where the pilot can see you, and hold up an improvised wind flag (such as streamers), or position yourself with the wind behind your back, and point with both arms at the landing site. If there is

a danger at the last minute before landing, signal "don't land" to the helicopter pilot by lifting your arms from a horizontal (to-the-side) outstretch to straight overhead several times. Remember that waving your arms and hands frantically is the universal "wave-off" instruction! If the landing area is on snow, place some large markers, such as backpacks, near the landing spot to offer the pilot some depth perception. At night, create a landing area at least half again as large as during the daytime, and position lights or small fires in the corners, pointing down at the ground rather than up into the air. Never shine a flashlight directly at a helicopter, to avoid blinding the crew. If fires are used, remember that the helicopter may scatter embers, so watch carefully for unintended fire spread. Minimize the number of people approaching the helicopter.

2. To summarize hand signals for guiding a helicopter pilot into a landing: Stand with your back to the wind and extend both arms directly toward the landing area, which signifies where to land and that the wind is at your back. As the helicopter hovers over the proper landing site, extend your arms to the sides with clenched fists, which signifies to the pilot to hold the hover. As the helicopter begins to touch the ground, move your arms down at a 45-degree angle to the ground with hitchhiker thumbs pointing downward, signifying to the pilot to hold the ground position. When you want the rotors to be turned off, slice your hand across your neck with the palm pointed down.

3. Unless otherwise instructed, stay at least 150 ft (46 m) from a helicopter with rotors spinning. Look away as the ship lands, so as not to be struck in the face or eyes by flying debris. Protect the victim. Secure all loose objects or clear them from the landing area. Coil and secure all ropes. Because of the strong gusts from the approaching helicopter (up to 100 mph, or 161 km per hour), don't stand near the edge of a cliff! Don't stand in the landing zone if on snow, in case the helicopter settles.

4. Always approach or leave a helicopter at a 30- to 45-degree angle from the front, in sight of the pilot and crew (Figure 271). Never approach the helicopter from ground higher than the landing spot, to avoid walking into a rotor. Stay away from the tail rotor, because it is nearly invisible when rotating. All loading and unloading of a helicopter should occur on the downhill side of the aircraft, to avoid striking a rotor.

5. Keep your head down! You may not perceive that the rotor blade is dipping (up to 4 ft, or 1.2 m, from the center attachment) until it chops off your head. Don't hold any objects (particularly not your arms) above your head. Protect your eyes from dust kicked up by the rotor wash.

6. Don't smoke a cigarette near a helicopter.

7. Follow the pilot's and flight crew's instructions. Don't approach, enter, leave, or load a helicopter until you are given the command. Establish eye contact with the pilot and obey his signals.

8. Don't stand under or anywhere near a helicopter during takeoff or landing. Everyone near the landing site should stay at a safe distance in a single group, clearly visible to the pilot. At night, carry a light or wear a reflective object or clothing.

9. If a cable or rope is lowered, allow it to touch the ground before you handle it, to avoid a shock from static electricity. Never tie the rope or cable to an immovable object on the ground; this could cause a crash.

10. If a rescue device (e.g., litter) is being used, put the victim into the rescue device and take care to keep the hoist cable clear of looping around anyone in the area. Be certain that the victim is properly strapped into the rescue device before anyone signals the helicopter crew to haul up the cable.

11. All people should wear hard hats and eye protection, if available. Keep jackets zipped. Carry all packs, rather than wear them on your back.

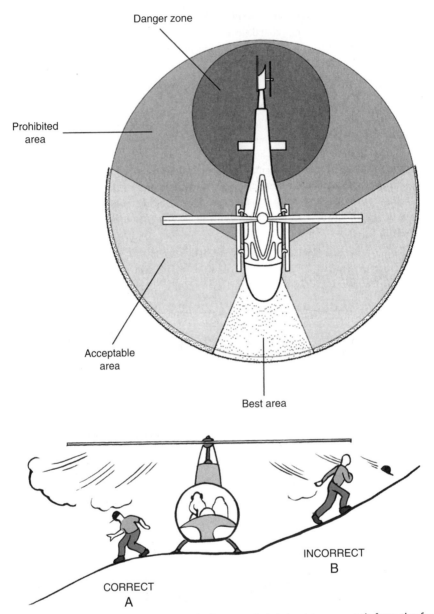

Figure 271. Approach zones around a helicopter. **A,** It is best to approach from the front. **B,** Don't walk uphill into the helicopter rotor blades.

GROUND-TO-AIR DISTRESS SIGNALS

If a party is trapped or lost, and helicopter or airplane search parties are likely to be in the region, it may help to attempt to signal the aircraft. One way that this can be done is by creating ground-to-air distress signals, either by marking an open field or a riverbank that's visible from the air by stamping out large (8 to 10 ft [2.4 to 3 m]) designs in the snow (in an open area), or by attracting attention with display patterns of clothing, rocks, fire rings, or the like. Figure 272 illustrates some standard ground markings for communication.

The three signals that are recognized (and remembered) by most pilots are: three of anything—"distress"; large X—"unable to proceed" or "need medical assistance"; and an arrow—"proceeding in this direction." Three fires (set 100 ft [31 m] apart) placed in a triangular configuration is a sign of distress to a passing pilot. Ground-to-air patterns should be large, composed of straight lines, and made up of colors that contrast sharply with the natural colors of the environment (royal blue is best). Small battery-powered emergency strobes are also useful. A heliograph mirror is a small signal reflector that can be accurately aimed to reflect sunlight at a distant object (such as an aircraft).

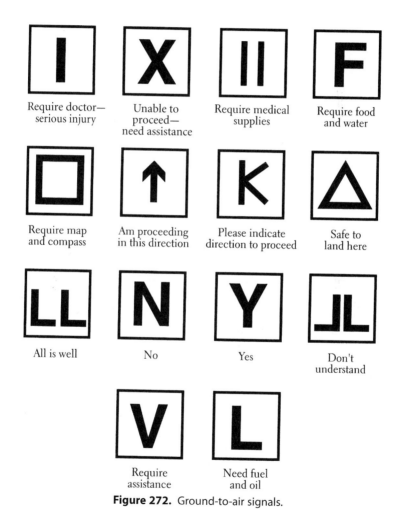

Figure 272. Ground-to-air signals.

LOST PEOPLE

People lost in the wilderness often act in a predictable manner. Rapid location of a lost person can make the difference between life and death. These general guidelines may assist you in a search:

1. Lost people tend to follow the path of least resistance (open fields, trails, roads, dry streambeds).
2. A person who is lost tends to travel downhill and to seek apparent shortcuts toward civilization or a familiar location.
3. People tend to avoid barriers and obstacles (lakes, large rivers, boulder fields, dense brush).
4. At night, a lost person tends to travel toward lights.
5. In bad weather, people tend to seek shelter with overhead protection.
6. Small children tend to seek shelter when tired.

PROCEDURES

INTRAMUSCULAR INJECTION

Intramuscular (into the muscle) injection of epinephrine is used to manage a severe allergic reaction. The injection may be performed with a preloaded syringe (already containing the medicine in the barrel—see page 460) or may require that the medicine be drawn up for administration. After you wash your hands, follow these instructions:

1. Select the proper syringe and needle. For the treatment of an allergic reaction, a syringe that holds at least 1 mL is necessary, equipped with a 21- or 23-gauge needle (the larger the gauge number, the smaller the diameter of the needle) sufficiently long to penetrate through the skin and fat into the muscle.
2. Never touch the metal of the needle with your hands.
3. Never share needles (never use the same needle to inject multiple people).
4. If the medication is in a preloaded syringe, be sure to see that the amount of medicine does not exceed the dose you want to administer. Be certain not to inject too much medicine.
5. If the medicine is in a glass vial, flick the vial a few times with your finger to drive the air bubble to the top, and then snap the vial open at the line marked on the glass at the neck (Figure 273, A and B). Draw the proper amount of medicine to be administered up into the syringe (see Figure 273, C). In the case of epinephrine, this will be 0.3 to 0.5 mL for an adult, and 0.01 mL/kg (2.2 lb) of body weight for a child, not to exceed 0.3 mL.
6. If the medication is in a glass bottle with a rubber top, wipe the top of the bottle with alcohol, stick the needle through the rubber, and draw up the desired amount of medication. If you cannot draw the medicine out of the bottle, you may need to inject some air into the bottle first (use the same entry into the bottle to inject air in and to draw medicine out).
7. Before injection, point the needle upward, tap the syringe a few times to float the air bubbles to the top, and squirt out any air that is in the syringe (see Figure 273, D and E). You should be left with only medicine. Try not to inject any air.

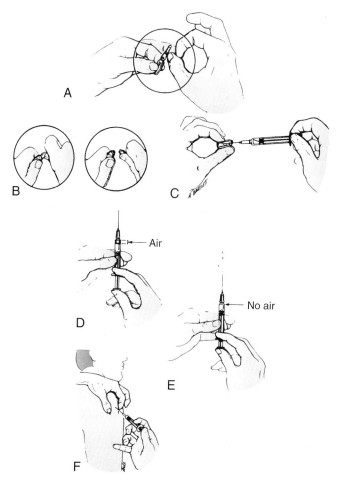

Figure 273. Administering an injection. **A,** Flick the air bubble to the top of the vial. **B,** Break of the top of the vial at the narrowing or line. **C,** Draw the medicine into the syringe. **D,** Holding the needle straight up, gently push the plunger until **(E)** no air is left. **F,** Pinch up a fold of skin and briskly stick the needle through the skin and into muscle at a 90-degree angle for an intramuscular injection, or just under the skin at a 15- to 30-degree angle for a subcutaneous injection.

8. Wipe off the skin with alcohol or with soap and water (if no alcohol is available) where you intend to administer the medicine. The easiest place to inject epinephrine is on the lateral arm at the shoulder.
9. Pinch the skin up between your fingers, and quickly plunge the needle in just under the skin at a 90-degree angle to the skin (see Figure 273, F). With the needle in the skin, gently pull back on the plunger, to see if blood enters the syringe. If it does, you have inadvertently entered a blood vessel, and you should draw back the needle until no blood is returned. If no blood is returned, firmly plush the plunger and inject the medicine. Quickly remove the needle from the skin, and gently massage the injection site.

Again, when administering an injection, *never* share needles between people.

SUBCUTANEOUS INJECTION

Subcutaneous (just below the skin) injection of epinephrine is sometimes used to manage a severe allergic reaction if an intramuscular injection is not available. After you wash your hands, follow the same instructions as for an intramuscular injection, with the exceptions of needle size and angle/depth of injection:

1. Select the proper syringe and needle. For the treatment of an allergic reaction, a syringe that holds at least 1 mL is necessary, commonly equipped with a 25- or 27-gauge needle (the larger the gauge number, the smaller the diameter of the needle).
2. Pinch the skin up between your fingers, and quickly plunge the needle in just under the skin at a 15- to 30-degree angle to the skin (see Figure 273, *F*). With the needle in the skin, gently pull back on the plunger, to see if blood enters the syringe. If it does, you have inadvertently entered a blood vessel, and you should draw back the needle until no blood is returned. If no blood is returned, firmly plush the plunger and inject the medicine. Quickly remove the needle from the skin, and gently massage the injection site.

FISHHOOK REMOVAL

If a fishhook enters the skin, gently scrub the skin surrounding the entry point with soap and water. After the skin is clean, apply gentle pressure along the curve toward the point while pulling on the hook. If the hook is not easily removed, this means that the barb is caught in the tissue (Figure 274, *A*).

  If the hook has a barbed shank, the hook can be removed by pushing it through the skin. This should be done (because of the increased risk of infection) if it will take more than 8 hours to get to a doctor. If the hook is a treble hook, carefully cut off the non-embedded barbs so that they will not inadvertently become embedded while you're handling the hook. Grasp the shank of the hook with a plier. With a steady, firm motion, push the hook through the skin so that the barb appears (see Figure 274, *B*). Cut off the shaft or the barb (take care to cover the area with a free hand to prevent the detached barb from flying into someone's eye) and then pull the remainder of the hook back out of the skin (see Figure 274, *C* and *D*).

  A popular method of fishhook removal is the "string-pull" or "press-and-yank" technique (see Figure 274, *E*). Attach (tie) a shoelace or 2 ft (60 cm) length of string, fishing line, or rolled

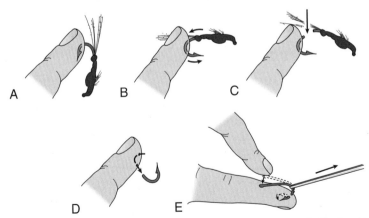

Figure 274. Fishhook removal. **A,** The barb is embedded in the finger. **B,** The hook and barb are pushed through the skin. **C,** The shaft of the hook is cut. **D,** Both pieces are easily extracted. **E,** "Press-and-yank" method of fishhook removal.

gauze around the bend of the hook. Push the shank of the hook down (toward the barb), parallel to the skin. This (hopefully) will disengage the barb from the tissue. Then use the string (at a 30-degree angle) to yank the hook from the skin in a snapping motion. Take care that the flying hook released from the skin does not impale anyone nearby. Wear eye protection or look away when you pull on the string to remove the hook.

Vigorously wash the wound and leave it open with a simple dry dressing. Don't seal in the dirt and bacteria with any grease or home remedies. If the hook was dirty (or was holding a dirty worm), begin the victim on dicloxacillin, penicillin, erythromycin, or cephalexin. If the victim suffers from a depressed immune system, use an antibiotic that's effective against germs acquired in an aquatic environment (see page 347). If a hook enters the skin anywhere near the eye, don't attempt removal. Tape the hook in place so that it cannot be snagged, and take the victim immediately to see a doctor.

SPLINTER REMOVAL

A splinter can be removed by gently cutting away the skin near its entry point, until a firm grasp can be made with a small tweezers or with the fingers. If a splinter enters the finger under the fingernail, cut a small V-shaped wedge out of the nail, so that the splinter can be grasped. Sometimes a splinter can be teased out a bit using a needle or sharp pin to allow the exposed end of the splinter to be grasped. This same technique can be done using a sharp-tipped scissors. Another method is to push a needle (bevel facing up) into the splinter end on for about $\frac{1}{8}$ of an inch and then push down on the hub, which elevates the needle tip and drags the splinter out from under the nail. If a splinter cannot be removed for more than 24 hours, begin the victim on penicillin, erythromycin, or cephalexin.

If a splinter lies in full view longitudinally under the skin, it may be easier to take a sharp blade and carefully cut down through the skin directly over the splinter along its entire length, to avoid fragmenting it by dragging the (usually) wood out of a small opening.

RING REMOVAL

A ring should be removed if swelling of a finger underneath will cause the ring to become an inadvertent tourniquet. This is particularly true with broken fingers, burns, crush injuries, stings, and bites. The easiest method is to lubricate the skin with soap, ointment, or something greasy, and then apply a circular motion with traction on the ring. Keep the hand or foot (for a toe ring) elevated and cool (cold water or ice pack for 10 minutes) to minimize the swelling.

If swelling prevents easy removal, wrap completely the entire portion of the finger beyond the ring very snugly with a strip of something elastic and leave the wrap in place for 5 minutes. This will hopefully squeeze blood and other tissue fluid out of the swollen part of the finger and back under the ring. Unwrap the finger, apply a lubricant, and see if the ring will now slide off the finger.

Another method is to use the "string-wrap" technique (Figure 275). Take a 20 inch (50 cm) string and pass it under the ring so that the long portion is left on the fingernail side of the ring. Wrap the long portion around the finger in a spiral fashion, starting next to the ring and working out toward the fingernail, keeping the loops close together. No tissue should bulge through between the loops. The string is then unwrapped by unwinding on the side closer to the hand, which pushes the ring little by little off the finger. The process is repeated over and over until the ring can be forced over the swollen finger joint(s), which may be a bit painful. Take care between wraps not to lose ground by inadvertently pushing the ring back toward the hand.

Some rings are made of metals (such as tungsten) that are extremely difficult to cut. It's sometimes possible to use a vice-grip wrench to make repeated forceful squeezes that create microfractures in the metal, eventually causing it to shatter and the ring to be removed.

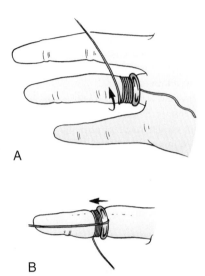

A

B

Figure 275. Ring removal. **A,** Thread a string under the ring. Wrap the long portion to compress the finger next to the ring. **B,** Unwrap the string to push the ring toward the end of the finger. The process is repeated until the ring is moved over the knuckle or swollen part of the finger.

ZIPPER REMOVAL

If skin gets caught in a zipper, the best way to solve the problem is to cut the diamond-shaped slider with a wire cutter so that the zipper falls apart (Figure 276). You also might be able to pop this piece apart using two well-placed small metal probes from, for instance, a pair of multitools. Another method is to cover the entire area with mineral oil, which hopefully will lubricate everything and free the skin from the zipper. Once the slider is removed, then pull apart the exposed zipper teeth, clean the affected skin, and apply an antiseptic ointment. Remember, if you keep trying to slide the zipper, you may entrap more skin, so that's not a good technique.

KNOTS AND HITCHES

One of the most useful wilderness skills is the ability to quickly tie a secure knot or hitch. This is particularly important when fashioning a litter or traction device. The following diagrams illustrate a selection of common useful knots, hitches, and bends: overhand knot (Figure 277), slip knot (Figure 278), figure-of-eight knot (Figure 279), half hitch and double half hitch (Figure 280), bowline (Figure 281), double bowline (Figure 282), loop knot and draw loop (Figure 283), round turn with double half hitch (Figure 284), single sheet bend (Figure 285), clove hitch (Figure 286), double carrick bend (Figure 287), Prusik hitch (Figure 288), and double fisherman's bend (Figure 289).

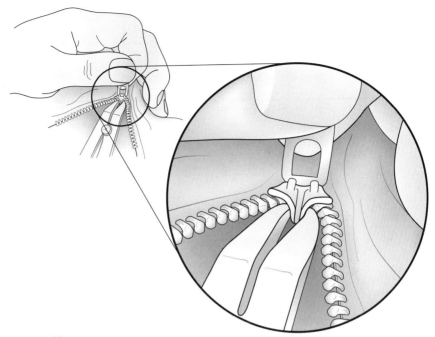

Figure 276. Zipper removal by cutting the diamond-shaped slider.

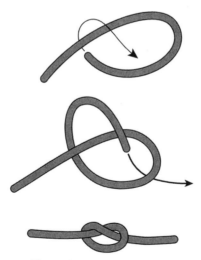

Figure 277. Overhand knot.

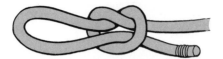

Figure 278. Slip knot.

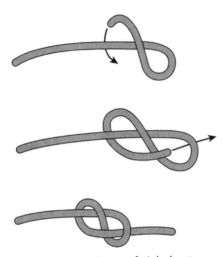

Figure 279. Figure-of-eight knot.

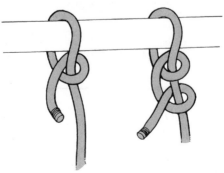

Figure 280. Half hitch and double half hitch.

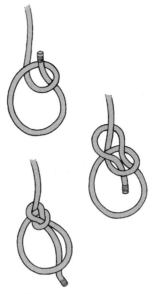

Figure 281. Bowline.

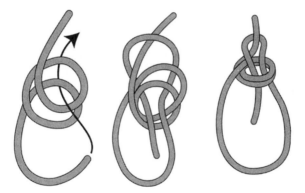

Figure 282. Double bowline.

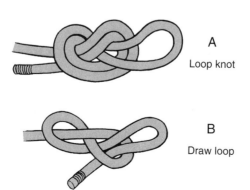

A

Loop knot

B

Draw loop

Figure 283. A, Loop knot. **B,** Draw loop.

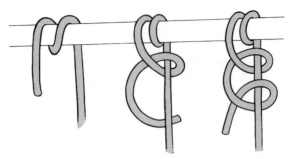

Figure 284. Round turn with double half hitch.

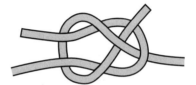

Figure 285. Single sheet bend.

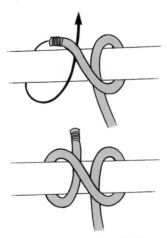

Figure 286. Clove hitch.

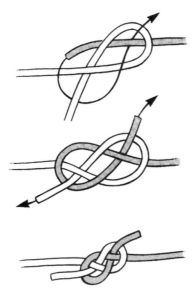

Figure 287. Double carrick bend.

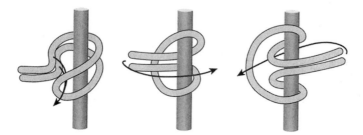

Figure 288. Prusik hitch.

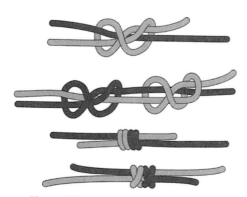

Figure 289. Double fisherman's bend.

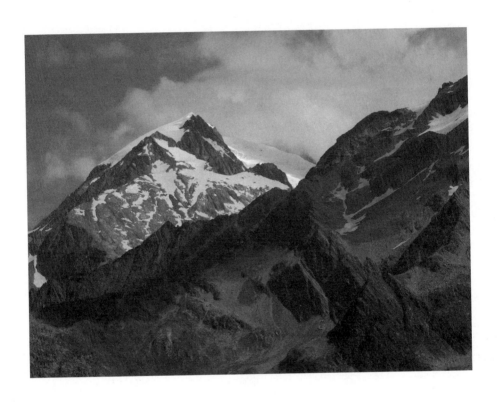

Appendices

This Appendix lists drugs that are mentioned in the book, and some that are not mentioned but that might be carried and taken by persons you may encounter.

Before administering any medication, ask the recipient if he suffers from allergy to it. If so, don't administer the drug or anything that you feel is similar to it. Use medications only if you have a reasonable understanding of what you are treating. Always have a doctor or pharmacist explain the actions and side effects of any drug you obtain to be carried with you. Exercise extreme caution and don't administer drugs to pregnant women, infants, or small children unless absolutely necessary. Drugs have many side effects. Some of the common ones are noted. Be familiar with the drugs you carry.

Many drugs are used to suppress symptoms (such as abdominal pain, nausea and vomiting, and headache) of potentially serious disorders. In these cases, don't overmedicate the victim if you need to watch for a worsening condition.

Drugs are listed here by purpose. I have listed some products that are available over-the-counter; however, many of the drugs require a prescription. This is not a comprehensive formulary, but rather emphasizes the medications most likely to be used or encountered.

Doses are listed in absolute amount (generally, for adults) or in amount to be given per body weight or per age (generally, for children). For determination of weight, 1 kilogram (kg) equals 2.2 pounds (lb). The drug should be administered orally unless otherwise specified.

Because children usually require a fraction of the dose used for adults, they may need to have the drug in special tablet or liquid form. The average weights for children, according to age, are as follows:

1 year—10 kg (22 lb)
3 years—15 kg (33 lb)
6 years—20 kg (44 lb)
8 years—25 kg (55 lb)
9 ½ years—30 kg (66 lb)
11 years—35 kg (77 lb)

Corticosteroids ("steroids") are interchangeable to a certain degree. If you must substitute, here is a rough measure of equivalence: 20 mg prednisone equals 16 mg methylprednisolone equals 3 mg dexamethasone.

Drugs are listed in the following order:

- For treatment of seizures (epilepsy) (page 464)
- For relief from pain (page 465)
- For relief from fever (page 466)
- For relief from muscle aches or minor arthritis; includes nonsteroidal antiinflammatory drugs (NSAIDs) (page 466)
- For relief from migraine headache (page 466)
- For relief from itching (page 466)
- For relief from toothache (page 467)
- For relief from motion sickness (page 467)
- For relief from nausea and vomiting (page 467)
- For relief from diarrhea (page 467)
- For relief from constipation (page 468)
- For relief from ulcer pain (page 469)
- For relief from indigestion or gas pains (page 469)
- For relief from heartburn (reflux esophagitis) (page 469)
- For relief from nasal congestion (page 470)
- For relief from cough (page 470)
- For relief from sore throat (page 470)
- Cold formulas (page 470)
- Skin medications (page 471)
- For sleep (page 472)
- Antibiotics (page 473)

DRUGS AND PREGNANCY

In general, it's best to avoid taking any medication when pregnant (particularly during the first trimester, or first third, of pregnancy) to avoid the risk of fetal malformation, or illness or injury in the newly born child. A pregnant woman should be discouraged from taking over-the-counter drugs. However, women can certainly become ill during pregnancy, so it's important to know what can be administered safely and what should be absolutely avoided. Fortunately, many of the drugs that are labeled "potentially hazardous" have only been proved hazardous in laboratory animals, frequently in relative doses that far exceed their common usage in humans. Furthermore, some drugs, such as diazepam and salicylates, formerly thought to cause malformation of the developing fetus, have since been proved safe when administered in normal therapeutic doses.

The following list reflects recommendations compiled from the current medical literature. Whenever possible, a pregnant woman contemplating use of a medication should seek advice *in advance* from her physician.

Antibiotic, Antifungal, Antiviral, Antimalarial
No Recognized Hazard
amoxicillin–clavulanate
ampicillin/amoxicillin
cephalosporins
clotrimazole
erythromycin
gentamicin topical eye medication
mefloquine (apparently safe)
miconazole
nystatin

paromomycin
penicillin
proguanil
terconazole
Avoid If Possible
acyclovir
chloramphenicol
chloroquine (apparently safe)
ciprofloxacin
fluconazole
gentamicin injection
metronidazole
nitrofurantoin
primaquine
quinacrine
quinine
trimethoprim–sulfamethoxazole
Hazardous
fleroxacin
norfloxacin
ofloxacin
tetracycline/doxycycline (causes staining of teeth and altered bone development in fetus)

Pain Medication
No Recognized Hazard
acetaminophen
hydrocodone
meperidine
oxycodone
Avoid If Possible
aspirin (during last 3 months of pregnancy)
codeine
ibuprofen and other NSAIDs (during last 3 months of pregnancy)
Hazardous
indomethacin

Vaccine
No Recognized Hazard
diphtheria toxoid
hepatitis A
hepatitis B (killed)
pooled serum immunoglobulin
tetanus immunoglobulin
tetanus toxoid
Avoid If Possible
cholera
influenza (inactivated virus)
meningococcal vaccine
pneumococcal vaccine
polio (oral and injection)

rabies vaccine (preexposure; must be used for postexposure)
tuberculosis (BCG)
typhoid
typhus
yellow fever
Hazardous
measles
mumps
rubella
smallpox
varicella

Antiallergy
No Recognized Hazard
cimetidine
dimenhydrinate
epinephrine (use only in a critical situation)
famotidine
loratadine
topical corticosteroids, decongestants (e.g., oxymetazoline)
Avoid If Possible
albuterol
chlorpheniramine
epinephrine (avoid in a noncritical situation)
hydroxyzine
prednisone
Hazardous
brompheniramine
cyclizine
dimenhydrinate
diphenhydramine (during first trimester)

Antinausea, Anti–Motion-Sickness, Antidiarrheal, Anticonstipation
No Recognized Hazard
bisacodyl
dimenhydrinate
docusate
meclizine
metoclopramide (apparently safe)
mineral oil
ondansetron
prochlorperazine
promethazine
psyllium fiber
trimethobenzamide
Avoid If Possible
anticholinergic drugs
scopolamine

Other
No Recognized Hazard
antacids
betamethasone
caffeine
casanthranol
cyproheptadine
dextromethorphan
kaolin-pectin
loperamide
omeprazole
oxymetazoline
prednisolone
prednisone
pyrethrins with piperonyl butoxide
ranitidine
simethicone
sucralfate
Avoid If Possible
acetazolamide
albuterol
amantadine
beclomethasone
bismuth subsalicylate
dexamethasone
diphenoxylate
furosemide
isoproterenol
lindane
loperamide
metaproterenol
nifedipine
theophylline
triazolam
Hazardous
captopril (and all other angiotensin-converting enzyme [ACE] inhibitors)
chlordiazepoxide
chlorothiazide
dapsone
diazepam
hydrochlorothiazide
isotretinoin
midazolam
phenacetin
phenytoin
thyroid inhibitors
tolbutamide

ALLERGIC REACTION TO A DRUG

If a person develops an allergic reaction to a drug (itching, shortness of breath, swollen tongue, difficulty talking, skin rash, hives, and so on), immediately discontinue the drug and follow the instructions on page 64.

FOR RELIEF FROM A SEVERE ALLERGIC REACTION

Epinephrine (adrenaline) 1 : 1,000 aqueous solution. Adult dose 0.3 to 0.5 mL injected
  intramuscularly (see page 444) into the lateral thigh. This may be repeated two times at
  20-minute intervals. The pediatric dose is 0.01 mL/kg (2.2 lb) of body weight,
  not to exceed 0.3 mL, injected intramuscularly into the lateral thigh. If the thigh
  is obese, whether in an adult or a child, such that the needle might not reach into
  muscle, then inject into the lower thigh. If obesity is extreme, consider injecting into
  the mid-calf. *Unless the situation is life-threatening, don't use epinephrine if the victim
  is older than 45 years, has a known history of heart disease, or is a pregnant
  female.*
  Side effects: Rapid heartbeat, nervousness.
  The only reason to administer the drug subcutaneously (see page 446) is if the equipment
    is not available for an intramuscular injection. The drug is available in preloaded
    syringes in certain allergy kits, which include the EpiPen autoinjector and EpiPen Jr.
    autoinjector, the Auvi-Q "talking" autoinjector (0.3 mg or 0.15 mg dose), and the
    Adrenaclick (0.3 mg or 0.15 mg dose). Other devices worldwide are the Jext,
    Emerade, Allerject, and Anapen. Instructions for use accompany the kits. For
    dosing purposes, a 0.3 mg autoinjector should be used for adults and children over
    66 lb (30 kg) in weight. Children 66 lb and under should be injected with a 0.15 mg
    autoinjector.
  Take particular care to handle preloaded syringes properly, to avoid inadvertent injection
    into an unintended location, such as a finger or toe. Don't intentionally inject
    epinephrine into the buttocks or a vein. Epinephrine should not be exposed to heat
    or sun, but does not need to be kept refrigerated. If clear (liquid) epinephrine turns
    cloudy or discolored, it should be discarded. When administering an injection, *never*
    share needles between people.
Diphenhydramine (Benadryl). Adult dose 25 to 50 mg every 4 to 6 hours; pediatric dose 1 mg/
  kg (2.2 lb) of body weight.
  Side effects: Drowsiness, paradoxical hyperactivity (children).
Albuterol (Ventolin) or metaproterenol (Alupent) metered-dose inhaler. Adult dose two puffs
  every 3 to 6 hours as needed.
  Side effects: Rapid heartbeat, nervousness ("jitters").
  The proper technique for using a metered-dose inhaler device is as follows:
  1. Shake the inhaler vigorously for 5 seconds before each use.
  2. Invert the inhaler so that the opening is downward if directed to do so. Hold the
     inhaler 4 cm (1.6 in) in front of an open mouth, or place a spacer on the opening,
     around which the lips will be sealed.
  3. Exhale fully. Close your lips around the spacer, or hold the device about 4 cm
     (1.6 in) from your mouth, or close your lips around the mouthpiece.
  4. Activate the inhaler at the beginning of inspiration.
  5. Inhale slowly and deeply to full lung capacity.
  6. Hold your breath for 10 seconds, then exhale slowly.
  7. Wait 1 minute before repeating all steps before the next puff. Shake the inhaler
     before each puff.

Prednisone. Adult dose 50 to 80 mg the first day. Each day, the dose is decreased by 10 mg. The pediatric dose is 1 mg/kg (2.2 lb) of body weight the first day, tapered every 4 days by halving the dose. Administer with food or with an antacid if possible. Corticosteroids are interchangeable to a certain degree. If you must substitute, here is a rough measure of equivalence: 20 mg prednisone equals 16 mg methylprednisolone equals 3 mg dexamethasone.

For a severe skin reaction to poison ivy, oak, or sumac, see the instructions on page 218.
For a severe sunburn, see the instructions on page 212.

Corticosteroids should always be taken with the understanding that a rare side effect is serious deterioration of the head ("ball" of the ball-and-socket joint) of the femur, the long bone of the thigh.

When corticosteroids are administered to a person for a sufficiently long period of time, the adrenal glands (which manufacture the same hormones) are suppressed. To allow the adrenal glands to recover, the following rules should be observed:

1. If someone has been receiving a high (non-tapered) dose of a corticosteroid for 5 days or less, then the medication can be abruptly discontinued without consideration for adrenal suppression.
2. If someone has been receiving a high (non-tapered) dose of a corticosteroid for 6 to 10 days, then the medication should be tapered over an additional 7 days.

FOR RELIEF FROM A MILD ALLERGIC REACTION OR HAY FEVER

Diphenhydramine (Benadryl). Same as "For Relief from a Severe Allergic Reaction."

Diphenhydramine (25 mg) with pseudoephedrine (60 mg) (Benadryl Decongestant). Adult dose one tablet every 8 hours.

Cetirizine hydrochloride (Zyrtec). Dose 5 to 10 mg every 24 hours; don't use in children under 6 years of age. Pediatric dose: children ages 6 to 11 years 5 or 10 mg every 24 hours; ages 6 months to 5 years 2.5 mg (½ teaspoon) every 24 hours.

Fexofenadine (Allegra). Adult dose 60 mg every 12 hours. In adults, it may also be administered as 180 mg once a day. Pediatric dose children ages 2 to 11 years 30 mg twice a day. Rarely causes drowsiness. Allegra-D: fexofenadine 60 mg with pseudoephedrine 120 mg extended-release tablet.

Loratadine (Claritin). Adult dose 10 mg every 24 hours. Pediatric dose children ages 2 to 6 years 5 mg every 24 hours. Rarely causes drowsiness. Claritin-D: loratadine 5 mg with pseudoephedrine 120 mg. Claritin-D 24 Hour: loratadine 10 mg with pseudoephedrine 240 mg.

Cyproheptadine (Periactin). Adult dose 4 mg every 8 hours. Pediatric dose: children 7 to 14 years 4 mg every 8 to 12 hours; ages 2 to 6 years 2 mg every 8 to 12 hours.

Prednisone. Adult dose 50 to 80 mg the first day for severe seasonal allergies that don't respond to other medications. Each day, the dose is decreased by 10 mg. The pediatric dose is 1 mg/kg (2.2 lb) of body weight the first day, tapered every 4 days by halving the dose. Administer with food or with an antacid, if possible. Corticosteroids should always be taken with the understanding that a rare side effect is serious deterioration of the head ("ball" of the ball-and-socket joint) of the femur, the long bone of the thigh. Corticosteroids are interchangeable to a certain degree. If you must substitute, here is a rough measure of equivalence: 20 mg prednisone equals 16 mg methylprednisolone equals 3 mg dexamethasone.

When corticosteroids are administered to a person for a sufficiently long period of time, the adrenal glands (which manufacture the same hormones) are suppressed. To allow the adrenal glands to recover, the following rules should be observed:

1. If someone has been receiving a high (non-tapered) dose of a corticosteroid for 5 days or less, then the medication can be abruptly discontinued without consideration for adrenal suppression.
2. If someone has been receiving a high (non-tapered) dose of a corticosteroid for 6 to 10 days, then the medication should be tapered over an additional 7 days.

Triprolidine with pseudoephedrine (Actifed). Adult dose 1 tablet every 8 hours; pediatric dose (6 to 12 years of age) half tablet every 8 hours.

Side effect: Drowsiness.

FOR RELIEF FROM SEVERE ASTHMA OR CHRONIC OBSTRUCTIVE PULMONARY DISEASE

Many asthma and chronic obstructive pulmonary disease (COPD) medications are administered by metered-dose inhaler. The proper technique for using this device is as follows:

1. Shake the inhaler vigorously for 5 seconds before each use.
2. Invert the inhaler so that the opening is downward if directed to do so. Hold the inhaler 4 cm (1.6 in) in front of an open mouth, or place a spacer on the opening, around which the lips will be sealed.
3. Exhale fully. Close your lips around the spacer, or hold the device about 4 cm (1.6 in) from your mouth, or close your lips around the mouthpiece.
4. Activate the inhaler at the beginning of inspiration.
5. Inhale slowly and deeply to full lung capacity.
6. Hold your breath for 10 seconds, then exhale slowly.
7. Wait 1 minute before repeating all steps before the next puff. Shake the inhaler before each puff.

Epinephrine (adrenaline) 1:1000 aqueous solution. Epinephrine (adrenaline) 1:1000 aqueous solution. Adult dose 0.3 to 0.5 mL injected intramuscularly (see page 444) into the lateral thigh. If the thigh is obese, whether in an adult or a child, such that the needle might not reach into muscle, then inject into the lower thigh. If obesity is extreme, consider injecting into the mid-calf. This may be repeated two times at 20-minute intervals. The pediatric dose is 0.01 mL /kg (2.2 lb) of body weight, not to exceed 0.3 mL, injected intramuscularly into the lateral thigh. If the thigh is obese, whether in an adult or a child, such that the needle might not reach into muscle, then inject into the lower thigh. If obesity is extreme, consider injecting into the mid-calf. *Unless the situation is life-threatening, don't use epinephrine if the victim is older than 45 years, has a known history of heart disease, or is a pregnant female. Don't use epinephrine for treatment of COPD.*

Side effects: Rapid heartbeat, nervousness.

The only reason to administer the drug subcutaneously (see page 446) is if the equipment is not available for an intramuscular injection. The drug is available in preloaded syringes in certain allergy kits, which include the EpiPen autoinjector and EpiPen Jr. autoinjector, the Auvi-Q "talking" autoinjector (0.3 mg or 0.15 mg dose), and the Adrenaclick (0.3 mg or 0.15 mg dose). Other devices worldwide are the Jext, Emerade, Allerject, and Anapen. Instructions for use accompany the kits. For dosing purposes, a 0.3 mg autoinjector should be used for adults and children over 66 lb (30 kg) in weight. Children 66 lb and under should be injected with a 0.15 mg autoinjector.

Take particular care to handle preloaded syringes properly, to avoid inadvertent injection into an unintended location, such as a finger or toe. Don't intentionally inject epinephrine into the buttocks or a vein. Epinephrine should not be exposed to heat or sun, but does not need to be kept refrigerated. If clear (liquid) epinephrine turns cloudy or discolored, it should be discarded. When administering an injection, *never* share needles between people.

Primatene Mist (inhaler) is a mixture of epinephrine and alcohol available over the counter. This preparation should not be used in substitution for injected epinephrine in cases of severe asthma.

Side effects: Rapid heartbeat, nervousness.

Terbutaline (Brethine) tablets. Adult dose 2.5 to 5 mg every 6 to 8 hours.

Terbutaline (Brethaire) metered-dose inhaler. Adult dose two puffs every 4 to 6 hours.

Flunisolide (Aerobid) metered-dose inhaler. Adult dose as directed.

Triamcinolone acetonide (Azmacort) metered-dose inhaler. Adult dose one puff twice a day for treatment of chronic asthma, equivalent to 10 mg per day of oral prednisone.

Albuterol (Ventolin) or metaproterenol (Alupent) metered-dose inhaler. Adult dose two puffs every 4 hours as needed.

Side effects: Rapid heartbeat, nervousness ("jitters").

Ipratropium bromide metered-dose inhaler. Adult dose two puffs every 4 hours.

Tiotropium bromide dry-powder inhaler. Adult dose one puff a day.

Combivent (ipratropium bromide and albuterol sulfate) metered-dose inhaler. Adult dose two puffs four to six times a day, not to exceed 12 puffs in 24 hours.

Bitolterol (Tornalate) metered-dose inhaler. Adult dose two puffs every 8 hours.

Pirbuterol (Maxair) metered-dose inhaler. Adult dose two puffs every 4 to 6 hours.

Salmeterol xinafoate (Serevent) or formoterol fumarate dry-powder inhaler. Adult dose one puff every 12 hours. Longer-acting beta-2 agonists, such as salmeterol, have been associated with a worsening of asthma episodes with or without the use of shorter acting beta-2 agonists, such as albuterol, so persons who take salmeterol should be watched carefully when they suffer an asthma attack.

Budesonide/formoterol fumarate dihydrate inhalation aerosol (Symbicort). Adult dose two inhalations twice daily.

Fluticasone propionate/250 micrograms plus salmeterol 50 micrograms (Advair Diskus). Adult dose one inhalation twice a day.

Metaproterenol (Alupent) tablets. Adult dose 20 mg every 4 to 6 hours; pediatric dose (6 to 9 years of age or less than 60 lb, or 27.2 kg, of body weight) 10 mg.

Albuterol (Ventolin) tablets. Adult dose 2 to 4 mg three to four times a day.

Cromolyn sodium (Intal) metered-dose inhaler. Adult and pediatric dose two puffs every 4 to 6 hours; not for use in children younger than 5 years of age.

Theophylline. Adult dose 100 to 200 mg every 6 to 8 hours; pediatric dose 4 mg/kg (2.2 lb) of body weight every 6 to 8 hours.

Prednisone. Adult dose 50 to 80 mg the first day. Each day, the dose is decreased by 10 mg. The pediatric dose is 1 mg/kg (2.2 lb) of body weight the first day, tapered every 4 days by halving the dose. Administer with food or with an antacid, if possible. Corticosteroids should always be taken with the understanding that a rare side effect is serious deterioration of the head ("ball" of the ball-and-socket joint) of the femur, the long bone of the thigh. Corticosteroids are interchangeable to a certain degree. If you must substitute, here is a rough measure of equivalence: 20 mg prednisone equals 16 mg methylprednisolone equals 3 mg dexamethasone.

When corticosteroids are administered to a person for a sufficiently long period of time, the adrenal glands (which manufacture the same hormones) are suppressed. To allow the adrenal glands to recover, the following rules should be observed:

1. If someone has been receiving a high (non-tapered) dose of a corticosteroid for 5 days or less, then the medication can be abruptly discontinued without consideration for adrenal suppression.

2. If someone has been receiving a high (non-tapered) dose of a corticosteroid for 6 to 10 days, then the medication should be tapered over an additional 7 days.

FOR RELIEF FROM MILD ASTHMA

In addition to drugs under "For Relief from Severe Asthma":

Ipratropium bromide (Atrovent) metered-dose inhaler. Adult dose two puffs every 4 to 6 hours as needed. Don't exceed 12 puffs in 24 hours. Don't use in children younger than 12 years of age.

Beclomethasone dipropionate (Vanceril) metered-dose inhaler. Adult dose 2 puffs every 4 to 6 hours, not to exceed 20 puffs in 24 hours; pediatric dose (6 to 12 years of age) 1 or 2 puffs every 6 hours, not to exceed 10 puffs in 24 hours. Rinse the mouth after each use.

Zafirlukast (Accolate). Adult dose 20 mg tablet twice a day taken 1 hour before or 2 hours following meals. Don't use in children younger than 12 years of age.

FOR TREATMENT OF CHEST PAIN (ANGINA)

Nitroglycerin $\frac{1}{150}$ grain (0.4 mg) or lingual aerosol (0.4 mg metered dose per spray). Adult dose one tablet dissolved under the tongue, or one spray under the tongue, for treatment of angina. This may be repeated every 10 minutes for two additional doses.

    Side effects: Dizziness (low blood pressure), headache. If a person uses nitroglycerin and becomes faint, he should lie down with his legs elevated until his skin color returns to normal and he feels better (usually, in a minute or two). If chest pain or weakness persists, this may indicate a heart attack (see page 47).

Nitroglycerin patch 0.4 to 0.6 mg. Apply for 12 to 24 hours.

Isosorbide mononitrate or dinitrate (short-acting formulation). Adult dose 20 to 60 mg by mouth twice daily.

Isosorbide mononitrate or dinitrate (sustained-release formulation). Adult dose 60 to 120 mg by mouth twice daily.

    Side effects: Headache, dizziness, nausea, irregular heartbeat (palpitations). This drug should not be given with medications for erectile dysfunction (e.g., sildenafil citrate [Viagra]).

Metoprolol (short-acting formulation). Adult dose 50 to 150 mg by mouth twice daily.

Metoprolol (sustained-release formulation). Adult dose 100 to 300 mg once daily.

    Side effects: Fatigue, shortness of breath, wheezing, weakness, dizziness. Should be used with caution in persons with chronic obstructive pulmonary disease, diabetes, depression, severe peripheral vascular disease, certain abnormal heart rhythms, or erectile dysfunction.

Nifedipine (sustained-release formulation). 30 to 90 mg by mouth once daily.

Verapamil (short-acting formulation). 20 to 120 mg 2 to 3 times by mouth daily.

Verapamil (sustained-release formulation). 180 to 240 mg by mouth once or twice daily.

Diltiazem (sustained-release formulation). 120 to 480 mg by mouth once daily.

FOR TREATMENT OF CONGESTIVE HEART FAILURE

Furosemide (Lasix) diuretic (promotes urination). Adult dose 1 to 4 tablets (20 to 80 mg) each day for the fluid retention associated with heart failure. Diuretics should not be used for fluid retention not associated with heart failure (such as that from high altitude) or for weight reduction.

Digoxin (Lanoxin). Adult dose 0.125 to 0.25 mg each day.

FOR TREATMENT OF SEIZURES (EPILEPSY)

Doses of antiseizure medications vary widely, depending on the age and size of the patient, whether or not other drugs are also being taken, any underlying chronic diseases, and other factors. Therefore, the doses for these medications are listed for reference only as possible maintenance doses.

Diphenylhydantoin (Dilantin). Adult dose 300 to 400 mg per day; pediatric dose 2.5 mg/kg (2.2 lb) of body weight twice a day.

Phenobarbital. Adult dose 60 to 120 mg three times per day; pediatric dose 1 to 1.5 mg/kg (2.2 lb) of body weight three times a day.

Carbamazepine (Tegretol). Adult dose 400 to 1200 mg a day in two to three divided doses; pediatric dose 10 to 20 mg/kg (2.2 lb) of body weight each day in two to three divided doses.

Levetiracetam (Keppra). Adult dose 500 to 1500 mg twice a day; pediatric dose 10 to 30 mg/kg (2.2 lb) of body weight twice a day.

Lamotrigine (Lamictal). Adult dose 100 to 200 mg once a day; pediatric dose children ages 2 to 12 years 1 to 5 mg/kg (2.2 lb) body weight in one or two divided doses.

Pregabalin (Lyrica). Adult dose 150 to 600 mg once a day.

Valproic acid (Depakote). Adult and pediatric (ages 10 years and older) dose 10 to 50 mg/kg (2.2 lb) body weight once a day.

Clonazepam (Klonopin). Adult dose 1.5 to 20 mg per day in three divided doses; pediatric dose (up to 10 years of age) 0.1 to 0.2 mg/kg (2.2 lb) of body weight in three divided doses.

Gabapentin (Neurontin). Adult dose 900 to 1800 mg per day in three divided doses; pediatric dose ages 3 to 12 years 25 to 40 mg/kg (2.2 lb) per day in three divided doses.

Trimethadione (Tridione). Adult dose 300 to 600 mg 3 or 4 times a day; pediatric dose 100 to 300 mg 3 or 4 times a day.

Primidone (Mysoline). Adult and pediatric (ages 8 years and over) dose 250 mg 3 or 4 times a day.

Ethosuximide (Zarontin). Adult and pediatric dose ages 3 years of age and older 20 mg/kg (2.2 lb) per day not to exceed 1.5 g daily.

FOR RELIEF FROM PAIN (SEE ALSO "FOR RELIEF FROM MUSCLE ACHES OR MINOR ARTHRITIS")

Acetylsalicylic acid (aspirin). Adult dose 325 to 1000 mg every 4 to 6 hours (maximum dose 4000 mg per day); pediatric dose 60 mg (1 grain) per year of age (not to exceed 600 mg) every 4 to 6 hours.

Side effect: Stomach irritation. Don't administer to a person with an ulcer or upset stomach. Take with food or an antacid, if possible. Enteric-coated aspirin (such as Ecotrin) helps prevent stomach irritation and should be used whenever possible. To avoid Reye syndrome (postviral encephalopathy and liver failure), don't use aspirin to control fever in a child under age 17 years.

Acetaminophen (Tylenol). Adult dose 500 to 1000 mg every 4 to 6 hours (maximum dose 4000 mg per day); pediatric dose: up to 1 year, 60 mg; 1 to 3 years, 60 to 120 mg; 3 to 6 years, 120 mg; 6 to 12 years, 240 mg. Acetaminophen taken in too high a quantity acutely or over time can cause liver failure, so it is very important to keep track of the amount ingested, including as part of combination medications.

Codeine. Adult dose 30 to 60 mg every 6 to 8 hours; pediatric dose 0.5 to 1 mg/kg (2.2 lb) of body weight.

Side effects: Codeine is a narcotic and has side effects of drowsiness and alteration of mental status. In addition, it may cause constipation.

Acetaminophen (Tylenol) 325 mg with codeine 30 mg. Adult dose one to two tablets every 4 to 6 hours.

Hydrocodone 5 mg with acetaminophen 500 mg (Vicodin). Adult dose one to two tablets every 4 to 6 hours. This is a narcotic drug and should not be taken in any situation in which altered mental status will be dangerous.

Ketorolac (Toradol) 10 mg. Adult dose one tablet every 6 to 8 hours. This is an antiinflammatory drug that is particularly useful for persons suffering kidney stones.

FOR RELIEF FROM FEVER

Acetylsalicylic acid (aspirin). Same as "For Relief from Pain." To avoid Reye syndrome (postviral encephalopathy and liver failure), don't use aspirin to control fever in a child under age 17 years.

Acetaminophen (Tylenol). Same as "For Relief from Pain."

Ibuprofen (Motrin, Advil, Nuprin). Adult dose 400 to 600 mg every 4 to 6 hours; pediatric dose 5 to 10 mg/kg (2.2 lb) of body weight, not to exceed 400 mg.

FOR RELIEF FROM MUSCLE ACHES OR MINOR ARTHRITIS

Acetylsalicylic acid (aspirin). Same as "For Relief from Pain."

Acetaminophen (Tylenol). Same as "For Relief from Pain."

Nonsteroidal antiinflammatory drugs ("NSAIDs"; should not be taken on an empty stomach; side effects are abdominal pain and diarrhea).

Ibuprofen (Motrin, Advil, Nuprin). Adult dose 400 to 800 mg every 6 to 8 hours.

Ketoprofen (Orudis KT, Actron). Adult dose 12.5 to 50 mg every 6 to 8 hours.

Naproxen (Naprosyn, Aleve). Adult dose 250 to 500 mg every 6 to 12 hours.

Naproxen sodium (Naprelan). Adult dose 375 or 500 mg sustained release every 24 hours.

Ketorolac (Toradol). Adult dose 10 mg every 8 to 12 hours; don't exceed 3 days' consecutive use.

Diclofenac/misoprostol (Arthrotec). Adult dose 50 to 75 mg (based on diclofenac) every 6 to 8 hours. This drug should not be given to women who are pregnant or who may become pregnant, because misoprostol may induce a miscarriage.

Celecoxib (Celebrex). Adult dose 10 to 200 mg twice a day. This is a COX-2 antagonist drug. *This drug is possibly associated with a higher incidence of heart attack in persons who use it.*

FOR RELIEF FROM MUSCLE SPASM

Metaxalone (Skelaxin). Adult dose 800 mg 3 or 4 times a day for relief from acute painful muscle spasms.

FOR RELIEF FROM MIGRAINE HEADACHE

Sumatriptan oral tablets. Adult dose 50 to 100 mg every 2 hours, not to exceed 200 mg/day.

Sumatriptan nasal spray. Adult dose 5 or 20 mg every 2 hours, not to exceed 40 mg/day.

Zolmitriptan oral tablets. Adult dose 2.5 to 5 mg every 2 hours, not to exceed 10 mg/day.

Zolmitriptan "melting" tablets. Adult dose 2.5 mg to dissolve under the tongue every 2 hours, not to exceed 10 mg/day.

Rizatriptan oral tablets. Adult dose 5 or 10 mg every 2 hours, not to exceed 30 mg/day. If propranolol is also taken, use the 5 mg dose.

Almotriptan oral tablets. Adult dose 6.25 or 12.5 mg every 2 hours, not to exceed 25 mg/day.

Naratriptan oral tablets. Adult dose 1 or 2.5 mg every 4 hours, not to exceed 5 mg/day.

Frovatriptan oral tablets. Adult dose 2.5 mg every 4 hours, not to exceed 5 mg/day.

Eletriptan oral tablets. Adult dose 20 or 40 mg every 2 hours, not to exceed 80 mg/day.

FOR RELIEF FROM ITCHING

Diphenhydramine (Benadryl). Same as "For Relief from a Mild Allergic Reaction."

Hydroxyzine (Atarax). Adult dose 25 to 50 mg every 8 hours; pediatric dose: up to 6 years 10 mg every 8 hours; 6 to 12 years 10 to 25 mg every 8 hours.

FOR RELIEF FROM TOOTHACHE

Benzocaine-phenol-alcohol (Anbesol). For topical application to the gums.
Oil of cloves. For topical application to the gums.

FOR RELIEF FROM MOTION SICKNESS

Dimenhydrinate (Dramamine). Adult dose 50 mg every 4 to 6 hours; pediatric dose (8 to 12
years of age) 25 mg every 4 to 6 hours.
Side effect: Drowsiness.
Meclizine (Antivert, Bonine). Adult dose 25 to 50 mg one to two times per day. Don't give this
drug to children under age 12 years.
Side effect: Drowsiness.
Cyclizine (Marezine). Adult dose 25 mg; pediatric dose 12.5 mg for ages 9 to 12.
Scopolamine (Transderm-Scōp Transdermal Therapeutic System). Adult dose: Apply 1 patch
(1.5 mg scopolamine) on the hairless area behind the ear. A single patch is good for 3
days. Take care to wash the hands carefully after application of the patch, to avoid getting
any medication in the eyes. Not approved for children under age 12.
Side effects: Blurred vision, dry mouth, decreased sweating, difficulty with urination,
propensity to heat illness, altered mental status. A diver who uses this preparation
should be alert to the danger of heat illness while out of the water encased in a
constrictive (heat-retaining) wet suit.

FOR RELIEF FROM NAUSEA AND VOMITING

Ondansetron (Zofran). Adult dose 4 or 8 mg tablet dissolved on the tongue every 8 hours;
pediatric dose 0.15 mg/kg body weight of the oral dissolving tablet every 8 hours. This
drug is also indicated for nausea and vomiting after surgery or associated with
chemotherapy. It appears to be safe in children and in the elderly.
Prochlorperazine (Compazine). Adult dose 5 to 10 mg by mouth every 8 to 12 hours (by
suppository 25 mg twice daily). Don't give this drug to children under age 12 years.
Side effects: Neck spasms, difficulty in swallowing and talking (inability to control the
tongue—it may stiffen and/or protrude from the mouth), restlessness, difficulty with
eye movement, and muscle stiffness. These side effects may occur in combination
("dystonic reaction"). If any of these occur, discontinue use of the drug and administer
diphenhydramine (Benadryl) 50 mg every 6 hours for four doses. If a child has a dystonic
reaction, the dose of diphenhydramine (Benadryl) to alleviate the side effects is 1 mg/kg
(2.2 lb) of body weight. Be certain that the victim is capable of purposeful swallowing.
Promethazine (Phenergan). Adult dose 25 mg every 6 to 8 hours (by suppository 12.5 to
25 mg every 12 hours); pediatric dose 0.25 to 0.5 mg/kg (2.2 lb) of body weight by mouth
or per rectum (suppository).
Side effects: Similar to those with prochlorperazine.
Trimethobenzamide (Tigan). Adult dose 250 mg by mouth or 200 mg by suppository every 6
to 8 hours.
Side effects: Similar to those with prochlorperazine.
Metoclopramide (Reglan). Adult dose 10 mg by mouth every 6 hours.
Side effect: Movement disorder.
Cyclizine hydrochloride (Marezine). Adult dose 25 to 50 mg every 6 to 8 hours.

FOR RELIEF FROM DIARRHEA

Loperamide (Imodium or Pepto Diarrhea Control caplets). Adult dose two pills (2 mg each)
initially, followed by one pill after each loose bowel movement, not to exceed eight pills.

With uncomplicated (no fever or blood in stools) watery diarrhea, this drug can be given to children age 2 years and older. The dose in children is 0.2 mg/kg (2.2 lb) of body weight every 6 hours. The liquid preparation contains 1 mg per 5 teaspoons (5 mL).

Diphenoxylate (Lomotil). Adult dose two tablets two to four times per day. Don't give this drug to children under age 18 years.

Bismuth subsalicylate (Pepto-Bismol). Adult dose 2 tablespoons (30 mL) or two tablets every 30 to 60 minutes, not to exceed 8 to 10 doses; pediatric dose: 3 to 6 years, 1 teaspoon (5 mL) or ½ tablet; 6 to 10 years, 2 teaspoons (10 mL) or one tablet; 1 to 14 years, 4 teaspoons (20 mL) or 1½ tablets; may repeat dose in children every 1 hour, not to exceed four doses. This drug should not be given to people who are sensitive to aspirin-containing products, have kidney disease or gout, or who are taking anticoagulants, probenecid, or methotrexate.

Side effects: Black discoloration of the tongue and bowel movements, ringing in the ears, nausea, and constipation.

Kaolin-pectin (Kaopectate). Adult dose 4 to 8 tablespoons (60 to 120 mL) after each loose bowel movement; pediatric dose: 3 to 6 years 1 to 2 tablespoons (15 to 30 mL); 6 to 12 years 2 to 4 tablespoons (30 to 60 mL); older than 12 years 4 tablespoons (60 mL) after each loose bowel movement. This drug is of limited value; it does not shorten the course of diarrheal illness, and acts only to add a little consistency to stools.

FOR RELIEF FROM CONSTIPATION

Mineral oil. Adult dose 1 to 2 tablespoons (15 to 30 mL); pediatric (older than 5 years) dose 1 to 2 teaspoons (5 to 10 mL). This drug is a mild laxative.

Docusate sodium (Colace). Adult dose 100 mg twice a day; pediatric dose 0.3 mg/kg (2.2 lb) of body weight once or twice a day. The dose should be adjusted to the response. This drug is a stool softener.

Docusate sodium (stool softener) with casanthranol (laxative) (Peri-Colace). Adult dose one capsule once or twice a day.

Docusate sodium (stool softener) 5 mL microenema. Adult dose 200 mg (one enema) once a day as necessary.

Docusate calcium (stool softener) (Surfak Stool Softener Gel Cap). Adult dose 240 mg once or twice a day.

Senna extract (Senokot). Two tablets a day at bedtime. This drug is a mild laxative.

Magnesium hydroxide (Phillips' Milk of Magnesia). Adult dose 1 to 2 tablespoons (15 to 30 mL) once or twice a day. This drug is a mild laxative.

Magnesium citrate (Evac-Q-Mag). Adult dose 10 to 20 tablespoons (150 to 300 mL) as needed.

Lactulose syrup, USP (Duphalac). Adult dose 1 to 2 tablespoons (15 to 30 mL) daily. This drug is a mild laxative.

Bisacodyl (Dulcolax). Adult dose two 5 mg tablets or one 10 mg suppository. This drug is a moderate laxative. A child age 6 to 12 years may take one 5 mg tablet.

Cascara sagrada 150 mg; aloe 100 mg (Nature's Remedy) (laxative). Adult dose two tablets a day.

Psyllium mucilloid (Metamucil, Perdiem, Fiberall). Adult dose titrate up to 20 g per day. These natural psyllium fiber products increase the bulk of the stool, and should be ingested with at least a quart (liter) of liquid.

Methylcellulose (Citrucel). Adult dose titrate up to 20 g per day.

Polycarbophil (Fibercon, Equalactin, Konsyl). Adult dose titrate up to 20 g per day.

Lactulose. 10 mg/15 mL of syrup. Adult dose 15 to 30 mL per day, up to 60 mL per day.

Polyethylene glycol solution (MiraLax). 17 g powder (1 heaping tablespoon) dissolved in 8 oz (240 mL) water, taken once per day for up to 4 days to produce a bowel movement.

FOR RELIEF FROM ULCER PAIN

Mylanta II. Adult dose 2 tablespoons (30 mL) or two tablets (chewed) 1 and 3 hours after meals, at bedtime, and as needed. This is a mixture of aluminum hydroxide, magnesium hydroxide, and simethicone.

Rolaids. Adult dose one to two tablets (chewed) after meals as necessary. These contain dihydroxy-aluminum sodium carbonate. Because of the relatively high sodium content, these should not be used routinely by people with congestive heart failure (see page 44).

Cimetidine (Tagamet). Adult dose 300 mg three times a day with meals and at bedtime. This H2RA (antagonist to histamine H2 receptor) drug decreases the secretion of gastric acid.

Ranitidine hydrochloride (Zantac). Adult dose 75 to 150 mg two times a day. This H2RA drug decreases the secretion of gastric acid.

Famotidine (Pepcid). Adult dose 20 mg twice a day or 40 mg at bedtime for 4 weeks to treat an active duodenal ulcer, then 20 mg at bedtime for 2 to 4 weeks for suppression therapy to diminish the secretion of gastric acid. This H2RA drug decreases the secretion of gastric acid.

Propantheline bromide (Pro-Banthine). Adult dose 7.5 to 15 mg three times a day before meals and at bedtime. This drug is used to control gastric acid secretion and to reduce bowel activity (decrease cramping).

Sucralfate (Carafate). Adult dose one tablet (gram) 1 hour before meals and at bedtime. This drug binds to the ulcer crater and therefore requires the presence of acid to work properly. Thus, antacids should not be ingested within 30 minutes before or after the ingestion of sucralfate.

Omeprazole (Prilosec). Adult dose one capsule (20 mg) a day given 30 minutes before a meal. This proton (acid) pump inhibitor (PPI) drug diminishes gastric acid secretion.

Rabeprazole (Aciphex). Adult dose 20 mg once a day. This PPI (proton [acid] pump inhibitor) drug diminishes gastric acid secretion.

FOR RELIEF FROM INDIGESTION OR GAS PAINS

Antacid (such as Mylanta II). Same as "For Relief from Ulcer Pain."

Simethicone (Mylicon-80). Adult dose one to two tablets (chewed) after meals and at bedtime.

FOR RELIEF FROM HEARTBURN (REFLUX ESOPHAGITIS)

Omeprazole (Prilosec). Adult dose 10 to 20 mg once a day.

Antacid (such as Mylanta II). Same as "For Relief from Ulcer Pain."

Ranitidine hydrochloride (Zantac). Adult dose 75 mg every 12 hours as needed. This H2RA (antagonist to histamine H2 receptor) drug decreases the secretion of gastric acid.

Cimetidine (Tagamet HB). Adult dose 200 mg (two 100 mg tablets) 30 to 60 minutes before a meal, not to exceed twice in a 24-hour period. This H2RA drug decreases the secretion of gastric acid.

Famotidine (Pepcid AC). Adult dose 10 to 20 mg as 10 mg chewable tablet or gelcap twice a day for up to 6 weeks.

Gaviscon or Gaviscon II. Adult dose one to two tablets (chewed) or 1 to 2 tablespoons (15 to 30 mL) (liquid preparation) after each meal and at bedtime. This is a mixture of aluminum hydroxide, magnesium trisilicate, sodium bicarbonate, and alginic acid.

Metoclopramide hydrochloride (Reglan). Adult dose 10 mg up to four times a day, 30 minutes before meals and at bedtime.

Side effects: Rarely, neck spasms, difficulty in swallowing and talking (inability to control the tongue—it may stiffen and protrude from the mouth), difficulty with eye movement, and muscle stiffness. These side effects may occur in combination ("dystonic reaction"). If any of these occur, discontinue use of the drug and administer diphenhydramine (Benadryl) 50 mg every 6 hours for four doses. Be certain that the victim is capable of purposeful swallowing.

FOR RELIEF FROM NASAL CONGESTION

Pseudoephedrine (Sudafed). Adult dose 30 to 60 mg every 6 to 8 hours; pediatric dose 1 mg/kg (2.2 lb) of body weight. **The U.S. Food and Drug Administration recommends that this drug not be used in children under 6 years of age.**

Phenylephrine hydrochloride 0.25% nasal spray (Neo-Synephrine ¼%). Adult dose two to three drops or sprays twice a day; pediatric dose (older than 6 years) 0.125% two drops twice a day. Don't use this drug for more than 3 consecutive days, to avoid "rebound" swelling of the nasal passages from chemical irritation and sensitization to the medicine.

Oxymetazoline hydrochloride 0.05% (Afrin). Adult dose two to three drops or sprays twice a day; pediatric dose (older than 6 years) two 0.025% (half-strength) drops twice a day. Don't use this drug for more than 3 consecutive days, to avoid "rebound" swelling of the nasal passages from chemical irritation and sensitization to the medicine.

FOR RELIEF FROM COUGH

A U.S. Food and Drug Administration advisory panel in 2007 recommended that there is no evidence that over-the-counter cold and cough medicines work in children and that the products should not be given to children younger than 6 years of age.

Glyceryl guaiacolate (Robitussin) expectorant. Adult dose 1 teaspoon (5 mL) every 3 to 4 hours.
Robitussin A-C: Plus codeine (cough suppressant).
Robitussin-DAC: Plus codeine, pseudoephedrine (decongestant).
Robitussin-PE: Plus pseudoephedrine.
Robitussin-DM: Plus dextromethorphan (cough suppressant).

Codeine. Adult dose 15 to 30 mg every 4 to 6 hours. This is a potent cough suppressant.

CoTylenol Liquid Cold Formula. Adult dose 2 tablespoons (30 mL) every 6 hours; 2 tablespoons (30 mL) contains dextromethorphan hydrobromide 30 mg (for cough), acetaminophen 650 mg (for fever, aches), chlorpheniramine maleate (antihistamine) 4 mg, and pseudoephedrine hydrochloride (decongestant) 60 mg.

Dextromethorphan hydrobromide–guaifenesin (Vicks Cough Syrup). Adult dose 2 to 3 teaspoons (10 to 15 mL) every 4 to 6 hours.

Dextromethorphan hydrobromide–guaifenesin–phenylpropanolamine (Naldecon cough syrup). Adult dose 1 teaspoon (5 mL) every 4 hours.

Buckwheat honey. Dose 1 to 2 teaspoons for children ages 2 to 18 years. *It is not advised to feed honey to infants or children younger than 12 months of age because of the risk for infant botulism.*

Mucinex (guaifenesin 600 mg). This drug is taken every 12 hours and works to help loosen phlegm (mucus) and thin bronchial secretions to rid the bronchial passageways of bothersome mucus and make coughs more productive.

FOR RELIEF FROM SORE THROAT

Benzocaine-hexylresorcinol (Sucrets antiseptic throat lozenges).
Benzocaine-cetylpyridinium (Cēpacol lozenges, Vicks lozenges).

COLD FORMULAS

A U.S. Food and Drug Administration advisory panel in 2007 recommended that there is no evidence that over-the-counter cold and cough medicines work in children and that the products should *not* be given to children younger than 6 years of age.

SKIN MEDICATIONS
Antiseptic Ointments, Solutions, and Scrubs
Apply ointments thinly to the skin twice a day.

Bacitracin antiseptic ointment.

Bacitracin–polymyxin B sulfate (Polysporin) ointment.

Mupirocin (Bactroban) 2% ointment.

Mupirocin (Bactroban) calcium 2% cream.

Bacitracin–polymyxin B sulfate–neomycin (Neosporin, triple antibiotic, or Mycitracin) ointment.

Neomycin-gramicidin (Spectrocin) ointment.

Neomycin (Myciguent) ointment.

Retapamulin 1% (Altabax) ointment.

Povidone–iodine 0.5% (Betadine First Aid) cream.

Silver sulfadiazine (Silvadene) cream. Soothing antiseptic cream for burns; apply to the skin once or twice a day. Don't use in children younger than 2 years. Avoid use on the face.

Benzalkonium chloride (Zephiran) antiseptic solution (1:750 dilution in water). May be used full strength to clean unbroken skin, but should be diluted 1:2 or 1:3 with water to swab an open wound or animal bite (to kill rabies virus).

Hexachlorophene scrub (pHisoHex). Use as a scrubbing soap on cuts, scrapes, and infected skin. Don't use on children under 1 year of age.

Povidone–iodine (Betadine) antiseptic solution. Use in a 1:10 dilution with water to gently scrub cuts and scrapes.

Anti-Itch, Anti-Sting
Campho-Phenique. Topical anti-itch gel medication consisting of camphorated phenol in mineral oil.

Campho-Phenique Maximum Strength ointment or Neosporin Plus ointment or Mycitracin Plus ointment. Topical anti-itch and antiseptic medication consisting of lidocaine hydrochloride, bacitracin zinc, neomycin sulfate, and polymyxin B sulfate.

Lidocaine hydrochloride 2.5% anesthetic ointment. Use for relief from pain due to scrapes; apply to the skin and leave in place for 10 minutes before scrubbing. Don't apply if the area to be covered is greater than 5% of the total body surface area (an area approximately four to five times the size of the victim's palm).

Benzalkonium chloride 0.13%; lidocaine hydrochloride 2.5% (Bactine solution). Very mild antiseptic–anesthetic combination available over the counter. May be used to swab animal bites if Zephiran is not available.

Calamine lotion. Apply thinly as a drying agent two to three times a day to skin affected with poison ivy, oak, or sumac.

Phenolated (1%) calamine lotion. Apply thinly as a drying agent two to three times a day to skin affected with poison ivy, oak, or sumac.

Calamine–pramoxine hydrochloride 1% (Caladryl). Apply thinly as a drying agent two to three times a day to skin affected with poison ivy, oak, or sumac.

Hydrocortisone and pramoxine (Pramosone). Topical anti-itch medication for skin rashes due to plant allergy, insect bites, or sunburn. Apply two to three times a day.

Antifungal Cream, Lotion, Pill, Spray and Powder
Apply to the skin two to three times a day for athlete's foot or jock itch.

Tolnaftate 1% (Tinactin, Aftate)

Terbinafine 1% cream or spray (Lamisil)

Clotrimazole 1% (Lotrimin, Mycelex)

Clotrimazole oral

Zinc undecylenate (Desenex)

Miconazole nitrate 2% (Micatin)

Naftifine (Naftin) 2%

Nizoral cream. Apply thinly once or twice a day to treat yeast or fungal infection.

Nizoral. 400 mg one oral dose for tinea versicolor (harmless yeast overgrowth on the skin); induce mild sweating 2 to 4 hours after dose; don't shower for 8 hours after dose (the drug is excreted in sweat).

Spectazole cream. Apply thinly once or twice a day to treat yeast or fungal infection.

Anti-Mites

Permethrin 5% cream (Elimite). Apply to entire skin, leave on for 8 hours, and then shower for treatment of scabies; appears to be safe in pregnant women and children over 2 months of age.

Permethrin 1% creme rinse (Nix). Apply to washed and towel-dried hair, leave on for 10 minutes, and then rinse thoroughly and comb out nits for treatment of head lice.

Malathion (Ovide). Apply to dry hair, leave on without occlusion for 8 to 12 hours, and then shampoo and rinse thoroughly and comb out nits for treatment of head lice.

Crotamiton (Eurax). For topical use only. To treat scabies, take a bath or shower. Apply the medication over the whole body from the chin down. Rub in gently, paying special attention to skinfolds and creases. Trim fingernails and apply the medication under the nails. Change all clothing and bed linens the next morning and wash them in the hot cycle of the washing machine. A second application of the medication should be done in 24 hours. Take a good cleaning bath or shower 48 hours after the last application. To relieve dry skin, apply a small amount of the medication to the affected area and rub it in gently until it disappears. Avoid use on open, irritated, or inflamed skin. Avoid use near the eyes, mouth, or vagina.

Spinosad (Natroba) 0.9% suspension. For topical use only. Apply as a liquid to the affected scalp and hair to treat head lice. Shake the suspension well right before each use to mix the medication evenly. Cover the face and eyes with a towel and keep eyes closed during treatment. Apply spinosad suspension to dry hair and scalp area. Use enough suspension to cover the entire scalp area first and then apply upward toward the ends of the hair to cover all of the hair. Keep the suspension on the hair and scalp for 10 minutes. After 10 minutes, rinse the suspension from the scalp and hair with warm water. You should not use a shower or bathtub to rinse the suspension away because you do not want to get the suspension over the rest of your body. Anyone who helped apply the suspension should wash his hands carefully after the application and rinsing steps. Shampoo the hair after rinsing the suspension from the scalp and hair. Repeat the procedure in 1 week if lice are still present.

Topical Steroids

Hydrocortisone 1% cream, 2.5% cream (Hytone). Safe for infants, face, perianal area, skinfolds.

Triamcinolone 0.1% ointment. Often mixed with Eucerin cream 1:1; moisturizer increases penetration—too potent for face, genitalia, or infants.

FOR SLEEP

Diphenhydramine (Benadryl, Sominex, Nytol). Adult dose 50 mg at bedtime.

Triazolam (Halcion). Adult dose 0.125 to 0.25 mg at bedtime. This is short-acting and may be a better choice at high altitude.

Side effects: Short-term memory loss, bad dreams.

Zolpidem tartrate (Ambien). Adult dose 5 to 10 mg, or 6.25 mg or 12.5 mg extended release, at bedtime. There have been rare reports of hallucinations in people who took higher doses; elders may be prone to such a reaction. Cautions to users should include information that impaired performance (e.g., driving) may be present the morning after using zolpidem, particularly extended-release forms of the medication.

Zaleplon (Sonata). Adult dose 5 to 10 mg at bedtime. The dose is 5 mg for elderly, debilitated, or liver-impaired adults.

Eszopiclone (Lunesta). Adult dose 1, 2, or 3 mg at bedtime. A dose of 3 mg can cause impairment to motor skills (such as driving), memory, and coordination that can last more than 11 hours after taking an evening dose, so it is best to begin with a dose of 1 mg at bedtime.

Ramelteon (Rozerem). Adult dose 8 mg at bedtime.

Temazepam (Restoril). Adult dose 15 to 30 mg at bedtime.

Flurazepam (Dalmane). Adult dose 15 to 30 mg at bedtime.

Melatonin. The hormone melatonin is endogenously produced by humans in the pineal gland from the precursor tryptophan. Melatonin levels in the blood increase and are highest during normal hours of sleep, decreasing toward morning.

Sold over the counter, melatonin is considered a "dietary supplement" and thus does not come under the scrutiny of the U.S. Food and Drug Administration. The science supporting its use to induce sleep, decrease wakefulness during sleep, and decrease jet lag is preliminary and suggests that it might be beneficial, without any obvious adverse effects. The doses cited range from 1 mg to 5 mg administered orally 1 to 2 hours before going to bed. Recommendations for its use to treat jet lag are found on page 413.

ANTIBIOTICS

If not otherwise specified, the default initial duration for administration of an antibiotic is 7 days. *When a pediatric dose is calculated (based on age and/or body weight), do not exceed the adult dose.*

Amoxicillin. Adult dose 250 to 500 mg every 8 hours; pediatric dose 10 to 15 mg/kg (2.2 lb) of body weight every 8 hours (three times a day).

Amoxicillin–clavulanate (Augmentin). Adult dose 500 to 875 mg two times a day; pediatric dose 25 to 45 mg/kg (2.2 lb) of body weight in two divided doses per day. For otitis media in children, use the higher dose.

Ampicillin. Same dose as phenoxymethyl penicillin (see later).

Azithromycin (Zithromax). Adult dose 500 mg day 1, then 250 mg per day for 4 additional days; pediatric dose 10 mg/kg (2.2 lb) of body weight day 1, then 5 mg/kg body weight for 4 additional days. CAUTION: Azithromycin can cause abnormal changes in the electrical activity of the heart that may lead to a potentially fatal irregular heart rhythm. Persons at particular risk for this complication include those with existing "prolonged QT interval," low blood levels of potassium or magnesium, a slower than normal heart rate, or use of certain heart medications.

Cefadroxil (Duricef). Adult dose 500 mg to 1 g twice a day. For pharyngitis, to eradicate the group A streptococcus, an acceptable dose is 1 g once a day for 10 days. Pediatric dose: for skin infections, 30 mg/kg (2.2 lb) of body weight per day in two divided doses; for pharyngitis, administer in a single dose or two divided doses for 10 days.

Cefdinir. Adult dose 300 mg twice per day; pediatric dose 7 mg/kg (2.2 lb) of body weight twice per day.

Cefixime. Adult dose 400 mg per day; pediatric dose 8 mg/kg (2.2 lb) of body weight once per day; no refrigeration needed—discard 14 days after the dry powder is reconstituted with water.

Cefuroxime axetil. Adult dose 500 mg twice a day; pediatric dose 30 mg/kg (2.2 lb) of body weight in two divided doses a day.

Cefpodoxime (Vantin). Adult dose 200 to 400 mg twice a day for pneumonia; pediatric dose 10 mg/kg (2.2 lb) body weight in two divided doses.

Cefprozil (Cefzil). Adult dose 500 g once a day; pediatric dose 15 to 30 mg/kg (2.2 lb) of body weight twice per day.

Ceftibuten (Cedax). Adult dose 400 mg once a day; pediatric dose 9 mg/kg (2.2 lb) of body weight once per day.

Cephalexin (Keflex). Adult dose 250 mg every 4 to 6 hours or 500 mg every 12 hours; pediatric dose the same as for phenoxymethyl penicillin. *Avoid use* in a person with penicillin allergy, because 5% to 10% of those allergic to penicillin are also allergic to cephalosporins.

Ciprofloxacin (Cipro). Adult dose 500 mg twice a day for 3 days to treat infectious diarrhea. This drug should not be given to pregnant women or children under age 18 years. This drug should not be administered to someone with myasthenia gravis, because of the possibility of a prolonged myasthenic crisis. Ciprofloxacin is in a class of antibiotics known as fluoroquinolones. These may cause tendon weakening and rupture. The tendon rupture problem is largely a problem of adults, and in particular those over the age of 60 years. It typically affects the Achilles tendon, with onset of symptoms within the first few weeks (typically about a week) after the initiation of antibiotic therapy. Other tendons, including those of the upper extremity, may be involved. It is perhaps the large forces placed upon the Achilles tendon that makes it so prominent in this particular medical situation. If any tendon becomes tender, but does not rupture, discontinue the antibiotic and expect recovery within approximately 10 weeks. During that period, cease stressing the tendon.

Clarithromycin (Biaxin). Adult dose 500 mg twice a day; pediatric dose 15 mg/kg (2.2 lb) of body weight in two divided doses per day. *This drug should optimally not be given to a person taking atorvastatin, simvastatin, or lovastatin, to avoid the possible side effect of breaking down muscle tissue.*

Clindamycin (Cleocin). Adult dose 300 mg three times a day; pediatric dose 30 mg/kg (2.2. lb) of body weight in three or four divided doses per day.

Dicloxacillin. Same dose as phenoxymethyl penicillin (later).

Doxycycline (Vibramycin). Adult dose 100 mg twice a day for treatment, or once a day for prevention, of infectious diarrhea. Don't give to pregnant women or children up to age 7 years, because this drug may cause permanent dark discoloration of the teeth. Children above age 7 years may take 2 to 4 mg/kg (2.2 lb) of body weight in two or four divided doses.

Erythromycin. Same dose as phenoxymethyl penicillin (see later). Common side effects are stomach upset and diarrhea. This drug is the first alternative to penicillin in penicillin-allergic individuals. *This drug should not be taken in combination with nitroimidazole antifungal agents (ketoconazole, itraconazole, fluconazole), diltiazem, verapamil, or troleandomycin because of a potential interaction that might cause a serious abnormal heart rhythm associated with sudden death. This drug should optimally not be given to a person taking atorvastatin, simvastatin, or lovastatin, to avoid the possible side effect of breaking down muscle tissue.*

Fleroxacin. Adult dose 400 mg once a day for 3 days for the treatment of infectious diarrhea. This drug should not be administered to someone with myasthenia gravis, because of the possibility of a prolonged myasthenic crisis. This is a fluoroquinolone antibiotic. See the precautions for ciprofloxacin.

Levofloxacin. Adult dose 250 to 500 mg once a day. This drug should not be administered to someone with myasthenia gravis, because of the possibility of a prolonged myasthenic crisis. This is a fluoroquinolone antibiotic. See the precautions for ciprofloxacin.

Linezolid (Zyvox). Adult dose 400 to 600 mg twice a day for methicillin-resistant *Staphylococcus aureus* (MRSA) infection; pediatric dose 30 mg/kg (2.2 lb) of body weight in three divided doses.

Loracarbef (Lorabid). Adult dose 200 to 400 mg every 12 hours; pediatric dose 7.5 to 15 mg/kg (2.2 lb) of body weight every 12 hours.

Metronidazole (Flagyl). Adult dose 250 mg three times a day. Don't drink alcohol when taking this medication and for 3 days afterward; the interaction would cause severe abdominal pain, nausea, and vomiting.

Moxifloxacin (Avelox). Adult dose 400 mg once a day. This drug should not be administered to someone with myasthenia gravis, because of the possibility of a prolonged myasthenic crisis. This is a fluoroquinolone antibiotic. See the precautions for ciprofloxacin.

Noroxin. Adult dose 400 mg every 12 hours. This drug should not be administered to someone with myasthenia gravis, because of the possibility of a prolonged myasthenic crisis. This is a fluoroquinolone antibiotic. See the precautions for ciprofloxacin.

Ofloxacin. Adult dose 300 to 400 mg every 12 hours. This drug should not be administered to someone with myasthenia gravis, because of the possibility of a prolonged myasthenic crisis. This is a fluoroquinolone antibiotic. See the precautions for ciprofloxacin.

Phenoxymethyl penicillin (Penicillin VK). Adult dose 250 to 500 mg every 4 to 6 hours; pediatric dose: 2 to 6 years, 125 mg every 6 to 8 hours; 6 to 10 years, 250 mg every 6 to 8 hours. For pharyngitis, to eradicate the group A *Streptococcus*, an acceptable adult dose is 1 g twice a day for 10 days. Swelling of the lips, eyes, and mucous membranes occurs in about 1 per 10,000 courses of penicillin.

Rifampin (Rifadin). Adult and pediatric dose 20 mg/kg (2.2 lb) of body weight per day in two or four divided doses, not to exceed 600 mg per day.

Rifaximin. Adult (ages 12 years and older) dose 200 mg three times a day for traveler's diarrhea.

Sparfloxacin (Zagam). Adult dose 400 mg day 1, then 200 mg each day. *This drug should not be administered to someone with myasthenia gravis, because of the possibility of a prolonged myasthenic crisis.* This is a fluoroquinolone antibiotic. See the precautions for ciprofloxacin.

Sulfisoxazole (Gantrisin). Pediatric dose 150 mg/kg (2.2 lb) of body weight in four to six divided doses a day, not to exceed 6 g per day.

Telithromycin (Ketek). Adult (ages 13 years and older) dose 800 mg once a day.

Tetracycline. Adult dose 500 mg four times a day. Don't give to pregnant women or children up to age 7, because this drug may cause permanent dark discoloration of the teeth.

Tinidazole (Tiniba, Fasigyn). Adult dose 2 g in a single dose; pediatric dose 50 mg/kg (2.2 lb) of body weight in a single dose.

Trimethoprim–sulfamethoxazole (Bactrim or Septra DS [double strength]). Adult dose one pill (80 mg trimethoprim with 400 mg sulfamethoxazole) twice a day for infectious diarrhea or bladder infection; one pill once a day for prevention of traveler's diarrhea. The pediatric dose for an ear infection, MRSA infection, or severe infectious diarrhea (caused by *Shigella* bacteria) is 1 teaspoon (5 mL) of the pediatric suspension per 10 kg (22 lb) of body weight every 12 hours (twice a day), not to exceed 4 teaspoons (20 mL) (the adult dose) per dose. More precisely, the pediatric dose is 4 mg/kg/dose trimethoprim (TMP) with 20 mg/kg/dose sulfamethoxazole (SMX). *It is possible that elder patients who take TMP-SMX may be at increased risk for high blood level of potassium.*

Trovafloxacin (Trovan). Adult dose 200 mg once a day for 10 days to treat acute sinusitis. *This drug should not be administered to someone with myasthenia gravis, because of the possibility of a prolonged myasthenic crisis.* This is a fluoroquinolone antibiotic. See the precautions for ciprofloxacin.

APPENDIX TWO:
CONVERSION TABLES

FAHRENHEIT AND CENTIGRADE (CELSIUS) TEMPERATURE CONVERSION

To convert degrees Fahrenheit (°F) into degrees centigrade (°C, or Celsius), subtract 32, then multiply by 5, then divide by 9. To convert degrees C into degrees F, multiply by 9, then divide by 5, then add 32. For extrapolation into "subzero" (below 0°F) range, be aware that 1 Fahrenheit degree represents the temperature change of $\frac{5}{9}$ of a centigrade degree, or 1 centigrade degree represents 1.8 times the temperature change of a Fahrenheit degree. For example, to obtain the centigrade number equivalent to 0°F, subtract 32 from 0° (which yields −32), then multiply by $\frac{5}{9}$, which yields −17.8 centigrade. However, recall that when most people use the phrase *17 below*, they are referring to below 0 on the Fahrenheit scale.

Degrees Centigrade	Degrees Fahrenheit
−17.8	0
−17	1.4
−16	3.2
−15	5.0
−14	6.8
−13	8.6
−12	10.4
−11	12.2
−10	14.0
−9	15.8
−8	17.6
−7	19.4
−6	21.2
−5	23.0
−4	24.8
−3	26.6
−2	28.4
−1	30.2
0	32.0
1	33.8
2	35.6

Degrees Centigrade	Degrees Fahrenheit
3	37.4
4	39.2
5	41.0
6	42.8
7	44.6
8	46.4
9	48.2
10	50.0
11	51.8
12	53.6
13	55.4
14	57.2
15	59.0
16	60.8
17	62.6
18	64.4
19	66.2
20	68.0
21	69.8
22	71.6
23	73.4
24	75.2
25	77.0
26	78.8
27	80.6
28	82.4
29	84.2
30	86.0
31	87.8
32	89.6
33	91.4
34	93.2
35	95.0
36	96.8
37	98.6
38	100.4
39	102.2
40	104.0
41	105.8

Continued

Degrees Centigrade	Degrees Fahrenheit
42	107.6
43	109.4
44	111.2
45	113.0
46	114.8
47	116.6
48	118.4
49	120.2
50	122.0
100	212.0

MEASURES OF LENGTH

Unit	U.S. Equivalent	Metric Equivalent
Inch	1 inch	0.0254 m; 2.54 cm
Foot	12 inches; 0.333 yd	0.3048 m; 30.48 cm
Yard	3 ft; 36 inches	0.914 m
Fathom	6 ft; 72 inches	1.83 m
Rod	16.5 ft; 5.5 yd	5.029 m
Mile	5280 ft; 1760 yd	1608.64 m; 1.609 km
Millimeter	0.03937 inch	0.001 m
Centimeter	0.3937 inch	0.01 m
Decimeter	3.937 inch	0.1 m
Meter	39.37 inches; 3.28 ft	1 m
Decameter	10.93 yd	10 m
Hectometer	328.08 ft; 109.36 yd	100 m
Kilometer	0.6214 miles	1000 m

MEASURES OF VOLUME (CAPACITY)

Unit	U.S. Equivalent	Metric Equivalent
Minim	$\frac{1}{60}$ fluidram	0.061610 mL
Drop	0.017 fluid oz	0.5 mL
Fluidram	60 minims	3.696 mL
Teaspoon	0.170 fl oz	5 mL
Tablespoon	3 tsp; 0.51 fl oz	15 mL
Fluid ounce	8 fluidrams	29.573 mL
Gill	4 fl oz	118.291 mL
Cup	8 fl oz; 16 tbsp	236.58 mL
Pint	2 cups	0.473 liter

Unit	U.S. Equivalent	Metric Equivalent
Quart	2 pints; ¼ gallon	0.946 liter
Gallon	4 quarts	3.785 liters
Barrel	31.5 gallons	119.23 liters
Hogshead	2 barrels; 63 gallons	238.46 liters
Milliliter	0.034 fl oz	0.001 liter
Centiliter	0.338 fl oz	0.01 liter
Deciliter	3.38 fl oz	0.1 liter
Liter	1.05 quarts	1 liter; 1000 mL
Kiloliter	1050 quarts; 262.5 gallons	1000 liters

MEASURES OF WEIGHT

Unit	U.S. Equivalent	Metric Equivalent
Grain	0.002083 oz (apothecary)	0.0648 g; 64.8 mg
Gram	0.04 oz; 0.002 lb	1 g
Ounce (avoirdupois)	437 grains	28.349 g
Pound (avoirdupois)	16 oz; 7000 grains	0.453 kg; 454 g
Ton (short)	2000 lb	0.907 metric ton

CONVERSION BETWEEN FEET AND METERS
Feet to Meters

Feet	Meters
1	0.30
10	3.05
100	30.48
1,000	304.8
2,000	609.6
3,000	914
4,000	1,219
5,000	1,524
6,000	1,829
7,000	2,134
8,000	2,438
9,000	2,743
10,000	3,048
11,000	3,353
12,000	3,658
13,000	3,962

Continued

Feet	Meters
14,000	4,267
15,000	4,572
16,000	4,877
17,000	5,182
18,000	5,486
19,000	5,791
20,000	6,096
21,000	6,401
22,000	6,705
23,000	7,010
24,000	7,315
25,000	7,620
26,000	7,925
27,000	8,230
28,000	8,534
29,000	8,839

Meters to Feet

Meters	Feet
1	3.28
10	33
100	328
1,000	3,281
2,000	6,562
3,000	9,842
4,000	13,123
5,000	16,404
6,000	19,685
7,000	22,966
8,000	26,247
9,000	29,528

APPENDIX THREE:
GUIDELINES FOR PREVENTION OF DISEASES
TRANSMITTED VIA HUMAN BLOOD AND
OTHER BODILY FLUIDS

Human fluids commonly encountered by laypeople during medical or recreational activities that would be considered high risk for the transmission of disease include blood, semen, vaginal secretions, saliva, and any fluid contaminated by blood, feces, and urine. Not all fluids are of equal risk, depending on the infectious agent. For instance, feces, nasal secretions, respiratory secretions, sweat, tears, urine, and vomitus don't appear to appreciably transmit the human immunodeficiency virus (HIV), but it's usually very difficult to tell if these fluids are contaminated with blood. Therefore, it's safest to assume that any bodily fluid can transmit disease, and to avoid unprotected contact with any moist human body substance.

There are some situations in which caution should be very high for a possible infectious disease. These include fever greater than 102°F (38.9°C), unexplained bleeding, jaundice, deep purple spotted rash, reddened eyes, swollen/tender/bruised lymph nodes, "pox" rash, severe cough, rapidly progressive severe illness, and multiple persons stricken ill during a tight time period who have been in close proximity.

To minimize the transmission of infectious disease, a medical rescuer should take the following precautions:

- Be careful with sharp objects, such as knives and needles. Obtain all available useful immunizations (including hepatitis; see page 425).
- Use personal protective equipment, such as disposable nitrile gloves (any liquid-impermeable gloves or even a thin plastic bag will do in a pinch; avoid latex gloves because of the risk for latex allergy), goggles (eye shields, glasses, ski goggles), pocket face mask or barrier shield (for rescue breathing), and gown or overclothing. A properly fitted N95 face mask may be worn if an airborne or contagious droplet-spread germ is suspected. If a face mask is not available, a bandana may provide some protection. In cold weather, thin glove liners can be worn under disposable gloves.
- After any victim contact, even if gloves are worn, wash your hands thoroughly with soap and water. If a glove breaks during contact with a victim, remove it and wash your hands immediately.
- Unbroken skin is very protective. However, if broken or unbroken skin is exposed to a victim's bodily fluid, it should be washed immediately with soap and water. If soap and water aren't available, use waterless antiseptic hand cleanser, plain water, or snow.
- Carry materials contaminated by bodily fluids in clearly labeled nonpermeable containers, such as heavy plastic bags. Carry "sharps" (e.g., used needles) in impenetrable containers.
- If equipment (such as a litter) has been contaminated by a bodily fluid and must be reused, it should be cleaned by washing with soap and water, and then scrubbing with a minimum 1:10 dilution of household bleach (sodium hypochlorite) in water. Alternative minimum dilutions (in water) for disinfection include 0.3% hydrogen peroxide, 25% ethyl alcohol, 35% isopropyl alcohol, 0.5% Lysol, and 0.25% povidone-iodine (Betadine). Wear gloves while cleaning the equipment. Eyeglasses can be washed with soap and water.

Sometimes it will be necessary to create the chlorine-based cleansing solution for disinfection of floors, clothes, bedding and equipment; or bodily fluids, particularly if someone has suffered diarrhea. Household bleach containing sodium hypochlorite usually has a 5% concentration of chlorine, but when preparing any solution, take care to note the precise original concentration. Because bleach loses its concentration of chlorine over time, be certain that the bleach has the odor of chlorine. Do not use "thick bleach" preparations. Use clear water to dilute the bleach.

1. Use clear water to dilute the bleach.
2. If possible, prepare the disinfection solution daily. Use a plastic container, not metal.
3. The goal is a 1:100 dilution (0.05% chlorine). A 1:10 dilution (0.5% chlorine) is caustic, and must be kept away from skin and eyes. The 1:10 dilution is used to disinfect spilled excrement, dead bodies, spills of blood and bodily fluids, and as the initial solution to create the 1:100 dilution.
4. The 1:10 dilution is made by adding one volume of household bleach to nine volumes of clean water.
5. The 1:100 dilution is made by adding one volume of the 1:10 dilution to nine additional volumes of clean water. An alternative is to take the original household bleach (5% chlorine) and add it to 99 volumes of clean water.
6. Use the 1:100 dilution to clean surfaces, bedding, gloves intended for reuse (not optimal, but sometimes necessary), contaminated waste intended for disposal, and clothing *before it is laundered*. It can be used to clean medical equipment, but if safely used, the 1:10 dilution is much more effective at attaining disinfection (see earlier).
7. When possible, rinse items and surfaces decontaminated with any chlorine-based solution with disinfected water if it is available.
8. Clean hands with soap and water washing and/or a commercial hand disinfectant. *Don't use the chlorine solution, even at a 1:100 dilution, for cleaning hands or other skin, because this can be dangerous.*

The purpose of educating you about precautions is not to discourage you from helping another in need. Rather, it is to support the notion that with just a moment of thought and the initiation of proper precautions, needless transmission of infectious diseases can be prevented, and a medical rescue can proceed without harm to the rescuer.

HUMAN IMMUNODEFICIENCY VIRUS POSTEXPOSURE PROPHYLAXIS

Despite efforts to avoid a dangerous exposure to HIV-contaminated blood, it sometimes occurs that a person is punctured by a needle or blade, or undertakes a high-risk sexual encounter. In this circumstance, it's very important to seek immediate medical attention and counseling. Highly active antiretroviral (oral drug) therapy (HAART), while most effective in preventing acquired immunodeficiency syndrome (AIDS) if initiated within 2 hours of exposure, may still have a beneficial effect if begun up to 72 hours after exposure. If a person is going to be isolated from medical care and responsible for his or her own postexposure prophylaxis, then seek advance education from a physician, from whom a prescription will be obtained. Some of the drug combinations that are recommended as of the time of this writing are zidovudine plus lamivudine (low exposure risk/low risk of drug resistance), or zidovudine plus lamivudine plus lopinavir with a ritonavir "boost" (high exposure risk/high risk of drug resistance).

APPENDIX FOUR: COMMONLY USED APPLICATIONS OF THE SAM SPLINT

This information is adapted with permission from the SAM Splint User Guide. SAM Splints (Sam Medical Products) are available in the following sizes:

Standard—$4\frac{1}{4}$ inches × 36 inches; 4 oz; roll or flatfold

Junior—$4\frac{1}{4}$ inches × 18 inches; 2.4 oz; flatfold

Wrist—$4\frac{1}{4}$ inches × 9 inches; 1.1 oz; flat

XL—$5\frac{1}{2}$ inches × 36 inches; 5.9 oz; flatfold

Finger—1.8 inches × $3\frac{3}{4}$; 0.2 oz; flat

GENERAL

The standard SAM Splint has a thin core of aluminum alloy and is closed-cell foam padded, reusable, not affected by ambient temperature or altitude, cuts with regular scissors, and is waterproof. Radiographs (x-rays) can be taken through the SAM Splint. The strength of the applied splint is derived from how it is shaped with proper angles and bends by the user.

The closed pore foam will not flash when exposed to flame, but will begin to melt and eventually ignite after approximately 8 seconds. The SAM Splint is easily cut with ordinary scissors. Cutting exposes the thin aluminum core. Unless serrated scissors have been used, the now-exposed aluminum is usually not very sharp. To prevent any injury from the exposed edge, we recommend folding the edge on itself 1 to 2 times. Covering the edge with tape is also effective.

Whether cut or used intact, the splint can be cleaned with antiseptic soap and water or with almost any protocol cleaning solution, such as an inexpensive 1:9 mixture of commercially available bleach and water. The closed-pore polyurethane foam does not absorb or allow passage of air or perspiration. This does not present a problem during short-term use. If, however, the splint is to be maintained for prolonged periods (hours to days), some absorbent material such as cotton cloth or cast padding should be placed between the splint and patient to prevent skin maceration and odor. If prolonged use is anticipated (more than a few hours), place absorbent material, such as cotton cloth, between the splint and the skin to prevent skin irritation and odor. Also, to prevent uncomfortable pressure points during prolonged use, place soft padding (such as gauze pads) around all bony prominences.

The splint is nonsterile. To reuse the SAM Splint, wash thoroughly with disinfectant before repacking.

THE CONCEPT: THE BASIC BEND

A SAM Splint without any bends (e.g., rolled in the package) is completely malleable. When a curve or fold is placed anywhere across its longitudinal axis, it becomes rigid and suitable for splinting almost any bone on the body. Always use curves to add strength and rigidity to the SAM Splint.

The **basic C-curve** (Figure 290) meets most splinting needs. To create the C-curve, place both thumbs in the center of the SAM Splint. Using your thumbs as a brace, pull the edges of the splint toward you to create a shallow C-curve. This curve immediately adds strength and rigidity to the splint. For greater strength, deepen the bend.

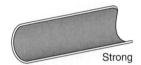

Figure 290. SAM Splint basic C-curve.

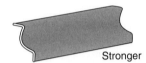

Figure 291. SAM Splint reverse C-curve.

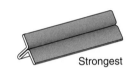

Figure 292. SAM Splint T-curve.

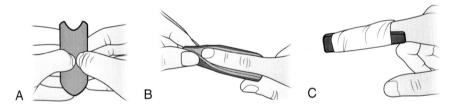

Figure 293. SAM Splint finger splint.

The **reverse C-curve** is stronger. First, form a C-curve. Then add additional strength by bending the edges of the C-curved splint back in the reverse direction (Figure 291).

The **T-curve** is yet stronger. This bend adds exceptional strength to the splint. To create the T-curve, fold the outer edges of the splint together. Next, bend half of each side of the fold in the opposite direction to create a T-shaped beam (Figure 292).

FINGER SPLINT (FOR FINGERTIP INJURIES, BROKEN OR DISLOCATED FINGER, CUT FINGER)

Step 1: To create a simple finger splint or fingertip guard, first form a SAM Finger Splint into the C-curve (Figure 293, *A*).

Step 2: Place the finger in the curved surface of the splint. Squeeze the end of the splint to create a fingertip guard (Figure 293, *B*).

Step 3: Secure with your wrap of choice (Figure 293, *C*).

VOLAR (UNDERNEATH) WRIST SPLINT (FOR BROKEN WRIST, CUT WRIST, CARPAL TUNNEL SYNDROME)

Step 1: Roll over the end of a 9-inch (for children) or 18-inch (for adults) SAM Splint to provide comfort for fingers (Figure 294, *A*).

Step 2: Apply a C-curve (Figure 294, *B*).

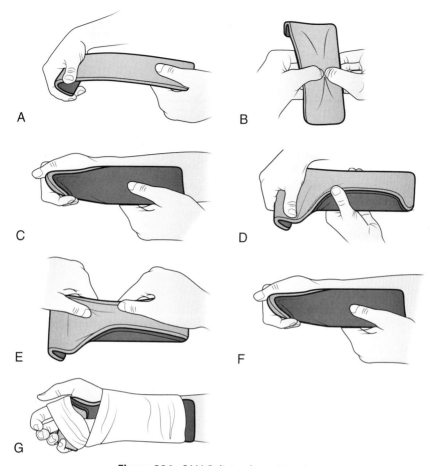

Figure 294. SAM Splint volar wrist splint.

Step 3: Using your own right or left hand and wrist as a template, mold the splint into the position of function (Figure 294, *C*).

Step 4: Be sure to create a generous curve for the base of the thumb (Figure 294, *D*).

Step 5: Obtain additional strength by folding up the ulnar (little finger) side of the splint (Figure 294, *E*).

Step 6: Apply to patient (Figure 294, *F*).

Step 7: Make fine adjustments as necessary. Secure with your wrap of choice (Figure 294, *G*).

THUMB SPICA SPLINT (FOR NAVICULAR [SCAPHOID] FRACTURE, BROKEN OR DISLOCATED THUMB, ULNAR COLLATERAL LIGAMENT SPRAIN)

Step 1: Using your own right or left thumb and wrist as a template, mold the thumb spica shape into the selected SAM Splint. A 9-inch splint works well for this (Figure 295, *A*).

Step 2: Be sure to create a generous curve for the base of the thumb (Figure 295, *B*).

Step 3: You may add reverse C-curves on the edges as needed for additional strength (Figure 295, *C*).

Step 4: Apply to the patient. Make fine adjustments as needed (Figure 295, *D*).

Step 5: Secure with your wrap of choice (Figure 295, *E*).

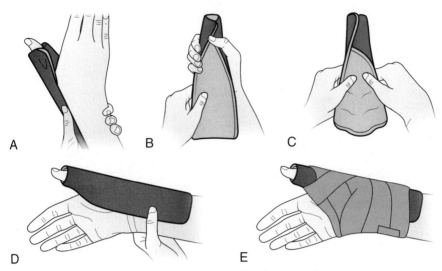

Figure 295. SAM Splint thumb spica splint.

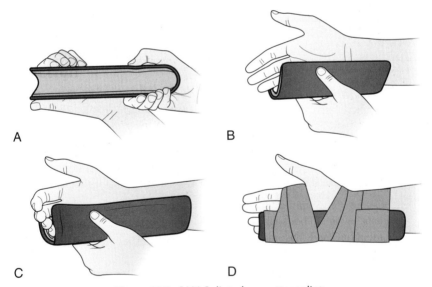

Figure 296. SAM Splint ulnar gutter splint.

ULNAR GUTTER SPLINT (FOR BROKEN OR DISLOCATED FOURTH OR FIFTH FINGER)

Step 1: Fold a 9-inch SAM Splint length-wise (Figure 296, *A*).

Step 2: Using the ulnar side of your own hand and wrist as a template, mold the splint into the desired shape (Figure 296, *B*).

Step 3: Apply to the patient (Figure 296, *C*).

Step 4: Make fine adjustments as needed and secure with your wrap of choice (Figure 296, *D*).

DOUBLE LAYER WRIST SPLINT (FOR SPRAINED OR BROKEN WRIST, CUT WRIST)

Step 1: Fold a 36-inch SAM Splint in half upon itself (Figure 297, *A*).

Step 2: Roll over the end to provide more comfort for the fingers (Figure 297, *B*).

Step 3: Add strength by creating a C-curve (Figure 297, *C*).

Step 4: Using your own right or left arm as a template, mold the splint to the general shape of the wrist and forearm (Figure 297, *D*).

Step 5: Make adjustments to fit the injury and apply to the patient. Only small adjustments should be made once the splint is in place. Secure with your wrap of choice (Figure 297, *E*).

UPPER ARM SPLINT (FOR BROKEN UPPER ARM)

Step 1: Fold one third of a 36-inch SAM Splint upon itself to create a 12-inch section of double-layered splint (Figure 298, *A*).

Step 2: Curve the double layer into a fishhook shape and secure the double layer with your wrap of choice (Figure 298, *B*).

Step 3: Form a C-curve along the shank of the fishhook for strength and fit (Figure 298, *C*).

Step 4: Apply the splint to the patient. Fold any excess splint over the patient's shoulder or back upon itself (Figure 298, *D*)

Step 5: Secure with your wrap of choice. Apply a sling and swath for additional support (Figure 298, *E*).

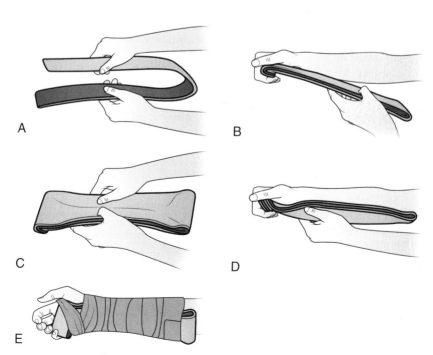

A

B

C

D

E

Figure 297. SAM Splint double-layer wrist splint.

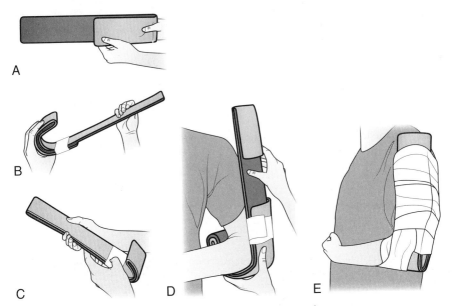

Figure 298. SAM Splint upper arm splint.

"SUGAR TONG" SPLINT (FOR DISLOCATED OR BROKEN ELBOW)

Step 1: Fold a 36-inch SAM Splint in half (Figure 299, *A*).

Step 2: To obtain the correct length, use the patient's arm as a template. Place the folded splint around the elbow so the end of the top half stops at the knuckles. Fold the bottom half down even with the top (Figure 299, *B*).

Step 3: Form a C-curve in each half. Extend the C-curve no further than two-thirds the distance down each half. If you extend the curve farther, it will limit your ability to fold the splint around the elbow (Figure 299, *C*).

Step 4: Using your own right or left arm as a template, shape the splint to fit (Figure 299, *D*).

Step 5: Pad any bony prominences about the wrist and elbow (Figure 299, *E*).

Step 6: Fit the splint to the patient (Figure 299, *F*).

Step 7: Secure the splint with your wrap of choice (Figure 299, *G*).

ELBOW SPLINT (FOR DISLOCATED OR BROKEN ELBOW)

Step 1: Using the patient's non-affected arm, extend a 36-inch SAM Splint from just below the patient's armpit to the knuckles (Figure 300, *A*).

Step 2: Fold over any portion of the splint that extends beyond the knuckles (Figure 300, *B*).

Step 3: Form a C-curve down the entire length of the splint (Figure 300, *C*).

Step 4: Using your own right or left arm as a template, shape the splint to fit (Figure 300, *D*).

Step 5: You may create reverse C-curve bends on the edges as needed for strength (Figure 300, *E*).

Step 6: Apply the splint to the patient (Figure 300, *F*).

Step 7: Secure with your wrap of choice (Figure 300, *G*).

ADJUSTABLE CERVICAL (NECK) COLLAR (FOR SUSPECTED NECK INJURY)

Step 1: Fold a 36-inch SAM Splint five inches from the end (Figure 301, *A*).

Step 2: Bracing your thumbs on each side of the fold, pull the upper edges toward you to create a V-shaped chin rest (Figure 301, *B*).

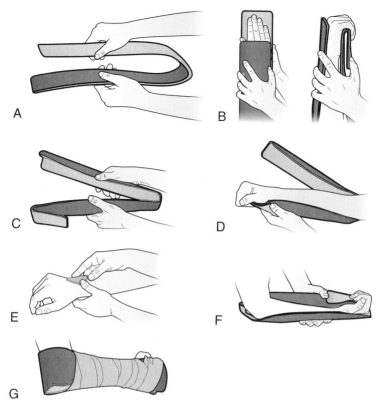

Figure 299. SAM Splint sugar tong splint.

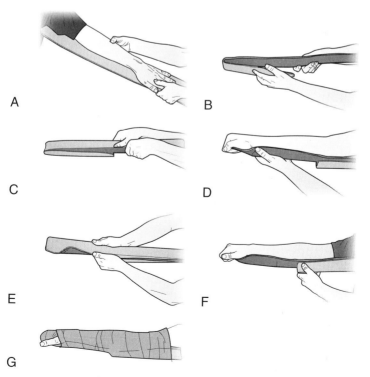

Figure 300. SAM Splint elbow splint.

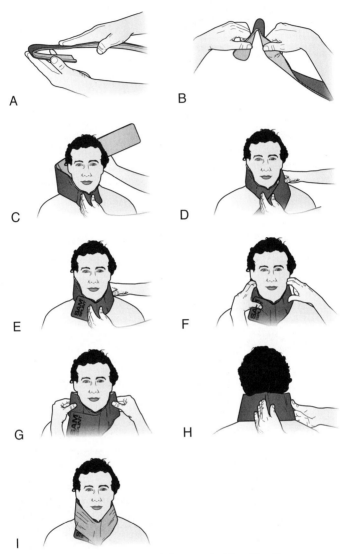

Figure 301. SAM Splint cervical (neck) collar.

Step 3: Place the chin rest beneath the patient's chin and lower jaw. Be careful to avoid pressure on the front of the neck. Loop the remaining portion of the splint loosely around the neck (Figure 301, *C*).

Step 4: Bring the end forward and down in an oblique direction until it touches the chest. This creates the correct chin-to-chest distance for the chin post (Figure 301, *D*).

Step 5: While continuing to support the chin, bring the chest portion of the splint around the original chin rest to create a chin-post. Squeeze to deepen the chin-post (Figure 301, *E*).

Step 6: Insert your index fingers in each side of the looped splint. Pull outward (Figure 301, *F*).

Step 7: Squeeze to create two side or lateral posts and ensure a snug fit (Figure 301, *G*).

Step 8: If the patient is sitting, you can form a back or posterior post in a similar manner (Figure 301, *H*).

Step 9: Fold up any excess splint. Secure with tape or your wrap of choice (Figure 301, *I*).

ANTERIOR DISLOCATION OF THE SHOULDER

In this common dislocation, the patient's arm is typically most comfortable when supported in the abducted (sitting away from the body) position. The arm can be supported in this manner with a rolled ski parka, blanket, pillow or SAM Splint "triangle." To create a "triangle," the splint is first folded into thirds. This produces three equal 12 inch sections of splint.

Step 1: Fold the outer sections along the longitudinal axis, leaving the middle section flat. Hook the outer folded ends together, producing a triangle. A more rounded, gentler curve or half-circle is then folded along the longitudinal axis of the flat section of the triangle. This curve is formed to the contour of the arm (Figure 302, *A*).

Step 2: The triangle is then placed in the axilla and used to support the abducted arm. The arm triangle is held in place by the patient or secured to the patient's trunk with your wrap of choice (Figure 302, *B*).

ANKLE STIRRUP SPLINT (FOR SPRAINED, BROKEN, OR DISLOCATED ANKLE; FOR BROKEN LOWER LEG)

Step 1: If footwear is removed or when the ankle is exposed, place padding above and around the bony prominences on each side of the ankle (Figure 303, *A*).

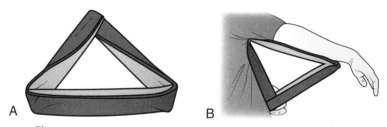

A   B

Figure 302. SAM Splint anterior shoulder dislocation prop splint.

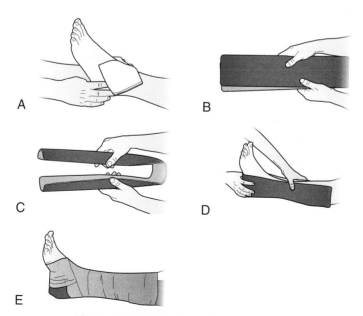

A   B

C   D

E

Figure 303. SAM Splint ankle stirrup splint.

Step 2: Fold a 36-inch SAM Splint to create two equal halves (Figure 303, *B*).

Step 3: Apply C-curves two thirds of the distance down each half. Add reverse C-curves on the edges if needed for strength. Don't extend the curves further or they will stiffen the splint and limit your ability to fold it around the foot and ankle (Figure 303, *C*).

Step 4: Fold the stirrup splint around the foot and ankle (Figure 303, *D*).

Step 5: Secure with your wrap of choice (Figure 303, *E*).

FIGURE-EIGHT ANKLE SPLINT (FOR SPRAINED, BROKEN, OR DISLOCATED ANKLE)

Step 1: If footwear is removed or when the ankle is exposed, place padding above and around the bony prominences on each side of the ankle (Figure 304, *A*).

Step 2: Lay a 36-inch SAM Splint flat. Place the patient's foot in the middle of the splint so that the splint lies just forward of the heel (Figure 304, *B*).

Step 3: Conform half of the splint snugly around the ankle (Figure 304, *C*).

Step 4: Fold the second half of the splint around the first in a figure-of-eight position. Crimp as necessary to fit (Figure 304, *D*).

Step 5: Secure with your wrap of choice (Figure 304, *E*).

COMBINATION ANKLE STIRRUP AND FIGURE-OF-EIGHT SPLINT (FOR SPRAINED, BROKEN OR DISLOCATED ANKLE WHERE MAXIMUM IMMOBILIZATION IS NEEDED)

Step 1: First apply a figure-of-eight splint (see previous steps) (Figure 305, *A*).

Step 2: Next, prepare an ankle stirrup splint (see previous steps) (Figure 305, *B*).

Step 3: Apply the ankle stirrup splint over the figure-of-eight splint (Figure 305, *C*).

Step 4: Secure with your wrap of choice and crimp as needed to fit (Figure 305, *D*).

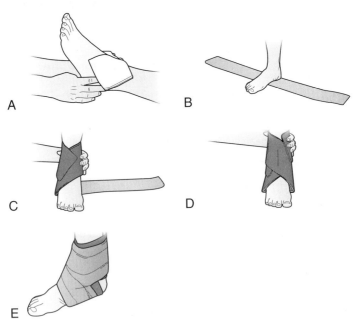

Figure 304. SAM Splint figure-of-eight ankle splint.

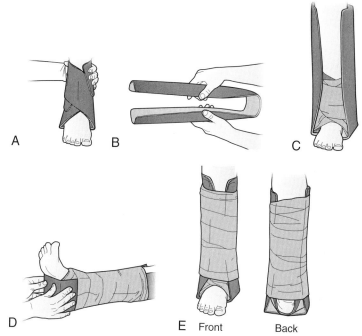

Figure 305. SAM Splint combination stirrup and figure-of-eight ankle splint.

SINGLE LONG LEG SPLINT (FOR BROKEN LOWER LEG)

Step 1: If footwear is removed or when the ankle is exposed, place padding above and around the bony prominences on each side of the ankle (Figure 306, *A*).

Step 2: Apply a C-curve to approximately 30 inches of a 36 inch SAM Splint. Leave the last 6 inches of the splint flat and soft to fold under the foot (Figure 306, *B*).

Step 3: For extra strength, apply reverse C-curves on the edges where necessary (Figure 306, *C*).

Step 4: Place the splint against the outside of the leg and fold the soft portion of the splint under the foot to create a footplate (Figure 306, *D*).

Step 5: Adjust splint to fit the leg (Figure 306, *E*).

Step 6: Secure with your wrap of choice (Figure 306, *F*).

DOUBLE LONG LEG SPLINT (FOR BROKEN LOWER LEG WHERE MORE IMMOBILIZATION IS NEEDED)

Step 1: If footwear is removed or when the ankle is exposed, place padding above and around the bony prominences on each side of the ankle (Figure 307, *A*).

Step 2: Create a long leg splint as shown previously (Figure 307, *B*).

Step 3: Apply the long leg splint to the outer aspect of the leg (Figure 307, *C*).

Step 4: Prepare a second splint, identical to the first. Apply this splint to the inner aspect of the leg (Figure 307, *D*).

Step 5: Fold the soft, flat end over the first footplate (Figure 307, *E*).

Step 6: Secure both splints to leg with your wrap of choice (Figure 307, *F*).

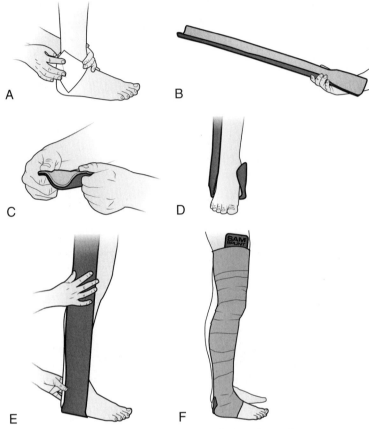

Figure 306. SAM Splint single long leg splint.

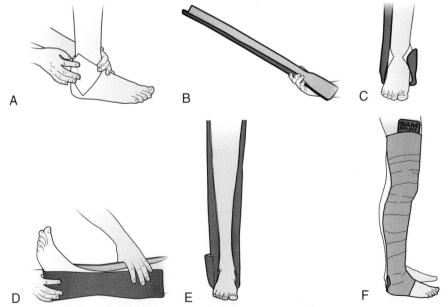

Figure 307. SAM Splint double long leg splint.

KNEE IMMOBILIZER SPLINT (FOR KNEE INJURIES)

Step 1: Fold a 36-inch SAM Splint in the center to create two equal halves. Spread the halves to produce a fan-shaped splint, wider at the top for the thigh and narrower at the bottom for the calf (Figure 308, *A*).

Step 2: Apply tape to the top and middle portions of the splint to maintain the fan shape (Figure 308, *B*).

Step 3: Apply a second fan-shaped splint (Figure 308, *C*).

Step 4: Form a C-curve in each SAM Splint (Figure 308, *D*).

Step 5: The C-curves should appear as shown (Figure 308, *E*).

Step 6: Place one splint on each side of the knee and make fine adjustments to fit (Figure 308, *F*).

Step 7: Secure with your wrap of choice.

HALF-RING SPLINT FOR FEMUR FRACTURE (FOR BROKEN FEMUR)

Step 1: First create the "foot support" by cutting an 8 inch section from an old ski pole. Drill 2 holes 6 inches apart through this foot support section. The hole should be sized with a larger entry hole and a smaller exit hole to tightly accommodate the tapered end of the ski pole. Keep the "foot support" section in your pack along with duct tape, safety pins, and strong cord (to be used for traction as desired). To create the "half-ring hip support," place

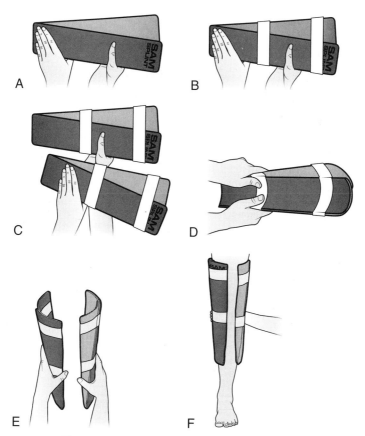

Figure 308. SAM Splint knee immobilizer splint.

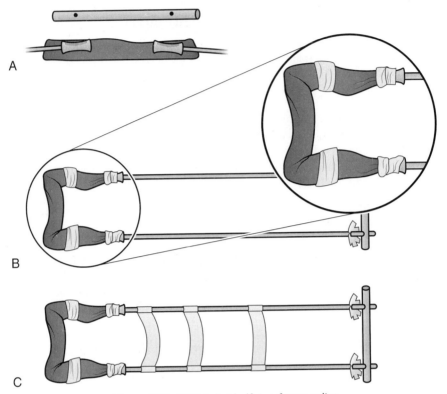

A

B

C

Figure 309. SAM Splint half-ring femur splint.

two ski poles, handle facing handle, each on the outer third of a 36-inch flat SAM Splint (Figure 309, *A*).

Step 2: Roll each end of the splint tightly around the handles and secure the splint with duct tape. The rolled middle third of the SAM Splint is then folded as the ski poles are aligned parallel to each other. The position of the ski poles is maintained by firmly fitting the tips of the poles into the tapered holes in the "foot support." The rolled "hip support section" of the SAM Splint between the two ski poles handles is now contoured to resemble a Thomas half-ring (Figure 309, *B*).

Step 3: Duct tape thigh and calf supports are then applied and may be reinforced with cloth or elastic wraps (Figure 309, *C*).

IMPALED OBJECT PROTECTOR

Step 1: Cut a section of a SAM Splint to the desired length.

Step 2: Make a series of parallel cuts along one margin of the splint to create a number of flaps.

Step 3: Fold these flaps to 90 degrees so they lie at the correct angle to the uncut margin of the splint.

Step 4: Roll the splint on itself and secure with tape.

Step 5: Place this device over the impaled object and secure to the body with tape or gauze (Figure 310).

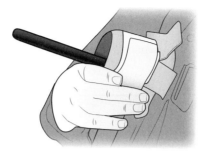

Figure 310. SAM Splint impaled object protector.

APPENDIX FIVE:
PERSONAL SAFETY IN AN AGE OF GLOBAL
CONFLICT, KIDNAPPING, AND TERRORISM

We live in an age of global conflict. Persons who travel outside of the United States to seek outdoor experiences are subject to criminal behavior, including acts of piracy, kidnapping, terrorism, and war. So, it's wise to be cautious, safe, and prepared to react to situations in which you may become a victim. As with any other adverse event, avoidance is key.

SAFE TRAVEL
General Crime Avoidance
1. Don't flaunt expensive items, such as jewelry, luggage, and cameras.
2. If you're in a hotel room with an electronic safe, use it to store valuables. Don't leave precious items unprotected. Lock all windows and doors when you are not in the room. Leave a light on in the room when you're not present.
3. Avoid unsafe neighborhoods. Use common, well-lighted routes.
4. Avoid arguments with strangers.
5. Travel in groups.
6. Be particularly careful at night. Don't walk alone at night.
7. Don't accept rides from strangers. Don't hitchhike. If you're going to be met at an airport, be informed ahead of time about who is picking you up, preferably with a name, photo, and vehicle license plate number.
8. Don't accept medicine or drugs from strangers.
9. Carry money in a travel money belt.
10. Don't become intoxicated in public.
11. Plan for an emergency evacuation.
12. Be cautious at checkpoints and military barriers.

KIDNAPPING AND HOSTAGE BEHAVIOR
Prevention of Kidnapping
1. Travel in groups.
2. Avoid unsafe neighborhoods. Use common, well-lighted routes.
3. Don't flaunt money or jewelry.

4. Don't accept rides from strangers. Don't hitchhike. If you're going to be met at an airport, be informed ahead of time about who is picking you up, preferably with a name, photo, and vehicle license plate number.

Proper Hostage Behavior

A person may be taken hostage by a kidnapper or as part of a larger conflict. If this occurs, proper hostage behavior can make the difference between life and death.

1. Do not resist.
2. Avoid sudden or threatening movements.
3. Do not try to be a hero.
4. Cooperate as best possible and follow orders.
5. Do not be belligerent and avoid complaining.
6. Keep answers to questions short. Don't volunteer information.
7. Try to relax.
8. Prepare yourself emotionally for a long ordeal.
9. Avoid direct eye contact and do not be obvious about observing your captor's activities.
10. Don't drink alcohol.
11. Eat what you are given. Do not overeat.
12. Attempt to establish rapport with your captors if the situation is prolonged.
13. Avoid discussions about politics and religion.
14. Get into a daily routine.
15. Be as positive as possible and avoid despair.

Avoiding Acts and Consequences of Terrorism

1. Don't congregate in public areas.
2. Avoid demonstrations, crowds, and protests.
3. Schedule direct flights and avoid stops in high-risk airports.
4. Minimize time spent in public areas of airports.
5. Refuse unknown luggage or packages.
6. Avoid shopping malls, nightclubs, and tourist destinations.
7. Note the location of police stations, hotels, and hospitals.
8. Have an escape plan.
9. Take taxicabs at random and compare the face of the driver with the posted license.
10. Drive with windows closed in crowded areas.
11. If you hear or witness shooting, take cover and drop to the ground. Move by crawling.
12. Do not attempt to assist rescuers or handle weapons unless you have been properly trained.

PIRACY

Pirates are thieves who board boats in order to steal, rob, kidnap, or worse. They are frequently armed. Unquestionably, safe boating practices are essential to lessen the chance of being pirated. Boating organizations and expert seagoers offer the following advice.

How to Lessen the Risks Associated with Pirates

1. Travel with other boats. Avoid high-risk areas. Register your itinerary with proper authorities and be in regular communication.
2. Bring your dinghy on board or along the toe rail at night, to lessen its attraction to pirates.
3. Keep the transom boarding ladder lifted to make it more difficult to board your boat.
4. Maintain an infrared alarm that emits a loud shrieking noise in the cockpit.

5. Keep the companionway hatch and other cabin hatches closed tightly when you perceive there to be a pirating risk.
6. Have internal hatches open toward the companion hatch, and jam toward the cabin.
7. Stow knives and other implements that might be used as weapons.
8. Keep valuables in a hidden safe.
9. Keep fake valuables, worthless credit cards, and cash available to give to pirates.
10. If anchored, have a quick get-away course charted and kept near the wheel. Be prepared and checked out to leave at a moment's notice.
11. Keep watch for pirates.
12. Have a red parachute flare easily available to fire out of a hatch as an alarm.

BLAST INJURIES

Blast injuries occur from explosions, often caused by improvised explosive devices (IEDs). They can release enormous quantities of energy. Other causes include land mines and other ordinance, such as grenades. Some bombs that have survived conflicts from many years ago, such as World War II, may still be active and can be triggered by unsuspecting curious persons.

Blast injuries are categorized, with a fair amount of overlap, as:

1. Primary: Injuries caused by the air pressure wave ("blast wave") caused by the explosion. This affects organs such as the eardrum (rupture—see page 166), lung (bruising, bleeding, and torn tissue leading to air embolism—see page 360), brain (see page 59), and bowel (often a torn colon, because gas-filled structures are very prone to effects from the pressure wave).
2. Secondary: Injuries caused by bomb fragments and flying debris, such as nails, which cause cuts and bleeding (see page 240), bruises (see page 237), amputations (see page 107), and penetrating injuries akin to gunshot wounds (see page 57).
3. Tertiary: Injuries caused by the victim being thrown by the blast wave, such as broken bones (see page 67), head injuries (see page 59), penetrating injuries (impalement), and internal injuries (see page 57).
4. Quaternary: All other injuries, such as crush injuries (see page 69), burns (see page 108), asphyxia (see page 22), toxic exposures (such as to chemicals or radiation), and worsening of a chronic disease(s), such as asthma.

How to Avoid Blast Injuries

1. Don't handle weapons or ordinance, regardless of its age or appearance.
2. Don't stray from frequently used paths in areas that are known to have been possible sites for land mines.
3. If there is a perceived risk for terrorist or war activities, don't congregate in public areas.

APPENDIX SIX:
EMERGENCY CANINE MEDICINE

Dogs may accompany you in the outdoors. A few basic problems for which there are simple or obvious interventions are mentioned here. In preparation for an adventure outdoors with a dog, be certain that the animal has had all of its immunizations, is at least 1 year of age, and is not expected to carry more than 30% of its body weight in a pack. Bathe the animal with a pyrethrin (insecticide)-containing shampoo and carry flea-tick-lice powder. Give heartworm preventive medication if mosquito bites are a possibility. Consider using a flea and tick preventive

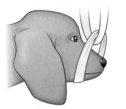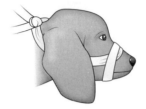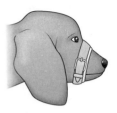

Figure 311. Improvised dog muzzle created from a rolled gauze or strap.

medication, which can be obtained from a veterinarian. Each day, inspect the animal and properly remove all ticks.

When treating a dog, use a muzzle if possible. An improvised muzzle can be created using a rolled gauze or strap (Figure 311).

The normal resting temperature of a dog is 100 to 102.5° F (37.8 to 39.2° C), and after exercise is 103 to 106° F (39.4 to 41.1° C). Resting heart rate is 60 to 80 beats per minute and depends on the size of the animal. After exercise, it is up to 130 beats per minute. The pulse is appreciated most easily by feeling one of the femoral arteries, which are found on the inside of a dog's rear thighs. The breathing rate is 10 to 40 breaths per minute, not counting panting. Dogs can certainly become dehydrated. Signs and symptoms of dehydration are shortness of breath, decreased skin elasticity, skin that "tents" (does not return to normal position) when pinched and pulled, dry gums, sunken eyes, increased abdominal efforts with breathing, coarse breath sounds, and deeply red-colored mucous membranes.

Heat exhaustion and heat stroke afflict dogs. Heat stroke is life-threatening. In addition to the symptoms of dehydration, the dog may show altered mental status (tired, uncooperative, confused, weak), weak pulses, vomiting, diarrhea, collapse, incoordination, and seizures. Treat the animal immediately by spraying with cool water and fanning to promote cooling by evaporation. If a body of cool water is available, immerse the animal. The goal is to reduce the body temperature to 103° F (39.4° C) as soon as possible. Any time an animal is this sick, if possible, get to a veterinarian, who may use more aggressive cooling measures and intravenous or subcutaneous rehydration.

Pay close attention to your dog in the heat. Allow sufficient rest in the shade and access to drinking water. If the weather is hot and the situation permits, allow the animal to immerse in cool or cold water.

Dogs will eat just about anything, so be alert to various poisonings, such as plants and mushrooms, certain toads, insect repellent (DEET), grapes, raisins, rodenticides, insecticides, lead, antifreeze, etc. If you have access to a phone, call the ASPCA poison control telephone number at 888-426-4435. There is a $65 fee for service.

A dog may be "quilled" by a porcupine. If only a few quills are present, the treatment is to muzzle the animal, cover its eyes, grasp the quills individually with pliers as close to the skin as possible, and pull. The same treatment holds true for humans. If the quill has been in the skin for a long time, it may have absorbed fluid and swelled. If need be, the skin can be nicked to allow the trapped barb to pass.

A dog sprayed with skunk musk is an unhappy animal. Instructions for treatment are found on page 370.

A dog may be bitten by a rattlesnake. Fundamentally, the treatment is the same as advised for a human (see page 318). Try to minimize the dog's activity and bring the dog promptly to medical attention, because administration of antivenom may be necessary. If the bite is near the nose and mouth, swelling can compromise breathing. The venom's effects can cause low blood pressure, increased bleeding, and shock. If the animal survives the bite, the local tissues may die, leaving a large sore that requires meticulous wound care. There is no effective first aid in the field. Snakebite kits have not been proved effective. If you're traveling in snake country, prevention is essential. Unleashed dogs wander, and their curiosity leads them directly to snakes. If you hear a snake, keep your dog close until the danger is passed. Snakes move around more at night. The same way that you would not reach under a rock or log, don't allow your dog to do this. If your dog is sniffing in tall grass or bushes that might be harboring a snake, move the dog away. Don't use an animal to flush out a snake or to provide combat protection. The snake will win.

A dog may suffer from high-altitude illness, including pulmonary edema (see page 310). Signs and symptoms include decreased appetite, weak and tired behavior, reduced activity, dusky tongue color, pale gums, pink or brownish fluid from the mouth and nose, coarse and difficult breathing. Dogs may be administered dexamethasone 4 mg by mouth for suspected high-altitude illness.

Dogs will occasionally eat poisonous plants. Signs and symptoms include seizures, weakness, confusion and lethargy up to coma, muscle spasm, vomiting, and apparent pain.

GLOSSARY (INCLUDING ACRONYMS AND ABBREVIATIONS)

A

ABC: airway, breathing, and circulation.

abdomen: the part of the body between the chest and the pelvis.

abrasion: a scraped area of skin.

abscess: a localized collection of pus, usually surrounded by inflamed tissue.

acclimatize: to adapt to a new altitude, climate, environment, or situation.

acidotic: in a state of abnormally reduced alkalinity; overwhelmed by acid; related to decreased pH.

acute: sudden in onset.

adrenaline: epinephrine.

AED: automated external defibrillator.

airway: passage for air into the lungs, including the mouth, nose, pharynx, larynx, trachea, and bronchi.

alkaline: having the properties of a base; related to high pH.

allergy: exaggerated reaction (sneezing, runny nose, itching, skin rash, difficulty in breathing) to substances that don't affect other individuals.

ALS: advanced life support.

alveoli: microscopic air spaces in the lung where oxygen is exchanged for carbon dioxide.

ambulatory: able to walk.

amnesia: loss of memory.

amniotic fluid: liquid that surrounds unborn child within the membranes inside the uterus.

amputate: to cut from the body.

AMS: altered mental status.

analgesia: relief from pain.

anaphylaxis: hypersensitivity to substances following prior exposure, resulting in a severe allergic reaction.

anemia: deficiency in red blood cells.

anesthesia: loss of sensation.

aneurysm: abnormally dilated blood vessel.

angina pectoris: episodic chest pain caused by insufficient oxygen supply to the heart.

antibiotic: drug used to kill bacteria.

antibody: body substance, produced by specialized cells, that combines with and neutralizes foreign substances or toxins.

antiemetic: drug used to control nausea and vomiting.

antihistamine: drug used to inactivate histamine.

antiinflammatory: drug used to prevent or correct inflammation.

antiseptic: substance that limits or stops the growth of microscopic germs.

antivenom: drug used to inactivate the effects of animal or insect venom.

anus: posterior opening from the intestine to the outside world.

aorta: the large artery that carries oxygenated blood from the heart to be distributed to the body.

aortic: pertaining to the aorta.

appendectomy: surgical removal of the appendix.

appendicitis: inflammation of the appendix.

appendix: wormlike appendage of the bowel, located in the right lower quadrant of the abdomen.

aqueous: mixed with or related to water.

arachnoid: middle layer of membranes that cover the brain and spinal cord.

argasid: related to soft ticks.

arrest: sudden stop.

arterial: pertaining to an artery.

arteritis: inflammation of an artery.

artery: muscular- and elastic-walled blood vessel that carries oxygenated blood from the heart to the body.

arthritis: inflammation of the joints.

arthropod: invertebrate animal with jointed limbs belonging to the phylum Arthropoda; insect, spider, or crustacean.

aspirate: to draw by suction; to inhale into the lungs.

asthma: labored breathing caused by narrowing of the smaller air passages (past the bronchi) in the lungs, associated with shortness of breath, wheezing, cyanosis, and coughing.

atherosclerosis: hardening of the arteries.

atrial: pertaining to the atrium.

atrium: one of two smaller chambers of the heart.

aura: a sensation of lights or sounds that occurs before a migraine headache or seizure.

B

barotitis: disorder of the ear due to increased or decreased atmospheric pressure.

BID: twice a day.

bile: green fluid produced by the liver and stored in the gallbladder, where it is released into the duodenum to aid in the digestion and absorption of fats.

bilirubin: a pigment formed from the destruction of red blood cells.

biopsy: the process of removing tissue from living creatures for diagnostic examination.

blister: fluid-filled elevation of the epidermis.

BLS: basic life support.

borrelial: related to microorganisms of the genus *Borrelia*, which transmit diseases such as Lyme disease.

bowel: intestine.

BP: blood pressure.

brainstem: part of the central nervous system between the spinal cord and brain that controls certain critical functions, such as breathing.

breech: buttocks first, as in breech birth.

bronchitis: inflammation of the bronchial tree.

bronchoconstriction: narrowing of small airways, often caused by smooth muscle contraction.

bronchodilator: drug used to relax and widen the bronchi.

bronchus: main passageway from the trachea to the smaller air passages in the lungs.

bruise: injury that does not break the skin, with rupture of small blood vessels that causes blue or purplish discoloration.

bursa: fluid-filled sac that allows smooth motion of muscles or tendons over a bone or joint.

bursitis: inflammation of a bursa.

buttocks: the seat of the body; the rump.

C

calorie: the amount of energy necessary to raise the temperature of 1 g of water by 1° C; 1 food calorie ("kilocalorie") is equal to 1000 energy calories.

cancer: malignant tumor; uncontrolled growth of cells that invade normal body tissues for no reason and serve no purpose.

canker sore: small, painful ulcer of the mouth.

cannula: small tube for insertion of fluid or air.

capillary: microscopic blood vessel that connects an artery to a vein.

carbonaceous: rich in carbon; black like soot.

carbon dioxide: gas that combines with water to form carbonic acid; formed by the combustion and decomposition of organic substances.

cardiac: pertaining to the heart.

cardiopulmonary: pertaining to the heart and lungs.

carotid artery: chief artery that travels up the neck and carries blood to the head and brain.

carpal: relating to the wrist.

cartilage: elastic tissue that is transformed into bone.

cartilaginous: composed of cartilage.

cataract: opacity in the lens of the eye.

caustic: corrosive; capable of destroying by chemical action.

cellulitis: inflammation of tissue, such as the skin.

central nervous system: the brain and spinal cord.

cerebral: pertaining to the brain.

cervical: pertaining to the neck.

chilblain: inflammation, swelling, and blistering of the skin caused by exposure to cold.

cholecystitis: inflammation of the gallbladder.

cholelithiasis: condition of having stones present in the gallbladder.

chronic: of long duration.

CNS: central nervous system.

CO: carbon monoxide.

colic: acute pain caused by spasm, obstruction, or twisting of a hollow organ.

colitis: inflammation of the colon.

colon: the large intestine.

coma: a state of profound unconsciousness.

comatose: in a coma.

comminuted: in multiple pieces; shattered.

compound fracture: broken bone accompanied by torn skin.

conjunctiva: membrane that covers the insides of the eyelids and extends over the whites of the eyes.

convulsion: seizure; abnormal involuntary contraction or series of contractions of the muscles.

COPD: chronic obstructive pulmonary disease, caused by scarred lung tissue.

core: center; involving the abdomen and chest organs.

cornea: the transparent covering of the eyeball over the iris and pupil that allows light to enter the eye.

corticosteroid: one of a number of hormones produced by the adrenal glands.

costochondritis: inflammation of the cartilage that attaches the ribs to the sternum.

CPR: cardiopulmonary resuscitation, with artificial breathing and chest compressions.

cravat: triangular cloth bandage folded into a longitudinal strap.

crepitus: a crackling sound or feeling.

culture: to grow in a prepared laboratory medium.

cyanosis: blue or purple discoloration of the skin due to inadequate oxygen in the blood.

cyst: an abnormal sac containing gas, fluid, or solid material.

D

debridement: surgical removal of torn, contaminated, or devitalized tissue.

decompression: loss of pressure; contributes to diving-related bends.

DEET: active ingredient of many insect repellents; N,N-diethyl-3-methylbenzamide.

dehydration: depletion of bodily fluids.

dermatitis: inflammation of the skin.

dermis: layer of skin just underneath the epidermis that contains sensitive nerve endings, blood vessels, and hair follicles.

diagnose: to identify a disease.

diaphragm: muscular wall that separates the chest from the abdomen.

dilation: stretching to normal or beyond normal dimensions.

dinoflagellate: marine plankton.

discharge: liquid released from an organ or tissue surface.

dislocation: displacement of bones at a joint.

disseminated: spread over a wide area.

distal: at the end of; in the area farthest from the center of the body.

diuretic: drug that promotes urination.

diverticulitis: inflammation of a diverticulum.

diverticulum: small outpouching from a hollow organ (such as the large intestine).

dressing: bandage; covering for a wound.

duodenum: first part of the small intestine.

E

ectopic: at a remote site; in the wrong place.

edema: swelling caused by the accumulation of fluid.

electrolyte: soluble inorganic chemical (such as sodium or potassium) found in bodily fluids.

embolism: sudden obstruction of a blood vessel by an embolus.

embolus: abnormal particle (such as a blood clot or air bubble) circulating in the bloodstream.

encephalopathy: disease of the brain that often results in abnormal mentation.

encyst: to completely surround with a membrane.

endemic: native to.

endotracheal: through the trachea.

envenom: to poison with venom.

epidermis: outermost layer of the skin.

epigastrium: area lying over the stomach; central upper area of the abdomen.

epiglottis: soft tissue pillar in the throat that covers the vocal cords and keeps food and liquid from entering the trachea during swallowing.

epiglottitis: inflammation of the epiglottis.

epilepsy: disorder associated with disturbed electrical discharges in the central nervous system that cause convulsions.

epinephrine: most potent hormone that stimulates increased heart rate and force of contraction, relaxation of smooth muscle in the airways that causes bronchoconstriction (during asthma or an allergic reaction), and constriction of microscopic blood vessels.

epistaxis: nosebleed.

eruption: a breaking out, particularly the appearance of redness, rash, blisters, sores, or other lesions of the skin.

erythema: redness.

esophageal reflux: return of food and acid from the stomach into the esophagus; major cause of heartburn.

esophagitis: inflammation of the esophagus.

esophagus: muscular tube from the pharynx to the stomach.

eustachian tube: a tube of bone and cartilage that connects the middle ear with the upper throat and allows equalization of pressure on both sides of the eardrum.

exhale: to breathe out.

expectoration: sputum, phlegm, or mucus; the act of spitting out saliva or mucus from the air passages via the mouth.

extend: lengthen; reach out.

extremity: arm and hand (upper extremity) or leg and foot (lower extremity).

F

facial: pertaining to the face.

fallopian tube: small tube that conducts the egg from the ovary to the uterus.

fascia: tough, fibrous tissue that surrounds muscle bundles.

fasciitis: inflammation of the fascia.

feces: solid human bodily waste discharged through the anus.

feculent: pertaining to or resembling feces.

femoral artery: large artery that carries blood to the leg.

femur: large bone of the thigh.

fetus: unborn young after it has taken form in the uterus.

fibrillation: unsynchronized quivering.

flagellate: possessing a flagellum.

flagellum: whiplike organelle (tail) for locomotion.

flail chest: series of detached ribs that cannot move properly to assist with breathing.

flatulence: the presence of excessive gas in the bowel.

flatus: gas generated in the digestive tract and discharged via the anus.

flex: bend; fold.

fluorescence: the reemission of light (usually lower frequency) following its absorption; this is usually most apparent when the absorbed light is in the (invisible) ultraviolet range and the reemitted light is in the visible range.

fluorescent: possessing fluorescence.

follicle: skin cavity in which a root of hair lies.

fracture: to break; a broken object.

frostbite: freezing of the tissues.

G

gallbladder: muscular, hollow organ that stores bile produced by the liver.

gangrene: tissue death due to loss of blood supply; may be caused by injury or infection.

gastroenteritis: inflammation or irritation of the stomach and intestine.

gastrointestinal: pertaining to the stomach and intestine; digestive system.

gauge: the diameter of a hypodermic needle expressed as a standard number.

genitals: external organs of reproduction.

GI: gastrointestinal.

gland: a specialized group of cells that selectively removes substances from the blood, concentrates or alters substances in the blood, and/or creates and releases special substances into the blood.

glaucoma: disease of the eye associated with increased pressure within the eyeball.

glucose: type of sugar used by the body for energy.

gonorrhea: sexually transmitted disease caused by the bacterium *Neisseria gonorrhoeae*.

graft (skin): piece of skin taken from one area of the body to cover a defect or burn in another area.

grain: a measure of weight equal to 0.0648 g.

gram: a measure of weight equal to 15.432 grains.

grand mal seizure: convulsion manifested by violent generalized muscle contractions, clouded consciousness, and a period of confusion after the event.

GU: Genitourinary.

H

HACE: high-altitude cerebral edema.

hallucinate: to see visions or experience lack of reality.

hallucination: imaginary perception.

HAPE: high-altitude pulmonary edema.

heartburn: burning discomfort behind the sternum related to irritation or spasm of the lower portion of the esophagus.

Heimlich maneuver: technique for removal of a foreign object caught in the upper airway.

helminth: intestinal worm-shaped parasite.

hemoglobin: iron-containing, oxygen-carrying pigment in red blood cells.

hemorrhage: bleeding.

hemorrhoid: dilated vein found at the anal margin.

hepatitis: inflammation of the liver.

hernia: protrusion of part or all of an organ through a wall of the space in which it is normally contained.

hiatal hernia: protrusion of part of the stomach through the diaphragm.

histamine: chemical compound that plays a major role in allergic reactions.

HIV: human immunodeficiency virus.

hives: raised red skin wheals associated with allergic reactions.

hormone: chemical substance formed in the body that is carried in the bloodstream to affect another part of the body; an example is thyroid hormone, produced by the thyroid gland in the neck, which affects growth, temperature regulation, metabolic rate, and other body functions.

HR: heart rate.

hydrate: to cause to take up water.

hygiene: the science or practice of preserving health.

hyper- (prefix): excessive.

hyperbaric: pertaining to increased atmospheric pressure.

hyperextension: accentuated extension or straightening of a limb.

hypertension: elevated blood pressure.

hyperthermia: elevated core body temperature.

hypertrophy: enlargement of; excessive size.

hyphema: collection of blood in the chamber of the eye between the lens and the cornea (anterior chamber).

hypo- (prefix): insufficient; underneath.

hypodermic: under the skin.

hypoglycemia: low blood sugar.

hyponatremia: low blood sodium.

hypothermia: low core body temperature.

I

ileum: the last (and longest) segment of the small intestine.

ileus: profoundly decreased physiologic activity (motility) of the bowel, characterized by dilation, abdominal pain, and vomiting.

iliac: pertaining to the ilium.

ilium: the upper bone that forms the side of the pelvis.

IM: intramuscular.

immobilize: to prevent freedom of movement.

immune: not susceptible to.

immunity: condition of being able to resist a certain entity or disease.

immunization: the process of developing immunity; often refers to an injection.

impetiginize: to involve with impetigo.

impetigo: contagious skin disease caused by *Staphylococcus* or *Streptococcus* bacteria, characterized by weeping, crusting, and areas of pus formation.

incarcerate: to confine; to entrap.

infarction: area of tissue death caused by obstruction of blood circulation.

inflammation: response to cell injury that involves dilation of small blood vessels, redness, warmth, pain, and migration of white blood (pus) cells to the region; part of the healing process that removes noxious substances and damaged tissue; can be destructive as a primary disease process.

infrared: light that lies outside of the visible spectrum, with wavelengths longer than those of red light.

inhale: to breathe in.

inspiration: the act of breathing in.

intestine: the digestive tube that passes from the stomach to the anus; the small intestine (bowel) consists of the duodenum, jejunum, and ileum; the large intestine (bowel) consists of the cecum (with attached appendix), colon (ascending, transverse, descending, and sigmoid), and rectum.

intoxication: state of poisoning.

intravenous: into a vein.

irrigate: to rinse.

ischemic: in a condition of lowered blood flow; lacking sufficient oxygen to sustain function.

-itis (suffix): inflammation of.

IV: Intravenous.

J

jaundice: yellow pigmentation of the tissues and bodily fluids.

jejunum: the segment of the small intestine that follows the duodenum and precedes the ileum.

K

ketoacidosis: condition of excessive ketones in the bloodstream, associated with increased systemic acidity; a life-threatening condition of diabetics.

ketone: acid by-product of metabolism.

kg: kilogram.

kilo- (prefix): one thousand of something.

kilocalorie: 1 food calorie, or 1000 energy calories; the energy necessary to raise the temperature of 1 kg of water by 1° C.

kilogram: 1000 g; 2.2 lb.

L

lacerate: to tear or cut roughly.

larva: wormlike form of an insect that issues from the egg; e.g., grub, maggot, or caterpillar.

larynx: the portion of the trachea that contains the vocal cords; the voice box.

lateral: away from the midline; outer.

lb (abbreviation): pound.

lethargy: drowsiness or aversion to activity, caused by disease.

ligament: fibrous connective tissue that attaches bone to bone.

liter: volume of water that weighs 1 kg; 1.0567 quarts.

localized: confined to a specific area.

lumbar: pertaining to the lower back.

lymph: amber nutrient fluid that contains white blood cells; it circulates in the lymphatic system and is involved with injuries, infections, and cancers.

lymphatic: related to lymph glands, cells, or fluid; small vessel that transports lymph fluid.

lymph node: collection of lymph cells that function as a gland; node (colloquial).

M

malleolus: rounded bony prominence, such as occurs on either side of the ankle.

mandible: lower bone of the jaw.

manipulate: to move mechanically, usually with the hands.

melena: dark-colored, tarry stools (feces), due to the presence of blood altered by intestinal fluids.

meningitis: inflammation of the covering of the brain and upper spinal cord.

menses: periodic hemorrhage from a woman's uterus that occurs most commonly at 4-week intervals.

menstrual: related to menses.

menstruation: periodic discharge of bloody fluid from the uterus.

mental status: condition of alertness and comprehension.

metabolism: the energy-producing and energy-using processes that occur in the human body.

mg: milligram.

micron: measure of length equal to one one-millionth of a meter.

microorganism: small life form that requires a microscope to be seen.

microscopic: very tiny; requires a microscope to be seen.

migraine: recurrent severe headaches generally accompanied by an aura (classic migraine), nausea, vomiting, and dizziness.

milli- (prefix): one one-thousandth.

milligram: 1/1000 of a gram.

milliliter: 1/1000 of a liter.

mL (abbreviation): milliliter.

mononucleosis: infectious disease characterized by an abnormal increase in monocytes (a type of white blood cell) in the blood, weakness, fever, sore throat, and enlargement of the spleen and lymph nodes in the neck.

mottled: covered with colored spots or blotches.

mucus: slippery secretion created by mucous glands associated with mucous membranes (such as those that line the nose, throat, and mouth) for lubrication and some protection against bacteria.

myocardial: pertaining to the heart muscle.

myoglobin: iron-containing, oxygen-carrying pigment present in muscle tissue.

myoglobinuria: condition of having myoglobin present in the urine.

N

nanometer: one one-billionth of a meter.

narcosis: altered mental status ranging from confusion to coma.

nebulize: to reduce to a fine spray.

neurologic: pertaining to the nervous system.

nm (abbreviation): nanometer.

nonsteroidal: not containing steroids.

NSAID: nonsteroidal antiinflammatory drug.

O

organ: part of the body with a specific function.

OTC: over-the-counter.

otitis: inflammation or infection of the ear.

ounce: measure of weight equal to 28.35 g; 1/16 lb.

ovary: one of two reproductive glands in a female that produces the female sex cells ("eggs").

ovulation: release of an egg from the ovary.

oxygen: colorless, odorless gas necessary for combustion and life.

oxygenate: to supply with oxygen.

oz (abbreviation): ounce.

ozone: triatomic form of oxygen (O_3) that is formed by electric discharge through air.

P

pallor: pale skin color.

palpate: feel with the hands.

palpation: the act of feeling with the hands.

palpitation: abnormal beating of the heart felt by the victim.

pancreas: gland that produces and secretes digestive enzymes (juices) and the insulin hormone.

pancreatitis: inflammation of the pancreas.

parasite: an animal or vegetable that lives on or in another and that draws its nourishment from the host.

paroxysmal: sudden.

pediatric: pertaining to children.

pelvic: related to the pelvis.

pelvis: strong, basin-shaped bone structure that provides support for the spine, hips, and legs.

penile: related to the penis.

peptic: related to digestive fluids.

perineum: area of skin situated between the external genitalia and the anus; area between the thighs extending from the tailbone to the front of the pubis.

peristalsis: natural contractions of the muscular walls of the bowel that move bowel contents forward.

peritoneum: lining of the abdominal organs and cavity.

peritonitis: inflammation of the peritoneum.

petit mal seizure: form of epilepsy characterized by brief periods of confusion without major abnormal muscle activity.

pharyngitis: inflammation of the pharynx; sore throat.

pharynx: throat.

phlegm: mucus secreted in the respiratory passages.

photophobia: aversion to light.

photosensitivity: sensitivity to light, particularly to ultraviolet radiation.

pigment: coloring matter or stain.

placenta: organ implanted within the uterus that supports an unborn child, which is attached by the umbilical cord.

plankton: microscopic plant life found in natural bodies of water.

plantar: on the bottom.

platelet: cellular component of the blood that contributes to clotting.

pleura: lining that covers the lungs and the inside of the chest cavity.

pleural space: a small space between the pleura that covers the lung and that lines the inside of the chest wall; normally, this space is minuscule (cannot be seen) because it is filled with negative pressure, which allows the lung to expand with the chest wall.

pleuritis: inflammation of the pleura.

pneumonia: infection of the lung characterized by fever, cough, shortness of breath, and the production of purulent or bloody sputum.

pneumothorax: collapsed lung with air in the pleural space.

PO: by mouth.

potable: drinkable (preferably, disinfected).

prognosis: projected outcome.

prolapse: to fall or sink down.

prone: lying flat with the face down.

prophylactic: for the purpose of prophylaxis.

prophylaxis: measures designed to maintain health and to prevent disease.

protozoan: microscopic unicellular or acellular animal.

proximal: closer to starting point or center; nearest to central part of the body.

pubic: pertaining to the region of the pubis.

pubis: the lowermost and anterior bone of the pelvis.

pulmonary: pertaining to the lungs.

punctate: like a dot or small mark.

pupil: contractile round opening in the center of the iris of the eye through which light is transmitted to the lens.

purulent: foul.

pus: white, yellow-green, or beige creamy fluid that is formed by decomposing tissue, white blood cells, and tissue fluids.

pyelonephritis: inflammation of the kidney due to a bacterial infection.

Q

QD: every day (daily).

QID: four times a day.

quadrant: one of the four quarters into which a region can be divided.

R

radial artery: the main artery that travels through the wrist to supply the hand.

radiation: emission of energy in the form of waves or particles.

radiation of pain: pain that travels from one region to another, such as from the hand to the shoulder.

rebound tenderness: pain in the abdomen that is worse on release of pressure than it is on creation of pressure (compression); often indicates peritonitis.

recompression: the method whereby increased atmospheric pressure is used to treat victims of air embolism or decompression sickness (diving-related disorders).

reflux: backward flow.

reflux esophagitis (heartburn): inflammation of the esophagus caused by backward flow of acid from the stomach.

relapse: return of a disease after it has spent its course.

renal: related to the kidney.

respiratory: pertaining to the organs of breathing or the act of breathing.

resuscitate: to revive from death or unconsciousness.

retina: the posterior inside surface of the eye, which receives a light image refracted through the cornea and lens, and transmits it to the brain via the optic nerve.

rigor mortis: stiffening of the body that begins a few hours after death and that disappears from 1 to 5 days later, when decomposition begins.

RR: respiratory rate.

S

saline: salty (solution); normal saline (liquid compatible with most human tissues) is 0.9% sodium chloride in water.

saturate: to soak; to dissolve to the highest possible concentration.

sedate: to bring under the influence of a sedative.

sedation: the act of calming.

sedative: calming or quieting; a drug or other substances that decreases nervous excitement.

seizure: epileptic convulsion.

serum: the fluid component of blood after the cells are removed.

shock: a clinical state manifested by profound depression of all body functions, caused by insufficient blood and nutrient supply to the tissues; signs and symptoms include low blood pressure, cool and clammy skin, altered mental status, and collapse.

silica: silicon dioxide.

SL: sublingual (under the tongue).

soft tissue: body tissue that is not composed of bone or cartilage; generally refers to skin, muscle, and fat; generally excludes internal organs.

spasm: involuntary muscular contraction.

sphincter: muscular ring that serves as a junction between two tubes, such as the esophageal sphincter (between the esophagus and stomach).

spirochete: curled or spiraled microorganism capable of causing infectious disease.

sprain: incomplete stretching or tearing of ligaments.

sputum: phlegm composed of saliva and discharges from the respiratory passages.

SQ: subcutaneous (under the skin).

status: unchanging situation, such as status asthmaticus (severe, unchanging asthma), or status epilepticus (nonceasing convulsions).

STD: sexually transmitted disease.

sterile: uncontaminated by infectious agents.

sternocleidomastoid: prominent neck muscle that connects the mandible to the collarbone and sternum.

sternum: breastbone.

steroids: hormones, vitamins, body constituents, and drugs with a specific chemical structure.

strain: incomplete stretching or tearing of tendons or muscles.

stridor: harsh vibrating noise heard in the upper airway during breathing; commonly associated with an outflow obstruction during exhalation; may be inspiratory.

stroke: cerebral hemorrhage, thrombosis, vasospasm, or embolism characterized by some degree of paralysis; also called apoplexy.

sub- (prefix): underneath.

subarachnoid: under the arachnoid.

subconjunctival: under the conjunctivae.

subcutaneous: under the skin.

sublingual: under the tongue.

supine: lying flat with the face up.

supraventricular: above the level of the ventricles (lower chambers) of the heart.

suture: to sew with surgical thread or nylon; the thread or nylon used to sew a wound closed.

symphysis: a barely movable junction of two bone surfaces connected by a fibrous cartilage pad.

syndrome: a collection of signs and symptoms that, taken together, constitute a particular disease or abnormality.

synthesize: to create or compose.

syringe: device used to inject fluids into or remove them from the body.

systemic: affecting the entire body.

T

tachycardia: rapid heart rate (beat).

TBI: traumatic brain injury.

tendon: fibrous tissue that attaches muscle to bone.

tension pneumothorax: collapsed lung under pressure from air in the pleural space.

testicle: testis.

testis: one of two male reproductive glands located in the scrotum.

tetanus: an infectious disease caused by the bacterium *Clostridium tetani* and characterized by severe muscle contractions and inability to open the mouth (lockjaw); the bacterium that causes tetanus.

thermal: pertaining to heat.

thermoregulatory: in control of temperature.

thrombophilia: increased number of platelets.

thrombophlebitis: an inflammation of the veins that causes the formation of blood clots.

thrombosis: formation of a thrombus.

thrombus: clot formed in a blood vessel or in one of the cavities of the heart.

TID: three times a day.

tinnitus: noises, such as ringing, in the ears.

tissue: a group of cells that combine in the body to serve a specific function.

tourniquet: a device used to control blood flow by impeding or preventing circulation.

toxin: poisonous substance.

trachea: main passageway for air from the pharynx to the bronchi.

tracheostomy: surgical opening created in the neck into the trachea to allow breathing when the upper airway is obstructed.

trauma: mechanical injury.

traumatic: related to mechanical injury.

triage: sorting of patients by priority.

tubal: related to a tube.

tumor: abnormal growth of tissue that arises in the body without purpose; may be benign (noncancerous) or malignant (cancerous).

tympanic membrane: eardrum.

U

ulcer: erosion; open sore.

ultrasonic: beyond the normal range of sound waves.

ultraviolet: light outside of the violet end of the visible spectrum with a wavelength shorter than that of visible light.

umbilical: relating to the umbilicus.

umbilicus: navel; belly button; pit in the center of the abdominal wall where the umbilical cord was attached to the fetus before birth.

unconscious: unaware; unarousable.

ureter: muscular tube that carries urine from the kidney to the bladder.

urethra: passage that carries urine from the bladder to the external opening in the genital region.

URI: upper respiratory infection.

urogenital: genitourinary; pertaining to the urinary tract and genitalia.

urticaria: itchy, patchy, raised, and red skin rash, often associated with allergy.

uterus: muscular reproductive female organ in which a child develops; womb.

UTI: urinary tract infection.

UV: ultraviolet.

UVR: ultraviolet radiation.

V

vaccinate: to inject a special preparation for the purpose of achieving immunity from disease.

vaginitis: irritation of the vagina.

varicose: abnormally swollen or dilated.

vascular: pertaining to the blood vessels.

vasospasm: contraction of a blood vessel, often caused by microscopic muscle contraction.

vein: blood vessel that carries blood from the body back to the heart.

venom: poison secreted from venom glands in animals and insects; usually introduced into the victim with a bite or sting.

venous: pertaining to the veins.

ventricle: one of two large chambers of the heart.

ventricular: pertaining to the ventricle.

vertebra: one of the bony segments that form the spinal column (backbone).

vertigo: dizziness; sensation of whirling motion.

vessel: container; a blood vessel may be an artery, vein, or capillary.

VF: ventricular fibrillation.

vitreous: gelatinous fluid within the eye.

W

wheezing: labored breathing, usually noted on expiration, associated with lung disorders characterized by airway narrowing, such as asthma.

INDEX

Page numbers followed by f indicate figures; t, tables.

ABOUT THE AUTHOR

Dr. Paul S. Auerbach is the Redlich Family Professor of Surgery in the Division of Emergency Medicine at Stanford University School of Medicine. A founder and past president of the Wilderness Medical Society, Dr. Auerbach is editor of *Wilderness Medicine,* the definitive textbook for medical professionals, and author of the books *Field Guide to Wilderness Medicine, A Medical Guide to Hazardous Marine Life, Diving the Rainbow Reefs, An Ocean of Colors, Management Lessons from the E.R.,* and *Bad Medicine.* The nation's foremost authority on wilderness medicine, he serves on the Medical Committee of the National Ski Patrol System; is an advisor to the Divers Alert Network, Healthline Networks, and Redpoint Resolutions; and is a consultant or committee member for many other scientific, medical, and outdoor-related organizations. He is an elected member of the Council on Foreign Relations, was the first editor of the journal *Wilderness & Environmental Medicine* (formerly *Journal of Wilderness Medicine*), has been named a "Hero of Emergency Medicine," and is a recipient of numerous awards, including the Outstanding Contribution in Education Award from the American College of Emergency Physicians, Founders and Education Awards from the Wilderness Medical Society, DAN America and DAN Rolex Diver of the Year Awards from the Divers Alert Network, Diver of the Year Award for Science from Beneath the Sea, and NOGI Award for Science from the Academy of Underwater Arts and Sciences. In addition to his clinical work in emergency medicine at Stanford, Dr. Auerbach is engaged in research on frostbite, avalanche rescue, medical radiation exposure, and traumatic brain injury; assists early-stage biodesign and technology companies; is an active international medical volunteer involved in disaster response and prehospital care system design; and is highly sought after as a speaker and writer, both in the medical profession and in the popular media. He lives in Los Altos, California.